THE CANCER
CHEMOTHERAPY
HANDBOOK

NOTICE

Every effort has been made to ensure that the drug dosage schedules herein are accurate and in accord with the standards accepted at the time of publication. However, human errors can occur. In addition, as new research and experience broaden our knowledge, changes in treatment and drug therapy occur. Therefore the reader is advised to check the product information sheet included in the package of each drug to be administered to be certain that changes have not been made in the recommended dose or in the contraindications. This is of particular importance in regard to new or infrequently used drugs.

Cover image:
Bone marrow aspirate from 60-year-old male with multiple myeloma.

THE CANCER CHEMOTHERAPY HANDBOOK

a Mosby handbook

DAVID S. FISCHER, MD
Clinical Professor of Medicine,
Yale University School of Medicine;
Attending Physician,
Yale–New Haven Hospital,
New Haven, Connecticut

M. TISH KNOBF, RN, MSN
Associate Professor,
Yale University School of Nursing;
Clinical Nurse Specialist,
Yale–New Haven Hospital,
New Haven, Connecticut

HENRY J. DURIVAGE, PharmD
Director of Clinical Affairs,
Theradex Systems, Inc.,
Princeton, New Jersey

FIFTH EDITION

Mosby

St. Louis Baltimore Boston
Carlsbad Chicago Naples New York Philadelphia Portland
London Madrid Mexico City Singapore Sydney Tokyo Toronto Wiesbaden

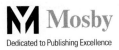

Mosby

Dedicated to Publishing Excellence

A Times Mirror
Company

Publisher: Anne S. Patterson
Editor: Susie Baxter
Developmental Editor: Ellen Baker Geisel
Project Manager: Carol Sullivan Weis
Production Editor: Karen M. Rehwinkel
Designer: Renee Duenow
Manufacturing Manager: David Graybill
Cover photo courtesy of David S. Fischer, MD

FIFTH EDITION

Printed in the United States of America
Composition by Accu-Color, Inc.
Printing/binding by R.R. Donnelley & Sons, Inc.

Mosby–Year Book, Inc.
11830 Westline Industrial Drive
St. Louis, Missouri 63146

International Standard Book Number ISBN 0-8151-3314-6

97 98 99 00 01 / 9 8 7 6 5 4 3 2 1

Contributors

Diane M. Komp, MD
Professor of Pediatrics,
Yale University School of Medicine;
Attending Physician,
Yale–New Haven Hospital,
New Haven, Connecticut

Edward L. Snyder, MD
Professor of Laboratory Medicine,
Yale University School of Medicine;
Director of the Blood Bank,
Yale–New Haven Hospital,
New Haven, Connecticut

Preface

The goal of the fifth edition of *The Cancer Chemotherapy Handbook* is to continue the previous edition's practical clinical value while incorporating large amounts of new material. We have maintained the original format for individual drugs and drug combinations so that the book will continue to serve as a practical reference and resource to all oncology professionals involved in prescribing, preparing, and administering therapy. Safety remains a critical element of cancer chemotherapy, and we strongly encourage each clinician to always check the original reference of listed protocols.

Additions to the current edition include three new chapters: Principles of Pediatric Cancer Therapy, by Diane M. Komp, MD, which provides a brief overview of this subspecialty; High-Dose Chemotherapy With Stem Cell Support, which recognizes the rapid progress of that therapeutic approach and highlights the potential significant risks and the importance of physicians being experienced and specially trained in that modality of therapy before employing it; and Blood Transfusion Therapy for the Cancer Patient, by Edward L. Snyder, MD. Finally, the appendix has been expanded to include special toxicity criteria associated with transplantation and an A to Z listing of acronyms and the possible drugs that they represent.

It was very gratifying to have our fourth edition translated into both Italian and Japanese. We welcome this opportunity to serve the international health profession and hope that our message goes out to the world: scientific progress and compassionate care are essential in the care of cancer patients and their families anywhere on the earth that we share as a common humanity, without regard to borders and boundaries.

David S. Fischer
M. Tish Knobf
Henry J. Durivage

Acknowledgments

In preparing this edition of *The Cancer Chemotherapy Handbook,* we are grateful to many people for their assistance. Debra Brandt, MD, and Stephen J. Windsor, MD, helped search the world literature for the new combination chemotherapy protocols, helped decide which to include and which to omit, and critiqued the introductions to the tumor sites in Chapter 6. We acknowledge the help of Dennis Cooper, MD, for review of the chapter on High-Dose Chemotherapy With Stem Cell Support; Constance Donovan, RN, for review of the chapter on Cancer Chemotherapy Administration; Diane M. Komp, MD, for writing the chapter on Principles of Pediatric Cancer Therapy; and Edward L. Snyder, MD, for writing the chapter on Blood Transfusion Therapy for the Cancer Patient. It has been a pleasure to work with Susie Baxter, Ellen Baker Geisel, and Karen Rehwinkel at Mosby–Year Book, Inc. on this fifth edition; we appreciate their support. We thank Drs. G. Bonadonna, S. Siena, and M. Bregni for translating our fourth edition into Italian and the Masson Company of Milan for publishing it. We thank the Igaku-Shoin MYTW Company of Tokyo for translating and publishing our fourth edition in Japanese. Finally, we wish to thank our respective spouses and children for putting up with the temporary neglect that is always the consequence of extensively revising this book.

David S. Fischer
M. Tish Knobf
Henry J. Durivage

Contents

1 Cancer Chemotherapy and Pharmacology, *1*
Cellular Kinetics, *2*
Cancer Chemotherapy, *2*
Drug Resistance, *3*
Antineoplastic Drugs, *4*
Drug Interactions With Antineoplastic Agents, *8*

2 Clinical Trials and Good Clinical Practice, *21*
Clinical Oncology Trials in the United States, *22*
Drug Development and the Phases of Clinical Trials, *25*
Conducting a Clinical Trial, *29*

3 Chemotherapy Drugs, *41*

4 Biological Response Modifiers, *219*
Antitumor Immunity, *220*
Clinical Development of the Biological Response Modifiers, *220*
Hematopoietic Growth Factors, *220*
Interferons, *221*
Interleukins, *222*
Prevention and Management of Toxicities, *222*

5 Cancer Chemotherapy Administration, *260*
Controlling Exposure to Antineoplastic Drugs, *261*
Drug Administration, *268*
Routes of Drug Administration, *274*
Intravenous Drug Delivery, *274*
Regional Drug Delivery, *295*
Ambulatory Infusion Pumps for Drug Delivery, *304*

6 Combination Chemotherapy, *307*
Adrenal Cortical Carcinoma, *310*
Anal Carcinoma, *311*
Bladder (Transitional Cell) Carcinoma, *312*
Brain Tumors, *316*

Breast Carcinoma, *317*
Carcinoid (Malignant) and Islet Cell Carcinoma, *327*
Carcinoma of Unknown Primary, *329*
Cervical Carcinoma, *330*
Colon Carcinoma, *332*
Endometrial Cancer, *336*
Esophageal Carcinoma, *337*
Gastric Adenocarcinoma, *339*
Gestational Trophoblastic Disease, *342*
Head and Neck Squamous Cell Carcinoma, *344*
Kaposi's Sarcoma, *347*
Leukemia: Acute Lymphoblastic, *349*
Leukemia: Acute Nonlymphocytic, *354*
Leukemia: Chronic Granulocytic (Myelocytic), *362*
Leukemia: Chronic Lymphocytic, *364*
Lung Cancer: Non–Small-Cell Carcinoma, *365*
Lung Cancer: Small-Cell Carcinoma, *370*
Lymphoma: Hodgkin's Disease, *375*
Lymphoma: Non-Hodgkin's Disease, *382*
Melanoma, *402*
Malignant Mesothelioma, *404*
Multiple Myeloma, *406*
Osteosarcoma, *409*
Ovarian Carcinoma, *411*
Ovarian Germ Cell Cancer, *417*
Pancreatic Carcinoma, *418*
Prostatic Carcinoma, *420*
Renal Cell Carcinoma, *423*
Sarcoma, *425*
Testicular and Extragonadal Germ Cell Cancer, *428*
Thymoma (Malignant), *432*
Thyroid Carcinoma, *434*

7 Ethical Considerations in Cancer, *436*
Major Principles of Medical Ethics, *436*
Managed Care, *437*
To Tell the Truth, *438*
"Do Not Resuscitate" Orders, *439*
Discontinuing Care, *440*
Advanced Directives, *441*
Hospice, *441*
Physician-Assisted Suicide, *442*

8 Cancer Pain Management, *448*
Underestimating Need, *448*
Assessment of Pain, *450*
Using Analgesics for Mild Pain, *451*
Using Analgesics for Moderate Pain, *454*
Using Analgesics for Severe Pain, *455*

Additional Measures for Pain Control, *458*
Pearls to Remember, *460*

9 High-Dose Chemotherapy With Stem Cell Support, *462*
Leukemias, *469*
Lymphomas, *470*
Multiple Myeloma, *472*
Breast Cancers, *473*
Germ Cell Tumors, *474*

10 Assessment and Management of Organ System Toxicity, *475*
Anemia, *475*
Neutropenia, *476*
Thrombocytopenia, *486*
Gastrointestinal Toxicity, *488*
Dermatological Toxicity, *514*
Renal Toxicity, *526*
Pulmonary Toxicity, *534*
Cardiac Toxicity, *537*
Neurological Toxicity, *539*
Gonadal Toxicity, *543*
Other Organ System Toxicity, *545*

11 Blood Transfusion Therapy for the Cancer Patient , *553*
Blood Components, *553*
Types of Donations, *554*
Platelets, *554*
Granulocytes, *556*
Plasma and Cryoprecipitate, *557*
Transfusion Reactions, *557*
Other Adverse Conditions, *561*
Administration of Blood Products, *562*

12 Principles of Pediatric Cancer Therapy, *564*
Clinical Cooperative Groups, *564*
Early Side Effects of Therapy, *565*
Delayed Consequences of Treatment, *566*
Ethical Considerations, *566*

Appendixes
Appendix A, *569*
Table A-1 Calculation of Body Surface Area, *569*
Table A-2 Calculation of Body Surface Area in Adult Amputees, *569*
Table A-3 Ideal Body-Weight Charts, *570*
Table A-4 Performance Scale, *571*
Table A-5 Methods Used to Calculate Creatinine Clearance, *572*

Table A-6 Carboplatin Dosing Calculations, *573*
Table A-7 National Cancer Institute Common Toxicity
           Criteria, *574*
Table A-8 Autologous Bone Marrow Transplant Studies,
           Supplemental Toxicity Criteria, *581*
Table A-9 Temperature Conversion Chart, *581*
Table A-10 Drug Acronyms, *582*
Appendix B General References, *585*

THE CANCER CHEMOTHERAPY HANDBOOK

1

Cancer Chemotherapy and Pharmacology

An adequate understanding of cancer and its treatment must begin with an appreciation of the fact that cancer is not a single disease but at least 100 different diseases, each with its own characteristics and natural history (DeVita, Hellman, and Rosenberg, 1993; Cadman and Durivage, 1990; Boyd, 1992). For example, choriocarcinoma is very different from basal cell carcinoma of the skin, and both differ substantially from melanoma, lung, or breast cancer. Even within a "single malignancy," such as breast cancer, major biological differences can exist. Recent evidence suggests that cancer is a process and that cancer cells are continually adapting and evolving (Schipper, Goh, and Wang, 1995). The process is thought to be potentially reversible and comprises an imbalance of regulatory factors that allow certain cells to proliferate. It is important for professionals to know this and counsel patients as to the nature of cancer, modern methods of therapy, and the importance of clinical research as a way to improve the treatment of future patients.

There is no single definition that describes all the malignancies. In general, cancer is a group of relatively normal cells growing without the controls that usually prevent cells from growing beyond their intended size, site, and nutritional base. Cancer cells have the capacity to extend beyond a capsule or other barrier, to invade normal tissues locally, and to metastasize via blood or lymphoid vessels to distant sites where they may take up residence and proliferate. Thus cancer cells overgrow normal cells, compete with them for space and nutrition, and ultimately cause their death and eventually that of the host.

There is no single cause for all cancers. However, cigarette smoking is the single most important identified cause of cancer in the United States. It is responsible for more than 100,000 deaths yearly from lung cancer, as well as additional morbidity and mortality from cancers of the oral cavity, pharynx, larynx, esophagus, pancreas, bladder, and pleura. The vast majority of these patients would not have developed this kind of cancer if they had not smoked. Viruses and occupational exposure to other substances, such as asbestos and carcinogenic chemicals, are better appreciated as potential causes of cancer.

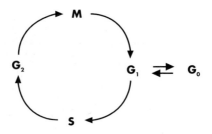

FIG. 1-1 Phases of the cell cycle. G_0, resting phase (nonproliferation of cells); G_1, pre-DNA synthetic phase (12 hours to a few days); *S*, DNA synthesis (usually 2 to 4 hours); G_2, post-DNA synthesis (2 to 4 hours; cells are tetraploid in this stage); *M*, mitosis (1 to 2 hours).

CELLULAR KINETICS

Most cancer cells are not characterized by rapid growth. For example, breast, lung, and colon cancer cells may take up to 100 days to double their population. The growth and division of normal and neoplastic cells occur in a sequence of events called the *cell cycle*. The cell cycle is divided into several different phases (Fig. 1-1). Many of the antineoplastic drugs have been and many continue to be classified based on whether their activity is cell cycle specific or nonspecific.

Synthesis of ribonucleic acid (RNA) and protein occurs during the G_1 *phase*. When cells are in G_1 for prolonged periods of time, they are often said to be in a *resting phase*, referred to as G_0. Synthesis of DNA occurs during S phase. During G_2, DNA synthesis halts, and RNA and protein synthesis continue. The final steps of chromosome replication and segregation occur during the mitotic, or *M phase*. The cell undergoes cell division and produces two daughter cells. The rate of RNA and protein synthesis slows during this phase as the genetic material is transferred into the daughter cells.

Drugs that exert their cytotoxic effects during a specific phase of the cell cycle (i.e., phase-specific agents) are usually not effective against cells that are predominantly in a dormant phase (G_0). In contrast, non–phase-specific agents are theoretically more likely to be effective against a tumor population that is not in a state of rapid division.

CANCER CHEMOTHERAPY

Since the first dose of cytotoxic chemotherapy was given in 1942, hundreds of thousands of chemical agents have been tested for their activity in destroying cancer cells. Relatively few of these drugs reach the stage of clinical testing in animals, and fewer still are found to be safe and effective enough to be tested in humans. A small number of those drugs that have been tested in humans are found to be useful for the treatment of patients with cancer. Since it is difficult for clinicians to have at their fingertips all their properties, modes of action, indications, doses, and toxicities, this book provides information taken from several sources to aid health care professionals in the day-to-day care of patients with cancer.

For anticancer drug treatment to be effective, several features must be present. The drug must reach the cancer cells, sufficiently toxic amounts of the drug (or its active metabolite) must enter the cells and remain there for a long enough period of time, the cancer cells must be sensitive to the effects of the drug, and all this must occur before resistance emerges (Chabner, 1990b; Cadman and Durivage, 1990). In addition, the patient must be able to withstand the adverse effects of treatment. Dose and dose intensity are important variables in the effective treatment of some cancers. For the more responsive malignancies (e.g., testicular cancer), it is important that "full doses" of chemotherapy be given "on schedule" for a short period of time. Low doses of chemotherapy given over a prolonged period of time favors the emergence of drug resistance.

DRUG RESISTANCE

The development of resistance to chemotherapeutic drugs by neoplastic cells is one of the major obstacles to the cure of many malignancies. Malignant cells may be intrinsically resistant or they may adapt after therapy by using various detoxification pathways to acquire resistance to cytotoxic agents (Moscow and Cowan, 1988; Ford and Hait, 1990; DeVita, 1990). To illustrate how cancerous cells acquire resistance to cytotoxic drugs, three of the myriad of known and potential mechanisms of drug resistance are described.

Multidrug Resistance

A transmembrane glycoprotein (called *P glycoprotein*, or *Pgp*), which is the product of the MDR-1 gene, is present in many cells that are resistant to vinca alkaloids, doxorubicin, and similar drugs. The type of drug resistance associated with Pgp has been called *typical multidrug resistance*. The hallmark of multidrug resistance is cross-resistance to several drugs after exposure to a single drug such as a vinca alkaloid, dactinomycin, or an anthracycline, but not to an alkylating agent, bleomycin, or an antimetabolite.

Pgp functions as a pump that is capable of ejecting cytotoxic agents from the cell (Moscow and Cowan, 1988). The activity of Pgp is under the influence of other cellular substances and is similar to bacterial peristaltic transport proteins. In the laboratory, several compounds have been tested for their ability to reverse or block the effects of Pgp. Some of these drugs have been tested clinically. Examples include verapamil, cyclosporine, cyclosporine analogues, and phenothiazines (Ford and Hait, 1990).

Atypical Multidrug Resistance, Topoisomerases

DNA is attached to the nuclear matrix at regular intervals. The sites where DNA is fixed to the nuclear matrix are called *domains*. During replication, the two DNA molecules and their domains are wound together like interlocked circles. For cell division to occur, separation and resealing of the DNA molecules must occur. This function and others are performed by DNA topoisomerase enzymes (Bender, Hamel, and Hande, 1990).

Several antineoplastic drugs exert their effects by inhibition of topo-isomerase enzymes (Liu, 1989; Sinha, 1995). Alterations in topoisomerase enzyme activity have been shown in cells resistant to topoisomerase inhibitors. Resistance to amsacrine, doxorubicin, teniposide, and etoposide may be acquired via decreased drug access to the enzyme, alteration of enzyme structure (and activity), or by other mechanisms.

Glutathione and Glutathione S-Transferase Isoenzymes

Glutathione (GSH) is a thiol that accounts for the majority of the intra-cellular nonprotein sulfhydryl content of most cells. It is regulated by other cellular processes and is essential for the synthesis of DNA precursors. GSH enzymes play important roles in detoxifying toxins, scavenging free radicals, and repairing DNA damage.

Glutathione S-transferase (GST) joins toxins with glutathione, forming a less toxic metabolite. Increased amounts of GST have been found in cancers of the head and neck, lung, and colon, but not in surrounding normal colon mucosa.

GST and GSH probably play some role in resistance to nitrogen mustard, melphalan, cisplatin, and nitrosoureas via inactivation of the drugs, through direct binding, increased metabolism, detoxification and/or DNA repair (Ford and Hait, 1990). Drugs that inhibit the activity of GSH and GST, such as buthionine sulfoximine (BSO) and ethacrynic acid, are being tested clinically for use in reversing resistance to alkylating agents.

ANTINEOPLASTIC DRUGS

The original use of the first cytotoxic chemotherapeutic agent, mechlorethamine, occurred at the New Haven Hospital. Studies began when two young investigators at Yale University, Goodman and Gilman, investigated a wartime agent with the code designation HN2. Investigation of this agent revealed that the drug caused depression of the white blood cell and platelet counts. Goodman and Gilman suggested to the thoracic surgeon, Lindskog, that this might be a useful drug for cancer treatment. A patient with inoperable and radiation-resistant lymphosarcoma was treated with HN2, subsequently known as *nitrogen mustard,* or *mechlorethamine,* and had a dramatic reduction of tumor size (Gilman, 1963). Although the response was brief and the patient relapsed shortly thereafter, it established the principle that drugs could shrink tumors and indicated the need for further research. Subsequent studies took place in this area with the progress that is now well known.

Anticancer drugs are classified in some respects by their cell-cycle activity and in other respects by their chemical derivation (Chabner, 1990b). We have chosen to assign the drugs into groups based on their presumed primary mechanism of action.

Alkylating and DNA Cross-Linking Agents

Alkylating agents are highly reactive compounds that easily attach to DNA and cellular proteins. The primary mode of action for most alkylating drugs is via cross-linking of DNA strands. Replication of DNA and transcription of RNA are prevented (Colvin and Chabner, 1990; Averbuch, 1990; Reed and Kohn, 1990).

Many alkylating agents have been developed (Table 1-1). Although these drugs have similar mechanisms of action, there are major differences in spectrum of activity, pharmacokinetic parameters, and toxicity. The alkylating agents are cell-cycle nonspecific. Alkylating agents play a significant role in the treatment of lymphoma, Hodgkin's disease, breast cancer, multiple myeloma, and other malignancies.

Alkylating agents often produce changes in testicular and ovarian function. In male patients these agents have produced oligospermia and azoospermia. Spermatogenesis may take several years to return to normal (Hansen, Berthelsen, and von der Maase, 1990). Amenorrhea occurs commonly and may be reversible in certain women (Bines, Oleske, and Cobleigh, 1996). Some alkylating agents are carcinogenic in humans (Colvin and Chabner, 1990). Cyclophosphamide has been associated with bladder malignancies (Wall and Clausen, 1975), and melphalan and semustine (methyl CCNU) have been associated with acute myelocytic leukemia (Karchmer et al, 1974).

TABLE 1-1
Alkylating Agents: Mechanisms of Action

Drug	Mechanisms
Altretamine	DNA cross-linking, binding to microsomal proteins
Amsacrine	DNA intercalation, inhibition of topoisomerase II
Busulfan	DNA cross-linking, alkylation of cellular thiols
Carboplatin	DNA cross-linking
Carmustine	DNA cross-linking; DNA polymerase repair, RNA synthesis inhibition
Chlorambucil	DNA cross-linking, alkylation of cellular thiols
Cisplatin	DNA cross-linking, intercalation, DNA precursor inhibition, alteration of cellular membranes
Cyclophosphamide	DNA cross-linking
Dacarbazine	DNA methylation, alkylation
Ifosfamide	DNA cross-linking and chain scission
Lomustine	DNA cross-linking; DNA polymerase repair, RNA synthesis inhibition
Mechlorethamine	DNA cross-linking
Melphalan	DNA cross-linking, alkylation of cellular thiols
Pipobroman	DNA alkylation
Procarbazine	DNA alkylation, inhibits methyl group incorporation into RNA
Streptozocin	DNA cross-linking, inhibits DNA repair enzyme guanine-O^6-methyl transferase
Temozolomide	DNA methylation, alkylation
Thiotepa	DNA cross-linking
Uracil mustard	DNA cross-linking

TABLE 1-2
Natural Products: Mechanisms of Action

Drug	Mechanisms
Aminocamptothecin	Inhibition of topoisomerase I
Asparaginase	Hydrolyzes the amino acid asparagine
Bleomycin	DNA strand scission by free radicals
Dactinomycin	DNA intercalation, inhibition of topoisomerase II
Daunorubicin	DNA intercalation, preribosomal DNA and RNA inhibition, alteration of cell membranes, free radical formation
Docetaxel	Promotes microtubule assembly, stabilizes tubulin polymers resulting in formation of nonfunctional microtubules
Doxorubicin	Same as daunorubicin
Epirubicin	Same as daunorubicin
Etoposide	Inhibition of topoisomerase II
Homoharringtonine	Inhibits synthesis of protein, DNA, and RNA by inhibiting chain initiation
Idarubicin	Same as daunorubicin
Irinotecan	Inhibition of topoisomerase I
Mitomycin	DNA cross-linking and depolymerization, free radical formation
Mitoxantrone	DNA intercalation, inhibition of topoisomerase II
Paclitaxel	Same as docetaxel
Plicamycin	DNA intercalation and adlineation, osteoclast inhibition
Suramin	Inhibition of growth factors (e.g., platelet-derived, epidermal) and DNA polymerases
Teniposide	Same as etoposide
Topotecan	Inhibition of topoisomerase I
Vinblastine	Tubulin binding (microtubule assembly inhibition and dissolution of mitotic spindle structure)
Vincristine	Same as vinblastine
Vinorelbine	Same as vinblastine

Antitumor Antibiotics

Antineoplastic drugs that are derived from microorganisms are called *antitumor antibiotics* (Table 1-2) (Chabner, 1990a; Myers and Chabner, 1990). Several of these drugs interfere with DNA through intercalation, a reaction whereby the drug inserts itself between DNA base pairs. Some of the antitumor antibiotics have other mechanisms to exert antitumor effects, such as inhibition of topoisomerase enzymes, antimitotic effects, and alteration of cellular membranes. Most of the antitumor antibiotics appear to be cell-cycle nonspecific agents.

Plant Alkaloids and Natural Products
Topoisomerase inhibitors

As mentioned earlier in this chapter, topoisomerases are enzymes that break and reseal DNA strands (Bender, Hamel, and Hande, 1990; Sinha, 1995). The plant alkaloid camptothecin and its analogues (e.g., topotecan, irinotecan [CPT-11], 9-aminocamptothecin) are specific inhibitors of topoisomerase I. Etoposide, teniposide, and drugs from other classes, such as amsacrine, doxorubicin, mitoxantrone, and daunorubicin, are inhibitors of topoisomerase II (Table 1-2). These drugs form a stable complex by binding to DNA and topoisomerase enzymes, resulting in DNA damage that interferes with replication and transcription.

Mitotic inhibitors

A group of mitotic inhibitors (e.g., vinblastine, vincristine, vinorelbine) exert their cytotoxic effects by binding to tubulin. This inhibits formation of microtubules, causing metaphase arrest (Bender, Hamel, and Hande, 1990). Their mechanisms of action and metabolism are similar, but the antitumor spectrum, dose, and clinical toxicities of vincristine, vinblastine, and vinorelbine are very different. Paclitaxel and docetaxel are also mitotic inhibitors. However, they differ from the vinca alkaloids by enhancing microtubule formation. As a result, a stable and nonfunctional microtubule is produced.

Enzymes

L-Asparaginase is an enzyme product that acts primarily by inhibiting protein synthesis by depriving tumor cells of the amino acid asparagine. Cells that have the ability to form their own asparagine, such as many normal cells, are not affected by L-asparaginase. L-Asparaginase is a foreign protein, is antigenic, and can cause serious hypersensitivity reactions.

Antimetabolites

A variety of agents interfere with the synthesis of DNA and RNA by mechanisms other than those described previously. Many of these drugs are called *antimetabolites* (Table 1-3) because they exert their effects largely in the synthetic phase of the cell cycle. Some antimetabolites are structural analogues of normal metabolites essential for cell growth and replication. This property allows them to be incorporated into DNA or RNA so that a false message is transmitted. Other antimetabolites inhibit enzymes that are necessary for the synthesis of essential compounds. In general, these agents have been most effective where cell proliferation is rapid. In addition, continuous infusion of antimetabolites (e.g., methotrexate, cytarabine) leads to enhanced toxicity. The antimetabolites traditionally are divided into the cytidine analogues (e.g., 5-azacytidine, cytarabine) (Chabner, 1990c), fluorinated pyrimidines (e.g., fluorouracil, floxuridine, tegafur) (Grem, 1990), purine analogues (e.g., mercaptopurine, thioguanine) (McCormack and Johns, 1990), ribonucleotide reductase inhibitors (e.g., hydroxyurea) (Donehower, 1990), adenosine deaminase inhibitors (e.g., pentostatin), and the folic acid antagonists (e.g., methotrexate, edatrexate) (Allegra, 1990).

Other Agents

Endocrine therapies, such as estrogens (e.g., diethylstilbestrol), androgens (e.g., fluoxymesterone), corticosteroids (e.g., prednisone, dexamethasone), progestins (megestrol acetate), and other drugs (e.g., tamoxifen, aminoglutethimide, leuprolide, goserelin, flutamide), have been used for many years. These and other "miscellaneous" drugs (e.g., mitotane, suramin) are discussed in Chapter 3.

TABLE 1-3
Antimetabolites: Mechanisms of Action

Drug	Mechanisms
Azacytidine	Competes for incorporation into nucleic acids, blocking production of cytidine and uridine
Cladribine	Deoxyadenosine analogue that accumulates in cells and blocks RNA synthesis
Cytarabine	Competitive inhibition DNA polymerase, an enzyme involved in conversion of cytidine to deoxycytidine, blocks DNA repair
Floxuridine	Inhibition of thymidylate synthesis
Fludarabine	Inhibition of DNA polymerase and ribonucleotide reductase
Fluorouracil	Inhibition of thymidylate synthase, an enzyme involved in conversion of deoxyuridylic acid to thymidylic acid
Edatrexate	Inhibits dihydrofolate reductase, thereby halting thymidylate and purine synthesis
Gemcitabine	Inhibits ribonucleotide reductase, competes with cytidine triphosphate for incorporation into DNA
Hydroxyurea	Inhibition of ribonucleoside reductase (inhibits conversion of ribonucleosides to deoxyribonucleosides), thymidine incorporation into DNA and DNA repair
Mercaptopurine	Competes with ribotides for enzymes responsible for conversion of inosinic acid to adenine and xanthine ribotides (inhibits purine synthesis)
Methotrexate	Inhibits dihydrofolate reductase, thereby halting thymidylate and purine synthesis
PALA	Inhibits aspartate carbamoylase, an enzyme that is important to the synthesis of uridine
Pentostatin	Inhibits adenosine deaminase, an enzyme that is important for the metabolism of purine nucleosides
Thioguanine	Competes with guanine in nucleotide (purine) synthesis pathways
Trimetrexate	Same as methotrexate
ZD1694 (Tomudex)	Thymidylate synthase inhibition

DRUG INTERACTIONS WITH ANTINEOPLASTIC AGENTS

A drug interaction is defined as a reaction that occurs when the effects and/or pharmacokinetics of a drug are altered by the prior use or coadministration of another drug. How quickly the reaction occurs varies. Acute-onset reactions (i.e., within 24 hours) may require immediate attention, whereas "slow" interactions may not require immediate action. There are many ways in which drugs may interact, some of which are listed in Box 1-1.

The outcomes of a drug interaction may be diverse. Drug interactions may be beneficial or adverse. A drug interaction may lead to a net increase or decrease in the anticipated pharmacological response, new effects

---

BOX 1-1
Mechanisms of Drug Interactions

Chemical or Physical Interactions
Acids and bases (protamine antagonizes the effects of heparin)
Adsorbent effects (charcoal and cholestyramine decreases absorption)
Incompatibilities of drugs in solutions

Altered Gastrointestinal Absorption
Reduced absorbing surface area and circulation site of absorption (cancer chemotherapy and digoxin tablets)
Reduced gastrointestinal flora (oral aminoglycosides can increase absorption of methotrexate)
Chelation complex

Protein-Binding Interactions
Displacement interactions (aspirin and other drugs displace warfarin, methotrexate, etc.); significance depends on percentage of drug that is protein bound and drug affinities for plasma proteins

"Receptor" Interactions
Agonists and antagonists (opioid analgesics and naloxone)
Additive pharmacological effects (anticholinergic effects)
Sensitization (general anesthetics sensitize the myocardium to the arrhythmogenic effects of catecholamines)
Masking (beta blockers may mask hypoglycemic symptoms of insulin)
Synergy (leucovorin and fluorouracil)
Reversal of cellular resistance (verapamil and doxorubicin)

Acceleration of Metabolism
Induction of hepatic microsomal enzymes (barbiturates, polycyclic hydrocarbons, or rifampin may increase the metabolism of other drugs to inactive compounds [e.g., quinidine, estrogens, methadone, propoxyphene] or may increase metabolism of other drugs [e.g., cyclophosphamide, meperidine] to active or toxic compounds)

---

may develop, or there may be no clinical changes despite changes in pharmacokinetic parameters. In many cases, such interactions may not be predictable.

The Nature of the Problem
Drug interactions are estimated to account for approximately 7% to 22% of all adverse drug reactions (Cramer et al, 1992). As the number of drugs taken by a patient increases, so does the likelihood of a drug interaction (May, Stewart, and Cluff, 1977). In patients taking 10 or more drugs, the prevalence of drug interactions may exceed 20%.

The outcome of a drug interaction is dependent on many factors. Some drug interactions may be clinically significant only if the patient has renal dysfunction or some other abnormality. Other drug interactions (e.g., allopurinol and mercaptopurine) require that a drug (e.g., mercaptopurine) be given orally, rather than intravenously.

Most drug interactions that have been reported are not of major clinical significance. However, antineoplastic agents and a few other drugs have a narrow therapeutic index. In the oncology patient population, there should be an increased amount of concern that a drug interaction may be clinically significant. The detection of an adverse drug interaction, however, may be difficult in oncology patients. Some degree of toxicity is expected from every antineoplastic drug; increased toxicity as a result of a drug interaction may be hard to detect. Evidence that a drug interaction reduces the effectiveness of an antineoplastic drug may be difficult to detect, especially when the treatment is effective in a minority of the patient population.

Specific Drug Interaction

A brief description of some drug interactions that have been reported with antineoplastic drugs follows. This section is organized alphabetically by the generic name of the antineoplastic drug. The more obvious additive drug interactions (e.g., additive nephrotoxicity with cisplatin, streptozocin, and other nephrotoxins; overlapping myelosuppression, etc.) are not included, nor are ex vivo drug interactions (i.e., drug incompatibilities). Table 1-4 is provided as a quick reference to the following discussions.

Altretamine

Altretamine administered in combination with a monoamine oxidase (MAO) inhibitor may potentiate orthostatic hypotension associated with the MAO inhibitor.

Aminoglutethimide

Aminoglutethimide increases the metabolic clearance of warfarin, probably as a result of induction of hepatic microsomal enzymes (Bruning and Bonfrer, 1983; Lonning, Kvinnsland, and Jahren, 1984; Lonning, Ueland, and Kvinnsland, 1986). In two patients taking aminoglutethimide, 250 mg 4 times a day, the plasma clearance of warfarin increased by 90% approximately 14 days after beginning treatment (Lonning, Kvinnsland, and Jahren, 1984).

Anticonvulsants

The observation that phenytoin serum concentrations decreased five-fold to tenfold in several patients during chemotherapy prompted a detailed pharmacokinetic study of one representative patient (Jarosinski et al, 1988). During induction therapy for acute lymphoblastic leukemia with high-dose methotrexate plus leucovorin rescue, prednisone, vincristine, L-asparaginase, and daunorubicin, the dose of phenytoin had to be increased from 8 mg/kg/day to 17 mg/kg/day to maintain a therapeutic serum concentration. Within 6 days after beginning the maintenance portion of treatment, which consisted of vincristine, high-dose methotrexate plus leucovorin rescue, mercaptopurine, and prednisone, phenytoin concentrations fell from 19.8 μg/mL to 3.6 μg/mL. During the second maintenance

TABLE 1-4
Drug Interactions With Antineoplastic Drugs

Drug A	Drug B	Potential outcome
Altretamine	MAO inhibitors	↑ Hypotension
Aminoglutethimide	Sedatives	Additive CNS depression
	Warfarin	↓ Prothrombin time
Asparaginase	Methotrexate	↓ Effects of methotrexate
	Vincristine	↓ Elimination of vincristine
Bicalutamide	Warfarin	↑ Prothrombin time
Bleomycin	Cisplatin	↓ Elimination of bleomycin
Carmustine (BCNU)	Cimetidine	↓ Metabolism of carmustine
	Digoxin	↓ Digoxin plasma levels
Cisplatin	Bleomycin	↓ Elimination of bleomycin
	Cytarabine	↑ Ototoxicity
CMF	Warfarin	↑ Prothrombin time, epistaxis, hematuria
C-MOPP	Digoxin	↓ Digoxin plasma levels
Cyclophosphamide	Succinylcholine	↑ Neuromuscular blockade
Cytarabine	Nephrotoxic drugs	↑ Neurotoxicity of cytarabine
Doxorubicin (with cisplatin)	Phenytoin, carbamazepine, valproate sodium	↓ Plasma levels of each anticonvulsant
Estramustine	Milk products, calcium	↓ Estramustine absorption
Floxuridine	Dexamethasone	↓ Floxuridine hepatotoxicity
Fluorouracil (5-FU)	Allopurinol	↓ 5-FU cytotoxicity
	Cimetidine	↑ 5-FU serum concentrations
	Sorivudine	↑ 5-FU toxicity
Interferon alfa	Theophylline	↓ Theophylline clearance
Leucovorin	Phenytoin	↓ Phenytoin plasma levels
Levamisole and 5-FU	Phenytoin	↓ Phenytoin plasma levels
	Warfarin	↑ Prothrombin time
	Ethanol	Disulfiram (Antabuse) reaction
Melphalan	Cyclosporine	↑ Acute renal failure
	Nalidixic acid	Hemorrhagic enterocolitis
Mercaptopurine (6-MP)	Allopurinol	↑ Oral bioavailability of 6-MP
	Nondepolarizing muscle relaxants	↓ Neuromuscular blockade
	Warfarin	↓ Prothrombin time
	Trimethoprim	↑ Myelosuppression

Continued

TABLE 1-4
Drug Interactions With Antineoplastic Drugs—cont'd

Drug A	Drug B	Potential outcome
Methotrexate (MTX)	Aspirin	↓ Renal elimination of MTX, ↑ toxicity
	Nonsteroidal antiinflammatory drugs	↑ MTX toxicity
	Probenecid	↓ Renal elimination of MTX, ↑ toxicity
	Sulfonamides	↑ MTX protein displacement, ↑ toxicity
	Trimethoprim	Additive enzyme inhibition, ↑ toxicity
Mitomycin	Vinblastine	Acute pneumonitis
Mitotane	Spironolactone	↓ Cytotoxicity of mitotane
	Warfarin	↓ Prothrombin time
Pentostatin	Fludarabine	↑ Fatal pulmonary toxicity
	Vidarabine	↑ Vidarabine toxicity
Procarbazine	Ethanol	Disulfiram (Antabuse) reaction
	Sympathomimetics	Hypertension
	Sedatives	Additive CNS depression
	Tyramine-containing foods	Hypertension
Tamoxifen	Warfarin	↑ Prothrombin time and hematuria
Tegafur	Sorivudine	↑ Tegafur toxicity
Teniposide	Phenytoin, Phenobarbital	↑ Elimination (twofold to threefold) of teniposide
Thiotepa	Pancuronium	↑ Neuromuscular blockade
Tretinoin	Ketoconazole	↓ Elimination of tretinoin
Vincristine	Filgrastim (G-CSF)	Atypical neuropathy
Combination chemotherapy*	Phenytoin	↓ Phenytoin plasma levels

CMF, cyclophosphamide, methotrexate, fluorouracil; *C-MOPP,* cyclophosphamide, vincristine, prednisone, procarbazine; *CNS,* central nervous system, *MAO,* monoamine oxidase.
Combination chemotherapy, methotrexate, leucovorin, vincristine, daunorubicin, asparaginase, mercaptopurine, prednisone.

treatment, phenytoin was administered by intravenous injection and its pharmacokinetics were studied. Peak phenytoin serum concentrations and phenytoin protein binding were no different before or during chemotherapy. However, the half-life of phenytoin decreased from 17 to 9 hours, the urinary elimination of phenytoin's major metabolite increased, and the phenytoin serum concentration fell to a low of 3.8 µg/mL by day 5 of treatment. All of the above is suggestive of accelerated metabolism of phenytoin as a result of one or a combination of the drugs.

In patients receiving cisplatin, vinblastine, and bleomycin (CVB), doubling the dose of phenytoin was required during chemotherapy. Phenytoin levels returned to normal between courses of therapy (Finchman and Schottelius, 1979; Sylvester et al, 1984). In one patient, the phenytoin serum concentrations decreased from 15 µg/mL to 2 µg/mL despite a recent increase in dose (Sylvester et al, 1984). Phenytoin absorption during the next course of chemotherapy with CVB was measured as 32%.

The phenytoin level in one patient receiving phenytoin and phenobarbital fell 50% after treatment with vinblastine and methotrexate. The phenytoin level remained low, presumably because of impaired oral absorption, for 10 days after chemotherapy.

One patient developed seizures after receiving doxorubicin and cisplatin. Plasma concentrations of carbamazepine, phenytoin, and valproic acid were markedly reduced. During a subsequent course of chemotherapy, phenytoin was given intravenously, and concentrations were reduced to 37% of the baseline levels. Serum concentrations of carbamazepine and valproic acid were also significantly reduced (Neef and Voogd-van der Straaten, 1988).

Increased plasma levels of phenytoin have been seen in patients receiving levamisole plus fluorouracil (Stevenson, 1991).

The anticonvulsants phenobarbital and phenytoin have been shown to increase the clearance of teniposide by twofold to threefold (Baker et al, 1992).

L-Asparaginase

L-Asparaginase pretreatment antagonizes the effects of methotrexate (Capizzi, 1975). Administration of L-asparaginase and methotrexate should be separated by at least 24 hours.

L-Asparaginase has been shown to inhibit the elimination of vincristine. It is recommended that vincristine be administered 12 to 24 hours before L-asparaginase.

Bicalutamide

Bicalutamide may displace warfarin from its protein binding sites. The potential for increased prothrombin times exists if bicalutamide is administered to patients already receiving warfarin.

Bleomycin

Cisplatin has been shown to inhibit renal elimination of bleomycin (Bennett, Pastore, and Houghton, 1980).

Carmustine

Cimetidine slows the metabolism of carmustine, presumably by decreasing liver blood flow. Enhanced myelosuppression has been observed in patients receiving cimetidine and carmustine (Volkin et al, 1982).

Cisplatin

Increased ototoxicity has been observed in patients receiving combination chemotherapy with cisplatin and high-dose cytarabine (Atkins et al, 1985).

Increased myelotoxicity has been observed when cisplatin is administered before paclitaxel compared with the reverse order of administration.

Cyclophosphamide

Cyclophosphamide inhibits cholinesterase enzyme activity up to 70%, leading to increased neuromuscular blockade and prolonged respiratory depression caused by succinylcholine. These effects are cyclophosphamide dose-dependent and may occur up to several days after cyclophosphamide therapy is stopped (Gurman, 1972; Dillman, 1987; Zsigmond and Robins, 1972).

Cytarabine

Nephrotoxic drugs may decrease elimination of cytosine arabinoside triphosphate (ara-CTP), a neurotoxic metabolite of cytarabine resulting in neurotoxic sequelae (i.e., confusion, lethargy, ataxia) (Damon, Mass, and Linker, 1989).

Digitalis glycosides

Mucosal defects decrease digoxin absorption in patients with malabsorption syndromes. Since the intestinal mucosa can be damaged by cytotoxic drugs, the effects of digoxin absorption have been studied (Kuhlmann, Zilly, and Wilke, 1981). In six patients with malignant lymphoma who received 0.8 mg beta-acetyldigoxin before and 24 hours after treatment with a combination of cyclophosphamide, vincristine (Oncovin), procarbazine, and prednisone (C-MOPP) or cyclophosphamide, Oncovin, and prednisone (COP), plasma digoxin concentrations were measured up to 8 hours after the dose and areas under the plasma concentration-time curves (AUCs) were calculated. In 15 patients receiving 0.3 mg of beta-acetyldigoxin daily, plasma glycoside concentrations and renal excretion were measured daily before and after the regimens already mentioned or those comprised of cyclophosphamide, vincristine, cytarabine, and prednisone, or doxorubicin, bleomycin, and prednisone. Steady-state digoxin plasma concentrations were significantly reduced 24 to 168 hours after the antineoplastic drug treatment. In addition, the time to achieve a peak digoxin concentration afterward was increased. To maintain adequate control of digoxin therapy in patients treated with antineoplastic drugs, plasma levels should be monitored.

Combination chemotherapy that included doxorubicin, bleomycin, and prednisone, or cyclophosphamide, vincristine, procarbazine, and prednisone, with or without cytarabine, apparently inhibited the absorption of digoxin tablets (Kuhlmann, Zilly, and Wilke, 1981). Plasma levels and AUC were decreased by 50%, arrhythmias recurred, and doubling the oral digoxin dose was required. The absorption of digitoxin tablets was not affected by chemotherapy regimens containing cyclophosphamide, vincristine, prednisone, or procarbazine (Kuhlmann, Wilke, and Rietbrock, 1982).

Estramustine

Milk, milk products, and calcium-rich foods or drugs have been shown to inhibit the absorption of estramustine.

Filgrastim

The combination of vincristine and filgrastim (granulocyte colony-stimulating factor [G-CSF]) is reported to induce a severe atypical neuropathy characterized by foot pain and severe motor weakness (Weintraub et al, 1996).

Floxuridine

Concomitant intrahepatic dexamethasone and floxuridine may reduce the hepatotoxicity of floxuridine (Kemeny et al, 1992).

Fluorouracil

Allopurinol inhibits activation of fluorouracil to one of its cytotoxic metabolites (Fox, Woods, and Tattersall, 1979; Fox et al, 1981; Howell et al, 1981). Allopurinol may decrease the effectiveness of fluorouracil.

Halogenated antiviral drugs (e.g., sorivudine, netivudine) inhibit dihydropyrimidine dehydrogenase, an important enzyme in the metabolism of fluorouracil. Concomitant administration of sorivudine and fluorouracil significantly increases the toxicity of fluorouracil (Peck et al, 1996).

Interferon alfa

Theophylline clearance has been shown to be reduced by 33% to 88% and theophylline half-life increased by 70% within 24 hours of an intramuscular injection of interferon alfa-2b (Williams, Baird-Lambert, and Farrell, 1987). The effect was greatest in fast metabolizers of theophylline (i.e., smokers). Theophylline serum concentrations should be monitored closely during and after discontinuation of interferon treatment.

Leucovorin

Leucovorin may adversely affect phenytoin serum levels. See the anticonvulsant section for a detailed description of this potential drug interaction.

Levamisole

Increased plasma levels of phenytoin have been seen in patients receiving levamisole in combination with fluorouracil (Stevenson, 1991).

Prolongation of the prothrombin time has been observed in patients receiving warfarin in combination with levamisole and fluorouracil (Stevenson, 1991).

Concomitant administration of ethanol and levamisole may precipitate a disulfiram (Antabuse) reaction.

Melphalan

Administration of cyclosporine and melphalan has resulted in acute renal failure after the first dose of each drug.

The combination of nalidixic acid and melphalan has been associated with an increased incidence of hemorrhagic enterocolitis.

Mercaptopurine

Allopurinol causes a 400% to 500% increase in the oral bioavailability of mercaptopurine because of decreased first-pass hepatic metabolism. Allopurinol inhibits xanthine oxidase, the enzyme that metabolizes mercaptopurine (Zimm et al, 1983; Coffey et al, 1972). The dose of oral mercaptopurine must be reduced by 75% if the patient is also taking allopurinol. Allopurinol does not significantly affect the pharmacokinetics of mercaptopurine administered by intravenous injection to patients with normal renal function (Zimm et al, 1985). Allopurinol may increase the amount of intravenous mercaptopurine that is excreted in the urine (from 21% to 42%), and this increase could be enough to enhance the toxicity of mercaptopurine if renal function is reduced.

Trimethoprim-sulfamethoxazole (Bactrim, Septra) may increase the myelo-suppression of mercaptopurine.

Methotrexate

Aspirin and other acetylated salicylates inhibit the renal elimination of methotrexate via competition for renal tubular secretion (Liegler et al, 1969). The potential for methotrexate toxicity is greatly enhanced when these drugs are given simultaneously.

Enhanced methotrexate toxicity has been observed when methotrexate and nonsteroidal antiinflammatory drugs (NSAIDs) are given simultaneously (Maiche, 1986; Singh et al, 1986; Gabrielli, Leoni, and Danieli, 1977; Ellison and Servi, 1985). Although the exact mechanisms are unknown, NSAIDs may reduce renal blood flow, decrease methotrexate clearance, or cause additive nephrotoxicity.

Probenecid has been shown to decrease the amount of methotrexate that is eliminated by renal tubular secretion (Aherne et al, 1978; Bourke et al, 1975; Lilly and Omura, 1985). The combination of methotrexate and probenecid may result in a threefold to fourfold increase in methotrexate concentrations. In one patient receiving methotrexate for rheumatoid arthritis, the concomitant administration of probenecid caused life-threatening pancytopenia (Basin, Escalante, and Beardmore, 1991).

Sulfonamides may displace methotrexate from protein-binding sites, causing enhanced methotrexate toxicity (Jeurissen, Boerbooms, and van de Putte, 1989).

Trimethoprim (a component of Bactrim, Septra) is also an inhibitor of dihydrofolate reductase. The combination of methotrexate and trimethoprim may enhance methotrexate toxicity (Jeurissen, Boerbooms, and van de Putte, 1989).

Mitomycin

The combination of vinblastine and mitomycin may be associated with acute pneumonitis (Luedke et al, 1985; Verweij et al, 1987).

Mitotane

Mitotane may accelerate the metabolism of warfarin and reduce prothrombin times.

Spironolactone may block the effects of mitotane (Wortsman and Soler, 1977).

Pentostatin

Concomitant administration of fludarabine and pentostatin has been associated with an increased incidence of fatal pulmonary toxicity.

Pentostatin has been shown to enhance the effects of vidarabine. Increased adverse effects of vidarabine and pentostatin are possible if the drugs are administered concomitantly.

Procarbazine

Concomitant administration of ethanol and procarbazine may precipitate a disulfiram (Antabuse) reaction (Spivack, 1974).

Procarbazine is a weak inhibitor of monoamine oxidase. The combined use of tricyclic antidepressants, sympathomimetic drugs (e.g., ephedrine), and/or tyramine-containing foods with procarbazine could increase blood pressure (Averbuch, 1990).

Tegafur

Halogenated antiviral drugs (e.g., sorivudine, netivudine) inhibit dihydropyrimidine dehydrogenase, an important enzyme in the metabolism of fluorouracil. Concomitant administration of sorivudine and tegafur significantly increases the toxicity of tegafur (Peck et al, 1996).

Teniposide

Phenobarbital and phenytoin have been shown to increase the clearance of teniposide by twofold to threefold (Baker et al, 1992).

Thiotepa

One patient experienced increased neuromuscular blockade, prolonged respiratory depression, and periods of apnea after the administration of intraperitoneal thiotepa given 90 minutes after pancuronium.

Tretinoin

Ketoconazole has been shown to inhibit the metabolism of tretinoin. A 72% increase in the area under the [plasma concentration] curve (AUC) was demonstrated when ketoconazole was administered with tretinoin.

Warfarin

A few cases of a drug interaction involving warfarin and cyclophosphamide have been reported (Seifter, Brooks, and Urba, 1985; Ward and Bitran, 1984). In each case, an increasing prothrombin time was observed after discontinuation of oral cyclophosphamide, 450 mg/day.

Increased doses of warfarin have been necessary in patients receiving treatment with mercaptopurine (Spiers and Mibashan, 1974).

In one patient taking warfarin 3 days after beginning tamoxifen, 10 mg twice daily, the prothrombin time (PT) was 39 seconds (baseline is 34 seconds). Three weeks later the PT was 206 seconds. A 40% decrease in the dose of warfarin was required to maintain the baseline PT (Lodwick, McConkey, and Brown, 1987).

Prolongation of the prothrombin time has been observed in patients receiving warfarin in combination with levamisole and fluorouracil (Stevenson, 1991).

DRUGS PRESENTED

In this revision, over 100 drugs and biological response modifiers are discussed. We have continued to list drugs and hormones alphabetically by their current generic name in Chapter 3. Biological response modifiers are also listed alphabetically and can be found in Chapter 4.

REFERENCES

Aherne GW et al: Prolongation and enhancement of serum methotrexate concentrations by probenecid, *Br Med J* 1:1097-1099, 1978.

Allegra CJ: Antifolates. In Chabner BA, Collins JM, eds: *Cancer chemotherapy, principles and practice*, Philadelphia, 1990, JB Lippincott, pp 110-153.

Atkins JN et al: Phase I study of high-dose cytarabine and cisplatin in patients with advanced malignancy, *Cancer Treat Rep* 69:897-899, 1985.

Averbuch SD: Non-classical alkylating agents. In Chabner BA, Collins JM, eds: *Cancer chemotherapy, principles and practice*, Philadelphia, 1990, JB Lippincott, pp 314-340.

Baker DK et al: Increased teniposide clearance with concomitant anticonvulsant therapy, *J Clin Oncol* 10:311-315, 1992.

Basin KS, Escalante A, Beardmore TD: Severe pancytopenia in a patient taking low dose methotrexate and probenecid, *J Rheumatol* 18:609-610, 1991.

Bender RA, Hamel E, Hande KR: Plant alkaloids. In Chabner BA, Collins JM, eds: *Cancer chemotherapy, principles and practice*, Philadelphia, 1990, JB Lippincott, pp 253-275.

Bennett WM, Pastore L, Houghton DC: Fatal pulmonary toxicity in cisplatin-induced acute renal failure, *Cancer Treat Rep* 64:921-924, 1980.

Bines J, Oleske DM, Cobleigh MA: Ovarian function in premenopausal women treated with adjuvant chemotherapy for breast cancer, *J Clin Oncol* 14:1718-1729, 1996.

Bourke RS et al: Inhibition of renal tubular transport of methotrexate by probenecid, *Cancer Res* 35:110-116, 1975.

Boyd NF: The epidemiology of cancer: principles and methods. In Tannock IF, Hill RP, eds: *The basic science of oncology*, ed 2, New York, 1992, McGraw-Hill, pp 7-22.

Bruning PF, Bonfrer JG: Aminoglutethimide and oral anticoagulant therapy, *Lancet* 2:582, 1983.

Cadman EC, Durivage HJ: Cancer chemotherapy. In Wilson JD et al, eds: *Harrison's principles of internal medicine*, ed 12, New York, 1990, McGraw-Hill, pp 1587-1599.

Capizzi RL: Improvement in the therapeutic index of methotrexate by L-asparaginase, *Cancer Chemother Rep* 6(part 3):37-41, 1975.

Chabner BA: Bleomycin. In Chabner BA, Collins JM, eds: *Cancer chemotherapy, principles and practice*, Philadelphia, 1990a, JB Lippincott, pp 341-355.

Chabner BA: Clinical strategies for cancer treatment: the role of drugs. In Chabner BA, Collins JM, eds: *Cancer chemotherapy, principles and practice*, Philadelphia, 1990b, JB Lippincott, pp 1-15.

Chabner BA: Cytidine analogues. In Chabner BA, Collins JM, eds: *Cancer chemotherapy, principles and practice*, Philadelphia, 1990c, JB Lippincott, pp 154-179.

Coffey JJ et al: Effect of allopurinol on the pharmacokinetics of 6-mercaptopurine (NSC 755) in cancer patients, *Cancer Res* 32:1283-1289, 1972.

Colvin M, Chabner BA: Alkylating agents. In Chabner BA, Collins JM, eds: *Cancer chemotherapy, principles and practice*, Philadelphia, 1990, JB Lippincott, pp 276-313.

Cramer RL et al: Drug interaction monitoring program in a community hospital, *Am J Hosp Pharm* 49:627-629, 1992.

Damon LE, Mass R, Linker CA: The association between cytarabine neurotoxicity and renal insufficiency, *J Clin Oncol* 7:1563-1568, 1989.

DeVita VT Jr: The problem of resistance. In DeVita VT Jr, Hellman S, Rosenberg SA, eds: *Principles and practice of oncology, PPO updates*, 4:1-12, 1990.

DeVita VT Jr, Hellman S, Rosenberg SA, eds: *Principles and practice of oncology*, ed 4, Philadelphia, 1993, JB Lippincott.

Dillman JB: Safe use of succinylcholine during repeated anesthetics in a patient treated with cyclophosphamide, *Anesth Analg* 66:351-353, 1987.

Donehower RC: Hydroxyurea. In Chabner BA, Collins JM, eds: *Cancer chemotherapy, principles and practice*, Philadelphia, 1990, JB Lippincott, pp 225-233.

Ellison NM, Servi R: Acute renal failure and death after sequential intermediate-dose methotrexate and 5-FU: a possible adverse effect due to concomitant indomethacin administration, *Cancer Treat Rep* 69:342-343, 1985.

Finchman RW, Schottelius DD: Decreased phenytoin levels in antineoplastic therapy, *Ther Drug Monit* 1:277-283, 1979.

Ford JM, Hait WN: Pharmacology of drugs that alter multidrug resistance in cancer, *Pharmacol Rev* 42:155-199, 1990.

Fox RM, Woods RL, Tattersall MHN: Allopurinol modulation of high-dose 5-FU toxicity, *Cancer Treat Rev* 6:143-147, 1979.

Fox RM et al: Allopurinol modulation of 5-FU toxicity, *Cancer Chemother Pharmacol* 5:151-155, 1981.

Gabrielli A, Leoni P, Danieli G: Methotrexate and non-steroidal antiinflammatory drugs, *Br Med J* 294:776, 1977.

Gilman A: The initial clinical trial of nitrogen mustard, *Am J Surg* 105:574-578, 1963.

Grem JL: Fluorinated pyrimidines. In Chabner BA, Collins JM, eds: *Cancer chemotherapy, principles and practice*, Philadelphia, 1990, JB Lippincott, pp 180-224.

Gurman GM: Prolonged apnea after succinylcholine in a case treated with cytostatics for cancer, *Anesth Analg* 51:761-765, 1972.

Hansen SW, Berthelsen JG, von der Maase H: Long-term fertility and Leydig cell function in patients treated for germ cell cancer with cisplatin, vinblastine and bleomycin versus surveillance, *J Clin Oncol* 8:1695-1698, 1990.

Howell SB et al: Modulation of 5-FU toxicity by allopurinol in man, *Cancer* 48:1281-1289, 1981.

Jarosinski PE et al: Altered phenytoin clearance during intensive chemotherapy for acute lymphoblastic leukemia, *J Pediatr* 112:996-999, 1988.

Jeurissen ME, Boerbooms AM, van de Putte LB: Pancytopenia and methotrexate with trimethoprim-sulfamethoxazole, *Ann Intern Med* 111:261, 1989.

Karchmer RK et al: Alkylating agents as leukemogens in multiple myeloma, *Cancer* 33:1103-1107, 1974.

Kemeny N et al: A randomized trial of intrahepatic infusion of fluorodeoxyuridine with dexamethasone versus fluorodeoxyuridine alone in the treatment of metastatic colorectal cancer, *Cancer* 69:327-334, 1992.

Kuhlmann J, Wilke J, Rietbrock N: Cytostatic drugs are without significant effect on digitoxin plasma level and excretion, *Clin Pharmacol Ther* 32:646-651, 1982.

Kuhlmann J, Zilly W, Wilke J: Effects of cytostatic drugs on plasma level and renal excretion of beta-acetyldigoxin, *Clin Pharmacol Ther* 30:518-527, 1981.

Liegler DG et al: The effect of organic acids on renal clearance of methotrexate in man, *Clin Pharmacol Ther* 10:849-857, 1969.

Lilly MB, Omura GA: Clinical pharmacology of oral intermediate-dose methotrexate with or without probenecid, *Cancer Chemother Pharmacol* 15:220-222, 1985.

Liu LF: DNA topoisomerase poisons as antitumor drugs, *Ann Rev Biochem* 58:351-375, 1989.

Lodwick R, McConkey B, Brown AM: Life threatening interaction between tamoxifen and warfarin, *Br Med J* 295:1141, 1987.

Lonning PE, Kvinnsland S, Jahren G: Aminoglutethimide and warfarin, a new important drug interaction, *Cancer Chemother Pharmacol* 12:10-12, 1984.

Lonning PE, Ueland PM, Kvinnsland S: The influence of a graded dose schedule of aminoglutethimide on the disposition of the optical enantiomers of warfarin in patients with breast cancer, *Cancer Chemother Pharmacol* 17:177-181, 1986.

Luedke D et al: Mitomycin and vindesine associated pulmonary toxicity with variable clinical expression, *Cancer* 55:542-545, 1985.

Maiche AG: Acute renal failure due to concomitant action of methotrexate and indomethacin (letter), *Lancet* 1:1390, 1986.

May FE, Stewart RB, Cluff LE: Drug interactions and multiple drug administration, *Clin Pharmacol Ther* 22:322-328, 1977.

McCormack JJ, Johns DG: Purine antimetabolites. In Chabner BA, Collins JM, eds: *Cancer chemotherapy, principles and practice*, Philadelphia, 1990, JB Lippincott, pp 234-252.

Moscow JA, Cowan KH: Multidrug resistance, *J Natl Cancer Inst* 80:14-20, 1988.

Myers CE, Chabner BA: Anthracyclines. In Chabner BA, Collins JM, eds: *Cancer chemotherapy, principles and practice*, Philadelphia, 1990, JB Lippincott, pp 356-382.

Neef C, Voogd-van der Straaten I: An interaction between cytostatic and anticonvulsant drugs, *Clin Pharmacol Ther* 43:372-375, 1988.

Peck R et al: Inhibition of dihydropyrimidine dehydrogenase by 5-propynyluracil, a metabolite of the anti-varicella zoster virus agent netivudine, *Clin Pharmacol Ther* 59:22-31, 1996.

Reed E, Kohn KW: Platinum analogues. In Chabner BA, Collins JM, eds: *Cancer chemotherapy, principles and practice*, Philadelphia, 1990, JB Lippincott, pp 465-490.

Schipper H, Goh CR, Wang TL: Shifting the cancer paradigm: must we kill to cure? *J Clin Oncol* 13:801-807, 1995.

Seifter EJ, Brooks BJ, Urba WJ: Possible interactions between warfarin and antineoplastic drugs, *Cancer Treat Rep* 69:244-245, 1985.

Singh RR et al: Fatal interaction between methotrexate and naproxen (letter), *Lancet* 1:1390, 1986.

Sinha BK: Topoisomerase inhibitors, a review of their therapeutic potential in cancer, *Drugs* 49:11-19, 1995.

Spiers ASD, Mibashan RS: Increased warfarin requirement during mercaptopurine therapy, *Lancet* 2:221-222, 1974.

Spivack SD: Procarbazine, *Ann Intern Med* 81:795-800, 1974.

Stevenson HC: Potential adverse levamisole interactions with phenytoin and also with coumarin, *NCI Warning Letter*, July 10, 1991.

Sylvester RK et al: Impaired phenytoin bioavailability secondary to cisplatin, vinblastine, and bleomycin, *Ther Drug Monit* 6:302-305, 1984.

Verweij J et al: Prospective study on the dose relationship of mitomycin C–induced interstitial pneumonitis, *Cancer* 60:756-761, 1987.

Volkin RL et al: Potentiation of carmustine–cranial irradiation-induced myelosuppression by cimetidine, *Arch Intern Med* 142:243-244, 1982.

Wall RL, Clausen KP: Carcinoma of the urinary bladder in patients receiving cyclophosphamide, *N Engl J Med* 293:271-273, 1975.

Ward K, Bitran JD: Warfarin, etoposide, and vindesine interactions, *Cancer Treat Rep* 68:817-818, 1984.

Weintraub M et al: Severe atypical neuropathy associated with colony-stimulating factors and vincristine, *J Clin Oncol* 14:935-940, 1996.

Williams SJ, Baird-Lambert JA, Farrell GC: Inhibition of theophylline metabolism by interferon, *Lancet* 2:939-941, 1987.

Wortsman J, Soler NG: Mitotane. spironolactone's antagonism in Cushing's syndrome, *JAMA* 238:2527, 1977.

Zimm S et al: Inhibition of first-pass metabolism in cancer chemotherapy: interaction of 6-mercaptopurine and allopurinol, *Clin Pharmacol Ther* 34:810-817, 1983.

Zimm S et al: Phase I and clinical pharmacological study of mercaptopurine administered as a prolonged intravenous infusion, *Cancer Res* 45:1869-1873, 1985.

Zsigmond EK, Robins G: The effect of a series of anti-cancer drugs on plasma cholinesterase activity, *Can Anaesth Soc J* 19:75-82, 1972.

2

Clinical Trials and
Good Clinical Practice

A clinical trial is a scientific study designed to answer important clinical and biological questions and is carried out by protocol, a written guideline for the study. Good clinical practice (GCP) is an international quality standard for the design, conduct, recording, analyses, and reporting of clinical trials that provides assurance that the data and reported results are accurate (ICH, 1995). The protocol defines the essential elements of the study and how it will be conducted. In the treatment of cancer, clinical trials provide the only scientific mechanism to test the effectiveness of new therapies and are a necessary corollary to laboratory research (Fisher, 1984; Levine, 1983). This chapter focuses on clinical oncology research, drug development in the United States, and the implementation and conduct of a clinical trial.

Clinical research is the foundation on which almost all accepted medical practices are based. The major advances made in the treatment of Hodgkin's and non-Hodgkin's lymphomas, testicular cancer, pediatric acute leukemia, hairy cell leukemia, bladder carcinoma, stage I-II breast cancer, and other malignancies could only be achieved through the conduct and completion of clinical trials. In the field of oncology almost all standard (i.e., commonly used and accepted) treatments for patients with cancer arose from clinical trials conducted by medical, surgical, and radiation oncologists. The chance of discovering successful anticancer therapies and building on current knowledge without the use of clinical trials is very unlikely. As Epictetus said, "It is impossible for a man to learn what he thinks he already knows" (Epictetus, 1978). Rapid improvement in the treatment of patients with cancer will only be achieved through the widespread participation of physicians and patients in clinical trials.

Clinical trials have undergone close scrutiny and critique because they influence and provide the basis for treatment selection by practicing oncologists. Criticism of clinical trials in medical oncology has touched on virtually every aspect from design to publication. Problems can occur because of poor design (Carpenter, 1993; Piantadosi, 1988), loose criteria for patient selection (Begg, 1988), lack of the ability to generalize results (Begg and Engstrom, 1987; Gail, 1985), journal bias for publishing "positive" results (Simes, 1986), and statistical inferences that often are of question-able clinical relevance.

Despite criticism, the clinical trial is the *only* mechanism to obtain answers to clinical questions with as little bias as possible. Treating patients with nonstandard or modified standard regimens (i.e., "ad hoc" treatments) or according to an ongoing clinical trial (Begg et al, 1983; Levine, 1983) does not contribute useful information about the safety or effectiveness of the treatment (Hanks, 1984). Furthermore, some would consider these practices to be potentially dangerous because the patients are not monitored as they would be if participating in a study, quality assurance measures are not in place, and serious adverse events not reported to a study center or principal investigator.

CLINICAL ONCOLOGY TRIALS IN THE UNITED STATES

When asked about clinical trials, the majority of patients and the public have favorable views regarding the values of clinical research (Cassileth et al, 1982). Patients participate in clinical trials with the hope of attaining therapeutic benefit (Daugherty et al, 1995). Patients may also participate in clinical trials to help other patients who will develop a similar medical condition in the future, to increase knowledge about their disease, to take advantage of increased monitoring as a part of a clinical study, to obtain a second opinion about their disease, and for many other reasons (Mattson et al, 1985; Cassileth et al, 1980). Patients most often refuse to take part in a clinical trial or withdraw from one because of real or per-ceived factors related to the treatment (Barofsky and Sugarbaker, 1979).

Although most oncologists believe they have an obligation to enroll patients onto clinical studies, currently only around 2% to 3% of the patients with cancer are enrolled onto clinical research protocols (Anon, 1988; Gelber and Goldhirsch, 1988; Friedman, 1987; Hunter et al, 1987; Wittes and Friedman, 1988). Moreover, only 1% to 2% of all patients with the most common malignancies (i.e., breast or colon cancer) participate in a clinical trial (Anon, 1988; Wittes and Friedman, 1988). In the United States the majority of patients with cancer (nearly 1 million per year) receive their treatment outside of a cancer center/university setting (Levine, 1983). Improved treatments will only be obtained through the participation of patients and their caregivers in clinical studies. Initial data from the National Cancer Institute (NCI) on the Community Clinical Oncology Program (CCOP) show that approximately 19% of the patients for whom there is a clinical trial actually enroll onto the study (Hunter et al, 1987). Cooperative oncology groups enroll approximately 10% to 30% of potentially eligible patients for whom there is a clinical trial (Wittes and Friedman, 1988; Martin et al, 1984; Levine, 1983; Begg et al, 1983). Since effective treatment does not exist for the majority of the adult malignan-cies, it should be clear that there is the need for substantial improvement in patient recruitment to clinical trials.

Medical schools teach students to be individual decision makers, that is, to use one's own clinical judgment to treat a patient. The randomization aspect of clinical trials philosophically opposes the teachings that support

---

BOX 2-1
Reasons for Not Enrolling Patients Onto a Clinical Trial

It may harm the doctor-patient relationship
Difficulty with informed consent
Dislike of open discussions about uncertainty
Conflict between roles of scientist and clinician
Limited staff and financial support for research activities
Practical difficulties with the protocol (e.g., procedures, data collection)
Concern with the design of the study
Not developed in collaboration with other participants
Significance of the scientific question is not important
Personal responsibilities if one of the treatments in a comparative trial is
    found to be unequal
Extra time involved to discuss protocol
Lack of third-party reimbursement

Modified from Taylor KM, Morgdese RG, Soskoline CL: Physicians' reasons for not entering eligible patients in a randomized clinical trial of surgery for breast cancer, *N Engl J Med* 310:1363-1367, 1984.

individual physician authority and power (Fisher, 1984). In practice, this speculation has been validated. Physicians participating in a cooperative group randomized clinical trial were surveyed to determine possible reasons for poor patient accrual (Taylor, Morgolese, and Soskoline, 1984). The reasons for not enrolling patients are shown in Box 2-1. This study was conducted with a group of surgeons who were asked to enroll women with primary breast cancer to a study comparing total mastectomy to segmental mastectomy with or without radiation therapy. This study has been criticized because patients and physicians had clear preferences to which therapy they preferred. Clinical equipoise (i.e., there is no preferred treatment because controversy exists in the medical community as to the best treatment) was not present in this study (Freedman, 1988). However, similar reasons (e.g., uncertainty with new treatment, loyalty to current practices, problems with study design, limited financial and staff support for research activities) have been cited by medical oncologists for not enrolling patients onto clinical trials (Matthews, 1995; Brennan, 1989; Taylor, 1985; Langley et al, 1987; Martin et al, 1984). The potential benefits of increasing patient accrual in clinical trials are expansion of the number of trials, rapid completion of the trial, and rapid transfer of results from the investigational stage to routine practice. A major goal of the National Cancer Institute (NCI) is to increase patient entry into clinical trials. The NCI-designated high-priority trials program is aimed toward this end (Wittes and Friedman, 1988). High-priority studies are those deemed to ask an important question and to have a reasonable chance of improving the survival of patients with a common disease (Wittes and Friedman, 1988).

The Physician's Data Query (PDQ) system is a major effort of the NCI that is directed at patients and health care providers. The PDQ database provides information on state of the art cancer treatments (updated monthly);

clinical research trials in the United States, Canada, and Europe; a directory of more than 1500 organizations with certified cancer programs; and more than 12,000 specialists for consultation or referral (Hubbard, Henney, and DeVita, 1987). Access to the PDQ database is available through the National Library of Medicine, MEDLARS, and commercial vendors (e.g., BRS/Saunders, DIALOG, Mead Data Control). Anyone who has a personal computer and a modem can access the PDQ database. In addition, the NCI network of Cancer Information Services* is a resource for information and questions on the PDQ system.

Institutions that wish to improve patient accrual to studies should consider each of the possible reasons why they have not been successful at enrolling patients onto clinical trials and develop strategies for overcoming these shortcomings. Examining the patient enrollment history from specific community-based medical oncologists will probably reveal that active participants remain active and inactive participants remain inactive. Priority should be given to invigorating the enthusiasm of previously and/or presently active community physicians, while spending little time and effort stimulating the enthusiasm of unlikely participants. Increased patient accrual from noninstitutional practitioners may be enhanced through awareness, availability, applicability, and collaboration (Hunninghake, Darby, and Probstfield, 1987). Several methods may be useful in enhancing public awareness of the studies available, primarily through mailings, news media, public appearances (e.g., tumor boards, grand rounds) and telephone calls (Gelber and Goldhirsch, 1988). Increased public relations efforts should be directed at surgeons and primary care physicians who refer patients with cancer for further treatment.

Studies should be made as applicable and as practical as possible (George, 1996; Begg, 1987). Actions such as elimination of extraneous testing procedures, reduction of the number of eligibility criteria, and elimination of nonessential data collection can make clinical trials more palatable to all participants and increase accrual to the clinical trial (Joseph, 1994). Reducing the number of eligibility criteria has been cited as a method for increasing patient enrollment, allowing broader generalizations of study results, and reducing the complexity and costs of patient participation (George, 1996). Relaxation of unnecessary restrictions on treating patients at the cancer center should be done if medically and logistically possible, provided that the quality of the data can be ensured. Institutions interested in increasing patient accrual from community participants should critically evaluate studies that require that patients be treated and/or evaluated solely at the main institution. Those who participate in a clinical trial need to be informed of its progress. Regular meetings among collaborators and frequent updates have been cited as positive influences on patient accrual to clinical trials (Taylor, Shapiro, and Skinner, 1987; Hunninghake, Darby, and Probstfield, 1987). Community-based practitioners who want to become involved in clinical research activities should also consider the topics described above and seek ways in which to become involved.

Reimbursement policies of insurance companies, health maintenance organizations (HMOs), and Medicare can adversely affect physician and

---

*NCI network of Cancer Information Services phone number: 1-800-4-CANCER.

BOX 2-2
Impact of Third-Party Reimbursement on Cancer
Clinical Investigations: A Consensus Statement
Coordinated by the National Cancer Institute

Third-party coverage be allowed for patient care costs of all nationally-approved (NCI or FDA) cancer treatment research protocols

Third-party coverage be allowed for all cancer treatment research protocols, provided these protocols have been approved by established peer-review mechanisms, such as:

    a. NCI and other designated cancer centers

    b. Recognized national or regional cooperative groups

    c. As a part of a peer-reviewed grant endeavor, or

    d. Protocols entered into the Physician Data Query (PDQ) system

---

Modified from McCabe M, Friedman MA: Impact of third-party reimbursement on cancer clinical investigations: A consensus statement coordinated by the National Cancer Institute, *J Natl Cancer Inst* 81:1585-1586, 1989.

patient participation in clinical trials (Wittes, 1987b; Antman, Schnipper, and Frei, 1988; McCabe and Friedman, 1989; Friedman and McCabe, 1992). Refusal to reimburse for the costs of a treatment that is offered as a part of a clinical study suppresses patient recruitment to clinical trials and slows the advancement of the field of oncology. Practitioners who find that insurance company or HMO policies impede their ability to enroll patients onto a study should notify the principal investigator. Efforts to remedy the situation should be undertaken by the principal investigator and appropriate cancer center/university personnel. A consensus conference was sponsored by the NCI to address this issue (McCabe and Friedman, 1989). It is recommended that third-party payers reimburse for the costs associated with the clinical care but not the research costs of NCI-approved and other, selected clinical trials (Box 2-2).

DRUG DEVELOPMENT AND THE PHASES OF CLINICAL TRIALS

In the United States, Canada, and many other countries, drugs and biological agents become commercially available only after careful preclinical testing (i.e., studies on animals or laboratory models) followed by clinical trials in man (Johnson and Temple, 1985). Major efforts have been made in recent years to standardize (or harmonize) the requirements of these stages of drug development (ICH, 1995). In the following section this process is briefly described. For a more detailed discussion of clinical trials development, design, and reporting of results, refer to other sources (Buyse, Staquet, and Sylvester, 1984; Piantadosi, 1988; Spilker, 1991; Simon, 1993; Johnson and Temple, 1985; Wittes, 1987a; Tannock and Murphy, 1983; Zelen, 1983).

Preclinical Evaluation of Drugs

The aim of preclinical testing is to evaluate the effectiveness and toxicity of a drug or biological agent before it is administered to humans.

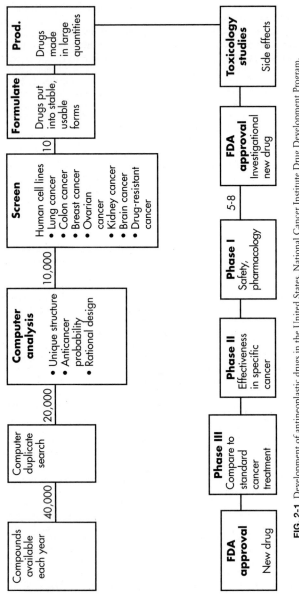

FIG. 2-1 Development of antineoplastic drugs in the United States. National Cancer Institute Drug Development Program. (From National Cancer Institute: *1989 NCI Budget Estimate*, 1987.)

The drug-development program of the NCI has changed from the traditional test system of in vivo animal screening to a panel of tumor cell lines derived from human malignancies (Boyd, 1989). Cell line screening helps identify new drugs but also allows target testing of drugs in patients with the same tumor type. Acceleration of the testing of treatments through large-scale national trials in specific cancers is the goal of these efforts (Fig. 2-1). In addition, as the data accumulate on the biochemical and genetic features of drug resistance, new lines with those features will be added to the drug screen. Also added will be new agents identified through the National Cooperative Drug Discovery Group that inhibit oncogene expression, growth factors, and DNA repair, and those that block other metabolic or regulatory pathways (Wittes, 1987a).

Preclinical toxicology studies are also done in at least two species (usually rat and dog). These studies are performed to determine dose-limiting toxicities, the extent of various toxicities, and the LD10 (i.e., dose of drug that is lethal to 10% of the animals). These studies are essential because they allow for the estimation of a safe starting dose for human studies (Grieshaber and Marsoni, 1986).

Phase I Trials

Because of their narrow therapeutic index, phase I trials of antineoplastic drugs differ from the phase I testing of other drugs by virtue of the fact that patients must be used instead of normal volunteers. In the field of oncology, phase I trials are conducted with therapeutic intent, although it is realized that a significant proportion of patients will not receive a biologically active dose. Therapeutic responses are not common (i.e., incidence is around 4%), and the majority of responses occur at or near the dose recommended for evaluation in future studies (Smith et al, 1996; Estey et al, 1986; Von Hoff and Turner, 1991). For many patients, however, the maintenance of hope, psychological benefits, and subjective responses to a therapy should not be underestimated (Daugherty et al, 1995). The major endpoints of a phase I trial are to evaluate acute toxicity, establish the maximum tolerated dose (MTD), and analyze pharmacological data (Von Hoff, Kuhn, and Clark, 1984). These endpoints usually need to be attained for each dosing schedule (e.g., once daily every 3 weeks, once daily for 5 days every 3 weeks). The initial drug dose is traditionally one tenth of the murine LD10. If at least three patients do not exhibit significant toxicity after the initial dose, additional patients are enrolled to the next dose level. Typically, a minimum of three patients are treated with each dose until dose toxicity is observed, and each subsequent dose producing dose-limiting toxicity requires six patients for evaluation. A commonly employed model for dose escalation is a modified Fibonacci method (Von Hoff, Kuhn, and Clark, 1984). This method allows for initial large-dose increments followed by smaller dose increments (Table 2-1). Even with this escalation method, approximately 60% of the patients are treated with doses below the MTD (Smith et al, 1996; Wittes, 1987a). Other methods by which to select a safe starting dose and to evaluate different treatment schedules for phase I trials have been proposed and/or evaluated (Ratain et al, 1993; Wittes, 1987a; EORTC, 1987; Gianni et al, 1990; Graham and Workman, 1992; Collins, Grieshaber, and Chabner, 1990).

TABLE 2-1
Modified Fibonacci Dose Escalation Schema*

Drug dose	% Increase above prior dose level
n*	—
2.0n	100
3.3n	67
5.0n	50
7.0n	40
9.0n	33
12.0n	33
16.0n	33

Modified from Von Hoff DD, Kuhn J, Clark GM: Design and conduct of phase I trials. In Buyse ME, Staquet MJ, Sylvester RJ, eds: *Cancer clinical trials: methods and practice,* New York, 1984, Oxford University Press, pp 210-220.
*Initial dose level, $n = mg/m^2$.

Phase II Trials

Phase II trials are intended to determine antitumor activity, gather information on dose response, and further evaluate the safety of the drug (Piantadosi, 1988). The chances of detecting an active drug are best when the phase II agent is administered before other treatments have been given. Patients who are eligible for phase II trials are, ideally, untreated patients. Most are patients with malignancies for which chemotherapy has shown little or no benefit, such as renal cell carcinoma, nonsmall cell lung cancer, melanoma, and pancreatic cancer. However, it has been shown in patients with metastatic breast cancer or small cell lung cancer that administering a phase II agent as the first therapy does not negatively affect survival (Evans et al, 1990). At the end of the phase II trial, specific knowledge regarding tumor activity, as well as administration techniques, precautions, modifications of dose and scheduling, predicted acute toxicity, and the necessary supportive care are more clearly defined.

Phase III Trials

Phase III trials aim at defining the role of a drug in a cancer-treatment regimen. For example, the effectiveness of a drug may be studied by comparing it with another treatment or combining it with a standard treatment regimen. In phase III comparative studies, patients are randomized to receive one of the treatments to be evaluated. Evaluation of the drug's impact on survival, assessment of rates of response, duration of response, toxicity, and quality of life are all elements that are used to determine the preferred treatment in a comparative study. When the study has been completed, it should be known whether the treatment is equal to or better than the standard therapy, whether it produces equivalent or less toxicity, whether demonstrates the potential for combination with other agents, and finally, whether it has a significant positive effect on the quality of life and survival of patients treated.

Phase IV Trials

Phase IV trials are postmarketing studies. Their endpoints are often aimed at defining new uses, dosing schedules, and additional information about long-term safety of a commercially available drug or biological agent.

CONDUCTING A CLINICAL TRIAL

"If clinical trials are worth doing, then they are worth doing well" (Wittes, 1986). Clinical trials are experiments that are no less important than a laboratory experiment. Thus to protect data quality, clinical trials must be designed and conducted with many of the same assurances that occur in the design and conduct of a laboratory experiment (Piantadosi, 1988). This is often referred to as *good clinical practice,* for which guidelines have been established (ICH, 1995). A clinical trial has many components, including the following:

1. Planning and development
2. Patient enrollment and treatment
3. Maintenance of source documentation
4. Prospective monitoring
5. Assessment of response
6. Assessment and reporting of adverse events
7. Data retrieval and management
8. Quality assurance
9. Analysis and reporting of results

Quality assurance mechanisms at every step are needed to make sure that potential problems do not interfere with the progress of the study or the quality of the data. Obviously, documentation of events in the medical record and data retrieval are vital components of clinical research. Most problems with data quality arise from lack of attentiveness, failure to maintain adequate source documentation (e.g., tumor measurements, adverse drug reactions, performance status), and lack of adherence protocol guidelines (Zepp and Mackintosh, 1996; van der Putten et al, 1987).

The quality of data generated from cooperative group studies has been questioned and debated. In multicenter studies, some researchers have shown that inferior quality data are obtained from participants who enroll small numbers of patients annually (Sylvester et al, 1981). It has been recommended that participants be required to enroll a predetermined number of patients or no patients at all (Sylvester et al, 1981). Some groups report similar problems (Thomas, 1982), but others refute those conclusions (Begg et al, 1982; Begg et al, 1983; deDombal, 1982; Koretz et al, 1983; Levine, 1983). There is general agreement among investigators, however, that data quality can be maintained through clearly written, unambiguous protocols; close communication with the administrative center; prestudy orientation of participants; minimal patient eligibility criteria; and cooperative, well-trained data managers. A discussion follows of some of the more important elements of the conduct of a clinical trial. For a more detailed discussion of clinical trials, see additional sources (ICH, 1995; Spilker, 1991; Buyse, Staquet, and Sylvester, 1984).

Protocol Development

Once the need for conducting a study has been established, the specific aims have been enumerated, and it has been determined that adequate resources are available, a plan for conducting the study must be written. There are many important issues to consider when writing a protocol, including but not limited to eligibility criteria, definitions of response, identification of study parameters, and details of treatment, including modifications and duration of treatment. In addition, data forms, data retrieval schedules, communication, and orientation with participating investigators should be part of the usual study development procedures (Hunninghake, Darby, and Probstfield, 1987). A protocol review checklist (Table 2-2) describes many of the questions that need to be addressed when writing a protocol.

The Protocol Team

Before initiation of patient enrollment, the principal investigator should assemble a group of individuals that will plan a strategy for monitoring the study (Evans, 1979; Spilker, 1991). This group—the protocol team—should review the protocol, all the activities required to carry out the study, and define the responsibilities of each member (Box 2-3). In addition, the protocol team should develop strategies for monitoring and correcting unplanned situations, such as severe adverse drug reactions, protocol modifications and deviations, slow accrual, and so on. As discussed later, the protocol team should meet regularly during the time frame of the study to monitor data, discuss potential problems, and so forth.

Formal patient registration procedures (i.e., eligibility checks) and data-collection procedures must be firmly established before study activation. Principal investigators must be actively involved in their studies by seeking information on protocol deviations and patient accrual status, reviewing patient data regularly, and getting involved in problem solving. In addition, quality assurance guidelines (i.e., reviewing response data, recording tumor measurements) must be clearly established before enrollment of patients begins.

Patient Enrollment

Most cancer centers and universities involved in the conduct of clinical trials have established a data-coordinating center whose responsibility is managing the data from clinical trials. In smaller centers, data managers may be employed but there may be no central data office. Whatever the case, there should be a designated group of people whose task it is to conduct data-retrieval activities for clinical trials. Their responsibilities should include the development and conduction of patient registration and quality control guidelines. Before activating a clinical trial, it is important to develop an eligibility checklist (i.e., a list of specific questions asked when patients are registered to clinical trials) to maximize the ratio of eligible to entered patients. Exceptions to eligibility criteria should not be necessary or allowed. The protocol should be amended if certain eligibility or exclusion criteria are found to be unnecessary. As each patient is enrolled onto the study, an eligibility check must be performed before treatment assignment is given or therapy is begun.

TABLE 2-2
Protocol Review Checklist

Protocol section	Issues to be addressed
Schema	Can you tell what the research plan is from the schema?
	Does the information provided coincide with information in other protocol sections?
Introduction and rationale	Does the introduction and background information provide convincing evidence that the study is worth doing?
	Has information been provided concerning preclinical studies and previous clinical trials in humans?
	Is the information provided accurate, current, and consistent with study objectives?
Objectives	Are these clearly stated? (i.e., what are the endpoints?)
	Do the objectives seem to be clinically relevant?
	Do these coincide with the background?
Patient selection	Are the selection criteria clearly stated?
	Are unnecessary criteria (e.g., life expectancy requirements and other subjective evaluations, obtaining prestudy tests within a particular time frame) excluded?
Patient registration	Is it clear how patient registration will be handled?
	Where applicable, are randomization procedures clearly described?
Treatment plan	Is the drug treatment schedule clear and concise?
	For drugs administered over consecutive days (e.g., daily for 5 days), is the daily dose clearly described?
	Are drug administration guidelines provided to include route of administration, infusion solutions and concentrations, rate of infusion, and concomitant medications/hydration?
	Are dose-rounding guidelines provided?
	Are other treatments (radiotherapy, surgery) clearly described? (i.e., can you discern the sequence of therapies given?)
	Are there guidelines that detail procedures to follow when drug is administered at a "satellite" institution or clinic?

Continued

TABLE 2-2
Protocol Review Checklist—cont'd

Protocol section	Issues to be addressed
Treatment plan (cont'd)	Are criteria for the use of colony-stimulating factors (e.g., G-CSF, GM-CSF) necessary/included and, if included, are the guidelines appropriate for the treatment regimen?
	Would sample drug orders be useful for clarifying drug administration guidelines and if so, are they available?
	For double-blind studies are there procedures for breaking the blind?
Drug dose modifications and adverse event reporting	Are adverse drug reaction reporting requirements included and are they consistent with current NCI or FDA policies?
	Can you modify drug doses with certainty based on the criteria given? (i.e., if dose modification is based on nadir blood counts, are nadir blood counts always obtained? If dose modification is based on toxicity grading, is the potential toxicity routinely assessed?)
	Are dose modifications required for adverse events thought to be unrelated to the treatment?
	Should additional criteria be added?
	Should any criteria described be deleted?
	What should be done when no criteria are listed for a particular toxicity?
	Are investigators allowed to administer an additional course of treatment after an initial assessment of response that may indicate progressive disease?
Measurement of effect	Are the response criteria clearly described?
	Do the response definitions apply to the patients under study? (i.e., is the evaluation of liver size by physical examination an inappropriate measure of response for some patients?)
	Are response assessments made at times that coincide with the definitions of response? (i.e., if two assessments 2 months apart are required for response categorization, are these assessments made as described?)

Study parameters	Is it clear when all the tests are due?
	Are all tests required for eligibility determination listed as being due "prestudy"?
	Are some tests unnecessary?
	Is the frequency of testing excessive for certain parameters?
	Does the testing schedule coincide with the treatment plan, or does it complicate matters?
	Are the required tests listed in one section of the protocol?
Drug information, formulation, and procurement	Is the information necessary for investigational drug procurement (dosage forms, availability) provided?
	Is the pharmaceutical information complete? (i.e., is information provided on storage requirements, admixture procedures, stability in dry form and in solution, and compatibility/incompatibility?)
	Is there an omission of new drug information (such as drug interactions) that should be provided in the protocol?
	Is the drug information provided complete and accurate?
	Is the drug information provided applicable to this particular protocol?
Statistical considerations	Is it clear how many patients are to be accrued over what period of time?
	Including the time necessary for follow-up, how long will it take to complete this study?
	Is information provided concerning handling of drop-outs, ineligible patients, stopping rules, and interim analyses?
Records to be kept	Are these described?
	Are the forms present for review?
	If a patient diary would be useful in documenting compliance with self-administered medications, is one available?
	Is the patient diary too complex, yet designed in a way to minimize omissions?
References	Are the references current and complete (i.e., retrievable)?
	Should any references not listed be included?
	Are all the references cited in the protocol listed?
Consent form	Are the essential elements present?
	Are all the adverse events provided by the sponsor or NCI described in the consent form?

BOX 2-3
Responsibilities of the Clinical Trials Team

PHYSICIANS
Protocol development
Patient assessment
Documentation of all interactions with patients in the medical record
Documentation in the medical record of the reasons for any deviation
   from the protocol
Recording tumor measurements and assessments of disease status in the
   medical record
Reporting adverse drug reactions
Analyzing and reporting study results

RESEARCH NURSES AND STUDY COORDINATORS
Assisting in protocol development and/or review
Screening patient before registration
Education of patients regarding study procedures, appointments, completion
   of diaries, etc.
Administration and collection of quality-of-life questionnaires
Review of physician's prescription
Ensuring protocol is followed
Reschedule tests, if necessary
Patient assessment and treatment
Documentation of all interactions and assessment of patients in the medical
   record
Prospective monitoring and data retrieval
Coordination of specimen collection for pharmacokinetic or laboratory
   research studies

In addition, the signed informed consent form should be retrieved and reviewed by the data coordinating center, and documentation of on-study parameters (i.e., laboratory reports) should be reviewed before initiation of treatment. Review of the signed informed consent form is intended to ensure that the patient and investigator have signed and dated the form, that the most up-to-date version of the form has been used, and, where applicable, the form has been signed and dated by a witness and/or parent/guardian.

Data-coordinating centers should maintain research (or shadow) charts that are separate from the medical record for all patients enrolled onto clinical trials. Elements of the research chart should include the completed eligibility checklist, registration information, signed consent form, operative/pathology reports, study flow sheets, patient diaries, physician and nurse progress notes, laboratory and radiology reports for all tests performed, and data forms.

Source Documents
Source documents are defined as original documents and records kept at the pharmacy, laboratories, and medical or technical departments involved

in the clinical trial (ICH, 1995; Zepp and Mackintosh, 1996). Source documents may include progress notes, laboratory records, memoranda, patient diaries or evaluation checklists, pharmacy dispensing records, microfiches, photographic negatives, x-ray films, radiology reports, and microfilm or magnetic media. The use of flow sheets is generally not considered to be adequate source documentation unless the flow sheets are signed, dated, and accepted as a part of the official institutional medical record. Source documents contain clinical trial information that allows its accurate reporting, interpretation, and verification. Source documents also support the accuracy of the data recorded on case report forms and reported to the sponsor of the clinical trial. With regard to documenting administration of drugs utilized in a clinical trial, the investigator is required to include information on each patient's exposure to the drug, including the date (and time if relevant) of each administration and the quantity administered (FDA, 1995; Zepp and Mackintosh, 1996). In addition, documentation of drug administration should be independent of the flow sheet. Documentation of each dose of an oral or injectable medication self-administered by the patient at home is often insufficient unless methods are in place to capture this information. In general, pharmacy dispensing records do not provide sufficient information to verify drug administration. Many institutions have found success in documenting patient self-administered medications by using patient diaries and frequent (i.e., weekly) communication with the patients.

Data Retrieval

Although data retrieval will often be retrospective in nature, every attempt should be made to retrieve data on a prospective basis (i.e., while the patient is in the clinic). Infrequent review of medical records does not lend itself to rapid dissemination of up-to-date information, prevention of errors in protocol adherence, maintenance of adequate source documentation, and so forth.

Data retrieval and quality control are key elements in the conduct of a successful clinical trial. If the clinician obtains the required study parameters, administers treatment on schedule, and documents adverse effects of treatment, assessment parameters, and all protocol deviations in the medical record, the elements for an assessable patient are in place. When problems with the documentation of events and protocol adherence arise, retrospective chart reviews will not correct the problem. In many centers, prospective monitoring and data retrieval have been put in place to prevent this deficiency.

Prospective Monitoring

Participation in clinical research must be made as painless as possible. Consideration should be given to methods that improve protocol adherence and source documentation and simplify the clinician's efforts. Difficulties following study parameters may be decreased by using protocol-oriented computer systems, protocol-specific flow sheets, study calendars, and/or road maps (Evans, 1979; Levine, 1983). Protocol-specific flow sheets and/or study calendars should highlight the tests and procedures to obtain and when to obtain them. Methods that improve documentation of events in the medical record should be devised. Standardizing the medical dictation format, utilizing patient diaries to collect information on self-administered medications and adverse events, and including nurses and pharmacists on the protocol team can help improve prospective monitoring and data retrieval. All of the methods described should be implemented via direct communication between cancer center or university personnel (e.g., protocol managers, principal investigator) and the participating clinician and his or her staff (Mowery and Williams, 1979). Prospective monitoring and data retrieval can become a reality at off-site institutions through the use of facsimile (FAX) machines. Investigators at these sites can send data (e.g., flow sheets and reports) as they are generated (i.e., before treatment decisions are made). As a result, questions regarding eligibility criteria and other elements of the protocol can be answered before problems arise.

Reporting Adverse Drug Reactions and Serious Adverse Events

Adverse drug reactions (ADRs) and serious adverse events occur frequently in patients receiving cancer chemotherapy. Reporting of serious adverse events (SAEs) is required by federal regulations for SAEs occurring as a part

TABLE 2-3
Investigational Agent Adverse Drug Reaction Reporting Guidelines from the National Cancer Institute, Division of Cancer Treatment

Phase I studies	
All life-threatening events (Grade 4) that may be caused by drug administration, all fatal events while on study, first occurrence of any *previously unknown* clinical event (regardless of grade)	Report by telephone to the NCI within 24 hours A written report must be submitted within 10 working days

Phase II and III studies			
PREVIOUSLY UNKNOWN REACTIONS		**PREVIOUSLY KNOWN REACTIONS**	
Grades 2-3	**Grades 4-5**	**Grades 1-3**	**Grades 4-5**
Written report to NCI within 10 working days	Report by telephone to NCI within 24 hours Written report to follow within 10 working days	Not to be reported as ADRs These toxicities should be submitted as a part of the study results	Written report to NCI within 10 working days Grade 4 myelo-suppression not to be reported but should be submitted as a part of the study results

of an investigational drug study or a study approved by the NCI or Food and Drug Administration (FDA). Serious adverse events must also be reported to the local institutional review board. What constitutes an SAE may vary slightly from study to study and be dependent on whether the study is sponsored by a drug company, the NCI, or the FDA. The current FDA definition of an SAE is an event that results in death, is life-threatening, results in hospitalization or prolongation of a hospital stay, is permanently disabling, is the result of an overdose, results in a congenital anomaly, or results in a second malignancy. Adverse events are usually graded according to a five-point scale, with "0" being no adverse event, to "4" being a life-threatening adverse event. Fatalities are usually labeled as grade "5" events. The NCI Common Toxicity Criteria scale or modifications of it are often used to grade adverse events (see Appendix A). For most studies sponsored by the NCI, the "NCI Guidelines for Reporting Adverse Drug Reactions" will apply (Table 2-3). For studies sponsored by a pharmaceutical firm, SAEs that are unexpected (i.e., previously unreported) and are possibly, probably, or definitely of undetermined relationship to the study drug must be reported to the FDA within 3 working days of becoming aware of the event (Table 2-4).

Quality Assurance

Mechanisms need to be put in place to ensure that the clinical trial is going smoothly and data are being retrieved, and to assess data recording and entry onto data forms and/or computer files. The protocol team should meet regularly during the course of a clinical trial to make sure that these items are done.

TABLE 2-4
Adverse Event Reporting Guidelines, U.S. Food and Drug Administration

	Unexpected* serious adverse events	Expected serious adverse events and nonserious unexpected adverse events
Fatal or life-threatening and possibly, probably, definitely, or of undetermined relationship to the drug	Report to the FDA by telephone within 3 working days Submit written report to the FDA within 10 working days	Submit to the FDA as a part of the annual report
Nonfatal or life-threatening, serious adverse events that are possibly, probably, definitely, or of undetermined relationship to the drug	Submit written report to the FDA within 10 working days	Submit to the FDA as a part of the annual report

*Unexpected, previously unidentified adverse event (i.e., not previously identified in nature, severity, or frequency).

SUMMARY

Further advancement in the field of oncology will be obtained by increasing the number of patients enrolled onto clinical studies, as long as the quality of the data is protected. Poor patient enrollment and/or the provision of poor data jeopardize the scientific merit of the study (Antman et al, 1985; Hunninghake, Darby, and Probstfield, 1987). Ineligible patients, major protocol violations, and failure to obtain vital information renders the data of a patient's clinical trial experience meaningless and can be considered a breach of informed consent. There is general agreement among investigators, however, that data quality can be maintained by use of clearly written protocols, close communication with the administrative center, prestudy orientation of participants, strict and clear patient selection criteria, and well-trained data managers.

REFERENCES

Anon: Recruiting patients for clinical trials (news), *J Natl Cancer Inst* 80:619-620, 1988.

Antman K, Schnipper LE, Frei E: The crisis in clinical cancer research: third-party insurance and investigative therapy, *N Engl J Med* 319:46-48, 1988.

Antman K et al: Selection bias in clinical trials, *J Clin Oncol* 3:1142-1147, 1985.

Barofsky I, Sugarbaker PH: Determinants of patient nonparticipation in randomized clinical trials for the treatment of sarcomas, *Cancer Clin Trials* 2:237-246, 1979.

Begg CB: Selection of patients for clinical trials, *Semin Oncol* 15:434-440, 1988.

Begg CB, Engstrom PF: Eligibility and extrapolation in cancer clinical trials, *J Clin Oncol* 5:962-968, 1987.

Begg CB et al: Participation of community hospitals in clinical trials: analysis of five years experience in the Eastern Cooperative Oncology Group, *N Engl J Med* 306:1076-1080, 1982.

Begg CB et al: Cooperative groups and community hospitals: measurement of impact in the community hospitals, *Cancer* 52:1760-1767, 1983.

Boyd MR: Status of the NCI pre-clinical antitumor drug discovery screen. In DeVita VT Jr, Hellman S, Rosenberg SA, eds: *Principles and practice of oncology, PPO updates*, 3:1-12, 1989.

Brennan MJ: Factors affecting patient's and doctor's decisions to participate in clinical trials in oncology, a thesis submitted to the Yale University School of Medicine in partial fulfillment of the requirements for the degree of Doctor of Medicine, 1989.

Buyse ME, Staquet MJ, Sylvester RJ: *Cancer clinical trials: methods and practice*, New York, 1984, Oxford University Press.

Carpenter LM: Is the study worth doing? *Lancet* 342:221-223, 1993.

Cassileth BR et al: Information and participation preferences among cancer patients, *Ann Intern Med* 92:832-836, 1980.

Cassileth BR et al: Attitudes toward clinical trials among patients and the public, *JAMA* 248:968-970, 1982.

Collins JM, Grieshaber CK, Chabner BA: Pharmacologically guided phase I clinical trials based upon pre-clinical drug development, *J Natl Cancer Inst* 82:1321-1326, 1990.

Daugherty C et al: Perceptions of cancer patients and their physicians involved in phase I trials, *J Clin Oncol* 13:1062-1072, 1995.

deDombal FT: Quality of institutional participation in multicenter trials, *N Engl J Med* 306:813-814, 1982.

EORTC Pharmacokinetics and Metabolism Group: Pharmacokinetically guided dose escalation in phase I clinical trials: commentary and proposed guidelines, *Eur J Cancer Clin Oncol* 23:1083-1087, 1987.

Epictetus: Discourses II, cited in Evans: *Dictionary of Quotations,* New York, 1978, Avenel Books, p 381.

Estey E et al: Therapeutic response in phase I trials of antineoplastic agents, *Cancer Treat Rep* 70:1105-1115, 1986.

Evans JT: Internal monitoring: patient and study management in the clinic, *Clin Pharmacol Ther* 25:712-716, 1979.

Evans WK et al: Phase II study of amonafide: results of treatment and lessons learned from the study of an investigational agent in previously untreated patients with extensive small-cell lung cancer, *J Clin Oncol* 8:390-395, 1990.

Fisher B: Clinical trials for the evaluation of cancer therapy, *Cancer* 54:2609-2617, 1984.

Food and Drug Administration: Information sheets for institutional review boards and clinical investigators, October, 1995.

Freedman B: Equipoise and the ethics of clinical research, *N Engl J Med* 317:141-145, 1988.

Friedman MA: Patient accrual to clinical trials, *Cancer Treat Rep* 71:557-558, 1987.

Friedman MA, McCabe MS: Assigning care costs associated with therapeutic oncology research: a modest proposal, *J Natl Cancer Inst* 84:760-763, 1992.

Gail MH: Eligibility exclusions, losses to follow-up, removal of randomized patients, and uncounted events in cancer clinical trials, *Cancer Treat Rep* 69:1107-1113, 1985.

Gelber RD, Goldhirsch A: Can a clinical trial be the treatment of choice for patients with cancer? *J Natl Cancer Inst* 80:886-887, 1988.

George SL: Reducing patient eligibility criteria in cancer clinical trials, *J Clin Oncol* 14:1364-1370, 1996.

Gianni L et al: Pharmacology and clinical toxicity of 4'-iodo-4'-deoxydoxorubicin: an example of successful application of pharmacokinetics to dose escalation in phase I trials, *J Natl Cancer Inst* 82:469-477, 1990.

Graham MA, Workman P: The impact of pharmacokinetically guided dose escalation strategies in phase I clinical trials: critical evaluation and recommendations for future studies, *Ann Oncol* 3:339-347, 1992.

Grieshaber CK, Marsoni S: Relation of preclinical toxicology to findings in early clinical trials, *Cancer Treat Rep* 70:65-72, 1986.

Hanks GE: The dangers of ad hoc protocols, *J Clin Oncol* 2:1177-1178, 1984.

Hubbard SM, Henney JE, DeVita VT Jr: A computer data base for information on cancer treatment, *N Engl J Med* 316:315-318, 1987.

Hunninghake DB, Darby CA, Probstfield JL: Recruitment experience in clinical trials: literature summary and annotated bibliography, *Control Clin Trials* 8(4 suppl):6S-30S, 1987.

Hunter CP et al: Selection factors in clinical trials: results from the Community Clinical Oncology Program physician's log, *Cancer Treat Rep* 71:559-565, 1987.

ICH, International Conference on Harmonisation: Draft guideline on good clinical practice, *Fed Regist* 60:42948-42957, 1995.

Johnson JR, Temple R: Food and Drug Administration requirements for approval of anticancer drugs, *Cancer Treat Rep* 69:1155-1159, 1985.

Joseph RR: Viewpoints and concerns of a clinical trial participant, *Cancer* 74:2692-2693, 1994.

Koretz MM et al: A comparison of the quality of participation of community affiliates and that of universities in the Northern California Oncology Group, *J Clin Oncol* 1:640-644, 1983.

Langley GR et al: Why are (or are not) patients given the option to enter clinical trials? *Control Clin Trials* 8:49-59, 1987.

Levine AS: Clinical trials and the community physician, *Cancer* 51(suppl 12):2498-2502, 1983.

Martin JF et al: Accrual of patients into a multihospital cancer clinical trial and its implications on planning future studies, *Am J Clin Oncol* 7:173-182, 1984.

Matthews J: NCI survey explores the M.D.'s perspective on ABMT trials, *J Natl Cancer Inst* 87:1510-1511, 1995.

Mattson ME et al: Participation in a clinical trial: the patient's point of view, *Control Clin Trials* 6:156-167, 1985.

McCabe M, Friedman MA: Impact of third-party reimbursement on cancer clinical investigations: a consensus statement coordinated by the National Cancer Institute, *J Natl Cancer Inst* 81:1585-1586, 1989.

Mowery RL, Williams OD: Aspects of clinic monitoring in large-scale multiclinic trials, *Clin Pharmacol Ther* 25:717-719, 1979.

Piantadosi S: Principles of clinical trial design, *Semin Oncol* 15:423-433, 1988.

Ratain MJ et al: Statistical and ethical issues in the design and conduct of phase I and II clinical trials of new anti-cancer agents, *J Natl Cancer Inst* 85:1637-1643, 1993.

Simes RJ: The case for an international registry for clinical trials, *J Clin Oncol* 4:1529-1541, 1986.

Simon RM: Design and conduct of clinical trials. In DeVita VT Jr, Hellman S, Rosenberg SA, eds: *Cancer principles and practices of oncology,* ed 4, Philadelphia, 1993, JB Lippincott, pp 418-440.

Smith TL et al: Design and results of phase I cancer clinical trials: three-year experience at M.D. Anderson Cancer Center, *J Clin Oncol* 14:287-295, 1996.

Spilker B: *Guide to clinical trials,* New York, 1991, Raven Press.

Sylvester RJ et al: Quality of institutional participation in multicenter clinical trials, *N Engl J Med* 305:852-855, 1981.

Tannock I, Murphy K: Reflections on medical oncology: an appeal for better clinical trials and improved reporting of their results, *J Clin Oncol* 1:66-70, 1983.

Taylor KM: The doctor's dilemma: physician participation in randomized clinical trials, *Cancer Treat Rep* 69:1095-1100, 1985.

Taylor KM, Morgolese RG, Soskoline CL: Physicians' reasons for not entering eligible patients in a randomized clinical trial of surgery for breast cancer, *N Engl J Med* 310:1363-1367, 1984.

Taylor KM, Shapiro M, Skinner HA: Some thoughts on the future of clinical trials groups in cancer, *Cancer Treat Rep* 71:434-435, 1987.

Thomas P: Quality of institutional participation in multicenter trials, *N Engl J Med* 306:814, 1982.

van der Putten et al: A pilot study on the quality of data management in a cancer clinical trial, *Control Clin Trials* 8:96-100, 1987.

Von Hoff DD, Kuhn J, Clark GM: Design and conduct of phase I trials. In Buyse ME, Staquet MJ, Sylvester RJ, eds: *Cancer clinical trials: methods and practice,* New York, 1984, Oxford University Press, pp 210-220.

Von Hoff DD, Turner J: Response rates, duration of response, and dose response effects in phase I studies of antineoplastics, *Invest New Drugs* 9:115-122, 1991.

Wittes RE: How we know what we (think we) know, *J Clin Oncol* 4:827-829, 1986.

Wittes RE: Current emphasis in the clinical drug development program of the National Cancer Institute. In DeVita VT Jr, Hellman S, Rosenberg SA, eds: *Principles and practices of oncology, PPO updates* 1:1-15, 1987a.

Wittes RE: Paying for patient care in treatment research: who is responsible? *Cancer Treat Rep* 71:107-113, 1987b.

Wittes RE, Friedman MA: Accrual to clinical trials, *J Natl Cancer Inst* 80:884-885, 1988.

Zelen M: Guidelines for publishing papers on cancer clinical trials: responsibilities of editors and authors, *J Clin Oncol* 1:164-169, 1983.

Zepp VO, Mackintosh DR: Source documentation: a key to GCP compliance in clinical trials, *App Clin Trials* 5:42-45, 1996.

3

Chemotherapy Drugs

M ore than 100 drugs are discussed in this edition, a number that is similar to the previous edition. However, several drugs have been removed from this edition, and many new experimental drugs have been included. In addition, all drug reviews have been updated. Many drugs that were investigational a few years ago have become commercially available, and all drug monographs have been updated to include new information, including adverse events, dosing and administration, and storage and stability. Drugs used to treat patients with HIV have been removed from this edition; refer to the previous edition or other sources for information on these agents. As in the previous edition, Chapter 4 is devoted to biological response modifiers, and all drugs and biologicals are listed alphabetically by their current generic name or the United States Adopted Name.

Separate chapters are devoted to the management of the more common side effects, such as gastrointestinal toxicity, dermatological toxicity, and myelosuppression. Some aspects of toxicity are highlighted in the discussion of specific drugs. For example, renal toxicity appears in the discussion of cisplatin, cardiac toxicity and its evaluation with left ventricular ejection fraction (LVEF) appears in the doxorubicin section, and so on. Additional resources for more detailed information on antineoplastic drug-induced toxicities, their prevention, and management are listed at the end of this chapter.

Each drug information section is divided into several subsections. Some general guidelines were followed in the preparation of each section, as described below:

1. **Classification.** Drugs are categorized based primarily on their mechanisms of action (e.g., antimetabolites) or derivation (e.g., plant alkaloids). Unless the drug has mechanisms of action that have not been previously discussed in Chapter 1, they will not be discussed in detail this chapter. Readers are referred to Chapter 1 for information on mechanisms of action.

2. **Indications.** Indications listed for each commercially available drug are from the manufacturer's package insert or one of the three compendia used to determine medicare reimbursement (i.e., *United States Pharmacopeia, AMA Drug Evaluations, American Hospital Formulary Service [AHFS] Drug Information)*, or from the primary literature. In some instances, indications will be listed for

the investigational drugs and these were taken from the primary literature. Much of this information is provided in Table 3-1.

3. **Dose.** Commonly used doses are listed, along with some dose regimens recently published. However, doses vary enormously for some drugs. In all cases, consult the specific protocol and/or the manufacturer for doses and dose-adjustment guidelines.

4. **Administration.** Routes of administration that have been used are listed, and recommended routes may be described. In all cases, consult the specific protocol and/or the manufacturer for guidelines.

5. **Toxicity.** Adverse drug reactions are listed by organ system. Effects that are dose limiting or rare are usually noted as such. The incidence figures cited refer to the incidents of toxicities that have been reported (regardless of relationship to the drug) after the use of recommended doses and routes of administration. Where possible, we have attempted to include toxicities thought to be possibly, probably, or definitely related to the drug. In addition, unless otherwise indicated, the incidence of toxicities noted herein includes all grades (i.e., mild, moderate, severe, and life threatening) of the particular toxicity. With all drugs, especially those that are investigational, unexpected effects may occur.

6. **Storage and Stability.** Information may include data that are not part of the official labeling of marketed drugs but have been described in the literature. In all cases, the expiration date on the drug container should be observed unless the clinician has been officially notified that the expiration date has been extended as a result of stability testing. Stability studies are ongoing for many investigational drugs. For parenteral drugs that do not contain a preservative, the customary recommendation is to discard any unused solution after 8 to 24 hours. It is suggested that each institution follow its own policy regarding products that are otherwise stable for longer periods of time.

7. **Preparation.** Methods for reconstitution and dilution are described. In some cases, methods of preparation will be discussed that are not a part of the official drug label but have been described in the literature.

8. **Incompatibilities and Compatibilities.** Mixtures that should be avoided or are known to be compatible or incompatible are described. In general, the compatibility information included in this chapter is brief and only notes information where chemical compatibility has been assayed. It is recommended that admixtures not be prepared unless stability is known and that a pharmacist be consulted for detailed information. In some cases, significant drug interactions will also be described under Incompatibilities. Drug interactions with antineoplastic agents are also described in Chapter 1.

9. **Availability.** Sources of the drugs are listed. For commercially available drugs, a pharmacist should be consulted for manufacturers or wholesalers. Most investigational drugs are obtained from the National Cancer Institute (NCI). Occasionally, marketed drugs are supplied by NCI, and the specific protocol should be consulted.

TABLE 3-1
Approved Indications for Drugs Used in the Treatment of Patients With Cancer

Drug	Indications*
Altretamine	Single-agent use for persistent or recurrent ovarian carcinoma
	Non-Hodgkin's lymphoma, cancers of the endometrium and cervix
Amifostine	Reduction of cisplatin-induced nephrotoxicity in patients with ovarian carcinoma
	Reduction of toxicities associated with radiation therapy or cyclophosphamide
Aminoglutethimide	Breast cancer, suppression of adrenal function in selected patients with Cushing's syndrome
	Prostate cancer, adrenocortical carcinoma, ACTH-producing tumors
Amsacrine	ANLL (group C investigational agent, available from the NCI)
Anastrozole	Advanced breast cancer (postmenopausal women who have received prior tamoxifen therapy)
Asparaginase	Acute lymphocytic leukemia
	ANLL, CLL, CML, Hodgkin's and non-Hodgkin's lymphomas, soft-tissue sarcoma
Azacytidine	ANLL (group C investigational agent, available from the NCI)
Bicalutamide	Advanced prostate cancer in combination with an LHRH analogue
Bleomycin	Squamous cell carcinoma (head and neck, skin, penis, cervix, vulva), Hodgkin's and non-Hodgkin's lymphoma,
	reticulum cell sarcoma, lymphosarcoma, testicular carcinoma (embryonal cell, choriocarcinoma, teratocarcinoma)

AIDS, acquired immunodeficiency syndrome; *ALL*, acute lymphocytic leukemia; *ANLL*, acute nonlymphocytic leukemia; *CLL*, chronic lymphocytic leukemia; *CML*, chronic myelogenous leukemia; *HIV*, human immunodeficiency virus; *LHRH*, luteinizing hormone–releasing hormone; *VIP*, vasoactive intestinal peptide.

*Roman typeface designates FDA-approved indications; italics represents compendia-based indications from the Association of Community Cancer Centers (ACCC) Compendia-Based Drug Bulletin, 5(2), 1996 and the three federally recognized compendia. To obtain additional information, contact the ACCC, 11600 Nebel St., Suite 201, Rockville, MD. 20852. The three compendia are (1) *United States Pharmacopeia, Drug Information (USP DI)*, The US Pharmacopeial Convention, Inc., 12601 Twinbrook Parkway, Bethesda, MD. 20852; (2) *AMA Drug Evaluations*, American Medical Association, Divison of Drugs and Toxicology, 535 N. Dearborn St., Chicago, IL. 60610; and (3) *American Society of Hospital Pharmacists (AHFS) Drug Information*, American Society of Hospital Pharmacists, Inc., 4630 Montgomery Ave., Bethesda, MD. 20814.

Continued

TABLE 3-1
Approved Indications for Drugs Used in the Treatment of Patients With Cancer—cont'd

Drug	Indications
Bleomycin	Endometrium, esophagus, Kaposi's sarcoma, osteosarcoma, ovary, kidney, bladder, melanoma, thyroid, soft tissue sarcoma, sclerosis of malignant pericardial or pleural effusions
Busulfan	CML
Carboplatin	ANLL, polycythemia vera, conditioning regimen for bone marrow transplantation
	Ovarian carcinoma
Carmustine	Cancers of the head and neck, endometrium, lung, testes, breast, brain, cervix
	Brain tumors, multiple myeloma, Hodgkin's and non-Hodgkin's lymphomas
	Melanoma; colorectal, stomach, and liver cancers; cutaneous T-cell lymphoma
Chlorambucil	CLL and malignant lymphomas (including lymphosarcoma, giant follicular lymphoma and Hodgkin's disease)
	Breast cancer, hairy cell leukemia, multiple myeloma; ovarian, testicular, trophoblastic neoplasms; Waldenström's macroglobulinemia
Cisplatin	Testicular carcinoma, ovarian cancer, transitional cell bladder cancer
	Cancers of the brain, adrenal cortex, breast, cervix, endometrium, head and neck, esophagus, and lung; melanoma; non-Hodgkin's lymphoma; osteosarcoma; prostate, skin, stomach, uterus, and trophblastic neoplasms
Cladribine	Hairy cell leukemia
	CLL, cutaneous T-cell lymphoma, Sézary syndrome, ANLL, low-grade non-Hodgkin's lymphoma, Waldenström's macroglobulinemia, autoimmune hemolytic anemia
Cyclophosphamide	Non-Hodgkin's lymphoma, Hodgkin's disease, myeloma, cutaneous T-cell lymphoma, neuroblastoma, adenocarcinoma of the ovary, adenocarcinoma of the breast
	ALL; ANLL; cancers of the bladder, cervix, and endometrium; CML; Ewing's sarcoma; head, neck, and lung cancers; osteosarcoma; cancers of the stomach, testes, uterus; Wilms' tumor; soft-tissue sarcomas; prostate cancer; rhabdomyosarcoma; retinoblastoma; trophoblastic neoplasms
Cyclosporine	Prophylaxis for organ rejection in kidney, heart, and liver transplantation
	Reversal of drug resistance

Cytarabine	ANLL, ALL, CML, meningeal leukemia
Dacarbazine	*Hodgkin's and non-Hodgkin's lymphoma* Melanoma, Hodgkin's disease
Dactinomycin	*Islet cell carcinoma, neuroblastoma, soft tissue sarcomas, osteosarcoma, renal cell carcinoma* Wilms' tumor, rhabdomyosarcoma, testicular carcinoma, choriocarcinoma, carcinoma of the uterus, Ewing's sarcoma, sarcoma botryoides
Daunorubicin	*ANLL, endometrium, Kaposi's sarcoma, melanoma, osteosarcoma, ovary, trophoblastic neoplasms* ANLL (adult and pediatric); Kaposi's sarcoma (liposomal formulation)
Daunorubicin, liposomal	*CML, erythroleukemia, Ewing's sarcoma, neuroblastoma, non-Hodgkin's lymphoma, Wilms' tumor* Kaposi's sarcoma
Dexrazoxane	Protective agent of doxorubicin-induced cardiotoxicity in patients with metastatic breast cancer who have received a cumulative dose of 300 mg/m^2 of doxorubicin
Diethylstilbestrol	Prostate and breast cancers
Docetaxel	Breast cancer *Ovarian, head and neck, and lung cancers*
Doxorubicin	ANLL, ALL, Wilms' tumor, neuroblastoma, soft tissue and bone sarcomas, breast carcinoma, ovarian carcinoma, transitional cell bladder carcinoma, thyroid carcinoma, Hodgkin's disease, non-Hodgkin's lymphoma, gastric carcinoma; small-cell lung cancer; Kaposi's sarcoma (liposomal formulation) *CLL; cancers of the cervix, endometrium, esophagus, head and neck, pancreas, prostate, and testes; Ewing's* *sarcoma; islet cell carcinoma; Kaposi's sarcoma; myeloma; rhabdomyosarcoma; trophoblastic neoplasms*
Doxorubicin, liposomal	Kaposi's sarcoma
Estramustine	Prostate cancer
Etoposide	Refractory testicular tumors, small-cell lung cancer *ALL; ANLL; cancers of the breast, brain, adrenal cortex, bladder, prostate, stomach; Ewing's sarcoma; Kaposi's* *sarcoma; neuroblastoma; Hodgkin's and non-Hodgkin's lymphoma, non-small-cell lung cancer, trophoblastic* *neoplasms*

Continued

TABLE 3-1
Approved Indications for Drugs Used in the Treatment of Patients With Cancer—cont'd

Drug	Indications
Finasteride	Benign prostatic hypertrophy
	Early stage prostate cancer
Floxuridine	GI adenocarcinoma metastatic to the liver (administration by continuous intraarterial infusion)
	Breast, ovary, cervix, bladder, kidney, prostate cancers
Fludarabine	Relapsed or refractory B-cell chronic lymphocytic leukemia
	Low-grade non-Hodgkin's lymphoma, Hodgkin's disease, cutaneous T-cell lymphoma, hairy cell leukemia, prolymphocytic leukemia, macroglobulinemic lymphoma
Fluorouracil	Carcinoma of the stomach, colon, rectum, breast, pancreas
	Bladder, cervix, endometrium, esophagus, head and neck, islet cell, liver, lung, ovary, prostate, skin (topical) cancers
Fluoxymesterone	Breast cancer, hypogonadism in males
Flutamide	Metastatic prostatic carcinoma (in combination with an LHRH analogue)
Gallium nitrate	Symptomatic cancer-related hypercalcemia that has not responded to adequate hydration
Gemcitabine	Carcinoma of the pancreas
	Breast cancer
Goserelin acetate	Palliative treatment of advanced carcinoma of the prostate, endometriosis
	Breast cancer
Hydroxyurea	Melanoma; head and neck cancer; resistant CML; recurrent, metastatic, or inoperable carcinoma of the ovary
	Cervix and prostate cancer, trophoblastic neoplasms, polycythemia vera
Idarubicin	ANLL
Ifosfamide	Third-line therapy of germ cell testicular cancer
	ANLL, ALL, breast cancer, Ewing's sarcoma, Hodgkin's and non-Hodgkin's lymphoma; cancers of the lung, ovary, stomach, pancreas; osteosarcoma; soft tissue sarcoma; trophoblastic neoplasms

Irinotecan	Metastatic colorectal carcinoma
	Cancers of the lung, cervix, ovary
Leucovorin	Rescue agent after high-dose methotrexate (for osteosarcoma) and trimethoprim, advanced colorectal carcinoma in combination with fluorouracil
	Breast, head and neck, lung, stomach, pancreas cancers; non-Hodgkin's lymphoma; trophoblastic neoplasms (in combination with fluorouracil or methotrexate); megaloblastic anemia
Leuprolide	Palliative treatment of advanced prostatic carcinoma, management of endometriosis (including pain relief and reduction of endometriotic lesions)
	Breast, islet cell cancers
Lomustine	Brain tumors, Hodgkin's disease (secondary therapy in combination with other approved drugs)
	Breast, lung, colorectal, kidney cancers; melanoma; myeloma; non-Hodgkin's lymphoma
Mechlorethamine	Hodgkin's and non-Hodgkin's lymphoma, lymphosarcoma, CML, CLL, polycythemia vera, cutaneous T-cell lymphoma, lung cancer, palliative treatment of metastatic carcinoma resulting in effusion (peritoneal, pleural, or pericardial)
	CML
Medroxyprogesterone	Palliative treatment of inoperable, recurrent, and metastatic endometrial or renal carcinoma
Megestrol acetate	Advanced carcinoma of the breast or endometrium, anorexia associated with cancer or HIV infection
Melphalan	Multiple myeloma, nonresectable epithelial carcinoma of the ovary
	Breast, testes, thyroid cancers; melanoma (isolated limb perfusion); conditioning regimens for bone marrow transplantation
Mercaptopurine	Remission induction and maintenance therapy of ALL, ANLL
	CML, non-Hodgkin's lymphoma, polycythemia vera, inflammatory bowel disease, severe psoriatic arthritis
Mesna	Prevention of hemorrhagic cystitis caused by ifosfamide or cyclophosphamide
Methotrexate	Choriocarcinoma, hydatidiform mole, ALL, prophylaxis and treatment of meningeal lymphocytic leukemia, breast cancer, epidermoid cancers of the head and neck, lung cancer, non-Hodgkin's lymphoma, cutaneous T-cell lymphoma, osteosarcoma, psoriasis (severe, recalcitrant, disabling), rheumatoid arthritis (second- or third-line treatment)
	ANLL; cancers of the bladder, brain, cervix, esophagus, kidney, ovary, prostate, stomach, testis; myeloma; rhabdomyosarcoma

Continued

TABLE 3-1
Approved Indications for Drugs Used in the Treatment of Patients With Cancer—cont'd

Drug	Indications
Mitomycin	Disseminated adenocarcinoma of the stomach or pancreas (in combination with other drugs)
Mitotane	*CML; bladder, breast, cervix, esophagus, gallbladder, head and neck, colon, rectum, anus, lung cancers*
	Inoperable adrenocortical carcinoma of both functional and nonfunctional types
	Cushing's syndrome
Mitoxantrone	ANLL, prostate cancer
	Breast cancer, non-Hodgkin's lymphoma, hepatocellular carcinoma
Octreotide	Control of symptoms associated with carcinoid and VIP-secreting tumors
	Carcinoma of the pancreas, control of AIDS-associated diarrhea
Paclitaxel	Ovarian and breast cancer
	Lung, head and neck, stomach, prostate cancers
Pamidronate	Hypercalcemia of malignancy, osteolytic bone metastases associated with multiple myeloma
	Paget's disease
Pentostatin	Hairy cell leukemia
	Non-Hodgkin's lymphoma, cutaneous T-cell lymphoma
Pipobroman	CML, polycythemia vera
Plicamycin	Malignant tumors of the testis, hypercalcemia and hypercalciuria associated with a variety of advanced neoplasms
	Accelerated phase of CML
Porfimer sodium	Esophageal cancer (as a part of photodynamic therapy)
Procarbazine	Hodgkin's disease (stages III and IV)
	Brain tumors, lung cancer, melanoma, myeloma, non-Hodgkin's lymphoma, polycythemia vera
Streptozocin	Metastatic islet cell carcinoma of the pancreas
	Carcinoid tumors, Hodgkin's disease, pancreatic carcinoma

Tamoxifen	Breast cancer (adjuvant and metastatic)
	Melanoma (in combination with other drugs); breast cancer prevention; cancers of the pancreas, endometrium, liver
Teniposide	ALL in children (in combination with cytarabine)
	ALL in adults, small cell lung cancer
Thioguanine	Remission induction, consolidation and maintenance therapy of ANLL
	ALL, CML
Thiotepa	Adenocarcinoma of the breast, adenocarcinoma of the ovary, intracavitary effusions, superficial papillary bladder cancer, Hodgkin's and non-Hodgkin's lymphoma
	Lung cancer, conditioning regimens before bone marrow transplantation
Topotecan	Ovarian cancer
Toremifene	Advanced breast cancer
Tretinoin	Acute promyelocytic leukemia
Trimetrexate	Pneumocystis carinii infection (patients intolerant of or refratory to trimethoprim-sulfamethoxazole)
	Lung, colorectal, head and neck cancers
Uracil mustard	CLL, CML, non-Hodgkin's lymphoma, cutaneous T-cell lymphoma, polycythemia vera, thrombocytosis
	Ovarian carcinoma
Vinblastine	Hodgkin's disease, non-Hodgkin's lymphoma, mycosis fungoides (advanced stages), carcinoma of the testis, Kaposi's sarcoma, histiocytosis X, choriocarcinoma, breast cancer
	CML; cancers of the bladder, cervix, head and neck, kidney, lung, ovary; melanoma; neuroblastoma
Vincristine	ANLL, ALL, Hodgkin's and non-Hodgkin's lymphoma, rhabdomyosarcoma, Wilms' tumor, neuroblastoma, Ewing's sarcoma
	Cancers of the bladder, cervix, colorectal, head and neck, kidney, lung, ovary, thyroid; CLL; CML; Kaposi's sarcoma; melanoma; myeloma; osteosarcoma; soft-tissue sarcomas; trophoblastic neoplasms
Vinorelbine	Non-small-cell lung cancer
	Breast cancer

A

10. **References.** Each drug information section is followed by a short list of references taken from the primary literature. A lot of other information from the primary literature was used to compile these sections. Additional readily available sources are listed at the end of this chapter.

ALTRETAMINE
Other Names
Hexalen, Hexastat, hexamethylmelamine, HMM, HXM, NSC-13875.

Indications
FDA approved as a single agent for the treatment of persistent or recurrent ovarian carcinoma. Altretamine may be a useful treatment for patients with non-Hodgkin's lymphoma and cancers of the lung, endometrium, and cervix.

Classification and Mechanism of Action
Alkylating agent. Altretamine is activated by the liver to metabolites that are thought to bind with nucleic acids or microsomal proteins. Altretamine inhibits DNA and RNA synthesis by inhibiting their uptake into cells.

Pharmacokinetics
Well absorbed (75% to 89%) by mouth and reaches peak plasma levels 0.5 to 3 hours after dosing. Extensively metabolized in the liver (by microsomal enzymes) on first pass. Methylated metabolites appear to accumulate in the central nervous system. Elimination half-life is 4 to 13 hours. The pharmacokinetics of altretamine are not altered in patients with ascites. Phenobarbital could enhance and cimetidine could slow the metabolism of altretamine. Less than 1% is eliminated in the urine as unchanged drug.

Dose
The approved dose for advanced ovarian carcinoma is 260 mg/m^2/day in four divided doses for 14 to 21 days of a 28-day treatment cycle. When altretamine is combined with other myelosuppressive drugs, a dose of 150 mg/m^2/day for 14 days is commonly administered. Oral dosage ranges from 4 to 12 mg/kg/day in four divided doses for periods up to 3 to 6 weeks have been utilized. Higher doses (240 to 320 mg/m^2/day for 21 days) have been administered every 6 weeks.

Administration
Oral, usually taken after a meal.

Toxicity
Hematological. Leukopenia and thrombocytopenia are common (20% to 40% incidence) but usually mild. Nadir blood counts usually occur 3 to 4 weeks after beginning treatment, and recovery occurs 2 to 3 weeks thereafter. Anemia occurs frequently.

Gastrointestinal. Nausea and vomiting are common and occasionally dose limiting. These toxicities may worsen with continued therapy. Taking the drug with food or at bedtime may lessen these effects. Abdominal cramps, anorexia, and diarrhea occur occasionally.

Neurological. Neurological adverse effects occur infrequently and may include paresthesias, hyperesthesia, hyperreflexia, motor weakness, decreased sensory sensations, decreased proprioceptive sensations, agitation, anxiety, hallucinations, confusion, lethargy, depression, or coma.

Other. Weight loss, hepatic toxicity, cystitis, skin rash, pruritus, and alopecia are uncommon. Second malignancies (leukemia) have been reported.

Storage and Stability
The capsules should be stored in tightly sealed bottles at room temperature. Each bottle bears an expiration date.

Incompatibilities
Altretamine may potentiate orthostatic hypotension if administered with monoamine oxidase inhibitors.

Availability
Commercially available in 50-mg capsules.

Selected Readings
Foster BJ et al: Hexamethylmelamine: a critical review of an active drug, *Cancer Treat Rev* 13:197-217, 1986.
Hansen LA, Hughes TE: Altretamine, *DICP Ann Pharmacother* 25:146-152, 1991.

AMIFOSTINE
Other Names
Ethyol, WR-2721, ethiofos, ethanethiol, 2-[(3-aminopropyl)amino]-, dihydrogen phosphate (ester), gammaphos, NSC-296961.

Indications
Amifostine is FDA approved as a treatment to reduce the nephrotoxicity of cisplatin in patients with ovarian carcinoma and non–small-cell lung cancer. Amifostine may also reduce the toxicity of radiation and cyclophosphamide.

Classification and Mechanisms of Action
Amifostine is an organic sulfhydryl compound that protects (in laboratory animals) normal tissues against the cytotoxicity of radiation and alkylating agents. The mechanism by which this occurs appears to be in part related to the differential absorption of amifostine in normal and malignant tissues.

Pharmacokinetics
Amifostine is 30% to 40% absorbed by mouth (in experimental animals). The drug is preferentially distributed to normal tissues (such as bone

marrow, gastrointestinal mucosa, and skin) but not to tumor tissue. Amifostine is almost totally metabolized and is undetectable in the plasma approximately 6 minutes after IV administration. Approximately 0.7% to 2.5% of a dose is excreted in the urine unchanged.

Dose

The recommended dose of amifostine is 910 mg/m^2 starting 30 minutes before initiating treatment with a cisplatin-containing chemotherapy regimen.

Administration

Amifostine has been given as an IV infusion (as a 10 mg/mL solution in 5% dextrose or normal saline) over a 15-minute period. Longer infusions increase the likelihood of hypotension and vomiting.

Toxicity

Gastrointestinal. Nausea and vomiting may be severe and usually require antiemetic premedication. The manufacturer suggests the use of dexamethasone (20 mg via IV) and a 5-HT$_3$ receptor antagonist before administration of amifostine.

Neurological. Somnolence.

Cardiovascular. Transient hypotension, usually asymptomatic; concomitant administration of drugs that could exacerbate the hypotensive effects of amifostine (e.g., benzodiazepines) should be avoided. The manufacturer recommends monitoring of blood pressure every 5 minutes during the 15-minute IV infusion and 5 minutes after completion of the infusion. If the systolic blood pressure drops below a threshold level defined below, the infusion should be stopped, the patient should be placed in the Trendelenburg position, and hydration with normal saline should be initiated. If blood pressure returns to normal within 5 minutes, the infusion of amifostine may be resumed; if it does not, treatment with amifostine should be discontinued.

The infusion of amifostine should be interrupted if the baseline systolic blood pressure is 100 mm Hg and decreases by 20 mm Hg or more, if a baseline reading of 100 to 119 mm Hg decreases by 25 mm Hg or more, if a baseline blood pressure of 120 to 140 mm Hg decreases by 30 mm Hg or more, if a baseline blood pressure of 140 to 180 mm Hg decreases by 40 mm Hg or more, or if a baseline systolic blood pressure equal to or greater than 180 mm Hg decreases by 50 mm Hg or more.

Other. Sneezing, hypocalcemia (rare), flushing.

Storage and Stability

Amifostine is stable at refrigeration temperatures for at least 15 months. Reconstituted and dilute solutions of amifostine (5 to 40 mg/mL) are stable for at least 5 hours at room temperature and at least 24 hours in the refrigerator.

A

Preparation
The 500-mg vial is reconstituted with 9.5 mL of normal saline so as to result in a 50 mg/mL solution. The desired dose is further diluted with normal saline to a concentration of 5 to 40 mg/mL.

Availability
Amifostine, 500 mg per vial, is commercially available.

Selected Readings
Glick JH et al: Phase I clinical trials of WR-2721 with alkylating agent chemotherapy, *Int J Radiat Oncol Biol Phys* 8:575-580, 1982.

Glover D et al: Phase I/II trials of WR-2721 and cis-platinum, *Int J Radiat Oncol Biol Phys* 12:1509-1512, 1986.

Spencer CM, Goa KL: Amifostine: a review of its pharmacodynamic and pharmacokinetic properties, and therapeutic potential as a radioprotector and cytotoxic chemoprotector, *Drug Evaluation* 50:1001-1031, 1995.

AMINOCAMPTOTHECIN

Other Names
9-aminocamptothecin, 9-AC, NSC-603071.

Indications
Aminocamptothecin is an investigational drug undergoing evaluation in several malignancies.

Classification and Mechanisms of Action
Topoisomerase I inhibitor. Topoisomerase I relaxes supercoiled DNA by incision and is necessary for DNA and RNA synthesis. Resealing of DNA is prevented by the binding of camptothecin to the DNA-enzyme complex, resulting in the accumulation of reversible enzyme-DNA cleavable complexes.

Dose
Several doses have been evaluated. As a 72-hour IV infusion, 9-aminocamptothecin has been administered at doses of 35 to 59 µg/m²/hr repeated every 2 to 3 weeks. A phase II dose of 35 µg/m²/hr as a 72-hour infusion has been recommended. Combined with a colony-stimulating factor, the phase II dose may be increased to 47 µg/m²/hr repeated every 2 to 3 weeks.

Administration
Aminocamptothecin is usually administered as a continuous IV infusion over 72 hours. If administered at concentrations greater than 1 µg/mL, it is recommended that the solution be administered directly into a central venous catheter that has been flushed with a small volume of the PEG/phosphoric acid diluent to displace any aqueous solution.

Toxicity
Hematological. Leukopenia and thrombocytopenia are common and may be dose limiting. When 9-aminocamptothecin is administered with

a colony-stimulating factor, thrombocytopenia is usually dose limiting. Anemia has also been observed.

Gastrointestinal. Nausea and vomiting (38% grade II, 8% grade III), diarrhea (30% grade II, 8% grade III), mild stomatitis (33%).

Dermatological. Alopecia is common. Skin rash.

Hepatic. Liver function test abnormalities.

Neurological. Peripheral neuropathy has been reported in patients who had received prior treatment with cisplatin. Mild hearing loss and tinnitus have been reported.

Other. Fatigue (58% grade II, 8% grade III), flulike symptoms (headache, fever, malaise), facial and neck swelling.

Storage and Stability

Ampules of aminocamptothecin in dimethylacetamide (DMA) are stored in the refrigerator (2° C to 8° C). When mixed with the supplied diluent, the drug is stable for 72 hours at room temperature. The drug is also stable for 72 hours in CADD pump cassettes. The drug is unstable in 5% dextrose.

Preparation

Aminocamptothecin concentrate, 5 mg/mL in a 1-mL ampule, is added to 49 mL of the PEG/phosphoric acid diluent to yield a 100 µg/mL solution. It is recommended that aminocamptothecin concentrate be drawn into a glass syringe unless the contact time with a plastic syringe will be less than 1 minute. The aminocamptothecin concentrate should not be filtered. Additional PEG/phosphoric acid diluent may be used to prepare the desired concentration of aminocamptothecin.

Incompatibilities

Aminocamptothecin is not soluble in many common intravenous fluids. Dilution with infusion fluids will result in precipitation at concentrations greater than 1 µg/mL. It is unstable in aqueous media; therefore evacuated containers are not suitable containers for further dilution.

Availability

Aminocamptothecin is available from the NCI in two formulations, DMA and CD. The drug formulations and the diluents provided are not interchangeable. The DMA formulation is provided by the NCI as a 1-mL ampule containing a sterile concentrate of 5 mg/mL aminocamptothecin in DMA and 49 mL of sterile diluent containing PEG/phosphoric acid.

Selected Readings

Dahut W et al: Phase I and pharmacologic study of 9-aminocamptothecin given by 72-hour infusion in adult cancer patients, *J Clin Oncol* 14:1236-1244, 1996.

Schettino PR: *Update on 9-AC formulations and pharmaceutical information*, Drug Management and Authorization Section, NCI, March 14, 1995.

AMINOGLUTETHIMIDE

Other Names
Cytadren, Elipten, BA-16038.

Indications
FDA approved for the treatment of breast cancer and suppression of adrenal function in selected patients with Cushing's syndrome. Aminoglutethimide may also be useful in the treatment of prostate and adrenal cortical carcinoma and ACTH-producing tumors.

Classification and Mechanisms of Action
Aminoglutethimide is an aromatase inhibitor. It inhibits aromatase enzymes necessary for conversion of androgens to estrogens. Aminoglutethimide also blocks adrenal steroid biosynthesis by interfering with the enzymatic conversion of cholesterol to delta-5 pregnenolone. The onset of adrenal suppression occurs 3 to 5 days after initiation of therapy; recovery occurs within 1.5 to 3 days after discontinuing the drug.

Pharmacokinetics
Aminoglutethimide is well absorbed (90%) by mouth and reaches peak serum concentrations approximately 1.5 hours after dosing. Approximately 20% to 25% of the drug is bound to plasma proteins. The drug is metabolized by the liver to at least eight metabolites and excreted in the urine primarily as unchanged drug (35% to 50%) and metabolites. Aminoglutethimide has an elimination half-life of approximately 7 to 9 hours. The half-life is longer (13 hours) at the start of treatment. Aminoglutethimide induces the metabolism of warfarin, theophylline, digoxin, medroxyprogesterone, and dexamethasone. Larger doses of these drugs may be needed.

Dose
Treatment is occasionally begun with a lower dose of aminoglutethimide (250 mg twice daily) and a higher hydrocortisone dose (100 mg/day) for 2 weeks before initiating full doses. The usual dose is 250 mg 4 times per day in combination with hydrocortisone, 40 mg/day in three divided doses (i.e., 10 mg in the morning, 10 mg at noon, and 20 mg at bedtime). Occasionally, a mineralocorticoid is also needed (e.g., fludrocortisone 0.1 mg/day). When aminoglutethimide therapy is discontinued, there is no need to taper the corticosteroid dose.

Administration
Aminoglutethimide is given orally in divided fractions 4 times a day.

Toxicity
Hematological. Leukopenia, agranulocytosis, and pancytopenia are rare.

Gastrointestinal. Mild nausea, vomiting, anorexia.

A

Dermatological. Frequently (33%), transient erythematous maculopapular eruptions are associated with fever. Both of these toxicities remit within 3 to 4 days without stopping administration of the drug. Pustular psoriasis, desquamation, and oral ulceration have been reported.

Neurological. Lethargy (40%), fatigue (common, transient), ataxia (10%), dizziness, nystagmus, drowsiness. Lethargy usually resolves slowly (after 4 to 6 weeks of treatment).

Other. Adrenal insufficiency. Postural hypotension and hyponatremia (caused by decreased aldosterone secretion). Virilization, myalgia, fever, weight gain, facial fullness, leg cramps. Rarely: hypothyroidism, a systemic syndrome resembling lupus erythematosus with cholestatic jaundice and hepatic enzyme elevations. Possible elevated serum cholesterol levels in patients with breast cancer may predispose to atherosclerosis, but the great variation in levels among patients returns to normal level within a few weeks after therapy is stopped.

Storage and Stability
Store at room temperature. Each bottle bears an expiration date.

Incompatibilities
Aminoglutethimide has been shown to increase the metabolic elimination of warfarin by as much as 90%.

Availability
Commercially available in 250-mg tablets.

Selected Readings
Cocconi G et al: Low-dose aminoglutethimide with and without hydrocortisone replacement as first-line endocrine treatment in advanced breast cancer: a prospective randomized trial of the Italian Oncology Group for Clinical Research, *J Clin Oncol* 10:984-989, 1992.

Santen RJ et al: A randomized trial comparing surgical adrenalectomy with aminoglutethimide plus hydrocortisone in women with advanced breast cancer, *N Engl J Med* 305:545-551, 1981.

AMSACRINE
Other Names
m-AMSA, 4'-(9-acridinylamino) methanesulfon-*m*-anisidide, AMSA, acridinylanisidide, NSC-249992.

Indication
Group C (investigational) agent for the treatment of acute nonlymphocytic leukemia.

Classification
Amsacrine is an intercalating agent that also inhibits topoisomerase II.

A

Pharmacokinetics

Amsacrine is poorly absorbed by mouth. After IV administration it is metabolized by the liver and excreted in the bile (50% as unchanged drug and metabolites) and urine (22% to 42% as unchanged drug). Approximately 2% of amsacrine reaches the cerebrospinal fluid. The drug has an elimination half-life of 6 to 7 hours.

Dose

For leukemia, the usual dose is 90 to 150 mg/m^2 daily for 5 days. The dose for the Group C protocol is 120 mg/m^2/day for 5 days. For solid tumors, doses of 90 to 120 mg/m^2 every 21 to 28 days have been studied.

Administration

Slow IV infusion in 500 mL or more of 5% dextrose over a period of 1 or more hours. *Do not use chloride-containing solutions.* Make sure that the potassium level is normal before administering amsacrine.

Toxicity

Hematological. Leukopenia (dose limiting), thrombocytopenia (usually mild), anemia.

Gastrointestinal. Mucositis (uncommon), nausea, vomiting (uncommon).

Dermatological. Phlebitis, pain at injection site. Slowing the infusion rate, further dilution of amsacrine and/or a cold pack at the injection site may be necessary. Urticaria, skin rash, and erythema are rare.

Hepatic. Elevation of liver function tests (bilirubin, transaminases, alkaline phosphatase), usually reversible.

Neurological. Rarely: seizures, neuropathy, headache, dizziness, central nervous system depression.

Cardiovascular. Congestive heart failure, ventricular arrhythmias, ECG changes. Cardiac arrests have been reported in a few cases, while the drug was infusing, *usually in the presence of hypokalemia.*

Other. Orange urine (common). Rarely, allergic reactions (urticaria, skin rashes, anaphylaxis).

Storage and Stability

Unopened vials are stored at room temperature. After preparation, the combined solution is stable for 48 hours at room temperature with room lighting. Further diluted in 500 mL of 5% dextrose plus 1 mEq NaHCO$_3$, its stability at room temperature is 96 hours.

Preparation

Add 1.5 mL from the ampule containing amsacrine, 50 mg/mL in anhydrous N,N-dimethylacetamide (DMA), to the vial containing 13.5 mL of diluent, 0.035M L-lactic acid. The resulting orange-red combined solution contains 5 mg/mL of amsacrine. Dilute the combined solution in 500 mL

A

of 5% dextrose. *Plastic syringes should not be used* to prepare this drug because of the presence of DMA. Use only glass syringes to handle the undiluted solution.

Incompatibilities
Amsacrine *should not be mixed with a sodium chloride injection or any sodium chloride–containing solutions*, including those often found in evacuated containers. This may cause precipitation.

Availability
Available from the NCI in 75 mg/1.5 mL ampules with 13.5 mL of 0.0353M L-LACTIC ACID DILUENT.

Selected Readings
Louie AC, Issel BF: Amsacrine (AMSA): a clinical review, *J Clin Oncol* 3:562-592, 1985.
Weiss RB et al: Amsacrine-associated cardiac toxicity: an analysis of 82 cases, *J Clin Oncol* 4:918-928, 1986.

ANAGRELIDE
Other Names
Agrelin, anagrelide hydrochloride, BMY26538-01, BL4126A.

Indications
Anagrelide is an investigational drug that is being evaluated in the treatment of patients with life-threatening thrombocythemia that is no longer responsive to standard treatment.

Classification and Mechanisms of Action
Anagrelide inhibits platelet aggregation and suppresses platelet concentrations.

Pharmacokinetics
Anagrelide is readily absorbed from the gastrointestinal tract and is extensively metabolized. Anagrelide may also be a useful treatment in patients with myelodysplastic syndromes, polycythemia vera, and chronic myelogenous leukemia.

Dose
The usual starting dose is 2 mg/day taken in four equally divided doses (i.e., 0.5 mg 4 times a day). Doses are adjusted in increments of 0.5 mg/day every 5 to 7 days to maintain platelet counts at a particular level. It has been recommended that platelet counts be quickly reduced to a level less than 600,000/mm^3 and maintained within 150,000 and 450,000/mm^3. The daily dose of anagrelide should not exceed 10 mg or an individual dose in excess of 3 mg. It is recommended that the starting dose be reduced by 50% for patients with abnormal liver or renal function (i.e., 0.5 mg twice daily). Patients with a cardiac history that puts them at risk for developing severe toxicity (described on p. 59) should begin treatment with 0.5 mg/day.

A

Administration
Oral.

Toxicity
Hematological. Mild anemia (36%), thrombocytopenia.

Gastrointestinal. Nausea (19%), vomiting (4%), gas or bloating (8%), pain or gastric distress (8%). Diarrhea has been reported to occur in approximately 15% of the patients, and it has been observed that use of a lactase supplement can prevent diarrhea in the majority of patients. Pancreatitis has been reported in a few patients.

Dermatological. Rash (infrequent), hyperpigmentation of lower extremities.

Hepatic. Elevation of hepatic transaminase levels has been reported rarely.

Neurological. Headache (30%, severe in 4% of the patients). Headache usually occurs within the first two weeks of treatment and can be controlled with acetaminophen. Dizziness has been reported in 8% of the patients and is usually mild or moderate in severity.

Cardiovascular. Hypotension, palpitations, and/or tachycardia (36%); angina, fluid retention, or edema (24%); congestive heart failure, atrial fibrillation (rare). Deaths possibly related to treatment with anagrelide have occurred, predominately in patients with known coronary artery disease.

Pulmonary. Pulmonary infiltrates that improve after treatment with corticosteroids.

Other. Anagrelide is contraindicated in pregnant women.

Storage and Stability
Anagrelide tablets are stored at room temperature.

Availability
Anagrelide is an investigational drug that is available in 0.5-mg tablets.

Selected Readings
Anagrelide Study Group: Anagrelide, a therapy for thrombocythemic states: experience in 577 patients, *Am J Med* 92:69-76, 1992.
Silverstein MN et al: Anagrelide: a new drug for treating thrombocytosis, *N Engl J Med* 318:1292-1294, 1988.

ANASTROZOLE
Other Names
Arimidex.

Indications
Anastrozole is FDA approved for the treatment of advanced breast cancer in postmenopausal women who have previously received tamoxifen therapy. Patients with estrogen receptor–negative disease and patients whose tumor did not respond to tamoxifen rarely benefit from treatment with anastrozole.

A

Classification and Mechanisms of Action
Anastrozole is a nonsteroidal aromatase inhibitor. The drug produces its antitumor effects by significantly reducing serum estradiol levels. It does not affect the formation of adrenal corticosteroids or aldosterone. Corticosteroid replacement therapy is not necessary in patients taking anastrozole.

Pharmacokinetics
Anastrozole is well-absorbed (85%) after oral administration. Food does not appear to affect the absorption of anastrozole. Approximately 40% of the drug is bound to plasma proteins after absorption. Most of the drug is metabolized by the liver, and its major metabolite is inactive. Approximately 11% of a dose is eliminated into the urine as unchanged drug. The elimination half-life is approximately 50 hours.

Dose
Anastrozole is administered as a daily 1-mg dose. Adjustment of dose in patients with renal and hepatic function impairment is not necessary.

Administration
Oral.

Toxicity
Hematological. Mild leukopenia and anemia were rarely observed.

Gastrointestinal. Nausea (16%), vomiting (9%), diarrhea (8%), constipation (7%), abdominal pain (7%), anorexia (7%), xerostomia (5%).

Dermatological. Rash (5%); pruritus and thinning hair (rare).

Hepatic. Rare elevations of hepatic serum enzyme levels.

Neurological. Headache (13%), dizziness (6%), depression (5%), and paresthesia (4%). Insomnia, anxiety, nervousness, confusion, and somnolence were rarely observed.

Cardiovascular. Peripheral edema (5%); hypertension and thrombophlebitis occurred in less than 2% of the patients treated with anastrozole.

Pulmonary. Dyspnea (9%).

Other. Asthenia (16%), hot flushes (12%), pain (10%), back pain (10%), bone pain (6%), pelvic pain (5%), chest pain (5%), vaginal hemorrhage (2%), diaphoresis (1.5%), and weight gain (1.5%). Flulike symptoms, fever, neck pain, breast pain, malaise, myalgia, arthralgia, infection, and weight loss were rarely observed.

Storage and Stability
Anastrozole tablets are stored at room temperature. Bottles contain expiration dates.

Availability
Anastrozole is commercially available in 1-mg tablets.

Selected Reading

Plourde PV et al: Arimidex: a new oral, once-a-day aromatase inhibitor, *J Steroid Biochem Mol Biol* 53:175-179, 1995.

ASPARAGINASE

Other Names

Escherichia coli–derived: Elspar, L-Asparaginase.

Erwinia carotovora–derived: *Erwinia* asparaginase, Porton asparaginase, NSC-106977.

PEG-modified (*E. coli–derived*): Oncaspar, PEG-asparaginase, pegaspargase.

Indications

E. coli and PEG-modified asparaginase are FDA approved for the treatment of acute lymphocytic leukemia. Asparaginase has also been used in the treatment of patients with acute nonlymphocytic leukemia, chronic lymphocytic leukemia, chronic myelogenous leukemia, soft-tissue sarcoma, and Hodgkin's and non-Hodgkin's lymphoma. *Erwinia* asparaginase is an investigational (Group C) agent that may be used in acute lymphocytic leukemia in patients who are sensitive to *E. coli* L-asparaginase.

Classification and Mechanisms of Action

Enzyme. Asparaginase hydrolyzes the amino acid asparagine. The drug is believed to inhibit protein synthesis by depriving tumor cells of asparagine. Tumor cells that require asparagine are most affected by asparaginase.

Pharmacokinetics

Asparaginase is not absorbed by mouth and undergoes metabolic degradation. After intramuscular (IM) injection, peak plasma levels occur within 14 to 24 hours. Approximately 30% of the drug is protein bound. The *E. coli* formulation of asparaginase has an elimination half-life of 40 to 50 hours. PEG-asparaginase has an elimination half-life of 3 to 5 days. Only trace amounts of the drug are excreted in the urine.

Dose

Test Dose. The manufacturer of the *E. coli*–derived preparation recommends that a 2-IU intradermal test dose be given with the first treatment and with subsequent treatments if more than 1 week separates successive doses. Observation of the patient for 1 hour before administering the full dose is also recommended.

As a single agent, 200 IU/kg intravenously daily for 28 days has been used. A commonly used dose regimen is 6000 to 10,000 IU/m^2 via IM injection for nine injections, given every 3 days after cytotoxic therapy. PEG-asparaginase is administered at a dose of 2500 IU/m^2 every 14 days in children whose body surface area (BSA) is >0.6 m^2 and 82.5 IU/m^2 every 14 days for children whose BSA is <0.6 m^2.

A

Administration

All preparations of asparaginase may be given intramuscularly or by IV infusion. The recommended route of administration is IM. For IV administration, an infusion in 50 to 100 mL normal saline or 5% dextrose over a 30-minute period is preferred. It is recommended that PEG-asparaginase be given intramuscularly or by IV in 100 mL of normal saline or 5% dextrose over a period of 1 to 2 hours. The test dose, if desired, is usually administered as an intradermal injection. The following precautions should be taken when the drug is administered:

1. Avoid giving the drug at night.
2. Two professionals (a registered nurse and a physican) must be directly accessible.
3. Have a running IV infusion in place.
4. Have syringes of epinephrine (Adrenalin) (1:1000, 1 mg), diphenhydramine (50 mg), and hydrocortisone (100 mg) readily available.
5. Monitor the patient's blood pressure every 15 minutes for 1 hour.

Toxicity

Hematological. Prolonged thrombin, prothrombin times. Decrease in protein synthesis (decreased fibrinogen and depression of clotting factors, in particular antithrombin III), resulting in thrombosis and/or pulmonary embolism. Myelosuppression is not common.

Gastrointestinal. Nausea and vomiting are common (50% to 60%) but usually controlled with antiemetics. Anorexia, abdominal cramps, weight loss (25%), diarrhea (rare), mucositis, malabsorption, and pancreatitis (<15%) also occur.

Hepatic. Hepatotoxicity (i.e., elevations in liver enzyme and alkaline phosphatase levels; depression of serum albumin levels, cholesterol, and/or plasma fibrinogen levels) is very common (50% to 100%) but rarely severe.

Neurological. EEG changes, depression, somnolence, lethargy, fatigue, seizures, coma, headache, confusion (25%), irritability, agitation, dizziness, and hallucinations, ranging from mild to severe.

Hypersensitivity reactions. Most hypersensitivity reactions occur within 30 minutes of an IV dose, usually longer than 30 to 60 minutes after an IM dose. Some clinicians believe the intradermal test dose is not predictive of who will develop a hypersensitivity reaction. Manifestations of a hypersensitivity reaction may include urticarial eruptions (may be controlled with antihistamines), laryngeal constriction, hypotension, diaphoresis, edema, asthma, and loss of consciousness. The most serious hypersensitivity reactions occur after several doses have been administered, but reactions have been reported after the first dose. The risk of developing a hypersensitivity reaction is greatest in patients *not* receiving vincristine and prednisone, if a 1-month or greater period of time has elapsed since the last dose was given, if the IgG3 level exceeds 100 AU, and if the drug is given by IV infusion rather than intramuscular injection. Patients who have had reactions to the *E. coli* product may be able to tolerate *Erwinia* or PEG-asparaginase.

Approximately 30% of patients who developed a hypersensitivity reaction to the *E. coli* preparation will develop a reaction to PEG-asparaginase.

Renal. Azotemia (68%), usually prerenal; rarely: severe renal failure.

Other. Hyperglycemia, chills, fever (25%); rare: hyperthermia.

Storage and Stability

Intact vials of all preparations are refrigerated. Reconstituted solutions of the *E. coli* and *Erwinia* formulations and those further diluted are stable for 8 hours at room temperature and 14 days in the refrigerator. Cloudy solutions should not be used. *Erwinia* asparaginase is incompatible with the rubber stopper on the vial; therefore the reconstituted solution should be used within 15 minutes. PEG-asparaginase should be used immediately and the remainder of the vial discarded. PEG-asparaginase must not be frozen as this destroys its activity.

Preparation

To the *E. coli* formulation, add 1 to 5 mL of sterile water or sodium chloride injection without preservative to each 10,000-IU vial of drug. This results in a concentration of 10,000 to 2000 IU/mL, respectively. Vigorous shaking of the vial may cause excessive foaming. A small number of gelatinous fiberlike particles that occasionally develop may be removed using a 0.5-μm filter. The desired dose may be further diluted in normal saline or 5% dextrose. Reconstitute the 10,000-IU vial of *Erwinia* preparation with 2 mL normal saline without preservative to yield a 5000 IU/mL solution.

Incompatibilities

Use of a 0.2-μm filter results in a loss of potency. Asparaginase pretreatment antagonizes the effects of methotrexate. Administration of asparaginase and methotrexate should be separated by at least 24 hours.

Availability

Available in 10,000-IU vials as lyophilized cake material from two natural sources. The *E. coli* preparation is commercially available. *Erwinia* asparaginase (10,000 IU/vial) is an investigational Group C agent available from the NCI. PEG-asparaginase is commercially available in 5-mL vials that contain 3750 IU (750 IU/mL).

Selected Readings

Evans WE et al: Anaphylactoid reactions to *Escherichia coli* and *Erwinia* asparaginase in children with leukemia and lymphoma, *Cancer* 49:1378-1383, 1982.
Land VJ et al: Toxicity of L-asparaginase in children with advanced leukemia, *Cancer* 30:399-347, 1972.

AZACYTIDINE

Other Names

5-azacitidine, ladakamycin, AZA-CR, 5-AZC, NSC-102816.

A

Classification
Antimetabolite (cytidine analogue).

Indications
Group C (investigational) agent for the treatment of refractory acute non-lymphocytic leukemia.

Pharmacokinetics
The drug is activated to azacytidine triphosphate and deaminated by the liver to 5-azauridine. Approximately 90% of the drug and its metabolic products are excreted in the urine (20% as unchanged drug) in 24 hours. Azacytidine has an elimination half-life of 3 to 6 hours.

Dose
Commonly used doses are 150 to 300 mg/m^2/day for 5 days, repeated every 3 weeks, and 150 to 200 mg/m^2 twice weekly for 2 to 8 weeks. Azacytidine, 750 mg/m^2/week, has also been given. Low-dose regimens of azacytidine, 25 mg/m^2 for 14 days, have also been used.

Administration
Usually administered as a continuous infusion. Has also been given as an IV bolus (in 50 mL or more of 5% dextrose or normal saline), as a short infusion over a period of 10 to 30 minutes, and by subcutaneous injection. Because of its short stability in solution, "fresh bags" must be prepared every 2 to 3 hours for long infusions.

Toxicity
Hematological. Leukopenia, dose related and dose limiting, occasionally prolonged; thrombocytopenia, less common; anemia.

Gastrointestinal. Nausea and vomiting, severe and dose limiting when given as an IV bolus but less common with continuous infusions; diarrhea (50%); stomatitis (infrequent).

Dermatological. Alopecia; rash (rare), pruritus (sometimes). Local injection site reactions may occur after subcutaneous injection.

Genitourinary. Azotemia (transient and reversible), renal tubular acidosis (rare), proteinuria (rare).

Hepatic. Elevations of liver enzyme, bilirubin, and/or alkaline phosphatase levels. Because of hepatic coma, some have warned against its use in patients with hypoalbuminemia (i.e., <3 g/dL).

Neurological. Progressive lethargy, confusion, and coma have been reported.

Cardiovascular. Hypotension after an IV bolus (rare).

Other. Hypophosphatemia, sometimes with myalgia, muscle weakness, restlessness, insomnia, fatigue, rhabdomyolysis (rare), conjunctivitis, fever.

Storage and Stability
The vials are stored in the refrigerator. It is stable for at least 2 years when stored at room temperature and for 4 years when refrigerated.

After reconstitution, the drug rapidly decomposes and must be further diluted within 30 minutes. Its stability in solution is concentration and fluid dependent. On further dilution to a concentration of 2 mg/mL, 10% of its potency is lost in 2.4 hours (normal saline), 3 hours (5% dextrose or Normosol-R), and 2.9 hours (lactated Ringer's solution). At a concentration of 0.2 mg/mL the drug loses 10% of its potency within 1.9 hours (normal saline, lactated Ringer's solution, or Normosol-R) and 0.8 hours (5% dextrose).

Preparation
The 100-mg vial is reconstituted with 19.9 mL sterile water to result in a 5-mg/mL solution. It may be further diluted in an appropriate fluid.

Incompatibilities
Electrolytes have a destabilizing effect and should not be added to azacytidine solutions.

Availability
Available as an investigational agent from the NCI in 100-mg vials of lyophilized powder.

Selected Readings
Cheung YW et al: Stability of azacytidine in infusion fluids, *Am J Hosp Pharm* 41:1156-1159, 1984.
Glover AB, Leyland-Jones B: Biochemistry of azacitidine: a review, *Cancer Treat Rep* 71:959-964, 1987.
Glover AB, Leyland-Jones BR, Chung HG: Azacitidine: 10 years later, *Cancer Treat Rep* 71:737-746, 1987.

BICALUTAMIDE
Other Names
Casodex, ICI 176,334.

Indications
FDA approved for the treatment of patients with advanced cancer of the prostate when combined with a luteinizing hormone–releasing hormone (LHRH) analogue (e.g., leuprolide, goserelin).

Classification and Mechanisms of Action
Nonsteroidal antiandrogen. Bicalutamide inhibits the effects of androgens by preventing their binding to cellular androgenic receptors. The drug may also inhibit androgen uptake in the pituitary gland.

Pharmacokinetics
Bicalutamide is slowly absorbed after oral administration and reaches peak plasma concentrations approximately 31 hours after administration. Food does not affect the absorption of bicalutamide from the gastrointestinal tract. The drug is metabolized in the liver to inactive metabolites and the

elimination half-life of approximately 6 days. The elimination of bicalutamide does not appear to be affected by renal or hepatic impairment.

Dose
Bicalutamide is administered as a daily dose of 50 mg in combination
with an LHRH analogue.

Administration
Oral. Bicalutamide may be administered with meals or on an empty stomach.

Toxicity
Hematological.   Anemia (7%), leukopenia (rare).

Gastrointestinal.   Nausea (11%), vomiting (3%), anorexia, constipation
(7% to 17%), diarrhea (10%), flatulence, xerostomia; rectal bleeding and
melena occur rarely.

Dermatological.   Rash (6%), diaphoresis (6%), dry skin, pruritus, alopecia (<5%).

Hepatic.   Increased liver enzymes levels (6%).

Endocrine.   Hot flushes (49%), breast pain (39%), gynecomastia (38%).
Impotence and diabetes mellitus have occurred in patients receiving bicalutamide and an LHRH analogue.

Genitourinary.   Nocturia (9%), hematuria (7%), urinary tract infection
(6%), impotence (5%), urinary incontinence (2%), urinary frequency,
impaired urination, dysuria, urinary retention, urinary urgency, increased
BUN and creatinine levels.

Neurological.   Dizziness (7%), paresthesia (6%), insomnia (5%), anxiety,
headache (4%), depression, decreased libido, hypertonia, confusion, neuropathy, somnolence, nervousness (<5%).

Cardiovascular.   Hypertension (5%), angina pectoris, peripheral edema
(8%), congestive heart failure (<5%).

Pulmonary.   Dyspnea, cough, pharyngitis, bronchitis, pneumonia, rhinitis,
lung disorder (<5%).

Musculoskeletal.   Myasthenia, arthritis, myalgia, leg cramps, pathological
fractures (<5%).

Other.   Generalized pain (27%), back pain (15%), pelvic pain (13%), asthenia (15%), infection (10%), flulike symptoms (4%), fever, chills, weight
loss (4%), hyperglycemia (5%).

Storage and Stability
Tablets are stored at room temperature, and each bottle bears an expiration date.

Incompatibilities
Bicalutamide may displace coumarin anticoagulants from protein-binding
sites and lead to prolongation of prothrombin times in patients taking warfarin or similar drugs.

Availability
Commercially available as a 50-mg tablet.

Selected Reading
Blackledge G: Casodex: mechanism of action and opportunities for usage, *Cancer* 72:3830-3833, 1993.

BLEOMYCIN
Other Names
Blenoxane, BLM, Bleo, NSC-125066.

Indications
FDA approved for the treatment of squamous cell carcinoma (head and neck, skin, penis, cervix, vulva), Hodgkin's and non-Hodgkin's lymphoma, reticulum cell sarcoma, lymphosarcoma, and testicular carcinoma (embryonal cell, choriocarcinoma, teratocarcinoma). Bleomycin is also useful as a sclerosing agent for pleural and pericardial effusions and may also be useful in the treatment of Kaposi's sarcoma, soft-tissue sarcoma, osteosarcoma, melanoma, and cancers of the bladder, kidney, endometrium, esophagus, ovary, and thyroid.

Classification
Antitumor antibiotic.

Pharmacokinetics
Bleomycin is poorly absorbed by mouth. Approximately 45% is absorbed into the systemic circulation after intracavitary administration. Less than 1% is bound to plasma proteins. Approximately 50% to 70% of the drug is excreted by the kidneys as unchanged drug that cannot be removed by hemodialysis. The remaining drug is metabolized by intracellular aminopeptidase (hydrolysis). Bleomycin has an elimination half-life of 2 to 5 hours in patients with normal renal function and up to 30 hours in patients with renal failure. The dose should be reduced in patients with reduced creatinine clearance (e.g., a 25% reduction for a creatinine clearance of 10 to 50 mL/min and a 50% to 100% reduction for a creatinine clearance less than 10 mL/min).

Dose
Common doses. 10 to 20 units/m² weekly or twice weekly via IM injection, intravenously, or subcuteneously, or as a continuous infusion over a period of 3 to 7 days at 15 to 20 units/m²/day. The intrapleural dose is usually 60 units/m².

Test Dose. Because anaphylactoid reactions can occur in patients with lymphoma (1% to 8% incidence), it has been recommended that a 2-unit test dose be given before the first treatment. The test dose is usually given intravenously (in 50 mL 5% dextrose or normal saline over 15 minutes) and followed by an observation period of 1 to 2 hours, although some advocate 6 to 24 hours before administering the full dose.

Total Lifetime Dose. Until predictive methods are available for the diagnosis of impending pulmonary damage, the total lifetime dose of bleomycin should *never* exceed 400 units. Many physicians limit the total dose to 300 units.

Administration

Bleomycin may be given via IM injection, by slow IV push, by IV infusion in 50 to 100 mL of normal saline or 5% dextrose over 15 minutes or longer, intraarterially, intratumorally, by bladder instillation, subcutaneously, or intracavitarily. The intrapleural dose is usually dissolved in 50 mL of normal saline and left in the pleural space for 8 to 24 hours.

Toxicity

Hematological. Myelosuppression is uncommon and mild.

Gastrointestinal. Anorexia is common. Mucositis occurs occasionally and mild nausea and/or vomiting are unusual.

Dermatological. Skin reactions are common (50%) and may include pruritus, hyperpigmentation, hyperkeratosis (mainly on the palms and fingers), edema, erythema, and thickening of nail beds. Skin peeling (especially on the fingertips), skin tenderness, urticaria, rash, and alopecia may also occur.

Pulmonary. Interstitial pneumonitis and pulmonary fibrosis are related to the total cumulative dose; doses greater than 400 units must be avoided. Signs and symptoms include dyspnea, cough, fine rales, radiographic findings resembling pneumonia, and altered pulmonary function status (e.g., reduced carbon monoxide diffusing capacity).

Hypersensitivity. Anaphylactoid reactions occur in about 1% (up to 8% in some series) of lymphoma patients and are often associated with a severe febrile reaction. Deaths have been reported.

Other. Fever with or without chills is common (25%), frequently occurs within 4 to 10 hours after administration, and lasts 4 to 12 hours or longer. The incidence may decrease with subsequent doses. Preventive treatment with acetaminophen (e.g., 650 mg every 4 to 6 hours for three to four doses) is recommended. Hypotension, pain at the injection site, phlebitis, headache, Raynaud's phenomena, lethargy, and unusual taste sensations have also been reported.

Storage and Stability

Bleomycin is stored in the refrigerator. After reconstitution the solution is stable for at least 28 days if refrigerated or for 14 days at room temperature.

Preparation

One to 5 mL of normal saline injection is added to the 15-unit vial to result in concentrations of 15 to 3 units/mL, respectively. A standard dilution of 3 mL to yield 5 units/mL is suggested. It may be further diluted in normal saline or 5% dextrose.

Incompatibilities
Bleomycin should not be mixed with solutions containing divalent or trivalent cations (especially copper) because of chelation. It is inactivated by hydrogen peroxide, methotrexate, mitomycin, and ascorbic acid.

Compatibilities
Reconstituted bleomycin in 5% dextrose solution with 100 to 1000 units/mL of heparin is stable for 24 hours at room temperature. Bleomycin is also compatible with cyclophosphamide, doxorubicin, mesna, vinblastine, and vincristine. A pharmacist should be consulted for more information.

Availability
Commercially available in 15-unit vials as a lyophilized powder.

Selected Readings
Comis RL: Detecting bleomycin pulmonary toxicity: a continued conundrum, *J Clin Oncol* 8:765-767, 1990.
Crooke ST et al: Effects of variations in renal function on the clinical pharmacology of bleomycin administered as an IV bolus, *Cancer Treat Rep* 61:1631-1636, 1977.
Ostrawski MJ: Intracavitary therapy with bleomycin for the treatment of malignant pleural effusions, *J Surg Oncol* 41(suppl):7-13, 1989.

BUSERELIN
Other Names
Buserelin acetate, HOE 766, Suprefact.

Indications
Investigational drug that may be a useful treatment for patients with advanced prostate cancer.

Classification and Mechanisms of Action
Buserelin is a luteinizing hormone–releasing hormone (LHRH) analogue. In men, the administration of pharmacological doses inhibits gonadotropin release and results in decreased serum concentrations of luteinizing hormone (LH), follicle-stimulating hormone (FSH), and testosterone (estradiol in women). After 1 to 2 weeks, down-regulation of LHRH receptors occurs, with reduced LH and FSH secretion and castration levels of testosterone or estradiol. With continued therapy the concentration of these hormones can be expected to remain at castration levels for over 2 years.

Dose
For the first week, 500 µg 3 times a day by subcutaneous injection followed by 200 µg/day by subcutaneous injection. Alternatively, 800 µg 3 times a day followed by 400 µg 3 times a day by intranasal inhalation.

B

Administration
Subcutaneous injection or intranasal inhalation.

Toxicity
Gastrointestinal. Infrequent nausea, vomiting, diarrhea, and constipation.

Dermatological. Local discomfort after injection. Rashes are rare.

Hepatic. Elevated levels of serum cholesterol.

Endocrine. Hot flashes (50%), decreased libido (80% to 90%), impotence (common), and gynecomastia in men; cessation of menses and spotting in women.

Tumor flare. Increased bone pain, urinary retention, or spinal cord compression may occur in the first 2 weeks of treatment. As with other LHRH agonists, this effect may be blocked by antiandrogens (e.g., flutamide, bicalutamide).

Other. Headache, muscle weakness (rare), depression (rare), hypertension (rare), increased serum creatinine levels (rare); pituitary adenomas have been reported to occur in rats treated with LHRH agonists.

Storage and Stability
The drug should be stored at room temperature. Freezing the drug must be avoided.

Availability
Available as an injectable solution (1 mg/mL) and as an intranasal spray (1 mg/mL in 10-mL containers).

Selected Reading
Presant CA et al: Buserelin treatment of advanced prostatic carcinoma, *Cancer* 59:1713-1716, 1987.

BUSULFAN
Other Names
Myleran, BSF, NSC-750.

Indications
FDA approved for the treatment of chronic myelogenous leukemia. Busulfan has also been used in the treatment of acute nonlymphocytic leukemia and polycythemia vera and as a part of chemotherapy regimens for bone marrow transplantation.

Classification
Alkylating agent.

Pharmacokinetics
Well absorbed by mouth with peak plasma levels occurring 0.5 to 2 hours after administration. The drug is metabolized to several metabolites that

B

are excreted into the urine. Approximately 25% to 35% of busulfan is eliminated via the kidneys as methanesulfonic acid. Busulfan has an elimination half-life of approximately 2.5 hours.

Dose
The usual adult dose for induction therapy is 4 to 12 mg/day. Maintenance doses are usually 1 to 3 mg/day but have ranged from 2 mg/week to 4 mg/day. Busulfan is usually given in a dose of 4 mg/kg/day (in divided doses) for 4 days before bone marrow transplantation.

Administration
Oral.

Toxicity
Hematological. Prolonged myelosuppression with slow recovery and severe thrombocytopenia; anemia, agranulocytosis (rare).

Gastrointestinal. Nausea and vomiting are not usually severe with standard doses but are commonly moderate to severe with the doses used in patients undergoing bone marrow transplantation. Diarrhea is uncommon, anorexia; moderate to severe mucositis with accompanying diarrhea can occur with high-dose therapy.

Dermatological. Hyperpigmentation (diffuse brown, bronze, dusky), dryness of skin and mucous membranes, alopecia, rashes, melanoderma, urticaria.

Hepatic. Abnormalities in hepatic enzymes, cholestatic jaundice, hepatic venoocclusive disease (transplant doses).

Neurological (associated with high-dose therapy). Dizziness, blurred vision, confusion, seizures.

Pulmonary. "Busulfan lung" (interstitial pulmonary fibrosis) with persistent cough, fever, rales, dyspnea, and respiratory insufficiency. Pulmonary fibrosis is rare and most often occurs after chronic therapy.

Other. Occasional gynecomastia, hyperuricemia, hyperuricosuria, Addison-like syndrome, asthenia, hypotension (rare), fatigue, impairment of fertility, cheilosis, impotence (rare), amenorrhea, hemorrhagic cystitis (rare), endocardial fibrosis (rare), cataracts, second malignancy.

Storage and Stability
Store tablets at room temperature. Containers bear expiration dates.

Availability
Commercially available in 2-mg scored tablets.

Selected Readings
Buggia I et al: Busulfan, *DICP Ann Pharmacother* 28:1055-1062, 1994.
Hassan M et al: Pharmacokinetic and metabolic studies of high-dose busulphan in adults, *Eur J Clin Pharmacol* 36:525-530, 1989.

O'Donnell MR et al: Busulfan/cyclophosphamide as a conditioning regimen for allogeneic bone marrow transplantation for myelodysplasia, *J Clin Oncol* 13:2973-2979, 1995.

B

BUTHIONINE SULFOXIMINE

Other Names
BSO, DL-buthionine-[S,R]-sulfoxime, buthionine sulfoxime, NSC-326231.

Indications
BSO is an investigational drug that is being studied for its role as a potentiator of alkylating agent (e.g., melphalan, chlorambucil) cytotoxicity.

Classification and Mechanisms of Action
BSO depletes cells of glutathione by inhibiting the enzyme gamma-glutamylcysteine synthetase. Since glutathione is involved in detoxifying alkylating agents, BSO may have a role in sensitizing malignant cells to the effects of various alkylating agents.

Pharmacokinetics
BSO is a mixture of R and S isomers. The elimination half-life of BSO is approximately 3.5 hours (no difference between isomers).

Dose
Six doses of 1500 to 3000 mg/m^2 every 12 hours. The alkylating agent (i.e., melphalan) has been administered 1 hour after the fifth dose of BSO.

Administration
BSO is administered as an IV bolus over a 5- to 10-minute period.

Toxicity
BSO is used in combination with antineoplastic drugs. The only toxicities attributable to BSO in phase I studies have been nausea and vomiting, which occurred in approximately 50% of the patients.

Storage and Stability
BSO is stored at room temperature. Further dilution of the injectable solution to a concentration of 0.1 mg/mL in normal saline or 5% dextrose (in a plastic or glass container) is stable for at least 14 days at room temperature.

Preparation
The injectable liquid should be diluted to a concentration of 0.1 mg/mL in 5% dextrose or normal saline before administration.

Availability
BSO is an investigational agent that is available as an injectable solution (100 mg/mL, 1000-mg vials) from the NCI.

Selected Reading

O'Dwyer PJ et al: Phase I trial of buthionine sulfoximine in combination with melphalan in patients with cancer, *J Clin Oncol* 14:249-256, 1996.

CARBOPLATIN

Other Names

Paraplatin, CBDCA, carboplatinum, JM-8, NSC-241240.

Indications

FDA approved for the treatment of ovarian carcinoma. Carboplatin has also been found to be useful in the treatment of neuroblastoma, refractory leukemias, and cancers of the bladder, brain, breast, testes, head and neck, endometrium, cervix, and lung.

Classification

Heavy metal alkylating-like agent.

Pharmacokinetics

After IV administration, carboplatin disappears rapidly from the bloodstream. It has an elimination half-life of approximately 2.5 to 6 hours. At least 60% to 70% of the drug is eliminated unchanged in the urine, necessitating dose attenuation in patients with impairment of renal function when dosing does not take into account renal function.

Dose

A common IV dose is 360 to 400 mg/m^2 every 4 weeks. Concomitant hydration is not necessary. Alternate dosing schemes, based on target area under the curve (AUC) plasma concentration, prediction of carboplatin clearance, or the desired nadir platelet count have been utilized. Doses of 400 to 550 mg/m^2 have been given by the intraperitoneal route. As a part of preparative regimens for bone marrow transplantation, carboplatin has been administered in higher doses (e.g., 1500 mg/m^2) in combination with other antineoplastic drugs.

The dose of carboplatin, based on target AUC, is calculated using the following formula:

$$\text{Dose (total mg)} = \text{Target AUC} \times (\text{GFR} + 25)$$

The patient's creatinine clearance, in mL/minute, is often used in place of GFR. A target AUC of 6 to 7 is often used depending on the patient's prior therapies and drug(s) that will be used in combination with carboplatin. A target AUC of 4 to 6 may be appropriate for patients who have received extensive prior treatment, and a higher target AUC may be appropriate for previously untreated patients.

Administration

Usually by IV infusion in 50 to 250 mL of 5% dextrose or normal saline over 15 to 30 minutes. Carboplatin has also been given intraperitoneally and intraarterially (intrahepatic and intracarotid).

C

Toxicity

Hematological. Thrombocytopenia is dose limiting (nadir, within 2 to 3 weeks; recovery, 1 to 2 weeks thereafter). Neutropenia occurs frequently but is usually not dose limiting. When doses are calculated based on mg/m^2, patients with impaired renal function will experience more pronounced myelosuppression unless the dose is attenuated. Clinically significant anemia is uncommon after treatment with carboplatin but may be cumulative.

Gastrointestinal. Nausea and vomiting occur frequently but are less severe when compared with cisplatin and usually preventable with antiemetic treatment. Symptoms usually begin 6 to 12 hours after administration and may last for 24 hours. Anorexia, constipation, and diarrhea have been reported.

Dermatological. Rash, urticaria, alopecia, mucositis (8%).

Hepatic. Abnormal liver function values occur in 20% to 30% of patients and are generally mild and transient. Hepatic venoocclusive disease has been reported after high-dose carboplatin therapy before bone marrow transplantation.

Neurological. Peripheral neuropathy is infrequent and more common in patients older than 65 years of age. This toxicity may be cumulative, especially in patients who have received prior treatment with cisplatin. Ototoxicity occurs in approximately 12% of the patients.

Renal. Elevations in serum creatinine and BUN levels and electrolyte loss (i.e., hypomagnesemia [61%], hyponatremia, hypokalemia) are uncommon; hematuria is rare.

Other. Pain at the site of injection, asthenia (44%), hearing loss, blurred vision, flulike syndrome, optic neuritis, hyperamylasemia.

Storage and Stability

Carboplatin vials are stored at room temperature. The reconstituted solution and 1 mg/mL solutions are stable for at least 24 hours at room temperature and 5 days in the refrigerator. When further diluted in glass or polyvinyl plastic to a concentration of 0.5 mg/mL, solutions have the following stability: in normal saline, 8 hours at room temperature, 24 hours in the refrigerator; in 5% dextrose (when reconstituted in sterile water), 24 hours at room or refrigeration temperatures.

Preparation

Add 5, 15, or 45 mL sterile water, normal saline, or 5% dextrose to the 50-, 150-, or 450-mg vial, respectively. The resulting solution contains 10 mg/mL. The desired dose is further diluted, usually in 5% dextrose.

Incompatibilities

Forms a precipitate when in contact with aluminum.

Compatibilities

Carboplatin (0.3 mg/mL) and etoposide (0.4 mg/mL) are chemically compatible in normal saline or 5% dextrose for at least 24 hours at room temperature.

Availability
Commercially available as a lyophilized powder in 50-, 150-, and 450-mg vials.

Selected Readings
Bunn PA et al: *Carboplatin (JM-8): current perspectives and future directions*, Philadelphia, 1990, WB Saunders.
Calvert AH et al: Carboplatin dosage: prospective evaluation of a simple formula based on renal function, *J Clin Oncol* 7:1748-1756, 1989.
Christian MC: Carboplatin. In DeVita VT Jr et al, eds: Principles and practice of oncology, *PPO Updates* 3:1-16, 1989.

CARMUSTINE
Other Names
BCNU, BiCNU, bis-chloronitrosourea, NSC-409962.

Indications
FDA approved treatment of brain tumors, multiple myeloma, Hodgkin's disease, and non-Hodgkin's lymphoma. Carmustine may also be a useful treatment for melanoma, cutaneous T-cell lymphoma, and cancers of the colon, rectum, stomach, and liver.

Classification
Alkylating agent of the nitrosourea class.

Pharmacokinetics
Carmustine rapidly distributes into the tissues after IV injection. Significant amounts of carmustine and/or its metabolites, some which are active, penetrate into the cerebrospinal fluid (up to 70% of plasma concentrations). Carmustine metabolites also distribute into breast milk. The drug is metabolized by the liver (microsomal enzymes may play a significant role), and approximately 80% of the drug and its metabolites are eliminated via the kidneys. Carmustine has a half-life of approximately 15 to 20 minutes; metabolites have longer half-lives. Carmustine is not hemodialyzable.

Dose
The usual dose as a single agent is 150 to 200 mg/m^2 every 6 weeks as a single dose or divided over a period of 2 days. As a preparative agent before bone marrow transplantation, doses are usually 300 to 600 mg/m^2. The higher dose has been associated with considerable toxicity (when used in combination with other drugs).

Administration
Usually administered in 100 mL or more of 5% dextrose or normal saline as a 1- to 2-hour infusion. Do not infuse over longer than 2 hours because of incompatibility with the IV tubing. Carmustine has also been given intraarterially, topically as a 0.2% solution or 0.4% ointment, and intratumorally as a biodegradable polymer (Gliadel wafer).

Toxicity

Hematological. Leukopenia and thrombocytopenia occur within 25 to 35 days, may last 60 days, and are cumulative. Anemia may also occur after treatment with carmustine.

Gastrointestinal. Nausea and vomiting are common but preventable with antiemetics. Diarrhea, anorexia, esophagitis, and dysphagia are infrequent side effects.

Dermatological. Alopecia, brown discoloration of the skin (more common with topical administration), skin rash, pruritus.

Hepatic. Reversible elevation of liver enzyme levels (25%), hyperbilirubinemia, venoocclusive disease after transplantation doses.

Pulmonary. Infiltrates and/or fibrosis, especially with prolonged therapy and higher doses. Pulmonary damage may not become evident until years after treatment has been discontinued. It has been recommended that a cumulative dose of 1400 mg/m^2 not be exceeded.

Cardiovascular. Hypotension (from rapid or concentrated infusion).

Renal. Azotemia, decrease in kidney size, and renal failure with large cumulative doses.

Other. Burning at the injection site and along the vein is common and can be lessened by the application of a cold compress above the site and/or by slowing the rate of the infusion. Facial flushing, dizziness, ataxia, and second malignancies have also been reported. Severe retinal toxicity, blindness, and seizures have been reported when given by intracarotid artery.

Storage and Stability

Intact vials are stored in the refrigerator. If exposed to heat, the powder becomes an oily liquid, and it should be discarded. The reconstituted solution is stable for 48 hours if refrigerated and 14 hours at room temperature when protected from light. After further dilution to 1 mg/mL or less in normal saline or 5% dextrose, it is stable for 16 hours in glass or polyolefin containers when protected from light at room temperature and for 48 hours when refrigerated. A 0.5 mg/mL solution mixed with absolute ethanol is chemically stable for at least 3 months in the refrigerator. Dilutions of carmustine, 0.2 mg/mL in 5% dextrose or normal saline, are stable for 48 hours at room temperature and 56 hours in the refrigerator. Freezing does not affect the potency of carmustine solutions.

Preparation

Each vial is reconstituted with 3 mL of the provided alcohol. After complete dissolution, 27 mL of sterile water is added to result in a concentration of 3.3 mg/mL. The desired dose is further diluted in 100 to 250 mL of 5% dextrose or normal saline. A stock solution of carmustine for topical administration may be prepared by dissolving 100 mg of carmustine in 50 mL of 95% ethanol. A 5-mL portion of the stock solution is diluted with 60 mL of tap water just before topical administration.

Incompatibilities
Incompatible with polyvinyl chloride infusion bags and with sodium bicarbonate. Cimetidine may slow the metabolism of carmustine and result in enhanced myelosuppression.

Compatibilities
Solutions of cisplatin and carmustine (0.86 and 1.5 mg/mL, respectively) are compatible for 4 hours in a glass container.

Availability
Commercially available as a duopak containing a 100-mg vial of carmustine and a 3-mL vial of absolute alcohol.

Selected Readings
Aronin PA et al: Prediction of pulmonary toxicity in patients with malignant gliomas, *N Engl J Med* 303:183-188, 1980.

Brem H et al: Placebo-controlled trial of safety and efficacy of intraoperative controlled delivery by biodegradable polymers of chemotherapy for recurrent gliomas, *Lancet* 345:1008-1012, 1995.

Weiss RB, Issell BF: The nitrosoureas: carmustine (BCNU) and lomustine (CCNU), *Cancer Treat Rev* 9:313-330, 1982.

CHLORAMBUCIL
Other Names
Leukeran, NSC-3088

Indications
FDA approved for the treatment of chronic lymphocytic leukemia and malignant lymphomas (including lymphosarcoma, giant follicular lymphoma, and Hodgkin's disease). Chlorambucil may also be a useful treatment for Waldenström's macroglobulinemia, breast cancer, hairy cell leukemia, multiple myeloma, and ovarian, testicular, and trophoblastic neoplasms.

Classification
Alkylating agent.

Pharmacokinetics
Chlorambucil is well absorbed (85% to 90%) by mouth with maximum plasma concentrations occurring 1 hour after administration. The presence of food slows the rate of absorption but does not affect overall bioavailability. Chlorambucil is almost entirely metabolized by the liver (to some active metabolites) and has an elimination half-life of 1 to 2 hours. Less than 1% of the drug is eliminated via the kidneys as unchanged chlorambucil or phenylacetic acid mustard, the primary active metabolite. Chlorambucil and phenylacetic acid mustard are not dialyzable.

Dose

Chlorambucil has been given in various dose schedules, including 0.1 to 0.2 mg/kg/day for 3 to 6 weeks (leukemia induction), 0.4 mg/kg every 2 to 4 weeks, and 16 mg/m²/day for 5 days every 4 weeks (lymphoma).

Administration

Oral.

Toxicity

Hematological. Leukopenia and thrombocytopenia are dose related. Cumulative, dose-limiting myelosuppression has been observed in some patients. Anemia occurs infrequently.

Gastrointestinal. Nausea, vomiting, anorexia, and diarrhea are relatively uncommon.

Dermatological. Alopecia and mucositis are uncommon. Dermatitis, rash, pruritus, urticaria, erythema multiforme, epidermal necrolysis, and Stevens-Johnson syndrome are rare.

Hepatic. Increased liver enzyme levels occur but are usually mild and transient.

Pulmonary. Cumulative pulmonary fibrosis (rare).

Neurological. Seizures (more common in patients with impaired renal function), confusion, agitation, tremors, ataxia, and peripheral neuropathy are rare side effects.

Ocular. Diplopia, papilledema, retinal hemorrhage, and keratitis are rare.

Other. Sterility (amenorrhea, azoospermia, oligospermia), possible secondary malignancy (i.e., leukemia), cystitis (rare), drug fever (rare).

Storage and Stability

Tablets are stored at room temperature. Bottles bear expiration dates.

Availability

Chlorambucil is commercially available in 2-mg sugar-coated tablets.

Selected Readings

Palmer RG, Denman AM: Malignancies induced by chlorambucil, *Cancer Treat Rev* 11:121-129, 1984.

Portlock CS et al: High-dose pulse chlorambucil in advanced, low-grade non-Hodgkin's lymphoma, *Cancer Treat Rep* 71:1029-1031, 1987.

CISPLATIN

Other Names

Platinol-AQ, Platinol, cis-platinum, cisdiamminedichloroplatinum (II), CDDP, DDP, DACP, platinum, NSC-119875.

Indications

FDA approved for the treatment of testicular carcinoma, ovarian cancer, and transitional cell bladder cancer. Cisplatin may be a useful treatment for cancers of the brain, adrenal cortex, breast, cervix, uterus, endometrium, head and neck, esophagus, lung, skin, prostate, and stomach; non-Hodgkin's lymphoma; osteosarcoma; and trophoblastic neoplasms.

Classification

Heavy metal alkylating-like agent.

Pharmacokinetics

Approximately 50% to 100% of cisplatin is absorbed into the systemic circulation after intraperitoneal administration. After IV administration, cisplatin rapidly distributes into tissues, including breast milk. Approximately 90% is bound to plasma proteins within 2 to 4 hours of dosing and 20% to 45% is eliminated unchanged via the kidneys. Although only 10% of cisplatin is measured in the plasma 1 hour after a dose, cisplatin has a long terminal half-life (i.e., 60 to 90 hours). Cisplatin is not hemodialyzable 1 to 1.5 hours after administration because of its extensive protein binding.

Dose

Doses may vary from 20 to 40 mg/m^2/day for 3 to 5 days every 3 to 4 weeks or from 20 to 120 mg/m^2 given as a single dose every 3 to 4 weeks. Intraperitoneal doses of 100 to 270 mg/m^2 have been given in combination with IV sodium thiosulfate. It has been recommended that doses be reduced by 25% and 50% in patients with creatinine clearances of 10 to 50 mL/min and less than 10 mL/min, respectively. Many physicians avoid using cisplatin when the creatinine clearance is less than 40 mL/min.

Administration

Usually administered by slow IV infusion in 100 to 500 mL of normal saline, over a 30-minute or longer period. Many believe that drug infusions should not exceed 1 mg/min. The drug has also been given intraarterially, intraperitoneally, by intravesical instillation, and by isolated limb perfusion.

Hydration. Concomitant hydration is necessary when doses of 40 mg/m^2 or greater are given as a short infusion. Prehydration with 1 to 2 L of normal saline (plus 20 mEq KCl and 8 mEq MgSO$_4$ per liter) is commonly given. Mannitol, 12.5 to 25 g, may be given before cisplatin but is not necessary if the patient is voiding. Furosemide or a similar diuretic may be added to increase diuresis, but most believe that it should not be used except to prevent fluid overload. In general, hydration should be adequate to maintain a urine output of 100 to 150 mL/hour before administration of the drug. Post-cisplatin hydration with 1 to 2 L of the same fluids is also commonly given. Treatment of testicular cancer patients with cisplatin, 20 mg/m^2/day for 5 days, requires only 1 L of hydration per day.

Toxicity

Hematological. Leukopenia and thrombocytopenia occur, but are rarely dose limiting. Anemia occasionally occurs after several treatments. Coombs-positive hemolytic anemia has been reported.

Gastrointestinal. Nausea and vomiting are common and may persist for up to 24 to 96 hours. Aggressive antiemetic treatment is required during the first 24 hours and for the next 4 days. Anorexia and diarrhea are common.

Dermatological. Alopecia and rash are uncommon.

Renal. Nephrotoxicity (elevated serum creatinine and BUN levels) is dose related and relatively uncommon with adequate hydration and diuresis. This can be cumulative, and careful assessment of kidney function is essential before each dose. Each patient should have BUN and serum creatinine levels, and when practical, a 24-hour urine creatinine clearance evaluated before treatment. Concomitant use of nephrotoxic drugs such as aminoglycosides, methotrexate, or amphotericin B should be undertaken with great caution.

Hepatic. Elevated hepatic enzyme levels (uncommon).

Neurological. Peripheral sensory neuropathies are common and dose limiting when the cumulative cisplatin dose exceeds 400 mg/m². Symptoms may become apparent after the administration of 210 mg/m². Treatment should be discontinued when numbness and tingling of the fingers and/or toes become bothersome, as continued dosing can be disabling. Symptoms may begin and/or progress after discontinuing therapy. The toxicity is reversible, but may take many months to resolve. Other neurological toxicities occur infrequently but may include seizures (possibly caused by hyponatremia or hypomagnesemia), dizziness, loss of taste, tetany, agitation, disorientation, paranoia, Lhermitte's sign, aphasia, and cortical blindness.

Otic. Ototoxicity, manifested initially by high-frequency hearing loss and/or tinnitus, occurs occasionally. It occurs more commonly in patients receiving higher doses of cisplatin (i.e., ≥100 mg/m²) by rapid infusion and may also be associated with high cumulative doses. Significant hearing loss occurs commonly when a single dose of cisplatin exceeds 150 mg/m².

Cardiovascular. Rarely reported cardiovascular toxicities include bradycardia, bundle branch block, congestive heart failure, and Raynaud's phenomenon.

Other. Hypomagnesemia is common, can be severe, and is difficult to correct in some patients. It is not known whether prophylactic magnesium supplementation during each treatment, as a part of the hydration regimen, is helpful at preventing this adverse effect. Other toxicities may include hyperuricemia, hypocalcemia, hyponatremia, syndrome of inappropriate antidiuretic hormone (SIADH), hypophosphatemia, vein irritation, papilledema (rare), retrobulbar neuritis (rare), blurred vision (rare), myalgia, fever, altered color perception (rare), anaphylaxis (rare), and fatigue (common).

Storage and Stability

Vials of cisplatin are stored at room temperature. When reconstituted as directed, the solution is stable at room temperature for 72 hours. When further diluted to less than 0.6 mg/mL with normal saline, it is stable for 96 hours at room or refrigerator temperature. Refrigeration may result in precipitation of solutions >0.6 mg/mL.

Preparation

Cisplatin lyophilized powder, 10- and 50-mg vials, should be reconstituted with 10 and 50 mL of sterile water, respectively, to result in a 1 mg/mL solution. The desired dose of cisplatin is often further diluted with 250 mL or more of 0.45% to 0.9% NaCl *and* 5% dextrose, normal saline, or 3% sodium chloride. *Do not use 5% dextrose.*

Incompatibilities

Cisplatin is less stable in solutions that do not contain chloride ions (i.e., 5% dextrose). Cisplatin may react with the aluminum found in some syringe needles or IV sets to form a black precipitate. Cisplatin is also incompatible with metoclopramide, sodium bicarbonate, sodium thiosulfate, fluorouracil, and mesna.

Compatibilities

Cisplatin is compatible with mannitol, magnesium sulfate, potassium chloride, carmustine, cyclophosphamide, and etoposide. Consult your pharmacist regarding specific concentrations, containers, and storage conditions.

Availability

Commercially available as a 1 mg/mL solution (50 and 100 mg/vial). The original manufacturer has discontinued the lyophilized powder for injection (10- and 50-mg vials), but these are likely to be available through other suppliers.

Selected Readings

Gregg RW et al: Cisplatin neurotoxicity: the relationship between dosage, time, and platinum concentration in neurologic tissues, and morphologic evidence of toxicity, *J Clin Oncol* 10:795-803, 1992.

Hutchison FN et al: Renal salt wasting in patients treated with cisplatin, *Ann Intern Med* 108:21-25, 1988.

Ries F, Klastersky J: Nephrotoxicity induced by cancer chemotherapy with special emphasis on cisplatin toxicity, *Am J Kidney Dis* 8:368-379, 1986.

CLADRIBINE

Other Names

Leustatin, chlordeoxyadenosine, 2-chlordeoxyadenosine, 2-chloro-2-deoxyadenosine, 2-CdA, CldAdo, NSC-105014.

C

Indications
FDA approved for the treatment of hairy cell leukemia. Cladribine may also be useful for the treatment of chronic lymphocytic leukemia, cutaneous T-cell lymphoma, Sézary syndrome, low-grade non-Hodgkin's lymphoma, acute nonlymphocytic leukemia, Waldenström's macroglobulinemia, and autoimmune hemolytic anemia.

Classification and Mechanisms of Action
Cladribine is an adenosine deaminase–resistant deoxyadenosine congener. The drug induces DNA strand breaks and blocks RNA synthesis. The phosphorylated metabolites of the drug accumulate in cells with high deoxycytidine kinase activity such as lymphocytes.

Pharmacokinetics
Approximately 37% to 55% of an oral dose of cladribine is absorbed. Cladribine rapidly distributes (initial half-life 36 minutes) after IV administration and is approximately 20% protein bound. The drug has been detected in significant concentrations in the cerebrospinal fluid after doses of 0.15 mg/kg/day. Cladribine has an elimination half-life of approximately 5 to 7 hours.

Dose
Patients with hairy cell leukemia receive a single 7-day treatment, 0.09 mg/kg/day (4 mg/m^2/day), as a continuous infusion. A second cycle of treatment has been given to some nonresponding patients. Patients with other malignancies have received 0.1 to 0.3 mg/kg/day for 7 days as a continuous infusion repeated every 4 to 5 weeks or the same dose daily for 5 days. Higher doses (0.4 to 0.5 mg/kg/day for 7 to 14 days) have been associated with more adverse effects. Daily doses of cladribine should not exceed 0.3 mg/kg/day. A dose of 0.05 mg/kg/day has been combined with chlorambucil, 10 mg/m^2 × 1.

Administration
Continuous IV infusion over a 7-day period. Outpatients may receive the full 7-day dose in 100 mL of bacteriostatic normal saline; inpatients may receive each daily dose in 500 to 1000 mL of normal saline. Cladribine has also been given as a 2-hour infusion and by subcutaneous injection.

Toxicity
Hematological. Neutropenia (20% to 43%), lymphopenia (100%), thrombocytopenia (recovery, 7 to 10 days after end of a 7-day infusion), mild anemia. Myelosuppression has been cumulative in some studies. Purpura, petechiae, and epistaxis have been reported in 5% to 10% of the patients.

Gastrointestinal. Nausea (18% to 28%) is usually mild and preventable with antiemetic drugs, vomiting (13%), anorexia (17%), diarrhea (10%), constipation (9%), abdominal pain (6%).

Dermatological. Skin reactions (i.e., cellulitis) at catheter site (9% to 18%), phlebitis (2%), rash (28%), pruritus, erythema (6%).

Neurological. Headache (13% to 22%), dizziness (9%), insomnia (7%), motor weakness, paresthesias, paraparesis, and quadriparesis have been reported.

Cardiovascular. Edema, tachycardia (6%).

Pulmonary. Cough, dyspnea.

Renal. Elevated serum creatinine levels and renal failure have been reported in patients receiving cladribine 0.4 to 0.5 mg/kg/day for 7 to 14 days.

Other. Asthenia (45% to 70%), fever (43%), chills (18%), fatigue (17% to 45%), myalgia (7%), arthralgia (5%), pancreatitis (rare), diaphoresis, malaise, and trunk pain (rare).

Storage and Stability
Cladribine is stored in a refrigerator. Diluted in 100 to 500 mL of normal saline, the drug is stable for at least 7 days at room temperature, although it is recommended that cladribine should be administered promptly or stored in the refrigerator for no more than 8 hours. Admixtures are stable for at least 7 days in Pharmacia Deltec medication cassettes. Freezing has no adverse effects on cladribine. If freezing occurs, the drug should be thawed at room temperature. A precipitate may form during freezing that can be resolubilized by allowing the solution to warm to room temperature or by shaking vigorously. Do not heat or microwave.

Preparation
The desired dose should be passed through the 0.22 µm filter before further dilution in 100 mL of bacteriostatic normal saline (for outpatient continuous infusion) or 500 to 1000 mL of normal saline (for inpatient administration).

Incompatibilities
Dextrose 5% in water is not recommended as a diluent because it increases cladribine degradation.

Availability
Cladribine is commercially available as a 1-mg/mL solution in 10 mL vials.

Selected Readings
Estey EH et al: Treatment of hairy cell leukemia with 2-chlorodeoxyadenosine (2-CdA), *Blood* 79:882-887, 1992.
Piro ID et al: Lasting remissions in hairy-cell leukemia induced by a single infusion of 2-chlorodeoxyadenosine, *N Engl J Med* 322:1117-1121, 1990.

CYCLOPHOSPHAMIDE
Other Names
Cytoxan, Cytoxan Lyophilized, Neosar, Procytox, Endoxan, CTX, CPM, NSC-26271.

Indications
FDA approved indications include non-Hodgkin's lymphoma, Hodgkin's disease, myeloma, cutaneous T-cell lymphoma, neuroblastoma, adenocarcinoma of the ovary, and adenocarcinoma of the breast. Other indications may include retinoblastoma, acute leukemias, chronic myelogenous leukemia, Ewing's sarcoma, osteosarcoma, Wilms' tumor, soft-tissue sarcomas, rhabdomyosarcoma, trophoblastic neoplasms, and cancers of the prostate, head and neck, lung, bladder, cervix, stomach, and uterus.

Classification
Alkylating agent.

Pharmacokinetics
At least 75% of cyclophosphamide is absorbed by mouth and reaches peak plasma levels 1 hour after administration. The drug is activated by hepatic microsomal enzymes. The liver is also involved in metabolizing cyclophosphamide metabolites to inactive compounds that are excreted by the kidney. The drug is distributed into breast milk. Approximately 12% and 50% to 75% of unchanged cyclophosphamide and its metabolites, respectively, are excreted into the urine. Dose reductions are not necessary for patients with severe renal impairment. Cyclophosphamide has an elimination half-life of 3 to 10 hours, and its principal active metabolite (phosphoramide mustard) has a half-life of 8 to 9 hours. Approximately 36% of an IV dose of cyclophosphamide can be removed by hemodialysis (9% per hour for a 4-hour hemodialysis treatment).

Dose
Cyclophosphamide may be given as a single dose or in several divided doses over a period of time. Some common doses are 500 to 1500 mg/m^2 intravenously every 3 weeks, 50 to 200 mg/m^2 orally each day for 14 days every 28 days, 400 mg/m^2 daily for 4 days every 4 to 6 weeks, or 60 mg/kg intravenously for 2 days for bone marrow transplant conditioning.

Administration
May be given orally or by IV push or infusion (in 100 mL or more of 5% dextrose; 5% dextrose in 0.9% sodium chloride; 5% dextrose in Ringer's injection, lactated Ringer's injection, or sodium chloride injection [0.45% sodium chloride]; or sodium lactate injection [1/6 molar sodium lactate]) over a 15-minute or longer period. It has been generally recommended that doses of cyclophosphamide be given in the morning or early afternoon because of the fear of allowing toxic metabolites to remain in the bladder overnight.

Hydration. It is recommended that patients receiving higher doses (>1000 mg) of cyclophosphamide receive hydration; 500 to 1000 mL of normal saline is commonly given.

Toxicity

Hematological. Leukopenia, with nadirs about 8 to 14 days after administration and recovery in 1 to 2 weeks thereafter. Thrombocytopenia occurs but is rarely significant. Anemia occurs occasionally.

Gastrointestinal. Nausea and vomiting are relatively common after administration of larger doses (i.e., >600 mg/m^2). Symptoms usually begin 6 to 10 hours after administration, which necessitates preventative antiemetic therapy through this time. When the drug is given orally, nausea can be chronic and extremely annoying. Eating small, frequent meals sometimes helps to relieve the nausea. Dividing the dose may also be helpful. Stomatitis, diarrhea, anorexia, and hemorrhagic colitis have occurred in patients receiving treatment with cyclophosphamide.

Dermatological. Alopecia (common), pigmented fingernails and/or skin (19%), dermatitis, rash, hives, pruritus.

Hepatic. Increased liver enzyme levels (uncommon); hepatitis and jaundice (rare).

Neurological. Headache, dizziness.

Pulmonary. Interstitial pulmonary fibrosis (rare).

Cardiovascular. Cardiac necrosis and/or acute myopericarditis with high-dose cyclophosphamide (rare).

Genitourinary. In conventional doses, cyclophosphamide rarely causes hemorrhagic cystitis. When cyclophosphamide is used in high doses (i.e., 50 to 60 mg/kg) as a part of a preparative regimen for bone marrow transplantation, hemorrhagic cystitis is more common and can be severe. Prevention includes hydration and treatment with mesna (see the mesna drug review for specific instructions on its use). Other, less common toxicities include bladder fibrosis (most often after long-term oral therapy), bladder carcinoma, syndrome of inappropriate antidiuretic hormone (SIADH) (more common with single doses greater than 2000 mg/m^2, especially if saline-poor solutions are used in the hydration regimen).

Other. Metallic taste during injection, nasal congestion, diaphoresis, faintness, facial flushing, blurred vision, cataracts (rare), hypothyroidism, hyperglycemia, testicular atrophy, amenorrhea, anaphylaxis, urticaria, angioedema, fever, second neoplasms (i.e., leukemia, bladder cancer). The risk of developing bladder cancer after treatment with cyclophosphamide is greatest when the total cumulative dose exceeds 20,000 mg. When the total cumulative dose exceeds 50,000 mg, the risk of developing bladder cancer is increased 14-fold.

Storage and Stability

Tablets and injectable powder are stored at room temperature. Containers bear an expiration date. Reconstituted parenteral solutions are stable for 7 days at room temperature or 14 days (20 mg/mL) to 28 days (4 mg/mL) if refrigerated. Frozen solutions are chemically stable for at least 19 weeks.

Preparation
Dissolve the 100-, 200-, 500-, 1000-, and 2000-mg vials with 5, 10, 25, 50, and 100 mL, respectively, of sterile water or normal saline to result in a 20 mg/mL solution.

Compatibilities
Cyclophosphamide (6 to 8 mg/mL) and doxorubicin (0.4 to 0.6 mg/mL) are compatible for 7 days at room temperature. Cyclophosphamide is also compatible with dacarbazine, bleomycin, cisplatin, mesna, and other drugs. A pharmacist should be consulted for additional information.

Availability
Commercially available in 25- and 50-mg tablets and as powder for injection in 100-, 200-, 500-, 1000-, and 2000-mg vials.

Selected Readings
Ayash LJ et al: Cyclophosphamide pharmacokinetics: correlation with cardiac toxicity and response, *J Clin Oncol* 10:995-1000, 1992.
Stillwell TJ, Benson RJ Jr: Cyclophosphamide-induced hemorrhagic cystitis: a review of 100 patients, *Cancer* 61:451-457, 1988.

CYCLOSPORINE
Other Names
Cyclosporin-A, CsA, Sandimmune, Neoral.

Indications
FDA approved for the prophylaxis of organ rejection in kidney, heart, and liver transplants. Investigationally used to reverse multidrug resistance.

Classification and Mechanisms of Action
Cyclosporine is an immunosuppressant that inhibits the function of T-lymphocytes (T-helper cells primarily). The precise mechanism by which cyclosporine alters the cytotoxicity of doxorubicin, vinblastine, and other drugs is not fully known. Biochemical modulation by cyclosporine may involve interaction with the transmembrane protein, P-glycoprotein. As a result, intracellular retention of doxorubicin, vinblastine, or other drugs in multidrug-resistant cells is enhanced.

Pharmacokinetics
Approximately 30% to 40% of a dose of cyclosporine is absorbed by mouth, reaching peak blood levels 3 to 3.5 hours after administration. Most (90%) of cyclosporine is protein bound (mostly to lipoproteins). The drug is widely distributed throughout the body, including breast milk. Cyclosporine is extensively metabolized by the liver and is excreted into the bile. Less than 1% is eliminated into the urine as unchanged drug. Cyclosporine is not hemodialyzable. The elimination half-life of cyclosporine is around 20 to 30 hours. Cyclosporine blood levels are monitored for prevention of organ rejection after transplantation. Concentrations of

cyclosporine in the blood, measured 24 hours after a dose, should be 250 to 800 ng/mL (50 to 300 ng/mL in the plasma). Higher levels are associated with increased toxicity, primarily nephrotoxicity.

Dose

When used in combination with etoposide, vinblastine, or other drugs cyclosporine has been given as a continuous infusion over 5 days (i.e., up to 18 mg/kg/day) and as a 1- to 3-hour infusion over a period of 3 or more days. For prevention of organ rejection, the initial dose (15 mg/kg/day orally, 5 to 6 mg/kg intravenously) is begun before organ transplantation and continued for 1 to 2 weeks. Thereafter the dose is tapered (5% per week) to a maintenance oral dose of 5 to 10 mg/kg/day.

Administration

IV infusion in a glass container (in 50 mL or more of 5% dextrose or normal saline) over a period of 2 to 3 hours or longer. Oral and intraperitoneal routes of administration have also been used.

Toxicity

Much is known about the toxicity of cyclosporine in patients undergoing organ transplantation. The adverse effects associated with cyclosporine given as an intermittent 5-day treatment regimen are generally less common and less severe than continuous cyclosporine therapy used for organ transplantation. The incidence figures shown in parentheses are for patients receiving cyclosporine for prevention of organ rejection.

Hematological. Leukopenia (2% to 6%), thrombocytopenia (<2%), anemia (<2%).

Gastrointestinal. Diarrhea (3% to 8%), anorexia (<2%), nausea and vomiting (2% to 10%), gastritis, hiccups (<2%), ulcers, constipation, pancreatitis (rare), mucositis (rare), gingival hyperplasia (4% to 16%).

Dermatological. Hirsutism (20% to 45%), acne (1% to 8%), brittle fingernails (<2%).

Hepatic. Transient elevations of hepatic transaminase and lactic dehydrogenase levels and hyperbilirubinemia are uncommon (4% to 7%) in transplant patients. Hyperbilirubinemia may be the dose-limiting toxicity in drug-resistance studies.

Neurological. Tremor (12% to 50%), headache (2% to 15%), paresthesia (≤3%), flushing (≤4%), confusion, seizures (≤5%), depression, ataxia, drowsiness, amnesia, mental disturbance, cortical blindness (rare).

Cardiovascular. Hypertension (common, 15% to 50%), hypotension (rare), edema.

Renal. Renal dysfunction is common (25% to 40%), dose related, and manifested as elevated serum creatinine levels, reduced creatinine clearance, and an elevated BUN concentration. Other toxicities may include hyperkalemia, hyperuricemia, and hypomagnesemia.

Ophthalmic. Conjunctivitis (<2%), visual disturbances (rare).

Hypersensitivity reaction. More common with IV use, believed to be caused by the Cremophor diluent. Reactions may consist of facial flushing, hypotension or hypertension, shortness of breath, wheezing, and tachycardia. The manufacturer recommends close monitoring of patients during the first 30 minutes of an IV infusion and at frequent intervals thereafter.

Other. Sinusitis (≤7%), gynecomastia (≤4%), myalgia (<2%), tinnitus (<2%), weight loss (rare), night sweats (rare), lymphoma (≤6%).

Storage and Stability

Ampules, bottles of oral solution, and capsules of cyclosporine bear expiration dates and are stored at room temperature and protected from light. Cyclosporine (2 mg/mL) is chemically stable in glass containers of normal saline (12 hours) and 5% dextrose (24 hours). In polyvinylchloride containers the drug is stable for 6 hours (normal saline) to 24 hours (5% dextrose) at room temperature.

Preparation

The desired dose of injectable cyclosporine may be further diluted in 250 to 500 mL of normal saline or 5% dextrose (in glass bottles). It is important to ensure that cyclosporine solution is adequately dispersed throughout the 250 to 500 mL injection bottle. Unmixed solutions may be associated with a higher incidence of anaphylactoid reactions caused by delivery of uneven concentration of Cremophor EL in the bottle. The oral solution may be mixed in warm milk, orange juice, or other beverages.

Incompatibilities

Cyclosporine is incompatible with magnesium sulfate and polyvinylchloride infusion equipment, causing leaching of plasticizers. Cyclosporine interacts with many drugs, including erythromycin, ketoconazole, fluconazole, and others. A pharmacist should be consulted for additional information.

Availability

Cyclosporine ampules (250 mg/5 mL), bottles of oral solution (5000 mg/50 mL), and capsules (25, 50, and 100 mg) are commercially available.

Selected Readings

Kahan BD: Cyclosporine, *N Engl J Med* 321:1725-1738, 1989.
Rodenburg CJ et al: Phase II study of combining vinblastine and cyclosporin-A to circumvent multidrug resistance in renal cell cancer, *Ann Oncol* 2:305-306, 1991.
Theis JGW et al: Anaphylactoid reactions in children receiving high-dose intravenous cyclosporine for reversal of tumor resistance: the causative role of improper dissolution of Cremophor EL, *J Clin Oncol* 13:2508-2516, 1995.

CYTARABINE
Other Names

Cytosar-U, Cytosar, Tarabine Pfs, Ara-C, cytosine arabinoside, NSC-63878.

Indications

FDA approved for the treatment of acute nonlymphocytic leukemia, acute lymphocytic leukemia, chronic myelogenous leukemia, and meningeal leukemia. Cytarabine may be useful in the treatment of Hodgkin's and non-Hodgkin's lymphoma.

Classification

Antimetabolite.

Pharmacokinetics

Cytarabine is poorly absorbed by mouth (i.e., 20%). After IV administration, it is rapidly distributed throughout the body and is rapidly deaminated within the bloodstream. Peak plasma concentrations after subcutaneous administration occur within 20 to 60 minutes. Less than 10% of the drug is eliminated in the urine as unchanged drug. However, one metabolite, uracil arabinoside (ara-U), has the ability to produce high concentrations of cytosine arabinoside triphosphate (ara-CTP) in patients with renal insufficiency. Accumulation of ara-CTP in the central nervous system may result and lead to nervous system toxicities. Cytarabine has an elimination half-life of 1 to 3 hours.

Dose

Some common doses are as follows:
1. 60 to 200 mg/m^2/day as a continuous IV infusion for 5 to 10 consecutive days.
2. 100 mg/m^2 intravenously or subcutaneously twice a day for 5 days every 28 days.
3. 10 to 30 mg/m^2 intrathecally up to 3 times per week.
4. 1000 to 3000 mg/m^2 intravenously over a period of 1 to 3 hours every 12 hours for 3 to 6 days.
5. 10 mg/m^2 subcutaneously every 12 hours for 15 to 21 days.

Administration

IV push, IV infusion in 50 mL or more of 5% dextrose or normal saline over a 30-minute or longer period. High-dose cytarabine is usually given in 250 to 500 mL of 5% dextrose or normal saline over a span of 1 to 3 hours. The drug has also been given subcutaneously, intrathecally, and intraperitoneally.

Toxicity

Hematological. Leukopenia and thrombocytopenia are expected, with the nadir occurring in 5 to 7 days and recovery in 2 to 3 weeks. Anemia is common. Hematological toxicity is more severe when cytarabine is given as a prolonged IV infusion versus administration as an IV bolus.

Gastrointestinal. Nausea, vomiting (dose related, common, and often prevented by antiemetic drugs), anorexia, diarrhea (potentiated with the addition of anthracycline), metallic taste, dysphagia, stomatitis, severe gastrointestinal ulceration, pancreatitis, peritonitis.

Dermatological. Transient skin erythema without exfoliation, alopecia (uncommon); rash, cellulitis, and thrombophlebitis are rare.

Ocular. Conjunctivitis, keratitis (usually on days 1 to 3 but reduced with prophylactic glucocorticoid eye drops), photophobia.

Hepatic. Transient, usually mild elevations of liver enzyme levels and/or hyperbilirubinemia.

Neurological. A 16% to 40% incidence (7% to 18% severe) with high-dose therapy (i.e., 2000 to 3000 mg/m^2 every 12 hours for 12 or more doses). Toxicity is usually cerebellar (i.e., lethargy progressing to confusion, ataxia, nystagmus, slurred speech). Symptoms begin on the fourth or fifth day of treatment and resolve 4 to 7 days thereafter. In most cases toxicity totally resolves, but in some cases it is irreversible or fatal. Toxicity is dose related (>48,000 mg/m^2 highest incidence) although it has been reported at lower doses. Age (>50 years), renal dysfunction (creatinine clearance less than 60 mL/min), gender (men more than women), infusion rate (1-hour infusion greater than a 3-hour infusion), and hepatic dysfunction have been implicated as factors that influence the incidence and severity of cerebellar toxicity. Treatment with pyridoxine (vitamin B$_6$) does not prevent neurotoxicity.

Rare neurotoxicities include expressive aphasia, peripheral and sensory neuropathies, brachial plexopathy, bilateral rectus muscle palsy, parkinsonism, dizziness, and somnolence. Dizziness and somnolence appear to be associated with rapid IV infusion.

After intrathecal administration, the most common side effects are nausea, vomiting, fever, and headache that are usually mild and self-limiting. Meningism, paresthesia, paraplegia, seizures, blindness, and necrotizing encephalopathy have rarely occurred.

Pulmonary. Rare syndrome of sudden respiratory distress, rapidly progressing to pulmonary edema and cardiomegaly.

Cardiovascular. Rare cardiomegaly, pericarditis with tamponade, thrombophlebitis.

Renal. Urinary retention (rare).

"Ara-C" syndrome. Bone and muscle pain, chest pain, fever, general weakness, reddened eyes, and skin rash. Generally occurs 6 to 12 hours after administration and may respond favorably to treatment with corticosteroids.

Other. Headache, hemorrhagic cystitis (rare), rhabdomyolysis, and hyperuricemia and hyperphosphatemia if tumor lysis syndrome develops.

Storage and Stability
Intact vials are stored at room temperature. After reconstitution, the solution is stable for 8 days (15 days in a plastic syringe) at room temperature and 15 days when refrigerated. Cytarabine, 20 to 80 mg/mL, is stable for 28 days in an Infusaid pump. Solutions with a slight haze should be discarded.

Preparation

For IV use, reconstitute the 100-mg vial with 5 mL bacteriostatic water for injection to achieve a concentration of 20 mg/mL. Add 10 mL of bacteriostatic water to the 500-mg vial to achieve a final concentration of 50 mg/mL. Add 10 and 20 mL of bacteriostatic water to the 1000- and 2000-mg vials, respectively, to achieve a final concentration of 100 mg/mL. For subcutaneous use, reconstitute the powder with sterile water or normal saline to a concentration of 50 to 100 mg/mL. For intrathecal use, mix with lactated Ringer's solution or normal saline *without* preservatives.

Incompatibilities

Cytarabine is incompatible with carbenicillin, fluorouracil, heparin sodium, oxacillin, penicillin G sodium, and nafcillin.

Compatibilities

Cytarabine (0.26 mg/mL), daunorubicin (0.03 mg/mL), and etoposide (0.4 mg/mL) are stable in 5% dextrose and 0.45% NaCl for 72 hours at room temperature. Cytarabine is also compatible with methotrexate, vincristine, hydrocortisone, sodium chloride, potassium chloride, calcium, and magnesium sulfate. Cytarabine and idarubicin are compatible at the "Y"-site. A pharmacist should be consulted for information on concentrations, containers, and storage conditions.

Availability

Commercially available as a lyophilized powder in 100-, 500-, 1000-, and 2000-mg vials and as an injectable solution in 100-, 500-, and 1000-mg vials containing 20 mg/mL.

Selected Readings

Baker WJ, Royer GL, Weiss RB: Cytarabine and neurologic toxicity, *J Clin Oncol* 9:679-693, 1991.

Damon LE, Mass R, Linker CA: The association between cytarabine neurotoxicity and renal insufficiency, *J Clin Oncol* 7:1563-1568, 1989.

Herzig RH et al: Cerebellar toxicity with high dose cytosine arabinoside, *J Clin Oncol* 5:927-932, 1987.

Rubin EH et al: Risk factors for high-dose cytarabine neurotoxicity: an analysis of a cancer and leukemia group B trial in patients with acute myeloid leukemia, *J Clin Oncol* 10:948-953, 1992.

DACARBAZINE

Other Names

DTIC, DTIC-Dome, DIC, imidazole carboxamide, dimethyl triazeno imidazole carboxamide, NSC-45388.

Indications

FDA approved for the treatment of melanoma and Hodgkin's disease. Dacarbazine may also be a useful treatment for soft tissue or bone sarcomas, renal cell carcinoma, neuroblastoma, and islet cell carcinoma.

Classification
Alkylating agent.

Pharmacokinetics
Dacarbazine is poorly absorbed after oral administration. The drug is activated to cytotoxic metabolites by hepatic microsomal enzymes and is not widely distributed throughout the body. Less than 15% penetrates into the cerebrospinal fluid. Approximately 30% to 50% of the active metabolite is excreted unchanged in the urine. Dacarbazine has an elimination half-life of 3 to 5 hours.

Dose
Some common doses are as follows:
1. 375 mg/m^2 on days 1 and 15 (as a part of the Adriamycin, bleomycin, vinblastine, and dacarbazine [ABVD] regimen for Hodgkin's disease).
2. 5-day course of 150 to 250 mg/m^2/day repeated every 3 to 4 weeks.
3. 400 to 500 mg/m^2 by IV push or rapid infusion on days 1 and 2 every 3 to 4 weeks.
4. 200 mg/m^2 daily as a continuous 96-hour infusion repeated every 3 to 4 weeks.
5. Single-dose regimen of 650 to 1450 mg/m^2 repeated every 3 to 4 weeks.

Administration
Usually administered by IV infusion in 100 mL or more of 5% dextrose or normal saline over a period of 30 to 60 minutes. The drug may also be given by IV push or by rapid infusion over a period of 15 minutes, but this may increase venous irritation compared with longer durations of IV infusion. Dacarbazine has also been given as a continuous IV infusion and by the intraarterial route.

Toxicity
Hematological. Leukopenia and thrombocytopenia are common and may be dose limiting. Nadir blood counts occur 2 to 4 weeks after treatment; recovery occurs 1 to 2 weeks thereafter. Anemia also occurs after administration of dacarbazine.

Gastrointestinal. Severe nausea and vomiting are common and prevented in some patients with aggressive antiemetic support. These symptoms tend to lessen with each subsequent daily dose. Also reported are anorexia, diarrhea (rare), and stomatitis (rare).

Dermatological. Alopecia (uncommon), facial flushing, skin rash, photosensitivity. Extravasation of the drug may result in severe pain but has not resulted in tissue damage. Rapid IV push causes pain along injection site more frequently compared with slower durations of IV infusion.

Hepatic. Increased liver enzyme levels, hepatic vein thrombosis (rare). Hepatic necrosis is a rare and fatal toxicity.

Cardiovascular. Thrombophlebitis.

Neurological. Facial paresthesia, confusion, lethargy, seizures, weakness, headache, polyneuropathy, and blurred vision have been reported.

Renal. Increased serum creatinine and BUN concentrations (rare).

Other. Flulike syndrome (with fever, malaise, sinus congestion, and myalgia) is rare, occurs about 7 days after treatment, and lasts 1 to 3 weeks. Other rare toxicities include anaphylaxis, fever, metallic taste, and cerebral hemorrhage.

D

Storage and Stability
Store vials under refrigeration and protected from light. In solution, dacarbazine is stable for 96 hours if refrigerated and for 24 hours at room temperature and protected from light. When further diluted in 500 mL of 5% dextrose or normal saline, it is stable for 24 hours if refrigerated and for 8 hours at room temperature.

Photodegradation. The manufacturer of dacarbazine states that the drug does not decompose when left at room temperature under normal lighting conditions for 8 hours.

NOTE: A change in the color of the solution from pale yellow to pink is indicative of decomposition of the drug.

Preparation
Dilute the 100- and 200-mg vials with 9.9, and 19.7 mL of sterile water, respectively, to result in a concentration of 10 mg/mL. Discard if solution turns pink or red. The drug can be further diluted in 100 to 500 mL of 5% dextrose or normal saline.

Incompatibilities
Dacarbazine is physically incompatible with allopurinol injection, hydrocortisone, and L-cysteine. Because of pH differences, the admixtures containing dacarbazine and sodium bicarbonate are not recommended. The compatibility of heparin and dacarbazine is dependent on the concentration of heparin.

Compatibilities
Dacarbazine is compatible with cyclophosphamide, doxorubicin, dactinomycin, vinblastine, methotrexate, and other drugs. A pharmacist should be consulted for additional information.

Availability
Commercially available as a lyophilized powder in 100- and 200-mg vials.

Selected Readings
Del Prete SA et al: Combination chemotherapy with cisplatin, carmustine, dacarbazine and tamoxifen in metastatic melanoma, *Cancer Treat Rep* 68:1403-1405, 1984.
Hochster H et al: Single-dose dacarbazine and dactinomycin in advanced malignant melanoma, *Cancer Treat Rep* 69:39-42, 1985.

DACTINOMYCIN

Other Names

Actinomycin-D, ACT-D, Actinomycin-C, Cosmegen, NSC-3053.

Indications

FDA approved for the treatment of Wilms' tumor, rhabdomyosarcoma, testicular carcinoma, choriocarcinoma, carcinoma of the uterus, Ewing's sarcoma, and sarcoma botryoides. Dactinomycin may be a useful treatment for acute nonlymphocytic leukemia, Kaposi's sarcoma, melanoma, osteosarcoma, trophoblastic neoplasms, and cancers of the endometrium and ovary.

Classification

Antitumor antibiotic.

Pharmacokinetics

Dactinomycin is poorly absorbed after oral administration. After IV administration, dactinomycin is widely distributed throughout the body, but only negligible amounts of drug penetrate into the cerebrospinal fluid. Dactinomycin is metabolized by the liver and eliminated in the bile (up to 50%) and urine (6% to 31%) as unchanged drug. Dactinomycin has an elimination half-life of 30 to 40 hours.

Dose

Common doses are 1 to 2 mg/m^2 every 3 weeks or 0.25 to 0.6 mg/m^2/day for 5 days every 3 to 4 weeks for adults and 0.25 to 0.5 mg/m^2/day for 5 consecutive days (not to exceed 0.5 mg each day) for children. As an isolated perfusion, dactinomycin has been administered at doses of 50 µg/kg (lower extremity) and 35 µg/kg (upper extremity).

Administration

With extravasation precautions, dactinomycin is given over a period of 2 to 3 minutes, preferably into the tubing of a free-flowing IV infusion of 5% dextrose or normal saline. Dactinomycin has been given by IV infusion in 50 mL of 5% dextrose or normal saline over a period of 20 to 30 minutes. The drug has been administered by isolated perfusion.

Toxicity

Hematological. Leukopenia and thrombocytopenia are expected and occur approximately 1 to 2 weeks after treatment, with the nadir at 3 weeks and recovery 1 to 2 weeks thereafter. Anemia occurs occasionally.

Gastrointestinal. Nausea and vomiting (often worsening with successive daily doses) occur about 1 hour after a dose and may last several hours. Mucositis, with ulcerative sores often under the tongue, occurs occasionally. Dysphagia, proctitis, cheilitis, anorexia, and diarrhea occur infrequently.

Dermatological. Acneiform changes, erythema, hyperpigmentation (especially in previously irradiated areas), rash, alopecia (may not be limited to scalp hair). Extravasation may result in severe pain, swelling, and necrosis.

Hepatic. Ascites, hepatomegaly, hepatitis, and elevated liver enzyme levels are rare toxicities.

Other. "Radiation recall" (skin irritation or even necrosis in previously irradiated areas). Rarely reported toxicities include anaphylaxis, hypocalcemia, fever, fatigue, lethargy, and secondary neoplasms.

Storage and Stability
Intact vials may be stored at room temperature. Reconstituted solutions are chemically stable for 2 months at room temperature.

Preparation
Add 1.1 mL preservative-free sterile water for injection to the 0.5-mg vial. The final concentration is 0.5 mg/mL (500 µg/mL).

Incompatibilities
Diluents containing preservatives. It has been shown that significant binding of dactinomycin occurs with 0.2-µm cellulose ester (Millex OR) and polytetrafluoroethylene (Millex-GV) filters.

Compatibilities
Dactinomycin is compatible with dacarbazine.

Availability
Commercially available in vials containing 500 µg (0.5 mg) lyophilized powder.

Selected Reading
Van Nagell JR et al: Adjuvant vincristine, dactinomycin, and cyclophosphamide therapy in stage I uterine sarcomas, *Cancer* 57:1451-1454, 1986.

DAUNORUBICIN
Other Names
Cerubidine, daunomycin, DNR, rubidomycin, NSC-82151. Liposomal formulation of daunorubicin (DaunoXome).

Indications
FDA approved for the treatment of acute nonlymphocytic leukemia (adults), acute lymphocytic leukemia (adults and children). Daunorubicin may also be a useful treatment for erythroleukemia, neuroblastoma, non-Hodgkin's lymphomas, Ewing's sarcoma, Wilms' tumor, and chronic myelogenous leukemia. The liposomal formulation of daunorubicin is FDA approved for the first-line treatment of HIV-associated Kaposi's sarcoma.

Classification
Anthracycline antitumor antibiotic.

Pharmacokinetics

Daunorubicin is widely distributed throughout the body after IV administration. Daunorubicin does not cross the blood-brain barrier. The drug is extensively metabolized by the liver to several metabolites, including the active metabolite daunorubicinol. Approximately 40% of the drug is eliminated by the biliary route. Approximately 15% to 25% is eliminated via the urine. Daunorubicin and daunorubicinol have elimination half-lives of 18 to 20 hours and 25 to 30 hours, respectively.

Dose

Usually given as a single IV injection or split into a 3- to 5-day schedule. A common regimen for induction treatment of acute leukemia uses 45 mg/m^2/day for 3 days. Liposomal daunorubicin is administered at a dose of 40 mg/m^2 intravenously every 2 weeks.

Administration

Using extravasation precautions, inject into a recently established patent IV site through the sidearm of a running IV over 2 to 5 minutes. Liposomal daunorubicin is administered intravenously over 60 minutes and has not been associated with severe tissue reactions after extravasation.

Toxicity

Hematological. Leukopenia is expected (nadir between 1 and 2 weeks, recovery 2 to 3 weeks thereafter); thrombocytopenia and anemia also occur. Liposomal daunorubicin, at the doses recommended for the treatment of Kaposi's sarcoma, induces Grades 3 and 4 neutropenia in 36% and 15% of the patients, respectively.

Gastrointestinal. Nausea and vomiting commonly occur 1 hour after a dose and may last for several hours but are usually prevented by antiemetics. Diarrhea (uncommon) and stomatitis (common) may also occur. Liposomal daunorubicin is associated with an 18% incidence of moderate to severe nausea and 13% incidence of moderate to severe vomiting. Diarrhea is reported to occur in 38% of the patients treated with liposomal daunorubicin.

Dermatological. Rash, urticaria, alopecia (common), chemical thrombophlebitis or local necrosis if extravasation occurs, pigmentation of fingernails. Alopecia occurs in approximately 8% of the patients treated with liposomal daunorubicin.

Hepatic. Transient elevations in serum bilirubin and liver enzyme levels.

Neurological. Neuropathies have been reported to occur in 13% of the patients receiving liposomal daunorubicin.

Cardiovascular. Arrhythmias, usually asymptomatic and transient, congestive cardiomyopathy (incidence becomes unacceptable after a total dose of 500 to 600 mg/m^2 has been given). See doxorubicin drug review for additional information. Cumulative cardiotoxicity after administration of liposomal daunorubicin at doses above 600 mg/m^2 is rare.

However, the manufacturer of liposomal daunorubicin recommends monitoring of the left ventricular ejection fraction after administration of cumulative doses 320 mg/m^2 and 480 mg/m^2, and every 240 mg/m^2 thereafter.

Other. Fever, chills, hyperuricemia, red urine (expected), anaphylaxis (rare). Within the first 5 minutes of an IV infusion of liposomal daunorubicin, 14% of the patients experienced back pain, flushing, and chest tightness. Interruption of the infusion and readministration at a slower rate tend to ameliorate these symptoms.

D

Storage and Stability
Vials of daunorubicin are stored at room temperature. Reconstituted solutions are stable for 72 hours when refrigerated and 48 hours at room temperature. Vials of liposomal daunorubicin are stored in the refrigerator. Diluted to a concentration of 1 mg/mL with 5% dextrose, liposomal daunorubicin is stable for at least 6 hours at room temperature.

Preparation
Each 20-mg vial is reconstituted with 4 mL of sterile water to give a final concentration of 5 mg/mL. The desired dose is drawn into a syringe containing 10 to 15 mL of normal saline. The liposomal formulation is diluted to a concentration of 1 mg/mL with preservative-free 5% dextrose.

Incompatibilities
Heparin sodium, 5-fluorouracil, and dexamethasone sodium phosphate. The liposomal formulation is incompatible with any solution other than preservative-free 5% dextrose. In-line filters should not be used when administering liposomal daunorubicin.

Compatibilities
Daunorubicin (0.03 mg/mL), cytarabine (0.26 mg/mL), and etoposide (0.4 mg/mL) are stable in D5/0.45% sodium chloride for 72 hours at room temperature.

Availability
Commercially available in 20-mg vials of lyophilized drug. The liposomal formulation is available at a concentration of 2 mg/mL in vials containing 50 mg.

Selected Readings
Gill PS et al: Phase I/II clinical and pharmacokinetic evaluation of liposomal daunorubicin, *J Clin Oncol* 13:996-1003, 1995.

Gottlieb AJ et al: Efficacy of daunorubicin in therapy of adult lymphocytic leukemia: a prospective randomized trial by cancer and leukemia group B, *Blood* 64:267-274, 1984.

Von Hoff DD et al: Daunomycin-induced cardiotoxicity in children and adults: a review of 110 cases, *Am J Med* 62:200-208, 1977.

DEXAMETHASONE

Other Names
Decadron, Hexadrol, Dexone, DXM, others.

Indications
FDA approved for the treatment of brain metastases with edema, breast cancer, acute and chronic lymphocytic leukemia, myeloma, non-Hodgkin's lymphoma, autoimmune hemolytic anemia, immunothrombocytopenia, rheumatic disorders, allergic disorders, dermatological rashes, and inflammation (intraarticularly). It is also frequently used as an antiemetic before cancer chemotherapy.

Classification and Mechanisms of Action
Dexamethasone is a potent adrenal corticosteroid that affects almost every body system. It has antiinflammatory, immunosuppressant, antineoplastic, and antiemetic properties and very little mineralocorticoid activity. As an antineoplastic agent, dexamethasone may bind to specific proteins within the cell, forming a steroid-receptor complex. Binding of the receptor-steroid complex with nuclear chromatin alters mRNA and protein synthesis within the cell.

Pharmacokinetics
Approximately 75% to 80% of dexamethasone is absorbed by mouth. The drug is metabolized by the liver to inactive metabolites and has an elimination half-life of 3 to 4 hours.

Dose
For multiple myeloma, 40 mg/day on days 1 to 4, 9 to 12, and 17 to 20 of each 28-day cycle is often administered as part of the vincristine, Adriamycin, dexamethasone (VAD) regimen. As an antiemetic, 10 to 20 mg intravenously is the usual dose. For neurological syndromes, 10 to 100 mg is used initially, followed by 4 to 8 mg every 6 to 12 hours.

Administration
Orally whenever possible; also IV push or as a short IV infusion in 50 to 100 mL of 5% dextrose or normal saline over a span of 10 to 20 minutes. Dexamethasone may also be administered topically, intraocularly, intranasally, and by intramuscular, intraarticular, and intralesional injection.

Toxicity
Hematological. Leukocytosis.

Gastrointestinal. Nausea, vomiting, anorexia, increased appetite, weight gain, pancreatitis, aggravation of peptic ulcers.

Dermatological. Rash, skin atrophy, acne, facial erythema, ecchymoses, poor wound healing, hirsutism.

Genitourinary. Menstrual changes (amenorrhea, menstrual irregularities).

Neurological. Insomnia, euphoria, headache, vertigo, psychosis, depression, seizures, muscle weakness.

Cardiovascular. Fluid retention and edema, hypertension; rarely, thrombophlebitis and thromboembolism.

Ocular. Cataracts, increased intraocular pressure, exophthalmos.

Metabolic. Hyperglycemia, decreased glucose tolerance, aggravation or precipitation of diabetes mellitus, adrenal suppression (with Cushingoid features), hypokalemia, sodium and fluid retention.

Other. Osteoporosis (and resulting back pain); aseptic necrosis of the femoral head; appearance of serious infections, including herpes zoster, varicella zoster, fungal infections, *Pneumocystis carinii*, and tuberculosis; muscle wasting; delayed wound healing; suppression of reactions to skin tests.

Storage and Stability
The drug is stored at room temperature in a dry place. When the injection is further diluted in 5% dextrose or normal saline, it is stable for at least 24 hours at room temperature.

Preparation
The injection may be further diluted in 50 to 100 mL of 5% dextrose or normal saline.

Availability
Commercially available in 0.25-, 0.5-, 0.75-, 1-, 1.5-, 2-, 4-, and 6-mg tablets; 0.1-mg/mL oral solution or syrup; and 4-, 10-, 20-, or 24-mg/mL solution for injection (dexamethasone sodium phosphate). It is also available as inhalers, ophthalmic solution, and dexamethasone acetate suspension for injection.

DEXRAZOXANE
Other Names
Zinecard, ADR-529, ICRF-187, NSC-169780.

Indications
Dexrazoxane is FDA approved as a protective agent for doxorubicin-induced cardiotoxicity in patients with metastatic breast cancer. The drug is approved for use in patients who have already received a total cumulative doxorubicin dose of 300 mg/m^2.

Classification and Mechanisms of Action
Dexrazoxane is an intracellular chelating agent that prevents iron from combining with doxorubicin to form free oxygen radicals.

Pharmacokinetics
After IV administration, dexrazoxane is rapidly distributed throughout the body. Only 2% to 3% of dexrazoxane is bound to plasma proteins.

The drug is metabolized by the liver, approximately 35% to 50% is eliminated in the urine unchanged, and the elimination half-life is 2 to 4 hours.

Dose

Dexrazoxane is to be administered at a dose of 500 mg/m^2 for every 50 mg/m^2 of doxorubicin (10:1 ratio). The drug is to be administered 30 minutes before administration of doxorubicin.

Administration

Dexrazoxane is given by IV infusion (in 50 to 100 mL of 5% dextrose or normal saline) over a period of 15 to 30 minutes. Infusions of 8 and 48 hours have been given investigationally.

Toxicity

In randomized studies dexrazoxane has been shown to enhance leukopenia slightly when administered with doxorubicin. The incidence and severity of all other toxicities were no different in patients receiving doxorubicin-containing chemotherapy compared with patients receiving chemotherapy plus dexrazoxane. Listed below are the toxicities reported in phase I and II trials of dexrazoxane.

Hematological. Leukopenia. Thrombocytopenia and anemia are uncommon.

Gastrointestinal. Mild nausea and vomiting, anorexia, stomatitis.

Dermatological. Alopecia.

Hepatic. Elevated liver enzyme levels, hyperbilirubinemia.

Cardiovascular. Hypotension, deep venous thrombosis.

Other. Mild, transient elevation of serum amylase levels, elevated serum triglyceride levels, fatigue, fever, seizure, respiratory arrest.

Storage and Stability

Store at room temperature. Containers bear expiration dates. Reconstituted dexrazoxane and solutions further diluted to 1.3 to 1.5 mg/mL in 5% dextrose or normal saline are stable for at least 6 hours at room and refrigeration temperatures.

Preparation

Add 50 mL of the diluent provided (preservative-free M/6 sodium lactate injection) to the 500-mg vial of dexrazoxane to yield a 10-mg/mL solution. The drug may be further diluted to a concentration of 1.3 to 5 mg/mL in normal saline or 5% dextrose.

Availability

Dexrazoxane is commercially available as a lyophilized powder in 250- and 500-mg vials.

Selected Readings

Levien T, Baker DE, Ballasiotes AA: Reviews of dexrazoxane and thalidomide, *Hosp Pharm* 31:487-510, 1996.

Seifert CF, Nesser ME, Thompson DF: Dexrazoxane in the prevention of doxorubicin-induced cardiotoxicity, *DICP Ann Pharmacother* 28:1063-1072, 1994.

Speyer JL et al: ICRF-187 permits longer treatment with doxorubicin in women with breast cancer, *J Clin Oncol* 10:117-127, 1992.

D

DIETHYLSTILBESTROL

Other Names

DES, diethylstilbestrol diphosphate, stilbestrol, Stilphostrol.

Indications

FDA approved for the treatment of prostate and breast cancer.

Classification and Mechanisms of Action

Diethylstilbestrol is an estrogen that elicits pharmacological effects similar to that of other estrogens, including development of female sex organs and maintenance of secondary sex characteristics. As an antineoplastic agent, diethylstilbestrol binds to specific intracellular receptors in hormone-sensitive tumors such as breast and prostate cancer. The estrogen-receptor complex binds to nuclear chromatin, resulting in altered mRNA and cytotoxic effects.

Pharmacokinetics

Diethylstilbestrol is well absorbed after oral administration, is metabolized by the liver to inactive compounds, and has an elimination half-life of approximately 24 hours.

Dose

The usual oral dose of diethylstilbestrol for breast cancer is 15 mg/day. For prostate cancer, the usual oral dose of diethylstilbestrol is 1 to 3 mg daily; the usual oral dose of diethylstilbestrol diphosphate is 50 mg 3 times daily, increasing to 200 mg 3 times daily if tolerated. The usual intravenous dose of diethylstilbestrol diphosphate is 500 mg on the first day, then 1000 mg daily for 4 or more days, and then 250 to 500 mg once or twice weekly.

Administration

Diethylstilbestrol is administered orally. Diethylstilbestrol diphosphate is administered orally or intravenously to patients who do not respond to high oral doses. Administer slowly (1 to 2 mL/min) for the first 10 minutes and give remainder over 1 hour.

Toxicity

Gastrointestinal. Nausea and vomiting (dose related), abdominal cramps, bloating.

Hepatic. Elevated liver function tests, cholestatic jaundice (rare).

Neurological. Headache, exacerbation of migraine headache, dizziness, mental depression, stroke.

Cardiovascular. Thromboembolic disorders (more common with doses >3 mg/day); sodium retention resulting in edema, hypertension, congestive heart failure, and myocardial infarction.

Genitourinary. In women, breakthrough bleeding, spotting, change in menstrual flow, premenstrual-like syndrome, amenorrhea, vaginal candidiasis, and cystitis-like syndrome with urinary incontinence. In men, feminization, including loss of libido and/or impotence. Painful gynecomastia can be prevented by low-dose breast irradiation.

Carcinogenicity and teratogenicity. Increased risk of endometrial cancer. In utero exposure: in women, infertility, cervicovaginal structural abnormalities, and increased risk of cervical and vaginal cancer; in men, genital abnormalities.

Endocrine. Increased bone pain, hypercalcemia on initiation of treatment, reduced carbohydrate tolerance.

Other. Chloasma or melasma, intolerance to contact lenses, optic neuritis, retinal thrombosis, weight changes, increased serum triglyceride levels, hirsutism, rash, pruritus.

Storage and Stability
Store tablets and ampules at room temperature. After reconstitution, diethylstilbestrol diphosphate is stable for 5 days at room temperature.

Preparation
Dilute the dose of diethylstilbestrol diphosphate with 250 to 500 mL of 5% dextrose or normal saline.

Availability
Diethylstilbestrol is commercially available as 0.5-, 1-, and 5-mg tablets. Diethylstilbestrol diphosphate is commercially available as 50-mg tablets and ampules containing 250 mg/5 mL.

Selected Readings
Abramson FP, Miller HC: Bioavailability, distribution and pharmacokinetics of diethylstilbestrol produced from stilphostrol, *J Urol* 128:1336-1339, 1982.

Graychack IT, Keeler TC, Kozlowski JM: Carcinoma of the prostate: hormonal therapy, *Cancer* 60(suppl):589-601, 1987.

Hendricksson P, Johansson SE: Prediction of cardiovascular complications in patients with prostatic cancer treated with estrogen, *Am J Epidemiol* 125:970-978, 1987.

DOCETAXEL
Other Names
Taxotere, RP 56976, NSC-628503.

Indications

FDA approved for the treatment of locally advanced or metastatic breast cancer after initial therapy. The drug also may be useful in the treatment of ovarian, lung, and head and neck cancers.

Classification and Mechanisms of Action

Antimicrotubule agent. Docetaxel promotes the assembly of tubulin and inhibits microtubule depolymerization. Bundles of microtubules accumulate and interfere with cell division.

Pharmacokinetics

After administration, docetaxel exhibits a triphasic elimination profile with an elimination half-life of approximately 11 hours. Docetaxel is extensively protein-bound (94% to 97%), is metabolized in the liver, and is eliminated from the body primarily in the feces. Less than 10% of a dose of the drug is eliminated unchanged in the feces. Docetaxel pharmacokinetics do not appear to be influenced by age or gender or pretreatment with dexamethasone. Although there is considerable interpatient variation concerning docetaxel elimination, patients with elevated hepatic transaminase and/or alkaline phosphatase levels tend to eliminate the drug slower than patients with normal liver function tests. The manufacturer does not recommend treatment with docetaxel in patients with hepatic transaminase levels greater than 1.5 times the upper limit of normal concurrent with alkaline phosphatase levels greater than 2.5 times the upper limit of normal.

Dose

For the treatment of advanced breast cancer the initial recommended dose is 100 mg/m² every 3 weeks. For patients who experience febrile neutropenia or other severe toxicities (e.g., peripheral neuropathy) a reduction in the dose to 75 mg/m² is recommended. Other doses have been evaluated, including 12 mg/m²/day for 5 days repeated every 3 weeks, 100 mg/m²/week for 2 doses repeated every 3 weeks, and 90 mg/m² as a 24-hour IV infusion repeated every 3 weeks. It is recommended that a 5-day course of dexamethasone be administered, starting one day before administration of docetaxel, to lessen the severity and likelihood of fluid retention and hypersensitivity reactions. Dexamethasone, 8 mg twice daily (16 mg/day), administered orally has been recommended.

Administration

Docetaxel is administered by IV infusion over a period of 1 hour. The drug is usually diluted in 250 mL of 5% dextrose or normal saline. Longer durations of IV infusion, including continuous infusion, have been administered.

Toxicity

The toxicities listed on p. 104 are those observed in patients with normal liver function tests receiving docetaxel at a dose of 100 mg/m² every 3 weeks. Patients with elevated liver function tests (i.e., transaminase levels >1.5

times the upper limit of normal *and* alkaline phosphatase levels >2.5 times the upper limit of normal) have been shown to experience a significantly higher incidence of many toxicities (e.g., myelosuppression, fluid retention, stomatitis).

Hematological. Neutropenia, often severe, is the primary dose-limiting toxicity. Grade 4 neutropenia has been reported to occur in 80% to 94% of the patients receiving doses of 75 to 100 mg/m^2, respectively. Grade 4 thrombocytopenia is rare, and anemia (hemoglobin less than 11 g/dL) has been reported in over 90% of the patients receiving doses of 75 to 100 mg/m^2. Febrile neutropenia was observed in 22% of the patients receiving 100 mg/m^2.

Gastrointestinal. Mucositis (56%, severe in 9%), nausea, vomiting, dysgeusia, anorexia, and diarrhea have been reported. Taste alterations are rare. Severe nausea, vomiting, and diarrhea are uncommon.

Dermatological. Alopecia is expected and total. Severe (Grade 3) skin rashes have been reported to occur in approximately 10% of the patients and may include desquamation after a localized pruriginous maculopapular eruption and erythema with edema. Extravasation reaction (erythema, swelling, tenderness, pustules), reversible peripheral phlebitis, hand-foot syndrome, and nail changes (hypopigmentation or hyperpigmentation) have been reported.

Neurological. Reversible dysesthesia or paresthesia (7%), peripheral neuropathy (13%), mild or moderate lethargy or somnolence, headache, seizure (rare).

Hepatic. Increased liver enzyme levels, hyperbilirubinemia, hepatic failure (rare).

Cardiovascular. Fluid retention (edema, pericardial effusion, pleural effusion, peripheral edema, ascites) occurs in 41% to 70% of the patients (severe in 3.4% to 10%) receiving docetaxel and the recommended premedications. Fluid retention may first appear as progressive weight gain followed by lower-extremity edema. Fluid retention is dose related and cumulative. The median time to significant fluid retention was 15 to 20 weeks in one study, the median cumulative dose of docetaxel was 705 mg/m^2. Up to 80% of the patients who received five or more courses of docetaxel developed significant fluid retention. Fluid retention slowly resolves over a median period of 29 weeks. A 5-day course of dexamethasone, beginning the day before administration of docetaxel, appears to be useful in delaying the onset of this toxicity. Hypotension requiring treatment has been reported in approximately 3% of the patients.

Pulmonary. Dyspnea with restrictive pulmonary syndrome, pleural effusions.

Hypersensitivity. Local or generalized rash, flushing, pruritus, drug fever, chills and rigors, low back pain; severe anaphylactoid reactions (flushing with hypotension or hypertension, with or without dyspnea). Hypersensitivity reactions have been reported in approximately 12% to 29% of the patients. Severe hypersensitivity reactions have been reported to occur in 0.9% of patients receiving the recommended 5-day course of dexamethasone.

Other. Fatigue, asthenia (63% to 80%, severe in 11%), conjunctivitis, arthralgia, myalgia (12% to 35%), and myopathy have been reported.

Storage and Stability

Docetaxel is stored in the refrigerator. The solvent vials may be stored at room or refrigeration temperatures. The 10 mg/mL solution is stable at room or refrigeration temperatures for at least 8 hours.

Preparation

Just before use, vials of docetaxel should be allowed to reach room temperature for 5 minutes. The entire contents of the diluent is added to the vial of docetaxel. The resulting solution contains 10 mg/mL of docetaxel. The desired dose of docetaxel is further diluted in 5% dextrose or normal saline to a maximum concentration of 0.9 mg/mL. Non–PVC-containing intravenous infusion bags and administration sets should be used to avoid patient exposure to the plasticizer DEHP.

Incompatibilities

Docetaxel is metabolized by cytochrome P450 3A4. Drugs that induce or inhibit this enzyme may adversely affect the metabolism of docetaxel and lead to enhanced toxicity or decreased efficacy. Drugs that may interact with docetaxel include cyclosporine, terfenadine, ketoconazole, erythromycin, and troleandomycin.

Availability

Docetaxel is commercially available as a concentrated solution (40 mg/mL) in 20- and 80-mg vials.

Selected Readings

Cortes JE, Pazdur R: Docetaxel, *J Clin Oncol* 13:2643-2655, 1995.

Dreyfuss AI et al: Docetaxel: an active drug for squamous cell carcinoma of the head and neck, *J Clin Oncol* 14:1672-1678, 1996.

Hudis CA et al: Phase II and pharmacologic study of docetaxel as initial chemotherapy for metastatic breast cancer, *J Clin Oncol* 14:58-65, 1996.

Ravdin PM et al: Phase II trial of docetaxel in advanced anthracycline-resistant or anthracenedione-resistant breast cancer, *J Clin Oncol* 13:2879-2885, 1995.

Trudeau ME et al: Docetaxel in patients with metastatic breast cancer: a phase II study of the National Cancer Institute of Canada-Clinical Trials Group, *J Clin Oncol* 14:429-433, 1996.

Valero V et al: Phase II trial of docetaxel: a new, highly effective antineoplastic agent in the management of patients with anthracycline-resistant metastatic breast cancer, *J Clin Oncol* 13:2886-2894, 1995.

DOXORUBICIN

Other Names

Adriamycin, Rubex, Adriamycin RDF, Adriamycin PFS, Adriamycin MDV, Adria, hydroxydaunorubicin, hydroxydaunomycin, NSC-123127. Doxorubicin hydrochloride liposomal injection (Doxil).

D

Indications
FDA approved for the treatment of acute nonlymphocytic leukemia, acute lymphocytic leukemia, Wilms' tumor, neuroblastoma, soft-tissue and bone sarcomas, breast carcinoma, ovarian carcinoma, transitional-cell bladder carcinoma, thyroid carcinoma, Hodgkin's disease, non-Hodgkin's lymphoma, gastric carcinoma, and small-cell lung cancer. Doxorubicin may also be a useful treatment for multiple myeloma, chronic lymphocytic leukemia, Ewing's sarcoma, Kaposi's sarcoma, rhabdomyosarcoma, trophoblastic neoplasms, and cancers of the cervix, endometrium, liver, esophagus, head and neck, islet cells, pancreas, prostate, and testes. The liposomal formulation of doxorubicin is approved for the treatment of AIDS-related Kaposi's sarcoma.

Classification
Anthracycline antitumor antibiotic.

Pharmacokinetics
Doxorubicin is poorly absorbed (5%) by mouth. After IV administration doxorubicin is widely distributed throughout the body, including breast milk. Approximately 70% of the drug is bound to plasma proteins. Doxorubicin does not penetrate into the cerebrospinal fluid. The drug is extensively metabolized by the liver to several metabolites, including the active metabolite doxorubicinol. Approximately 40% to 50% of doxorubicin and doxorubicinol is eliminated by the biliary route and 4% to 5% is eliminated via the urine. Doxorubicin and doxorubicinol have elimination half-lives of 18 to 30 hours.

Dose
The usual dose is 60 to 75 mg/m^2 as a bolus injection or continuous infusion over 2 to 4 days, repeated every 3 to 4 weeks. Higher bolus doses (80 to 90 mg/m^2) have also been used. Other dosage schedules are 20 mg/m^2 weekly and 30 mg/m^2 daily for 3 days, repeated every 3 to 4 weeks. It has been recommended that patients with serum bilirubin levels of 1.2 to 3 mg/dL should receive 50% of the usual dose and that patients with bilirubin levels greater than 3 mg/dL should receive 25% of the usual dose. The dose of liposomal doxorubicin is 20 mg/m^2 every 3 weeks.

Administration
Intravenously, either as a bolus injection (using extravasation precautions into a free-flowing IV line over 2 to 5 minutes) or as a continuous infusion in 50 mL or more of 5% dextrose or normal saline through a central venous line. Doxorubicin has also been given intraarterially to the liver, intravesicularly, and intraperitoneally.

Liposomal doxorubicin is not a vesicant and is usually mixed in 250 mL of 5% dextrose and administered over a period of 30 minutes.

Toxicity
Hematological. Leukopenia (dose limiting), also thrombocytopenia and anemia. Nadir blood counts occur in 10 to 14 days, recovery in 21 days.

In more than 700 patients with AIDS-associated Kaposi's sarcoma, the following hematologic toxicities have been reported after treatment with liposomal doxorubicin: neutropenia <1000/mm³ (50%), anemia (20%), thrombocytopenia (10%).

Gastrointestinal. Nausea and vomiting, sometimes severe, dose related and preventable with antiemetic prophylaxis. Anorexia, diarrhea, mucositis (especially with the 3 times daily schedule, 10% incidence after doses of 60 to 75 mg/m²); ulceration and necrosis of the colon have also been reported. In more than 700 patients with AIDS-associated Kaposi's sarcoma, the following gastrointestinal toxicities have been reported after treatment with liposomal doxorubicin: nausea (17%), vomiting (8%), diarrhea (8%), stomatitis (7%), oral moniliasis (5.5%).

Dermatological. Alopecia is usually total when doxorubicin is administered as a bolus injection every 3 to 4 weeks. Weekly injections of 10 mg/m² are associated with minimal or no hair loss. Hyperpigmentation of nail beds and dermal creases and radiation recall reactions occur occasionally. In more than 700 patients with AIDS-associated Kaposi's sarcoma, the following dermatological toxicities have been reported after treatment with liposomal doxorubicin: Palmar-plantar erythema (i.e., hand-foot syndrome, 3.4%), alopecia (9%). Rare toxicities of liposomal doxorubicin include: rash, skin ulcer, dermatitis, skin discoloration, erythema multiforme, psoriasis, urticaria, and skin necrosis.

Local effects. Vesicant if extravasated, flush along vein, facial flush, urticaria. Liposomal doxorubicin does not appear to be a vesicant.

Cardiovascular. Arrhythmias, ECG changes, rare sudden death. Congestive heart failure caused by cardiomyopathy is related to the total cumulative dose. The risk of developing significant cardiomyopathy is greatest when total doses exceed 550 mg/m² (7% incidence at 550 mg/m², 15% at 600 mg/m², 30% to 40% at 700 mg/m²). Other risk factors include mediastinal irradiation, preexisting cardiac disease, and old age. The risk of developing this serious toxicity is reduced by giving the drug on a weekly schedule or as a continuous infusion or concomitant administration of dexrazoxane. Serial monitoring of left ventricular ejection fraction (LVEF) by equilibrium radionuclide angiocardiography (ERNA) is mandatory. A baseline ERNA is done before beginning treatment and is repeated when the total dose of doxorubicin exceeds 250 to 300 mg/m² and again after 450 mg/m² has been given. If criteria for dose-limiting cardiotoxicity are not met, ERNA is repeated before each or every other subsequent treatment. Doxorubicin is discontinued when there is an absolute decrease in the LVEF of 10% or more that is associated with a decline to a level less than 50%. Reports of cardiomyopathy occurring years after discontinuing therapy suggest that the LVEF may give a false sense of security when doses exceed 550 mg/m². In over 700 patients with AIDS-related Kaposi's sarcoma who received treatment with liposomal doxorubicin, chest pain, hypotension, and tachycardia have been reported in 1% to 5%. Cardiomyopathy after liposomal doxorubicin treatment has occurred in less than 1% of the patients. However, experience is limited with long-term treatment of liposomal doxorubicin.

Other. Red urine, fever, chills, muscle weakness, lacrimation, conjunctivitis, anaphylactoid reaction; may enhance cyclophosphamide cystitis or mercaptopurine hepatotoxicity. Infusion-associated reactions have occurred in approximately 7% of the patients treated with liposomal doxorubicin. These reactions resolve within a day of the infusion and may consist of flushing, chills, dyspnea, facial swelling, headache, back pain, chest or throat tightness, and/or hypotension.

Storage and Stability
Rubex or Adriamycin RDF vials are stored at room temperature. Doxorubicin in liquid form is stored in the refrigerator. Reconstituted solutions are stable for 35 days at room temperature and 6 months under refrigeration temperatures or frozen. Adriamycin Pfs (0.05 to 2 mg/mL) is stable for at least 14 days at room temperature in plastic syringes, Travenol infusors, or PVC bags or bottles (diluted with normal saline).

Preparation
Add 5, 10, 25, 50, or 75 mL of preservative-free normal saline to the 10-, 20-, 50-, 100-, or 150-mg vials, respectively, to produce a solution containing 2 mg/mL.

Incompatibilities
Physically incompatible with heparin, fluorouracil, aminophylline, cephalothin, methotrexate, dexamethasone, sodium phosphate, diazepam, hydrocortisone sodium succinate, or furosemide.

Compatibilities
Stable with vincristine in normal saline for at least 5 days at room temperature and 7 days in the refrigerator. The manufacturer states that doxorubicin (1.4 mg/mL) and vincristine (0.33 mg/mL) in normal saline are chemically stable for 14 days at room temperature. Also compatible in solution with cyclophosphamide, dacarbazine, bleomycin, vinblastine, and other drugs. A pharmacist should be consulted for additional information.

Availability
Commercially available as a powder for injection in 10-, 20-, 50-, 100-, 150-mg vials, and as 2-mg/mL solution for injection in 10-, 20-, 50-, and 200-mg vials. Liposomal doxorubicin is available as a 2-mg/mL solution.

Selected Readings
Schwartz RG et al: Congestive heart failure and left ventricular dysfunction complicating doxorubicin therapy: seven year experience using serial radionuclide angiocardiography, *Am J Med* 82:1109-1118, 1987.

Steinherz LJ, Steinherz PG: Delayed anthracycline cardiac toxicity. In DeVita VT Jr, Hellman S, Rosenberg SA, eds: *Principles and practice of oncology, PPO updates* 5:1-15, 1991.

Uziely B et al: Liposomal doxorubicin: antitumor activity and unique toxicities during two complementary phase I studies, *J Clin Oncol* 13:1777-1785, 1995.

EDATREXATE

Other Names
10-EDAM, 10-ethyl-10-deaza-aminopterin, GGP 30693, NSC-626715.

Indications
Edatrexate is an investigational agent that has activity against non–small-cell lung cancer, cancers of the head and neck, and other malignancies.

Classification
Antimetabolite (antifol). Leucovorin will block the effects of edatrexate.

Pharmacokinetics
Edatrexate is metabolized in the liver to 7-hydroxy-edatrexate, a weak inhibitor of dihydrofolate reductase. Approximately 33% of the drug is eliminated in the urine. Renal tubular secretion is believed to play a role in the elimination of edatrexate. Edatrexate has an elimination half-life of about 12 hours. The clearance of edatrexate does not appear to correlate with either serum albumin levels or creatinine clearance.

Dose
The usual dose of edatrexate is 80 mg/m^2/week.

Administration
IV bolus, without further dilution, administered over a period of 1 to 2 minutes. Edatrexate has also been administered as an IV infusion over 15 to 30 minutes.

Toxicity
Hematological. Leukopenia, thrombocytopenia, elevated prothrombin and partial prothrombin times.

Gastrointestinal. Stomatitis is dose limiting. Leucovorin has been used with some success in averting this toxicity. Diarrhea, nausea, and vomiting are uncommon toxicities.

Dermatological. Skin rash; alopecia is uncommon and usually mild. Life-threatening exfoliative dermatitis has occurred in patients receiving treatment with edatrexate.

Hepatic. Elevated hepatic enzyme levels.

Renal. Elevated serum creatinine levels (uncommon).

Other. Fatigue, interstitial pneumonitis (rare).

Storage and Stability
Edatrexate is stored at room temperature. Each vial bears an expiration date. Undiluted solutions of edatrexate are stored in the refrigerator for

up to 24 hours. Solutions of 2 mg/mL are stable at room temperature for 7 days.

Preparation
Add 4 mL normal saline to the 50-mg vial to yield a concentration of 12.5 mg/mL. Doses of edatrexate are usually further diluted in 50-mL of normal saline.

Compatibilities
Edatrexate and sodium bicarbonate 50 mEq are compatible in 1000 mL of 5% dextrose.

Availability
Edatrexate is an investigational drug that is available as a lyophilized powder (50-mg/vial) from the National Cancer Institute.

Selected Readings
Kemeny N, Israel K, O'Hehir M: Phase II trial of 10-EDAM in patients with advanced colorectal carcinoma, *Am J Clin Oncol* 13:42-44, 1990.
Lee JS et al: Improved therapeutic index by the addition of leucovorin to an edatrexate, cyclophosphamide, and cisplatin regimen for non-small-cell lung cancer, *J Natl Cancer Inst* 84:1039-40, 1992.
Verweij J et al: Toxic dermatitis induced by 10-ethyl-10-deaza-aminopterin (10-EDAM), a novel antifolate, *Cancer* 66:1910-3, 1990.

EPIRUBICIN
Other Names
4'-epidoxorubicin, 4'-epiadriamycin, NSC-256942.

Indications
Epirubicin is an investigational drug in the United States and is currently approved in some European countries. Epirubicin has been shown to be a useful treatment for patients with acute nonlymphocytic leukemia, soft-tissue sarcomas, breast carcinoma, ovarian carcinoma, non-Hodgkin's lymphoma, and small-cell lung cancer.

Classification
Anthracycline antitumor antibiotic.

Pharmacokinetics
The drug is widely distributed in tissues. Excretion is primarily via the biliary route; approximately 10% is eliminated via the urine. Epirubicin has an elimination half-life of approximately 30 to 40 hours.

Dose
The usual dose is 90 to 120 mg/m^2 as a bolus injection repeated every 3 to 4 weeks. Epirubicin 90 mg/m^2 produces an equivalent degree of myelosuppression as doxorubicin, 60 mg/m^2.

Administration

Intravenously, either as a bolus injection (using extravasation precautions into a free-flowing IV line over 2 to 5 minutes) or as a continuous infusion through a central venous line.

Toxicity

Hematological. Leukopenia is dose limiting and expected. Thrombocytopenia and anemia occur less commonly.

Gastrointestinal. Nausea and vomiting are usually prevented with antiemetics. Anorexia, diarrhea (rare), and mucositis have been reported.

Dermatological. Alopecia is common but less pronounced than with doxorubicin. Hyperpigmentation of nail beds and dermal creases, dermatitis, and radiation recall occur frequently.

Local effects. If extravasated, epirubicin will cause local tissue damage. Flush along vein, facial flush, urticaria, phlebitis.

Cardiovascular. Arrhythmias and ECG changes occasionally occur but are rarely clinically significant. Congestive heart failure caused by cardiomyopathy may occur and is related to total cumulative dose. Mediastinal irradiation, preexisting cardiac disease, and advanced age increase risk; weekly or continuous infusion regimens decrease risk.

Other. Red urine (common), fever, anaphylactoid reaction, paresthesias, fatigue, headache.

Storage and Stability

Vials are stored at room temperature. The reconstituted 2-mg/mL solution is stable at room temperature for at least 48 hours.

Preparation

Add 5 or 25 mL of sterile water or normal saline to the 10- and 50-mg vials, respectively, to yield a 2-mg/mL solution.

Availability

Epirubicin is an investigational drug that is available as a powder for injection in 10- and 50-mg vials.

Selected Readings

Conley BA et al: Phase II trial of 4'-deoxydoxorubicin in advanced non-small-cell lung cancer, *Cancer Treat Rep* 71:861-862, 1987.

Perez DJ et al: A randomized comparison of single-agent doxorubicin and epirubicin as first-line cytotoxic therapy in advanced breast cancer, *J Clin Oncol* 9:2148-2152, 1991.

ESTRAMUSTINE

Other Names

Estramustine phosphate, Emcyt, Estracyt, NSC-89199.

E

Indications
FDA approved for the treatment of prostate cancer.

Classification and Mechanisms of Action
Estramustine has been classified as a hormone but may also be an antimicrotubule agent. Estramustine elicits some pharmacological effects that are similar to those of estrogens. Estramustine has been shown to bind to microtubule-associated proteins and disrupt the normal cytoskeletal structure of cells by depolymerizing microtubules. Distribution studies with radioactive estramustine have shown that the drug accumulates in cells that contain a binding site called *estramustine binding protein (EMBP)*. EMBP levels have been found to be increased in prostatic carcinoma, a disease for which estramustine is an active therapy.

Pharmacokinetics
Estramustine is well absorbed (75%) by mouth, is metabolized by the liver, and has an elimination half-life of approximately 20 hours. The majority of the drug is excreted in the feces as metabolites.

Dose
The usual oral *daily* dose of estramustine for the treatment of prostate cancer is 15 mg/kg (in three or four divided doses). The drug should be taken on an empty stomach because milk and milk products interfere with its absorption. Calcium supplements should not be taken with estramustine because calcium binds to estramustine and prevents its absorption.

Administration
Oral.

Toxicity
Hematological. Leukopenia and thrombocytopenia are rarely clinically significant.

Gastrointestinal. Nausea and vomiting are the major dose-limiting side effects of estramustine and occur in 20% to 50% of the patients. These symptoms usually lessen with continued dosing. Other gastrointestinal toxicities include anorexia and diarrhea (20% to 50%).

Dermatological. Skin rash, alopecia (rare), pruritus, dry skin.

Hepatic. Increased liver enzyme levels, hyperbilirubinemia, jaundice (rare), increased serum amylase and lipase levels (rare).

Neurological. Headache.

Cardiovascular. Thromboembolic disorders; cerebrovascular accident; sodium retention resulting in edema, hypertension, and congestive heart failure (rare).

Genitourinary. Decreased libido (20% to 50%), impotence.

Endocrine. Hypercalcemia.

Other. Gynecomastia (20% to 50%), breast tenderness, phlebitis, lacrimation.

Storage and Stability
Store intact capsules at refrigeration temperatures. The drug retains its potency for up to 30 days at room temperature.

Availability
Estramustine is commercially available as 140-mg capsules.

Selected Readings
Ahlgren JD, Schein PS, eds: Emcyt (estramustine phosphate sodium), *Semin Oncol* 10(suppl 3):1-47, 1983.

Gunnarsson PO et al: Impairment of estramustine phosphate absorption by concurrent intake of milk and food, *Eur J Clin Pharmacol* 38:189-193, 1990.

Pienta KJ et al: Phase II evaluation of oral estramustine and oral etoposide in hormone-refractory adenocarcinoma of the prostate, *J Clin Oncol* 12:2005-2012, 1994.

ETOPOSIDE

Other Names
VePesid, Toposar, VP-16, VP-16-213, EPEG, epipodophyllotoxin, NSC-141540, Etoposide phosphate (Etopophos).

Indications
FDA approved for the treatment of refractory testicular tumors and small-cell lung cancer. Etoposide also may be a useful treatment for acute leukemias, Hodgkin's and non-Hodgkin's lymphoma, Kaposi's sarcoma, Ewing's sarcoma, neuroblastoma, trophoblastic neoplasms, brain tumors, and cancers of the breast, lung (non–small-cell), adrenal cortex, bladder, stomach, and prostate. In high-dose chemotherapy regimens, the use of etoposide phosphate allows for the administration of etoposide in a smaller volume than would be necessary with etoposide. As a result, etoposide phosphate may shorten the time necessary to administer high-dose chemotherapy and reduce the volume of fluid that would otherwise be necessary.

Classification
Plant alkaloid (topoisomerase II inhibitor).

Pharmacokinetics
Oral absorption of etoposide varies from 25% to 75% (average 50%), and peak plasma levels occur approximately 1 to 1.5 hours after dosing (absorption half-life, 0.44 hours). There is no evidence of first-pass metabolism in the liver after oral administration. Etoposide has been measured in breast milk. Cerebrospinal fluid concentrations of etoposide rarely exceed 5% of the concurrent plasma concentration. The drug is extensively protein bound (96%), metabolized by the liver, and eliminated in the bile (10% to 15% as unchanged drug) and urine (30% to 40% as unchanged drug).

Etoposide is not hemodialyzable. The elimination half-life is 7 to 14 hours. Etoposide phosphate is rapidly converted to etoposide in plasma after IV administration. Etoposide and etoposide phosphate are bioequivalent when administered in molar equivalent doses.

Dose

Common doses are 50 to 120 mg/m²/day by IV for 3 to 5 days; larger doses (e.g., 400 mg/m²/day for 3 days) have been used before bone marrow transplantation. For the treatment of testicular cancer (in combination with cisplatin and bleomycin), the dose is 100 mg/m²/day for 5 days, repeated every 3 weeks. The oral dose is usually twice the IV dose. Daily oral doses of 50 mg/m² for 21 days have been used. Etoposide doses should be reduced if renal function is impaired. A 25% and 50% reduction has been recommended for creatinine clearances of 10 to 50 mL/min, and less than 10 mL/min, respectively. Doses of etoposide should not be reduced for elevated serum bilirubin concentrations. It has been recommended that doses of etoposide be reduced by 33% in patients with a serum albumin less than 3.5 g/dL.

Administration

Etoposide. Slow IV infusion as a 0.2 to 0.4 mg/mL solution in 5% dextrose or normal saline over *at least 30 minutes.* Capsules are administered orally.

Etoposide phosphate. IV infusion over a period of 5 minutes or longer. Etoposide phosphate does not require further dilution before administration, although it may be diluted to a concentration as low as 0.1 mg/mL in 5% dextrose or normal saline.

Toxicity

Hematological. Leukopenia, dose related, primarily granulocytopenia, nadirs within 7 to 14 days and recovery within 20 days of administration; significant thrombocytopenia and anemia are uncommon.

Gastrointestinal. Nausea and vomiting are relatively uncommon after IV dosing, but common with oral dosing. Anorexia occurs in 10% to 13% of patients, and stomatitis is rare with conventional doses (more common and more severe in patients who have received radiation to the head and neck and with high doses). Abdominal pain, diarrhea, aftertaste, parotitis, dysphagia, and constipation occur rarely.

Dermatological. Alopecia is generally mild and reversible and is reported to occur in 20% to 66% of the patients, although some patients develop total baldness. Other toxicities include rash (rare), severe pruritus (rare), radiation recall reactions (rare), phlebitis, local pain at injection site, and hyperpigmentation (rare).

Hepatic. Hyperbilirubinemia and increased transaminase levels, usually mild, transient, and more common when high doses are given.

Neurological. Peripheral neuropathy (1% to 2%), somnolence, fatigue, headache, vertigo, transient cortical blindness (all rare), transient confusion with high doses, perhaps caused by the alcohol-containing vehicle.

Cardiovascular. Transient hypotension associated with rapid administration, transient hypertension (rare), and other cardiovascular events (e.g., congestive heart failure) thought to be related to large amounts of sodium chloride administered with the drug. Rare reports of arrhythmias.

Hypersensitivity. Anaphylactoid reactions (bronchospasm, fever, chills, dyspnea, tachycardia) are rare.

Other. Rarely, fever, muscle cramps, metabolic acidosis, hyperuricemia, second malignancy (acute myeloid leukemia).

Storage and Stability
Etoposide. The injection should be stored at room temperature, the capsules must be refrigerated. Capsules are stable for 24 months when refrigerated. After dilution in normal saline or 5% dextrose to concentrations of 0.2 to 0.4 mg/mL, the drug is chemically stable for 96 and 72 hours at room temperature, respectively. Bristol-Myers data indicate that etoposide may be stable in 5% dextrose or normal saline for 24 hours (0.6 mg/mL), 4 hours (1 mg/mL), and 2 hours (2 mg/mL) at room temperature.

Etoposide phosphate. Etoposide phosphate is stored at refrigeration temperatures before reconstitution. After reconstitution or further dilution, etoposide phosphate is stable at room temperature for at least 24 hours.

Preparation
The desired dose of etoposide is usually diluted to a concentration of <0.4 mg/mL in normal saline or 5% dextrose. More concentrated solutions have been used but they have shorter stability *(and may precipitate).* Etoposide phosphate: add 5 or 10 ml of 5% dextrose, normal saline, or sterile water to the 100-mg vial to produce a solution containing 20 or 10 mg/mL, respectively. Etoposide phosphate may also be reconstituted with bacteriostatic water or saline containing benzyl alcohol.

Incompatibilities
Etoposide and idarubicin are not compatible in solution.

Compatibilities
Compatible with cisplatin 200 µg/mL in 5% dextrose and 0.45% NaCl or normal saline for 24 hours when protected from light. The addition of mannitol and/or potassium chloride reduces the stability to 8 hours in normal saline, but it remains stable for 24 hours in 5% dextrose and 0.45% NaCl. Also compatible with carboplatin, cytarabine, mesna, and daunorubicin. A pharmacist should be consulted for additional information.

Availability
Etoposide is commercially available as an injection in 100-, 150-, 500-, and 1000-mg (20-mg/mL) multiple-dose vials and in 50-mg capsules

for oral use. Etoposide phosphate is commercially available as a lyophilized powder in 100-mg vials.

Selected Readings

Joel SP et al: Predicting etoposide toxicity: relationship to organ function and protein binding, *J Clin Oncol* 14:257-267, 1996.

Johnson DH et al: Prolonged administration of oral etoposide in patients with relapsed or refractory small-cell lung cancer: a phase II trial, *J Clin Oncol* 8:1613-1617, 1990.

F

FINASTERIDE

Other Names

Proscar, MK-906.

Indications

FDA approved for the treatment of benign prostatic hypertrophy. Finasteride may also be a useful preventative therapy for patients with early stage prostate cancer.

Classification and Mechanisms of Action

5-alpha-reductase inhibitor. Finasteride inhibits the conversion of testosterone to dihydrotestosterone (DHT) but does not significantly affect serum testosterone levels. Hyperplasia of cells within the prostate is inhibited because DHT stimulates prostate cell growth.

Pharmacokinetics

Finasteride is well absorbed (63%) after oral administration. Absorption is not affected by food and peak plasma levels occur approximately 1 to 2 hours after administration of a single dose. After 2 weeks of dosing, peak plasma levels are approximately 50% higher. Approximately 90% of the drug is bound to plasma proteins. Finasteride is metabolized in the liver to compounds that retain approximately 20% of the potency of the parent compound. Metabolites are eliminated from the body in the feces (57%) and urine (39%). Dose adjustments are not recommended for patients with hepatic or renal dysfunction.

Dose

The FDA-approved dose for benign prostatic hypertrophy is 5 mg/day for 6 to 12 months. The drug can be taken with food. Finasteride tablets may be crushed, if necessary.

Administration

Oral.

Toxicity

Genitourinary. Impotence (3.7%), decreased libido (3.3%), decreased volume of ejaculate (2.8%).

Other. Finasteride may affect male fetal development if the film coating of the tablets is broken (e.g., crushed). Tablets should not be handled by a woman who is or may become pregnant.

Storage and Stability
Room temperature, protected from light. Containers bear an expiration date.

Availability
Commercially available in 5-mg tablets.

F

Selected Readings
Fair WR et al: Multicenter, randomized double-blind placebo controlled study to investigate the effect of finasteride (MK-906) on stage D prostate cancer, *J Urol* 145(suppl):317A, 1991.
Gormley GJ et al. The effect of finasteride in men with benign prostatic hyperplasia, *N Engl J Med* 327:1185-1191, 1992.
Thompson I, Feigl P, Coltman C: Chemoprevention of prostate cancer with finasteride. In Devita VT Jr, Hellman S, Rosenberg SA, eds: *Principles and practice of oncology, PPO updates* 10(3):1-18, 1996.

FLOXURIDINE
Other Names
FUDR, 5-FUDR, 5-fluoro-2'-deoxyuridine, NSC-27640.

Indications
FDA approved for the treatment of gastrointestinal adenocarcinoma metastatic to the liver (administration of floxuridine by continuous intraarterial infusion). Floxuridine may also be useful in the treatment of cancers of the breast, ovary, cervix, bladder, kidney, and prostate.

Classification
Pyrimidine antimetabolite.

Pharmacokinetics
Floxuridine is metabolized in the liver to its active metabolite FUDR-MP. Floxuridine is preferred over 5-fluorouracil (5-FU) for intrahepatic therapy because 90% of the drug is metabolized by the liver to inactive metabolites. Approximately 10% to 15% of a dose is eliminated in the urine as unchanged drug. Floxuridine has an elimination half-life of 0.3 to 0.6 hours.

Dose
FDA-approved doses include 0.1 to 0.6 mg/kg/day by intrahepatic infusion. Floxuridine has also been given intravenously in doses up to 60 mg/kg/week.

Administration
Floxuridine may be administered by intraarterial or IV infusion. Intraarterial infusions are usually administered continuously over a period of

7 to 14 days. IV infusions may be given in 100 to 500 mL of normal saline or 5% dextrose over a 15-minute or longer period. Circadian infusion regimens have also been used.

Toxicity

Hematological. Leukopenia and, less commonly, thrombocytopenia. These toxicities are dose and schedule related and occur more frequently with IV bolus dose regimens. Anemia occurs infrequently.

Gastrointestinal. Nausea (uncommon), vomiting (uncommon), anorexia, diarrhea (more common with continuous infusion), mucositis (dose related, more common with continuous IV infusions), gastritis and abdominal cramps (more common with intrahepatic administration), enteritis, and duodenal ulcer.

Dermatological. Alopecia occurs infrequently and is generally mild. Dermatitis, localized erythema, edema, rash, pigmentation, pruritus, excoriation, and maceration are rare toxicities.

Hepatic/biliary. Hyperbilirubinemia, increased transaminase levels, increased alkaline phosphatase levels (occasionally an early indication of biliary toxicity, i.e., biliary sclerosis, stenosis, stricture), jaundice, cholecystitis, cirrhosis (rare), all mild and transient with IV injection, but dose limiting with intraarterial infusion to the liver. Adding dexamethasone to intrahepatic floxuridine may decrease biliary toxicity.

Neurological. Rarely: ataxia, blurred vision, fatigue, headache, depression, vertigo, nystagmus, seizures, and hemiplegia.

Mechanical. A variety of catheter problems may occur, including leakage, ischemia of the artery, occlusion of the catheter, bleeding at the catheter site, thrombosis or embolism, perforation of the vessel, dislodgement of the catheter, or infection. Periodic radionuclide scans can detect alterations in flow distribution.

Other. Fever, dysuria, hiccups, excess lacrimation, lethargy, malaise, and weakness are rare.

Storage and Stability

Floxuridine is stored at room temperature. Reconstituted floxuridine (100 mg/mL) is chemically stable for at least 14 days at refrigeration and room temperatures. Further dilution to 0.5 mg/mL in 5% dextrose or normal saline results in a solution that is stable for at least 7 days at room temperature.

Preparation

Floxuridine lyophilized powder is reconstituted by adding 5 mL of sterile water to the 500-mg vial to result in a solution containing 100 mg/mL.

Compatibilities

Floxuridine (2.5 to 12 mg/mL) in bacteriostatic 0.9% sodium chloride with heparin (200 units/mL) is chemically stable for at least 14 days in an implantable infusion pump (Infusaid model 400). Floxuridine (1 to 4 mg/mL) and leucovorin calcium (0.03 to 0.96 mg/mL) are chemically stable in plastic containers for at least 48 hours at room and refrigerated temperatures. Floxuridine is also compatible with dexamethasone.

Availability
Commercially available as a lyophilized powder for injection in 500-mg vials and a 500 mg/10 mL preservative-free injection.

Selected Readings
Hohn D et al: Biliary sclerosis in patients receiving hepatic arterial infusions of floxuridine, *J Clin Oncol* 3:98-102, 1985.

Kemeny N et al: Intrahepatic or systemic infusion of fluorodeoxyuridine in patients with liver metastases from colorectal carcinoma, *Ann Intern Med* 107:459-465, 1987.

Kemeny N et al: A randomized trial of intrahepatic infusion of fluorodeoxyuridine with dexamethasone versus fluorodeoxyuridine alone in the treatment of metastatic colorectal carcinoma, *Cancer* 69:327-334, 1992.

FLUDARABINE

Other Names
Fludarabine phosphate, Fludara, 2-fluoroadenine arabinoside-5-phosphate, 2-fluoro-ara AMP, FAMP, NSC-312887.

Indications
FDA approved for the treatment of relapsed or refractory B-cell chronic lymphocytic leukemia. Fludarabine may also be a useful treatment for low-grade non-Hodgkin's lymphoma, Hodgkin's disease, cutaneous T-cell lymphoma, hairy cell leukemia, prolymphocytic leukemia, and macroglobulinemic lymphoma.

Classification
Purine antimetabolite.

Pharmacokinetics
Fludarabine is metabolized to an active metabolite, 2-fluoro-ara-A (2-FLAA). 2-FLAA is extensively bound to body tissues, is eliminated primarily by the kidneys (i.e., urinary elimination, 60% [range 24% to 86%]). 2-FLAA has an elimination half-life of 9 to 10 hours. A significant correlation between area under the curve (AUC) and absolute neutrophil count (ANC) has been demonstrated as well as a significant correlation between creatinine clearance and total body clearance (i.e., AUC). A 30% decrease in dose is suggested for patients with renal impairment (i.e., creatinine clearance less than 70 mL/min or serum creatinine level greater than 1.5 mg/dL).

Dose
Fludarabine has been given as a 5-day treatment, 25 mg/m^2/day every 4 weeks, for chronic lymphocytic leukemia and low-grade non-Hodgkin's lymphomas.

Administration
Usually administered by IV infusion (in 50 to 150 mL of 5% dextrose or normal saline) over a 30-minute or longer period.

Toxicity
Hematological. Leukopenia, primarily lymphopenia and granulocytopenia, and thrombocytopenia are dose related, may be cumulative, and are dose limiting. Significant anemia occurs less frequently.

Gastrointestinal. Nausea and vomiting occur in approximately 30% of the patients and are preventable with standard antiemetic drugs. Anorexia (7% to 34%), stomatitis (rare with conventional doses), diarrhea (13% to 15%); constipation, and abdominal cramps occur infrequently.

Dermatological. Alopecia (uncommon, mild), rash (15%), dermatitis (rare).

Hepatic. Increased hepatic enzyme levels, mild and transient; cholestasis (rare).

Neurological. Somnolence, confusion, weakness, agitation, fatigue (10% to 38%), and peripheral neuropathy (4% to 12%) are usually transient. Delayed demyelinating central nervous system toxicities, including mental status changes, cortical blindness, severe somnolence and coma, have occurred, usually with high doses (e.g., 150 to 200 mg/m^2/day for 5 days); seizures (rare). Visual disturbances and coma have been reported rarely in patients receiving conventional doses of fludarabine.

Cardiovascular. Hypotension (rare), chest pain (rare), edema (8% to 19%).

Pulmonary. Dyspnea and interstitial infiltrates have been reported in a few patients previously treated with chlorambucil. Cough (10% to 44%) and pneumonia (16% to 22%) have been reported.

Other. Fever (60% to 70%), chills (10% to 20%). Metabolic acidosis and lactic acidemia caused by rapid tumor lysis; myalgia (4% to 16%); fever (rare).

Storage and Stability
It is recommended that unreconstituted vials of fludarabine be stored in the refrigerator. At a concentration of 25 mg/mL and after dilution in normal saline or 5% dextrose to a concentration of 1 mg/mL, the drug is chemically stable for at least 16 days at room temperature. Solutions of 0.04 mg/mL in 5% dextrose or normal saline in glass bottles or PVC bags are chemically stable for at least 48 hours at room and refrigerated temperatures.

Preparation
Fludarabine, 50-mg/vial, is reconstituted with 2 mL of sterile water to result in a 25 mg/mL solution. The desired dose is further diluted to concentrations of 0.04 to 1 mg/mL in normal saline or 5% dextrose (50 to 100 mL).

Availability
Fludarabine, 50-mg/vial, is commercially available as a lyophilized powder.

Selected Readings

Cheson BD, ed: Fludarabine phosphate: an effective therapy for lymphoid malignancies, *Semin Oncol* 17(suppl 8):1-78, 1990.

Hochster HS et al: Activity of fludarabine in previously treated non-Hodgkin's low-grade lymphoma: results of an Eastern Cooperative Oncology Group study, *J Clin Oncol* 10:28-32, 1992.

Hood MA, Finley RS: Fludarabine: a review, *DICP Ann Pharmacother* 25:518-524, 1991.

FLUOROURACIL

F

Other Names

5-Fluorouracil, 5-FU, Adrucil, Efudex, Fluoroplex, NSC-19893.

Indications

FDA approved for the treatment of carcinoma of the stomach, colon, rectum, breast, and pancreas. 5-FU may also be useful for the treatment of cancers of the bladder, cervix, endometrium, esophagus, head and neck, islet cells, liver, lung, ovary, prostate, and skin (topically).

Classification and Mechanisms of Action

Pyrimidine antimetabolite.

Pharmacokinetics

5-FU is poorly absorbed (25% to 30%) by mouth. After IV administration, the drug is metabolized to active metabolites. Activation is inhibited to some extent by allopurinol. Less than 10% of 5-FU is protein-bound. Approximately 22% to 45% of a dose of 5-FU is metabolized by the liver and 15% is excreted unchanged into the urine. 5-FU has an elimination half-life of 10 to 20 minutes. Certain antiviral agents (e.g., sorivudine and netivudine) inhibit dihydropyrimidine dehydrogenase, an important enzyme in the metabolism of 5-FU. Concomitant administration of these drugs significantly increases the toxicity of 5-FU.

Dose

Several regimens have been used, including the following:

1. 300 to 450 mg/m^2/day intravenously for 5 days every 28 days
2. 600 to 750 mg/m^2 intravenously weekly or every other week
3. 1000 mg/m^2 intravenously, infused over a 24-hour period, for 4 to 5 days
4. 300 mg/m^2/day, infused intravenously indefinitely
5. 3000 mg/m^2 intravenously over a 24-hour period once each week

Administration

The drug may be given by IV push, by IV infusion in 50 mL or more of 5% dextrose or normal saline over a 10-minute period or longer (i.e., continuous infusion), by arterial infusion, intracavitarily, intraperitoneally, topically, or orally mixed in water, grape juice, or a carbonated beverage.

Toxicity

Toxicities associated with 5-FU are more common and more severe in patients with dihydropyrimidine dehydrogenase deficiency.

Hematological. Leukopenia, thrombocytopenia, anemia, any of which can be dose limiting, but less common with continuous infusion. Myelosuppression may be reversed by administration of uridine.

Gastrointestinal. Mucositis, more common with 5-day infusion and is occasionally dose limiting. Mucositis may occur as small, shallow ulcerations on the inner surface of the lower lip or buccal mucosa and may progress to include a painful, erythematous tongue, and generalized mouth sores. Allopurinol mouth wash does not prevent mucositis. Diarrhea, which can be a severe, cholera-like diarrhea when 5-FU is given with high doses of leucovorin. Life-threatening toxicity and fatalities have resulted from drug-induced diarrhea. Nausea, vomiting, and anorexia occur infrequently.

Dermatological. Dermatitis, nail changes, dry skin, erythema, photosensitivity, hyperpigmentation, pruritic maculopapular skin rash, hand-foot syndrome (paresthesia, erythema, and swelling of the palms and soles) with protracted infusions, alopecia (uncommon).

Hepatic. Hepatitis with hepatic infusion.

Neurological. Rare and more common with high doses: cerebellar syndrome (headache, cerebellar ataxia, nystagmus, confusion).

Cardiovascular. Myocardial ischemia and angina are rare.

Ocular. Eye irritation, nasal discharge, excessive lacrimation caused by tear duct stenosis (10% to 25%), blurred vision, photophobia.

Other. Anaphylaxis (rare), vein pigmentation, fever (rare), thrombophlebitis, epistaxis.

Storage and Stability

Stable for prolonged periods of time at room temperature if protected from light. Inspect for precipitate; if apparent, agitate vial vigorously or gently heat to not greater than 140° F in a water bath. Do not allow to freeze. Solutions in 5% dextrose, 10 mg/mL, are stable for at least 16 weeks in the refrigerator.

Preparation

5-FU is available as a ready-to-use injectable solution. The desired dose may be further diluted in 5% dextrose or normal saline.

Incompatibilities

Incompatible with daunorubicin, doxorubicin, idarubicin, cisplatin, cytarabine, and diazepam.

Compatibilities

5-FU (5 to 25 mg/mL) and leucovorin (1 mg/mL) are compatible for 14 days at room temperature. 5-FU is also compatible with heparin sodium, vincristine, methotrexate, potassium chloride, and magnesium sulfate. A pharmacist should be consulted for additional information.

Availability
Commercially available in 500 mg/10 mL vials, and 1000 mg/20 mL, 2500 mg/50 mL, and 5000 mg/100 mL vials.

Selected Readings
Harris BE, Carpenter JT, Diasio RB: Severe 5-fluorouracil toxicity secondary to dihydropyrimidine dehydrogenase deficiency, *Cancer* 68:499-501 1991.

International Multicentre Pooled Analysis of Colon Cancer Trials (IMPACT) Investigators: Efficacy of adjuvant fluorouracil and folinic acid in colon cancer, *Lancet* 345:939-944, 1995.

Pinedo HM, Peters GFJ: Fluorouracil: biochemistry and pharmacology, *J Clin Oncol* 6:1653-1664, 1988.

F

FLUOXYMESTERONE
Other Names
Halotestin, Ora-testryl.

Indications
Fluoxymesterone is used primarily in the treatment of breast cancer and hypogonadism in men (androgen replacement).

Classification and Mechanisms of Action
Androgens are steroidal derivatives of testosterone. The antitumor actions of androgens may be caused by a reduction of or competition with prolactin receptors. Other potential mechanisms include inhibition of estrogen synthesis (by inhibition of adrenal precursors), inhibition at the estrogen receptor, and/or estrogen production in vivo via peripheral conversion of androgenic substances.

Dose
For the treatment of breast cancer the usual dose is 10 to 40 mg/day orally (in two or three divided doses) for at least 2 to 3 months.

Administration
Oral.

Toxicity
Hematological. Erythropoiesis.

Gastrointestinal. Nausea and vomiting occur infrequently.

Dermatological. Patchy alopecia, acne.

Hepatic. Liver function abnormalities, usually reversible when treatment is discontinued; cholestatic jaundice with high doses; peliosis of the liver; hepatocellular carcinoma.

Metabolic. Hypercalcemia may occur, especially in immobilized patients with bony disease.

Cardiovascular. Edema caused by sodium retention.

Genitourinary. *In women*: hirsutism, amenorrhea, clitoral hypertrophy, increased libido, voice deepening, and hoarseness. *In men*: oligospermia, priapism.

Other. Gynecomastia occurs in some men at high doses; anaphylactoid reactions are rare.

Storage and Stability
Room temperature; containers bear expiration dates.

Availability
Commercially available in 2-, 5-, and 10-mg tablets.

Selected Readings
Ingle JN et al: Combination hormonal therapy with tamoxifen plus fluoxymes-terone versus tamoxifen alone in postmenopausal women with metastatic breast cancer: an updated analysis, *Cancer* 67:886-891, 1991.

Skeel RT et al: Combination chemotherapy of advanced breast cancer: comparison of dibromodulcitol, doxorubicin, vincristine, and fluoxymesterone to thiotepa, doxorubicin, vinblastine, and fluoxymesterone: an Eastern Cooperative Oncology Group Study, *Cancer* 64:1393-1399, 1989.

FLUTAMIDE
Other Names
Eulexin, Euflex.

Indications
FDA approved for the treatment of prostate cancer; to be used in combination with a luteinizing hormone–releasing hormone (LHRH) agonist (e.g., leuprolide, goserelin).

Classification and Mechanisms of Action
Flutamide is a nonsteroidal antiandrogen that blocks the activity of testosterone at the androgen-dependent accessory sex structures.

Pharmacokinetics
Flutamide is almost completely absorbed after oral dosing. Peak plasma concentrations of flutamide occur 0.5 to 2 hours after administration. The drug is almost totally metabolized to several metabolites, including 2-hydroxyflutamide, the metabolite principally involved in the action of the drug. 2-Hydroxyflutamide is metabolized by the liver, and approximately 50% is eliminated unchanged in the urine. 2-Hydroxyflutamide has an elimination half-life of 8 to 10 hours. Flutamide is unlikely to be dialyzable because of its extensive protein binding.

Dose
The usual dose is 250 mg 3 times daily, and it is usually given in conjunction with an LHRH agonist or orchiectomy.

Administration
Oral. For patients unable to swallow the capsule, it may be opened and the contents mixed with applesauce, pudding, or other soft foods. Mixing flutamide in a beverage is not recommended because the drug does not dissolve well in water.

Toxicity
When flutamide was administered in combination with an LHRH agonist, the adverse events described below were observed.

Hematological. Anemia (6%), thrombocytopenia (1%), leukopenia (3%), and methemoglobinemia have been reported (rare).

Gastrointestinal. Nausea and vomiting occurred in 11% of the patients, diarrhea in 12%.

Dermatological. Rash (3%), photosensitivity (rare).

Hepatic. Elevations of hepatic transaminase levels (fourfold or more above upper normal limits) occur in fewer than 1% of the patients. Hyperbilirubinemia, elevated alkaline phosphatase and lactic dehydrogenase levels, hepatitis, hepatic necrosis, and hepatic encephalopathy are rare. Hepatic abnormalities usually resolve on discontinuation of flutamide.

Endocrine. Hot flashes (61%), loss of libido (36%), impotence (15% to 33%), galactorrhea. Gynecomastia occurred in approximately 10% of the patients and was occasionally associated with breast tenderness.

Other. Myalgia.

Storage and Stability
Capsules are stored at room temperature. Containers bear expiration dates.

Availability
Commercially available as 125-mg capsules.

Selected Readings
Crawford ED et al: A controlled trial of leuprolide with and without flutamide in prostatic carcinoma, *N Engl J Med* 321:419-424, 1989.
Gomez JL et al: Incidence of liver toxicity associated with the use of flutamide in prostate cancer patients, *Am J Med* 92:465-470, 1992.

GALLIUM NITRATE
Other Names
Ganite, NSC-15200.

Indications
FDA approved for treatment of symptomatic cancer-related hypercalcemia that has not responded to adequate hydration.

Classification and Mechanisms of Action
Gallium nitrate is a heavy metal and its exact mechanisms of action are unknown. Its activity is probably related to its ability to concentrate in malignant tumors rather than in normal tissue or serum. After internalization, gallium nitrate appears to be intracellularly bound to calcium and magnesium binding sites. Gallium inhibits calcium resorption from bone, which is thought to occur through inhibition of osteoclast activity.

Pharmacokinetics
Gallium nitrate is not metabolized by the liver or kidneys, and approximately 70% to 90% is eliminated as unchanged drug via the kidneys. Gallium nitrate has an elimination half-life of approximately 24 hours, which increases to 72 hours or longer with prolonged infusion.

Dose
The usual dose is 300 mg/m^2/day for 7 days by continuous IV infusion. Doses of 100 to 300 mg/m^2/day for 5 to 7 days by continuous IV infusion have been utilized. The duration of action of gallium nitrate is approximately 6 days.

Administration
Gallium nitrate has been given by IV infusion (in 100 mL or more of 5% dextrose or normal saline over a 30-minute period or longer), continuous infusion (usually in 1000 mL of normal saline or 5% dextrose), and subcutaneous injection.

Toxicity
Hematological. Mild cases of thrombocytopenia, leukopenia, and anemia have been reported.

Gastrointestinal. Nausea, vomiting, anorexia, metallic taste, diarrhea, constipation, and/or mucositis occur infrequently and are rarely dose limiting.

Dermatological. Rash.

Neurological. Decreased consciousness, fatigue, changes of mood, headache, lethargy, confusion, dizziness, and peripheral paresthesia are rare.

Renal. Elevations in BUN and serum creatinine levels are the major dose-limiting adverse effects of gallium nitrate (12%). Adequate hydration (2 L/day) minimizes the severity of this toxicity. Albuminuria, glycosuria, hematuria, and bilirubinuria have been rarely reported.

Metabolic. Hypocalcemia occurs within 3 to 4 days of administration of drug in 35% to 40% of the patients and may be dose limiting. Transient hypophosphatemia is common (76%) and may require treatment. Decreased serum bicarbonate levels (asymptomatic) have been reported in up to 33% of the patients.

Pulmonary. Rales and rhonchi; rarely, pleural effusion, pulmonary infiltrates, respiratory distress.

Other. Hearing loss (rare), tinnitus, conjunctivitis, decreased vision, optic neuritis (associated with high doses), hypothermia, fever, hypotension, tachycardia, lower-extremity edema.

Storage and Stability
Unopened vials are stored at room temperature. Diluted solutions (220 or 600 mg/1000 mL) are stable for 14 days at room or refrigeration temperatures.

Preparation
Gallium nitrate is usually further diluted in 500 to 1000 mL of normal saline or 5% dextrose for infusion.

Incompatibilities
Concurrent administration of nephrotoxic drugs (e.g., amphotericin B, aminoglycosides) should be avoided. Concurrent administration of calcium-containing drugs or vitamin D must be avoided.

Availability
Commercially available as a 25 mg/mL solution in 20-mL (500-mg) vials.

Selected Readings
Hughes TE, Hansen LA: Gallium nitrate, *DICP Ann Pharmacother* 26:354-362, 1992.

Warrell RP et al: Gallium nitrate for acute treatment of cancer-related hypercalcemia: a randomized, double-blind comparison to calcitonin, *Ann Intern Med* 108:669-674, 1988.

Warrell RP et al: A randomized, double-blind study of gallium nitrate compared with etidronate for acute control of cancer-related hypercalcemia, *J Clin Oncol* 9:1467-1475, 1991.

GEMCITABINE
Other Names
Gemzar, gemcitabine hydrochloride, 2',2' difluorodeoxycytidine, dFdC, 2'-deoxy-2',2'-difluorocytidine monohydrochloride.

Indications
Gemcitabine is FDA approved for the treatment of advanced carcinoma of the pancreas. Gemcitabine may also be a useful treatment for patients with breast cancer.

Classification and Mechanisms of Action
Antimetabolite (nucleoside analogue). Gemcitabine is converted to gemcitabine diphosphate, which inhibits the activity of ribonucleotide reductase and production of cellular nucleotides. Gemcitabine triphosphate inhibits DNA synthesis by competing with cytidine triphosphate for incorporation into DNA.

Pharmacokinetics

Maximum serum concentration of gemcitabine occurs approximately 30 minutes after a short IV infusion. The pharmacokinetics of gemcitabine are influenced by the length of the IV infusion and the age and gender of the patient. Men appear to eliminate the drug from the body more rapidly than women, and younger patients tend to eliminate the drug more rapidly than older patients. The elimination half-life of gemcitabine is reported to range from 42 to 79 minutes in men who are 29 to 79 years of age, respectively. The elimination half-life of gemcitabine in women aged 29 to 79 years is reported as 49 to 94 minutes, respectively. Gemcitabine is not protein bound to any significant degree, is metabolized primarily to a single inactive metabolite, and is eliminated almost entirely into the urine. Approximately 10% of a dose of gemcitabine is detected in the urine as unchanged drug.

Dose

Gemcitabine is administered at a dose of 1000 mg/m^2 intravenously over a period of 30 minutes once weekly for 7 weeks, followed by one week of rest. Subsequent courses of treatment are administered at a dose of 1000 mg/m^2/week for 3 weeks, followed by one week of rest.

Administration

The drug may be administered as the reconstituted solution (40 mg/mL) or may be further diluted with normal saline at a concentration as low as 0.1 mg/mL.

Toxicity

Hematological. Mild to moderate neutropenia, thrombocytopenia, and anemia are common. The incidence of Grade 3 or greater hematologic toxicity is neutropenia 26%, thrombocytopenia 5% to 10%, and anemia 8% to 11%.

Gastrointestinal. Mild nausea and vomiting (28% to 66%), nausea and vomiting requiring therapy (6% to 20%) of patients but that is rarely dose limiting. Diarrhea (8% to 31%), constipation (6% to 30%), mucositis (7% to 11%).

Dermatological. Rash (10% to 28%), accompanied by pruritus (10%). Skin rashes are usually mild, respond to local therapy, and are rarely dose limiting. Desquamation, vesiculation, ulceration, and significant alopecia are rare adverse effects.

Hepatic. Elevations of hepatic transaminase levels occur in approximately 66% of the patients and are Grade 3 or greater in 10% to 17%). Hyperbilirubinemia has been reported in 26% of the patients and is Grade 3 or greater in 8% to 10%.

Neurological. Somnolence is an uncommon adverse effect, occurring in approximately 10% of the patients. Insomnia and paresthesias have been reported.

Cardiovascular. Peripheral edema (30%), mild to moderate facial edema (rare); hypotension, myocardial infarction, congestive heart failure, and arrhythmia have been reported in patients receiving treatment with gemcitabine.

Pulmonary. Mild and transient bronchospasm (less than 1%), but parenteral therapy may be required. Dyspnea (10% to 23%) usually occurs within a few hours of administration and rapidly resolves without treatment. Cough and rhinitis are rare adverse effects.

Renal. Proteinuria (32%), hematuria (23%), elevated levels of BUN (15%) and serum creatinine (6%).

Other. Malaise and diaphoresis are common. Flulike symptoms (i.e., fever, headache, back pain, chills, myalgia, asthenia) have been reported in approximately 16% to 28% of the patients.

Storage and Stability
Unreconstituted vials of gemcitabine are stored at room temperature. Reconstituted solutions are stable at room temperature for at least 24 hours. It is not recommended that reconstituted solutions of gemcitabine be refrigerated because crystallization may occur.

Preparation
Each 200- or 1000-mg vial is reconstituted with 5 or 25 mL preservative-free normal saline, respectively, to yield a solution containing 40 mg/mL.

Availability
Gemcitabine is available in 200- and 1000-mg vials of lyophilized powder.

Selected Readings
Carmichael J et al: Advanced breast cancer: a phase II trial with gemcitabine, *J Clin Oncol* 13:2731-2736, 1995.

Rothenberg ML et al: A phase II trial of gemcitabine in patients with 5-FU-refractory pancreas cancer, *Ann Oncol* 7:347-353, 1996.

GOSERELIN
Other Names
Zoladex, ICI 118630, NSC-606864.

Indications
FDA approved for the palliative treatment of endometriosis and advanced carcinoma of the prostate. Goserelin may also be a useful treatment for patients with breast cancer.

Classification and Mechanisms of Action
Goserelin is a luteinizing hormone–releasing hormone (LHRH) analogue. In men, administration of pharmacologic doses inhibits gonadotropin release, resulting in decreased serum concentrations of luteinizing

hormone (LH), follicle stimulating hormone (FSH), and testosterone (estradiol in women). After 1 to 2 weeks, downregulation of LHRH receptors occurs, with reduced LH and FSH secretion and castration levels of testosterone or estradiol. With continued goserelin therapy (every 28 days) the concentrations of these hormones can be expected to remain at castration levels for over 2 years. The drug also binds to LHRH receptors in breast cancer tissue.

Pharmacokinetics
Goserelin is slowly released from the implanted pellet over a 28-day period. Peak serum concentrations occur 12 to 15 days after administration. The drug is almost totally eliminated as unchanged goserelin in the urine; its elimination half-life is 4.2 hours. The half-life has been shown to be prolonged (to 12 hours) in patients with impaired renal function (i.e., creatinine clearance less than 20 mL/min); however, dose adjustments are not necessary.

Dose
Recommended doses are 3.6 mg injected subcutaneously every 28 days or 10.8 mg by subcutaneous injection every 12 weeks.

Administration
Subcutaneous injection of the depot pellet into abdominal fat after swabbing the site with alcohol. A local anesthetic, such as 0.2 mL of lidocaine 1%, may be administered intradermally before injection.

Toxicity
Gastrointestinal. Infrequent nausea (5%), vomiting, anorexia (5%), diarrhea, and/or constipation.

Dermatological. Local discomfort lasting up to 30 minutes occurs occasionally. Skin rash (7%), diaphoresis (6% men, 45% women). In women, acne (42%), seborrhea (26%), hirsutism (7%).

Hepatic. Elevated serum cholesterol levels.

Neurological. Dizziness (5%), insomnia (5% to 11%), depression (54% in women), lethargy (8%).

Endocrine Hot flashes (men, 62%; women, 96%), decreased libido (men, 21%), increased libido (women, 12%), impotence (18% to 21%), gynecomastia in men, cessation of menses, spotting, dyspareunia (14%), vaginitis (75%).

Tumor flare. In patients with carcinoma of the prostate or breast, tumor flare (consisting of increased bone pain, spinal cord compression, and other symptoms) may occur in up to 25% of the patients. Tumor flare reactions usually occur in the first 2 weeks of treatment and are blocked by antiandrogens (flutamide) in men.

Other. Headache (75% in women), muscle weakness (rare), fatigue (5% to 8%); pituitary adenomas have been reported in rats.

Storage and Stability
Store at room temperature. Each syringe bears an expiration date.

Availability
Commercially available in prefilled syringes containing 3.6 and 10.8 mg of goserelin.

Selected Readings
Ahmann FR et al: Zoladex: a sustained-release, monthly luteinizing hormone–releasing hormone analogue for the treatment of advanced prostate cancer, *J Clin Oncol* 5:912-917, 1987.

Kaufmann M et al: Goserelin: a depot gonadotrophin-releasing hormone agonist in the treatment of premenopausal patients with metastatic breast cancer, *J Clin Oncol* 7:1113-1119, 1989.

Williams MR et al: Use of an LHRH agonist (ICI 118,630, Zoladex) in advanced pre-menopausal breast cancer, *Br J Cancer* 53:629-636, 1986.

H

HOMOHARRINGTONINE

Other Names
Cephalotaxine, HHT, 4-methyl-2-hydroxy-2-(4-hydroxy-4-methylpentyl) butanedioate ester, NSC-141633.

Indications
Homoharringtonine is an investigational agent that is undergoing evaluation as a treatment for acute leukemias.

Classification and Mechanisms of Action
Plant alkaloid. Homoharringtonine inhibits biosynthesis of protein, DNA, and RNA by inhibition of chain initiation.

Dose
Doses of 2 to 7 mg/m^2/day for a period of 5 to 8 days by continuous IV infusion have been investigated.

Administration
Intravenously, usually by continuous infusion.

Toxicity
Hematological. Leukopenia and thrombocytopenia are expected.

Gastrointestinal. Mild nausea, vomiting, anorexia, diarrhea.

Dermatological. Alopecia.

Hepatic. Transient elevations of hepatic transaminase levels.

Neurological. Confusion, lethargy, agitation, depression.

Cardiovascular. Hypotension may be severe and can occur during administration of the drug or up to 12 hours after discontinuation of the IV infusion. Tachycardia and cardiac arrhythmias have been reported.

Other. Hyperglycemia.

Storage and Stability
The intact vials should be stored in the freezer ($-10°$ to $-20°$ C). Reconstituted solutions and solutions further diluted to concentrations of 0.05 mg/mL in normal saline or 5% dextrose are chemically stable for 96 hours at room temperature.

Preparation
The 10-mg vial is reconstituted with 4.9 mL of normal saline to result in a solution containing 2 mg/mL. The desired dose is usually further diluted in normal saline or 5% dextrose.

Availability
Homoharringtonine is available from the NCI as a lyophilized powder in 10-mg vials.

Selected Readings
O'Dwyer PJ et al: Homoharringtonine: perspectives on an active new natural product, *J Clin Oncol* 4:1563-1568, 1986.

Ohnuma T, Holland JF: Homoharringtonine as a new antileukemic agent, *J Clin Oncol* 3:604-605, 1985.

HYDROXYUREA
Other Names
Hydrea, hydroxycarbamide, SQ-1089, WR-83799, NSC-32065.

Indications
FDA approved for the treatment of melanoma; resistant chronic myelogenous leukemia; recurrent, metastatic, or inoperable carcinoma of the ovary; and head and neck cancer. Hydroxyurea may also be useful for polycythemia vera, trophoblastic neoplasms, and cancers of the cervix and prostate.

Classification
Antimetabolite (ribonucleotide reductase inhibitor).

Pharmacokinetics
Hydroxyurea is well absorbed (>80%) by mouth. Peak serum concentrations occur approximately 2 hours after dosing. Hydroxyurea is distributed into breast milk. Approximately 50% of the drug is metabolized by the liver to inactive compounds; the other 50% is excreted unchanged in the urine. Hydroxyurea has an elimination half-life of 2 to 5 hours. It has been recommended that the dose be reduced in patients with renal impairment (i.e., a 50% reduction for a creatinine clearance of 10 to 50 mL/min, a 75% reduction for a creatinine clearance less than 10 mL/min).

Dose

For the treatment of chronic myelocytic leukemia, a daily dose of 20 to 30 mg/kg has been used. For the treatment of solid tumors or in combination with radiation therapy for the treatment of patients with cancer of the head and neck, a recommended dose is 60 to 80 mg/kg (or 2000 to 3000 mg/m^2) as a single dose every third day. Alternatively, 1250 mg/m^2 every 8 hours for 5 doses has been given once weekly.

Administration

Oral. If the capsules cannot be swallowed, they may be opened and the drug may be dissolved in water. Some of the excipients in the capsules will not dissolve in water. The white powder floating on top of the water may be discarded. The injectable formulation has been administered as a slow IV push or as a prolonged IV infusion over a period of 8 hours or longer.

Toxicity

Hematological. Leukopenia is expected and is occasionally dose limiting. Thrombocytopenia, anemia, and megaloblastic erythropoiesis are frequent occurrences.

Gastrointestinal. Nausea and vomiting are uncommon. Diarrhea, constipation, mucositis, and anorexia are rare.

Dermatological. Maculopapular rash, facial erythema, hyperpigmentation, pruritus, alopecia (rare), radiation recall phenomenon (rare).

Hepatic. Transient elevation of hepatic transaminase levels; jaundice and hepatitis have been rarely reported.

Neurological. Headache, drowsiness, dizziness, disorientation, hallucinations, and seizures are rare events.

Renal. Hyperuricemia, dysuria, increased BUN and serum creatinine levels, proteinuria.

Other. Pulmonary edema (rare), flulike syndrome (fever, chills, malaise), acral erythema (rare).

Storage and Stability

Store oral capsules at room temperature. Bottles bear expiration dates.

Availability

Hydroxyurea is commercially available in 500-mg capsules. An injectable formulation of hydroxyurea is available from the NCI as a 2000-mg vial.

Selected Readings

Kennedy BJ: Hydroxyurea therapy in chronic myelogenous leukemia, *Cancer* 29:1052-1056, 1972.

Weppelmann B et al: Treatment of recurrent head and neck cancer with 5-fluorouracil, hydroxyurea, and reirradiation, *Int J Radiat Oncol Biol Phys* 22:1051-1056, 1992.

IDARUBICIN

Other Names
Idarubicin hydrochloride, Idamycin, Zavedos, 4-demethoxydaunoru-bicin, NSC-256439.

Indications
FDA approved for the treatment of acute nonlymphocytic leukemia.

Classification
Anthracycline antitumor antibiotic.

Pharmacokinetics
Idarubicin is poorly absorbed (approximately 20% to 30%) by mouth. Idarubicin is metabolized by the liver to several metabolites, including idarubicinol, which is active. Significantly more idarubicinol is formed after administration of idarubicin. The clinical significance of this observation is uncertain. Some of the drug penetrates into the cerebrospinal fluid (20% idarubicin, 10% idarubicinol). Approximately 25% of the drug is excreted unchanged in the bile, 2% to 3% in the urine. The elimination half-life of idarubicin is 13 to 26 hours; for idarubicinol, it is 38 to 63 hours.

Dose
The usual dose for leukemia induction therapy is 12 mg/m^2/day for 3 days (combined with cytarabine, 200 mg/m^2/day for 7 days). Single doses of 8 to 15 mg/m^2 every 3 weeks have also been used.

Administration
IV injection (using extravasation precautions) over a 1- to 5-minute period.

Toxicity
Hematological. Myelosuppression (leukopenia and thrombocytopenia) is expected. Leukopenia is usually more severe than thrombocytopenia. Anemia also occurs but is a less frequent complication.

Gastrointestinal. Nausea and vomiting are common (82%), usually mild to moderate in severity, and preventable with antiemetic treatment. Diarrhea (20% to 73%), mucositis (50%), and enterocolitis may also occur.

Dermatological. Alopecia is common but usually partial; extravasation reactions, hives, urticaria, and radiation recall reactions are uncommon.

Hepatic. Transient elevation of hepatic transaminase levels occur infrequently.

Cardiovascular. Transient arrhythmia; cardiomyopathy and congestive heart failure can occur after large cumulative doses have been administered. Idarubicin is less cardiotoxic than daunorubicin and doxorubicin, but the same monitoring criteria apply. At cumulative doses of 150 to 290 mg/m^2, cardiomyopathy occurred in 5% of the patients. The results from a retrospective study indicated that the probability of developing a 15% or greater decrease in left ventricular ejection fraction to a level less than or equal to 45% is 7% after a cumulative idarubicin dose of 150 mg/m^2.

Neurological. Headache (20%), peripheral neuropathy (7%), seizures (4%).

Storage and Stability
Idarubicin vials are stored at room temperature. The reconstituted solution is stable for 3 days at room temperature and 7 days under refrigeration.

Preparation
Each 5-, 10-, or 20-mg vial is diluted with 5, 10, or 20 mL, respectively, of preservative-free normal saline or sterile water for injection to yield a 1 mg/mL solution. The manufacturer does not recommend the use of diluents that contain preservatives.

Incompatibilities
Idarubicin is incompatible with fluorouracil, etoposide, dexamethasone, heparin, hydrocortisone, methotrexate, vincristine, and other drugs. Idarubicin is deactivated on prolonged contact with alkaline solutions. A pharmacist should be consulted for additional information.

Compatibilities
Idarubicin and cytarabine are compatible at the "Y"-site.

Availability
Commercially available as a lyophilized powder in 5-, 10-, and 20-mg vials.

Selected Readings
Anderlini P et al: Idarubicin cardiotoxicity: a retrospective study in acute myeloid leukemia and myelodysplasia, *J Clin Oncol* 13:2827-2834, 1995.

Fields SM, Koeller JM: Idarubicin: a second generation anthracycline, *DICP Ann Pharmacother* 25:505-517, 1991.

Mandelli F et al: A randomized clinical trial comparing idarubicin and cytarabine to daunorubicin and cytarabine in the treatment of acute non-lymphoid leukemia, *Eur J Cancer* 27:750-755, 1991.

Vogler WR et al: A phase III trial comparing idarubicin and daunorubicin combined with cytarabine in acute myelogenous leukemia: a Southeastern Cancer Group study, *J Clin Oncol* 10:1103-1111, 1992.

IFOSFAMIDE

Other Names
Ifex, isophosphamide, Mitoxana, Holoxan, Naxamide, NSC-109724.

Indications
FDA approved for the treatment of relapsed testicular carcinoma. Ifosfamide may be useful for Hodgkin's and non-Hodgkin's lymphoma, acute leukemias, Ewing's sarcoma, osteosarcoma, trophoblastic neoplasms, soft-tissue sarcomas, and cancers of the breast, lung, ovary, stomach, and pancreas.

Classification
Alkylating agent.

Pharmacokinetics
Similar to cyclophosphamide, ifosfamide must be activated by hepatic microsomal enzymes. However, since less of the drug is activated, higher doses must be given (as compared with cyclophosphamide). The drug is metabolized by the liver to inactive metabolites and approximately 15% to 56% of the drug is excreted unchanged in the urine. The chloroacetaldehyde metabolite of ifosfamide may be responsible for much of the neurotoxic adverse effects. The clearance of this metabolite is slowed in patients with renal dysfunction. Ifosfamide has an elimination half-life of 7 to 15 hours. Ifosfamide is believed to be more efficacious when given daily for 5 days as compared with a single dose. Pharmacokinetic changes between the two dosing schedules (decreased half-life and urinary recovery of unchanged drug associated with the 5-day schedule) suggest that a single dose of drug "activates" microsomal enzyme systems to activate subsequent doses. Ifosfamide has been detected in breast milk.

Dose
Ifosfamide, (1000 to 1200 mg/m^2/day) is often given over a span of 5 consecutive days and repeated every 3 to 4 weeks. Higher doses (e.g., 2500 to 4000 mg/m^2/day) have been given over a 2- to 3-day period. Mesna must also be given with ifosfamide. The usual dose of mesna is 20% of the ifosfamide dose, given just before and 4 and 8 hours after ifosfamide (the total mesna dose is 60% of the ifosfamide dose). Mesna has also been given as a continuous IV infusion concurrently with ifosfamide; a total dose of mesna equal to the total dose of ifosfamide is given, preceded by a loading dose of 6% to 10% of the total ifosfamide dose. Occasionally the last dose of mesna is given orally so that the patient may take the drug at home.

Administration
Administered intravenously in 250 mL or more of 5% dextrose or normal saline over a 30-minute period or longer. It is recommended that patients receive aggressive concomitant hydration (at least 2 L/m^2/day) during ifosfamide dosing to reduce the incidence of hemorrhagic cystitis. Concomitant uroprotective therapy with mesna, as described above, is also recommended.

Toxicity
Hematological. Myelosuppression is a major dose-limiting toxicity. The leukopenic nadir usually occurs 7 to 10 days posttreatment. Thrombocytopenia and anemia occur less frequently.

Gastrointestinal. Nausea and vomiting are common (58%), dose related, and preventable in the majority of patients when antiemetics are used. However, antiemetic therapy (with sedating drugs) may mask detection of somnolence sometimes caused by ifosfamide. Anorexia, constipation, diarrhea, salivation, and stomatitis occur occasionally.

Dermatological. Alopecia is common (83%). Rash, urticaria, nail ridging, dermatitis, and hyperpigmentation are uncommon.

Hepatic. Elevated hepatic transaminase levels and hyperbilirubinemia are usually mild, transient, and uncommon.

Neurological. Occasional (12%) episodes of somnolence, lethargy, ataxia, disorientation, confusion, dizziness, malaise, depressive psychosis, and coma have been reported. These toxicities occur more frequently when ifosfamide is given over a 1-day period (versus 5 days), in the presence of impaired renal function (caused by impaired clearance of the toxic metabolite chloroacetaldehyde), in patients with hypoalbuminemia, and when sedatives (e.g., lorazepam, opiates) are administered concomitantly. Myoclonus and seizures have been rarely reported.

Genitourinary. Ifosfamide-induced hemorrhagic cystitis (more than four rbc/hpf) occurs relatively frequently when uroprotective measures are not used. The incidence of hemorrhagic cystitis is dose and schedule related (more common with a single high-dose regimen versus multiple-dose regimens). The use of mesna (greater than 20% of the ifosfamide dose) given before and after each ifosfamide dose greatly reduces the incidence and severity of this adverse effect. Whether mesna reduces the risk of developing secondary bladder carcinoma is not known.

Renal. Elevated serum creatinine levels occur infrequently with standard doses of ifosfamide. However, with higher doses (e.g., 4000 mg/day for 3 days) renal toxicity may be dose limiting.

Other. Hyponatremia, hypokalemia, phlebitis, fever, and hypotension or hypertension.

Storage and Stability
Unreconstituted vials are stored at room temperature. Ifosfamide liquefies at temperatures above 35° C. Appropriately reconstituted ifosfamide and ifosfamide further diluted to 16 mg/mL or 0.6 mg/mL in 5% dextrose, 5% dextrose and Ringer's injection, 5% dextrose and normal saline, lactated Ringer's solution, 0.45% sodium chloride, normal saline, or 1/6 M sodium lactate are stable for 7 days at room temperature and 6 weeks under refrigeration. Ifosfamide, 10 to 80 mg/mL in normal saline, is stable for at least 8 days in PVC portable pump infusion cassettes.

Preparation
Reconstitute the 1000-mg and 3000-mg vials with 20 and 60 mL of sterile water, respectively, to yield a concentration of 50 mg/mL. Bacteriostatic water for injection may also be used to reconstitute ifosfamide.

Compatibilities
Ifosfamide and mesna (in equal concentrations) are chemically stable at room temperature for at least 24 hours in 5% dextrose or lactated Ringer's solution. Ifosfamide (2600 mg/L) and mesna (1600 mg/L) are stable for at least 7 hours at room temperature in 5% dextrose or 0.9% sodium chloride. Ifosfamide (500 mg/10 mL) and mesna (400 mg/10 mL)

combined in polypropylene syringes are compatible for at least 7 days at room temperature.

Availability
Ifosfamide is commercially available as a lyophilized powder in 1000- and 3000-mg vials.

Selected Readings
Dechant KL et al: Ifosfamide/mesna: a review of its antineoplastic activity, pharmacokinetic properties and therapeutic efficacy in cancer, *Drugs* 42:428-467, 1991.

Goren MP et al: Potentiation of ifosfamide neurotoxicity, hematotoxicity and tubular nephrotoxicity by prior cis-diamminedichloroplatinum(II) therapy, *Cancer Res* 47:1457-1460, 1987.

Le Cesne A et al: High-dose ifosfamide: circumvention of resistance to standard-dose ifosfamide in advanced soft-tissue sarcoma, *J Clin Oncol* 13:1600-1608, 1995.

Yarbro JW, Bornstein RS, Mastrangelo MJ, eds: Advances in ifosfamide chemotherapy, *Semin Oncol* 17(suppl 4):1-79, 1992.

Zalupski M, Baker LH: Ifosfamide, *J Natl Cancer Inst* 80:556-566, 1988.

IRINOTECAN

Other Names
Camptosar, CPT-11, camptothecin-11.

Indications
FDA approved for metastatic colorectal carcinoma after initial therapy with fluorouracil. The drug also may be useful in carcinoma of the lung, cervix, and ovary.

Classification
Topoisomerase I inhibitor.

Pharmacokinetics
Metabolized to 7-ethyl-10-hydroxycamptothecin (SN-38), which is 40 to 200 times as potent as irinotecan. Irinotecan has a triphasic elimination pattern with an elimination half-life of 16 to 18 hours. SN-38 has an elimination half-life of 7 to 14 hours.

Dose
Several regimens have been evaluated, including 100 to 125 mg/m^2/week for 3 weeks, repeated every 4 weeks; 125 to 150 mg/m^2/week for 4 weeks followed by a 2-week rest period; 150 mg/m^2 every other week; 200 to 240 mg/m^2 every 3 to 4 weeks; 40 mg/m^2/day for 5 days every 4 weeks; 20 mg/m^2/dose twice daily for 7 days every 4 weeks; 40 mg/m^2/day for 3 days every week; and 30 mg/m^2/day (continuous infusion) for 5 days every 4 weeks. When combined with cisplatin (80 mg/m^2 on day 1 every 4 weeks), the usual dose of irinotecan is 60 mg/m^2/week for 3 weeks (days 1, 8, and 15).

Administration
Irinotecan is given by IV infusion in 500 mL of 5% dextrose or normal saline over a period of 60 to 90 minutes or longer.

Toxicity

Hematological. Neutropenia is dose limiting, and there is a 25% incidence of Grade 3 or greater neutropenia with 100 mg/m^2/week. With the weekly for 3 weeks schedule, nadir blood counts occur around day 30 and recover by day 35. Other hematological toxicities include eosinophilia (30%), anemia (15%), and thrombocytopenia. In patients who are taking warfarin (Coumadin), an increase in prothrombin times has been observed after treatment with irinotecan.

Gastrointestinal. Diarrhea is dose limiting and occasionally severe and unpredictable. In some studies a 15% to 25% incidence of Grade 3 or 4 diarrhea occurred with irinotecan administered at a dose of 100 mg/m^2/week. In one study involving 72 patients, diarrhea was uncontrollable in 3 of 72 patients (4%). Diarrhea usually begins after the second or third dose. It has been recommended that treatment with an aggressive regimen of loperamide be initiated at the first sign of diarrhea (e.g., first loose stool or episode of two or more bowel movements in one day). The recommended loperamide dose is 4 mg at the first sign of diarrhea followed by 2 mg every 2 hours (4 mg every 4 hours during the night) until there are no signs of diarrhea for a period of at least 12 hours. Prophylactic use of loperamide is not recommended.

Moderate to severe nausea and vomiting occurs in 20% to 25% of the patients. Other gastrointestinal toxicities include anorexia (63%), abdominal pain (19%), mucositis (4%), constipation (13%), bloating, and heartburn. Flushing, cramping, and diarrhea were reported to be significantly reduced by premedication with ondansetron and diphenhydramine with or without atropine.

Dermatological. Alopecia (40% to 56% overall, 4% significant), skin rash (rare), hives, pigmentation.

Hepatic. Elevated liver enzyme levels (7% to 20%).

Renal. Elevated serum creatinine levels and hematuria are rare.

Pulmonary. Dyspnea on exertion and pulmonary infiltrates (3%). The onset of symptoms occurs in approximately 60 days (range 40 to 175 days) after beginning treatment with irinotecan. Pneumonitis has also been reported.

Other. Fever (7%), chills, diaphoresis, fatigue (25%), salivation (35%), lacrimation (26%), bradycardia (13%), elevated serum amylase levels.

Storage and Stability

Irinotecan is stored at room temperature where it is stable for at least 3 years from the date of manufacture. Mixed in glass bottles or plastic containers containing 500 mL of 5% dextrose or normal saline, the drug is stable at room temperature for at least 24 hours. Solutions of irinotecan should not be refrigerated; precipitation may occur.

Preparation

Irinotecan is further diluted in 500 mL normal saline or 5% dextrose.

Availability
Irinotecan is available as a 20 mg/mL solution in 2- and 5-mL vials.

Selected Readings

Abigerges D et al: Phase I and pharmacologic studies of the camptothecin analog irinotecan administered every 3 weeks in cancer patients, *J Clin Oncol* 13:210-221, 1995.

Conti JA et al: Irinotecan is an active agent in untreated patients with metastatic colorectal cancer, *J Clin Oncol* 14:709-715, 1996.

Fukuoka BM et al: A phase II study of CPT-11, a new derivative of camptothecin, for previously untreated non–small-cell lung cancer, *J Clin Oncol* 10:16-20, 1992.

Rothenberg ML et al: Phase II trial of irinotecan in patients with progressive or rapidly recurrent colorectal cancer, *J Clin Oncol* 14:1128-1135, 1996.

ISOTRETINOIN

Other Names
Accutane, Accutane Roche, 13-*cis*-retinoic acid, 13-CRA.

Indications
Investigational studies are evaluating the effectiveness of isotretinoin as a chemoprevention agent for myelodysplastic syndromes, cutaneous squamous cell cancers, melanoma, head and neck cancer, cutaneous T-cell lymphoma, and other malignancies.

Classification and Mechanisms of Action
Isotretinoin is a derivative of vitamin A. The drug binds to a cellular protein that facilitates the transfer of isotretinoin from cellular cytoplasm into the nucleus. Isotretinoin is believed to increase DNA, RNA, and protein synthesis and to affect cellular mitosis. Isotretinoin affects the function of lymphocytes and monocytes, which results in a modulation of the cellular immune response. Isotretinoin possesses some antiinflammatory activity.

Pharmacokinetics
Isotretinoin is a natural retinoic acid metabolite (basal concentrations, 3 to 4 ng/mL). After oral administration, peak plasma levels occur in approximately 3 hours. The oral bioavailability of isotretinoin is around 25%. The drug is almost totally bound to plasma albumin, is metabolized to 4-oxo-isotretinoin, and is eliminated in the urine and feces. Isotretinoin has an elimination half-life of 10 to 20 hours; 4-oxo-isotretinoin has an elimination half-life around 24 hours (range 10 to 50 hours). Because of the extensive protein binding of isotretinoin, dose adjustments are not necessary for patients undergoing dialysis.

Dose
As a chemoprevention treatment, isotretinoin has been given in doses of 0.5 to 2 mg/kg/day for 3 months or longer (oral leukoplakia), 2.5 to 4 mg/kg/day for 8 weeks, and 20 to 125 mg/m^2/day for up to 6 months

(myelodysplastic syndromes). For the treatment of severe cystic acne, doses of 0.5 to 2 mg/kg/day for 15 to 20 weeks are recommended.

Administration
Oral as a single daily dose.

Toxicity
Hematological. Elevated sedimentation rate (40%). Thrombocytopenia, thrombocythemia, and anemia occur rarely.

Gastrointestinal. Nausea, vomiting, and abdominal pain (20%); xerostomia (80%), anorexia (4%), stomatitis, inflammatory bowel disease (diarrhea, rectal bleeding, and abdominal pain), chelitis (common), glossitis (common), inflamed and/or bleeding gums (rare).

Dermatological. Almost all patients will develop cheilitis and dry skin with mild exfoliation. Pruritus (80%) and skin fragility (80%) are also common. Rash, thinning of hair, epistaxis, and nail brittleness occur infrequently (less than 10%). Photosensitivity (30%). Erythema nodosum, hypopigmentation or hyperpigmentation, urticaria, hirsutism, and skin infections occur in less than 5% of the patients.

Hepatic. Transient elevations of hepatic enzyme levels and/or hyperbilirubinemia occur in 10% to 20% of the patients and may persist for weeks after treatment is stopped. Hepatitis has been reported in some patients.

Neurological. Headache (5%), fatigue, lethargy, and mental depression occur infrequently. Pseudotumor cerebri (manifested as papilledema, headache, nausea, vomiting, and visual disturbances) has occurred in patients taking isotretinoin.

Ocular. Conjunctivitis occurs in 40% to 55% of the patients. Corneal erosion, blurred vision, decreased tolerance to contact lenses, papilledema, corneal opacities, cataracts, and photophobia occur occasionally. Dry eyes and night blindness (which may occur suddenly) are infrequent toxicities but may persist after stopping therapy.

Other. Isotretinoin is teratogenic. Fetal abnormalities (e.g., thymic aplasia, craniofacial malformation, hydrocephalus, cleft palate, cerebellar malformation) are likely if in utero exposure occurs. Bone pain, myalgia, and arthralgia may occur in up to 20% of the patients and in some may be dose limiting. These symptoms may persist after treatment is stopped. Elevated serum triglyceride levels occur in approximately 25% of the patients; mild to moderate decreases in high-density lipoproteins have been reported in 15% to 70% of patients taking isotretinoin. White cells in the urine (10% to 20%), proteinuria, hematuria (less than 10%), abnormal menses (less than 1%). Other uncommon toxicities that have been reported in patients taking isotretinoin include hyperglycemia, hyperuricemia, elevated creatinine phosphokinase and serum cholesterol levels (7%), and skeletal hyperostosis.

Storage and Stability
Isotretinoin is stored at room temperature protected from light. Each bottle bears an expiration date.

Compatibilities
In patients who are receiving treatment with carbamazepine, isotretinoin may decrease serum carbamazepine concentrations. Combined with ethanol, isotretinoin may cause disulfiram-like reactions.

Availability
Isotretinoin is commercially available as 10-, 20-, and 40-mg capsules.

Selected Readings
Benner SE et al: Toxicity of isotretinoin in a chemoprevention trial to prevent second primary tumors after head and neck cancer, *J Natl Cancer Inst* 86:1799-1800, 1994.

Hong WK et al: Prevention of second primary tumors with isotretinoin in squamous cell carcinoma of the head and neck, *N Engl J Med* 323:795-801, 1990.

Smith MA et al: Retinoids in cancer therapy, *J Clin Oncol* 10:839-864, 1992.

L

LEUCOVORIN CALCIUM

Other Names
Leucovorin, Wellcovorin, citrovorum factor, folinic acid, 5-formyltetrahydrofolate, LV, LCV, NSC-3590.

Indications
FDA approved as a rescue agent after high-dose methotrexate therapy for osteosarcoma, to counteract the effects of folic acid antagonists (e.g., trimethoprim or pyrimethamine), in combination with fluorouracil in the treatment of advanced colorectal carcinoma, and megaloblastic anemia when treatment with folic acid is not feasible. Leucovorin combined with fluorouracil may be a useful treatment for breast, head and neck, lung, stomach, and pancreatic cancers; non-Hodgkin's lymphoma; and trophoblastic neoplasms.

Classification and Mechanisms of Action
Leucovorin is a tetrahydrofolic acid derivative that acts as a biochemical cofactor for carbon transfer reactions in the synthesis of purines and pyrimidines. Leucovorin does not require the enzyme dihydrofolate reductase (DHFR) for conversion to tetrahydrofolic acid. The effects of methotrexate and other DHFR antagonists are inhibited by leucovorin.

Leucovorin can potentiate the cytotoxic effects of fluorinated pyrimidines (i.e., fluorouracil [5-FU], floxuridine, tegafur). After 5-FU is activated within the cell, it is accompanied by a folate cofactor and inhibits the enzyme thymidylate synthase, thus inhibiting pyrimidine synthesis. Leucovorin increases the folate pool, thereby increasing the binding of folate cofactor and active metabolites of 5-FU with thymidylate synthase.

Pharmacokinetics

Leucovorin is well absorbed (75% to 97%) by mouth and is readily converted to 5-methyltetrahydrofolate after administration. Peak serum concentrations occur approximately 1.7 to 2.5 hours after an oral dose. More of active *l*-isomer (versus the inactive *d*-isomer) is absorbed after oral dosing. Reduced accumulation of the *d*-isomer favors potentiation of fluorouracil-leucovorin synergy. Leucovorin is excreted into the urine as metabolites and has an elimination half-life of approximately 2 to 6 hours.

Dose

When used as a rescue agent for methotrexate, doses of 10 to 25 mg/m^2 orally or intravenously every 6 hours for 6 to 8 doses (beginning 6 to 24 hours after methotrexate) are most commonly used. Dose adjustments are made based on methotrexate serum levels and serum creatinine levels (Table 3-2). When combined with intrathecal methotrexate, smaller doses of leucovorin may be given immediately after dosing. When used to avert trimethoprim- or pyrimethamine-induced myelosuppression, a daily leucovorin dose of 5 mg is adequate. When used to potentiate the effects of fluorinated pyrimidines, doses ranging from 20 to 500 mg/m^2 orally or intravenously have been used. High-dose (500 mg/m^2) oral leucovorin is usually given in 125 mg/m^2 increments for 4 doses.

Administration

Leucovorin has been given orally, intramuscularly, intraperitoneally, and via IV push and IV infusion in 50 mL or more of 5% dextrose or normal saline over a period of several minutes or longer.

Toxicity

Hematological. Thrombocytosis.

Gastrointestinal. Nausea, upset stomach, diarrhea.

Dermatological. Skin rash.

Allergic. Skin rash, hives, pruritus.

Pulmonary. Wheezing (possibly allergic in origin).

Other. Headache; may potentiate the toxic effects of fluoropyrimidine therapy, resulting in increased hematological and gastrointestinal (diarrhea, stomatitis) adverse effects.

Storage and Stability

All dosage forms are stored at room temperature. The reconstituted parenteral solution, 10 mg/mL, is stable for at least 7 days at room temperature. Leucovorin (0.5 to 0.9 mg/mL) is chemically stable at room temperature for at least 24 hours in normal saline, 5% dextrose, 10% dextrose, Ringer's solution, or lactated Ringer's solution. The oral solution, 1 mg/mL, is stable for 14 days if refrigerated and 7 days at room temperature.

TABLE 3-2
Leucovorin Rescue Dosing Guidelines

MTX level at 24 hours (Molar)	Increase in serum creatinine at 24 hours	Leucovorin dose starting 24 hours after MTX (mg/m²)	Further actions
$\leq 5 \times 10^{-7}$	<50%	10 every 6 hours × 6 doses	None
$\leq 5 \times 10^{-7}$	≥50%	10 every 6 hours × 8 doses	Monitor 24-hour MTX next course
$>5 \times 10^{-7}$ but $<1 \times 10^{-6}$	<50%	10 every 6 hours × 10 doses	Monitor 24-hour MTX next course
$>5 \times 10^{-7}$ but $<1 \times 10^{-6}$	≥50%	10 every 6 hours until [MTX] $<1 \times 10^{-8}$	Monitor 24-hour MTX and serum creatinine daily until MTX $<1 \times 10^{-8}$
$\geq 1 \times 10^{-6}$	<50%	10 every 6 hours × 12 doses $<1 \times 10^{-8}$	Obtain 48-hour MTX; if $<5 \times 10^{-7}$, do nothing more; if $\geq 5 \times 10^{-7}$, continue leucovorin until MTX
$\geq 1 \times 10^{-6}$	≥50%	25 every 6 hours until [MTX] $<1 \times 10^{-8}$	Hydrate with 2 L NS daily until MTX $<1 \times 10^{-7}$; monitor MTX and serum creatinine daily; admit to hospital for hydration and IV leucovorin if necessary

MTX, methotrexate; *[MTX]*, methotrexate serum concentration; *NS*, normal saline.

Preparation

The 50- and 100-mg vials for injection are reconstituted with 5 and 10 mL of sterile water or bacteriostatic water, respectively, so as to result in a 10 mg/mL solution. The 350-mg vial is reconstituted with 17 mL of sterile water to result in a 20-mg/mL solution. The 60-mg bottle oral formulation is reconstituted with 60 mL of aromatic elixir provided to result in a 1 mg/mL solution.

Incompatibilities

Leucovorin is incompatible with sodium bicarbonate, foscarnet, and droperidol.

Compatibilities

Leucovorin (0.03, 0.24, and 0.96 mg/mL) is stable for 48 hours at room and refrigeration temperatures when admixed with floxuridine (1, 2, or 4 mg/mL) in normal saline. Leucovorin (1 mg/mL) is also compatible with fluorouracil (5 to 25 mg/mL) for 14 days at room temperature. Leucovorin and methotrexate are also compatible. A pharmacist should be consulted for additional information.

Availability

Commercially available as a tablet (5-, 10-, 15-, and 25-mg), powder for oral solution (60 mg/bottle), and in parenteral formulations (5-mg ampules; 50-, 100-, 200-, and 350-mg vials).

Selected Readings

Anonymous: *Leucovorin*, Lederle Laboratories, Pearl River, NY, 1987, Professional Services, American Cyanamid Co.

Arbuck SG: Overview of clinical trials using 5-fluorouracil and leucovorin for the treatment of colorectal cancer, *Cancer* 63:1036-1044, 1989.

Grem JL: 5-Fluorouracil plus leucovorin in cancer therapy. In Devita VT Jr, Hellman S, Rosenberg SA, eds: *Principles and practice of oncology, PPO updates* 2:1-12, 1988.

Poon MA et al: Biochemical modulation of fluorouracil with leucovorin: confirmatory evidence of improved therapeutic efficacy in advanced colorectal cancer, *J Clin Oncol* 9:1967-1972, 1991.

LEUPROLIDE ACETATE

Other Names

Lupron, Lupron Depot, Lupron Depot-3 Month, leuprorelin acetate.

Indications

FDA approved for the palliative treatment of advanced prostatic carcinoma and management of endometriosis (including pain relief and reduction of endometriotic lesions). Leuprolide may be useful in the treatment of breast and islet cell cancers.

Classification and Mechanisms of Action

Leuprolide is a gonadotropin-releasing hormone (GnRH) analogue that binds to GnRH receptors in the pituitary, resulting in an initial increase and later a substantial decrease in secretion of luteinizing hormone (LH) and follicle stimulating hormone (FSH). Decreases in LH and FSH result in castration levels of serum testosterone in men and postmenopausal estrogen and progesterone levels in women, which result in growth inhibition of hormone-responsive tumors. Leuprolide is usually administered in combination with an antiandrogen, such as flutamide or bicalutamide.

Pharmacokinetics
Leuprolide is not absorbed by mouth. After subcutaneous administration of the solution, approximately 95% is absorbed and 7% to 15% of the drug is bound to plasma proteins. Absorption of the depot suspension is 85% to 100% after intramuscular or subcutaneous injection. Leuprolide has an elimination half-life of 3 hours.

Dose
For prostate carcinoma, the usual dosage is 7.5 mg of the depot suspension once a month, 1 mg (0.2 mL) of the injectable solution once daily, or 22.5 mg of the lyophilized microsphere depot once every 12 weeks.

Administration
The depot suspension is injected subcutaneously or intramuscularly. The injectable solution is administered subcutaneously using the syringes provided by the manufacturer. Alternatively, a 0.5 mL, low-dose, disposable U-100 insulin syringe (filled to the 20-unit mark to obtain a 1-mg dose) may be used to administer the injectable solution.

Toxicity
Hematological. Leukopenia and anemia are rare.

Gastrointestinal. Anorexia, nausea, vomiting, constipation, taste change, diarrhea, xerostomia.

Dermatological. Dermatitis, local skin reaction, hair growth or loss, itching, pigmentation, other lesions.

Hepatic. Transient, mild elevation of hepatic transaminase levels is common.

Neurological. Insomnia, depression, dizziness, and headaches are uncommon toxicities. Paresthesias, anxiety, blurred vision, lethargy, memory disorder, mood swings, insomnia, nervousness, numbness, hearing disorder, and syncope are rare.

Cardiovascular. ECG changes (20%), ischemia, high blood pressure, peripheral edema (12%); thrombosis/phlebitis, angina, cardiac arrhythmias, myocardial infarction, hypotension, pulmonary embolus, transient ischemic attack/stroke.

Endocrine. Hot flashes (50% to 60%), impotence (common), gynecomastia, breast tenderness, decrease in libido (common), decreased testicular size. In women: amenorrhea (dose related, 98% after the second dose); hypoestrogenic symptoms, including headache, vaginitis, vaginal dryness, depression, emotional lability, decreased bone density, decreased libido, breast tenderness, myalgia, insomnia, acne, and increased serum cholesterol levels.

Other. Tumor flare, manifested as increased pain at tumor sites, sometimes causing spinal cord compression or urinary retention; myalgia, asthenia, leukopenia (rare), anemia, and urinary tract symptoms (dysuria, incontinence, bladder spasms occur infrequently). Elevated cholesterol (7%) and triglyceride concentrations (12%) occasionally occur after several months of treatment.

Storage and Stability
The injectable solution is stored in the refrigerator protected from light. However, the vial currently in use may remain at room temperature for several months. The powder for suspension and the depot formulation may be stored at room temperature. After reconstitution of the powder for suspension, it is stable for 24 hours.

Preparation
The powder for suspension is reconstituted with 1 mL of the provided diluent (the diluent ampule contains excess diluent). The vial should be shaken well to obtain a uniform suspension.

Availability
Commercially available in vials containing 3.75 and 7.5 mg of powder for suspension with a diluent ampule and syringe and as a 2.8-mL multidose vial containing 5 mg/mL, supplied with 14 (2-week kit) or 28 (4-week kit) syringes, or in packs of six vials. Lyophilized microspheres of leuprolide are commercially available in 7.5-, 11.25-, 15-, and 22.5-mg vials.

Selected Readings
Dowsett M et al: A dose-comparative endocrine study of leuprorelin in premenopausal breast cancer patients, *Br J Cancer* 62:834-837, 1990.
Sharifi R, Soloway M, Leuprolide Study Group: Clinical study of leuprolide depot formulation in the treatment of advanced prostate cancer, *J Urol* 143:68-71, 1990.

LOMUSTINE
Other Names
CeeNU, CCNU, NSC-79037.

Indications
FDA approved for the treatment of brain tumors and Hodgkin's disease (secondary therapy in combination with other approved drugs). Lomustine may also be useful for the treatment of melanoma, multiple myeloma, non-Hodgkin's lymphoma, and cancers of the breast, lung, colon, rectum, and kidney.

Classification
Alkylating agent of the nitrosourea class.

Pharmacokinetics

Lomustine is thought to be well absorbed by mouth and after topical administration. Peak plasma concentrations occur 3 hours (range 1 to 6 hours) after an oral dose. The drug is widely distributed throughout the body, including breast milk. Concentrations of active metabolites in the cerebrospinal fluid may exceed those measured in the plasma. Lomustine is rapidly metabolized by the liver to active metabolites that are eliminated by the kidneys (50% to 75%). Dose reductions are recommended if renal function is impaired (e.g., a 25% reduction for creatinine clearances of 10 to 50 mL/min, a 50% reduction if the creatinine clearance is less than 10 mL/min). The drug is not hemodialyzable. The elimination half-life is approximately 72 hours.

Dose

A common dose regimen is 100 to 130 mg/m^2 every 6 weeks.

Administration

Oral.

Toxicity

Hematological. Leukopenia and thrombocytopenia are expected, dose limiting, and cumulative. Nadir white blood cell and platelet counts occur approximately 4 to 6 weeks after a dose, and recovery occurs 1 to 2 weeks thereafter. Anemia occurs less frequently and is also cumulative.

Gastrointestinal. Nausea, vomiting, and anorexia occur occasionally. Nausea and vomiting usually begin 45 minutes to 6 hours after administration. Antiemetic premedication is warranted. Anorexia may persist for 2 to 3 days after the nausea and vomiting have subsided. Mucositis is uncommon.

Dermatological. Alopecia is uncommon and usually mild. Skin rash, pruritus, and darkening of the skin are infrequent toxicities.

Hepatic. Elevated hepatic transaminase levels and hyperbilirubinemia are uncommon.

Neurological. Disorientation, lethargy, ataxia, confusion, slurred speech, and dysarthria are uncommon.

Renal. Increased serum creatinine levels and decreased creatinine clearance are uncommon and related to the cumulative dose.

Pulmonary. With long-term administration, pulmonary dysfunction (shortness of breath, decreased diffusing capacity, fibrosis) can occur. Discontinue lomustine after a lifetime dose of 1100 to 1400 mg/m^2 has been given.

Other. Fatigue, tiredness, pallor, menstrual cycle irregularities (amenorrhea), second malignancy (leukemia).

Storage and Stability

Lomustine capsules may be stored at room temperature. Containers bear expiration dates.

Availability
Lomustine is commercially available as 10-, 40-, and 100-mg capsules.

Selected Readings
Hoogstraten B et al: CCNU in the treatment of cancer, *Cancer* 32:38-43, 1973.
Stone MD, Richardson MG: Pulmonary toxicity of lomustine, *Cancer Treat Rep* 71:786-787, 1987.

MECHLORETHAMINE
Other Names
Mustargen, nitrogen mustard, HN_2, NSC-762.

Indications
FDA approved for the treatment of Hodgkin's and non-Hodgkin's lymphomas, lymphosarcoma, chronic myelogenous leukemia, chronic lymphocytic leukemia, polycythemia vera, cutaneous T-cell lymphoma, lung cancer, palliative treatment of metastatic carcinoma resulting in effusion (peritoneal, pericardial, or pleural).

Classification
Alkylating agent.

Pharmacokinetics
Mechlorethamine is rapidly deactivated within the blood and is undetectable within minutes of IV administration. Less than 0.01% of a dose is excreted in the urine. The drug has an elimination half-life of 15 minutes.

Dose
The usual intravenous dose for Hodgkin's disease is 6 mg/m^2 on days 1 and 8 of a monthly treatment cycle (Mustargen-Oncovin-procarbazine-prednisone [MOPP] regimen). The usual intracavitary (i.e., intrapleural) dose is 0.4 mg/kg. A smaller dose (0.2 mg/kg) has been used when the drug is administered intrapericardially. The drug has also been given as a single agent in doses up to 0.4 mg/kg monthly. Mechlorethamine may be used topically in the treatment of mycosis fungoides in a 10 mg/60 mL solution or a petrolatum-based ointment (10-mg/dL). Topical treatment is often administered daily (or more often if necessary) for 6 to 12 months after a complete response is attained.

Administration
Usually administered intravenously over 1 to 5 minutes using extravasation precautions. May also be administered by intracavitary injection or applied topically. It is recommended that ECG monitoring be conducted when mechlorethamine is administered into the pericardial cavity because the drug can cause arrhythmias. Also, intracavitary instillation is usually painful, and patients should be given appropriate analgesia.

M

Intraperitoneal administration should be avoided because intestinal adhesions and obstruction may occur.

Toxicity

Hematological. Leukopenia and thrombocytopenia are expected and dose related.

Gastrointestinal. Nausea and vomiting are common, are often severe, and usually begin within 1 hour of IV administration. Aggressive antiemetic premedication is mandatory. Diarrhea, anorexia, and peptic ulcers occur infrequently.

Dermatological. Discoloration of infused vein, alopecia, tissue irritation, and necrosis if extravasation occurs during IV administration. Use of the antidote sodium thiosulfate is indicated if extravasation occurs, followed by ice compresses for 6 to 12 hours. When mechlorethamine is administered topically, erythema, dermatitis, hyperpigmentation, burning, and pruritus may occur. Contact allergy occurs in approximately 50% of the patients after use of mechlorethamine solution and 25% after use of the ointment formulation. Contact allergy may begin within 2 weeks or 12 months of initiating topical therapy.

Other. Metallic taste, jaundice, fever, precipitation of herpes zoster, peripheral neuropathy, amenorrhea, impaired spermatogenesis, tinnitus, hearing loss (rare), thrombophlebitis, angioedema, secondary neoplasms.

Storage and Stability

Intact vials are stored at room temperature. The manufacturer recommends that the reconstituted solution be used within 60 minutes because of its instability. Within 6 hours, solutions of 1 mg/mL lose 4% to 6% potency in the refrigerator and 8% to 10% potency at room temperature. The 10-mg/dL ointment has traditionally been given a 3-month expiration date.

Preparation

To a 10-mg vial add 10 mL of sterile water or normal saline to yield a solution of 1 mg/mL. It may be further diluted for topical administration. Mechlorethamine has also been dissolved in 95% alcohol (1 mL/10-mg vial × 5 vials) and 4.5 mL is incorporated into aquaphor (454 g) to make a 10-mg/dL ointment.

Incompatibilities

Because of its instability, mechlorethamine is incompatible with other antineoplastic agents and sodium thiosulfate.

Availability

Commercially available as a lyophilized powder in 10-mg vials.

Selected Reading

Hoppe RT et al: Mycosis fungoides: management with topical nitrogen mustard, *J Clin Oncol* 5:1796-1803, 1987.

MEDROXYPROGESTERONE ACETATE

Other Names
Provera, Depo-Provera, Cycrin, Amen, Curretab.

Indications
FDA approved for adjunctive therapy and palliative treatment of inoperable, recurrent, and metastatic endometrial or renal carcinoma.

Classification and Mechanisms of Action
Medroxyprogesterone is a potent progestational agent that also has androgenic activity. The drug has no estrogenic activity. The mechanism of its antineoplastic effects is unknown; it may directly inhibit tumor growth, suppress the release of gonadotropins from the pituitary and inhibit growth of hormone-sensitive tumors, or interact with other hormones. Recent evidence suggests that breast cancer tumors with high levels of androgen receptors respond to treatment more often than tumors without the receptor.

Pharmacokinetics
Medroxyprogesterone acetate (MDA) is absorbed by mouth, reaching peak plasma levels within 1 to 2 hours. Oral bioavailability is around 10% (as a result of inadequate absorption and extensive first-pass metabolism in the liver). After intramuscular injection, plasma levels of MDA remain steady from 1 to 2 hours to 7 days after injection. The elimination half-life of MDA is reported to range from 14 to 60 hours. MDA is metabolized in the liver; 20% to 40% is excreted as inactive metabolites in the urine and 5% to 15% is excreted in the feces.

Dose
Initially, 400 mg to 1000 mg intramuscularly weekly has been used for endometrial or renal carcinoma, with a maintenance dose of as little as 400 mg monthly in responding patients. For breast and prostate cancers, up to 1500 mg/day has been used for induction therapy, with maintenance doses of 500 mg 1 to 3 times weekly. The metabolism of MDA to inactive metabolites may be increased twofold by aminoglutethimide.

Administration
Oral or by intramuscular injection. The suspension for injection must be shaken well to ensure complete mixing of the drug.

Toxicity
Gastrointestinal.   Nausea, cholestatic jaundice.

Dermatological.   Alopecia, acne, hirsutism (all rare). Discoloration or sterile abscess at the site of injection.

Neurological.   Nervousness, insomnia, somnolence, fatigue, dizziness, depression, headache.

Cardiovascular. Edema (with weight gain), thrombophlebitis, pulmonary embolism.

Endocrine. Menstrual changes (i.e., breakthrough bleeding, spotting), amenorrhea, gynecomastia, breast tenderness, galactorrhea, hot or cold flashes.

Hypersensitivity. Urticaria, pruritus, angioedema, generalized rash, anaphylaxis (all rare side effects).

Other. Fatigue, flare reaction at initiation of treatment for prostate cancer characterized by increased tumor (bone) pain.

Storage and Stability
Both the parenteral suspension and the tablets are stored at room temperature. Each container bears an expiration date.

Preparation
Shake the suspension well just before administration.

Availability
Commercially available as 2.5-, 5-, and 10-mg tablets and as a 150-mg/mL (1-mL vial) or 400 mg/mL (2.5- and 10-mL vials) suspension for injection.

Selected Readings
Birrell SN et al: Medroxyprogesterone acetate therapy in advanced breast cancer: the predictive value of androgen receptor expression, *J Clin Oncol* 13:1572-1577, 1995.

Cavalli F et al: Randomized trial of low- versus high-dose medroxyprogesterone acetate in the induction treatment of postmenopausal patients with advanced breast cancer, *J Clin Oncol* 2:414-419, 1984.

Etienne MC et al: Pharmacokinetics and pharmacodynamics of medroxyprogesterone acetate in advanced breast cancer patients, *J Clin Oncol* 10:1176-1182, 1992.

MEGESTROL ACETATE
Other Names
Megace, megestrol.

Indications
FDA approved for the treatment of advanced carcinoma of the breast or endometrium and for the treatment of anorexia associated with cancer or human immunodeficiency virus (HIV) infection.

Classification and Mechanisms of Action
Megestrol is a progestin that has antiestrogenic properties. Megestrol interferes with the replenishment of cytoplasmic estrogen receptors, thereby decreasing the quantity of estrogen receptors. Megestrol also inhibits the release of luteinizing hormone (a stimulus for endometrial growth).

Pharmacokinetics
Megestrol is well-absorbed by mouth, reaching peak plasma levels 1 to 3 hours after dosing. The drug is metabolized by the liver and excreted in

the urine as steroid metabolites and inactive compounds (57% to 80% within 10 days). Megestrol has an elimination half-life of 15 to 20 hours.

Dose
When used for the treatment of breast cancer, 80 mg twice daily is commonly used. However, there is evidence to support daily administration (160 mg/day). For endometrial cancer, 40 to 320 mg/day have been used. As an appetite stimulant, higher doses (320 mg/day) are indicated.

Administration
Oral.

Toxicity
Gastrointestinal. Nausea, vomiting, and abdominal pain are uncommon. Diarrhea and constipation have been reported with high doses.

Dermatological. Alopecia (uncommon), rash.

Neurological. Headache, carpal tunnel syndrome.

Cardiovascular. Hot flashes, thrombophlebitis, thromboembolism, fluid retention, edema, hypertension with high doses, congestive heart failure (rare).

Genitourinary. Vaginal bleeding or discharge, menstrual changes, amenorrhea, urinary frequency.

Metabolic. Hypercalcemia with high doses; irreversible insulin-dependent diabetes mellitus developed in a woman 6 weeks after initiation of megestrol acetate, 160 mg/day. Megestrol may cause adrenal suppression when administered in doses of 800 mg/day, necessitating the administration of corticosteroids during times of acute illness.

Other. Hyperpnea, dyspnea, weight gain and increased appetite, tumor flare (with or without hypercalcemia). Megestrol is porphyrogenic in animals and may be unsafe in patients with porphyria.

Storage and Stability
Megestrol tablets are stored at room temperature; bottles bear expiration dates.

Availability
Megestrol is commercially available in 20- and 40-mg tablets and as a 40 mg/mL suspension in 240-mL bottles.

Selected Readings
Ettinger DS et al: Megestrol acetate vs. tamoxifen in advanced breast cancer: correlation of hormone receptors and response, *Semin Oncol* 13(Suppl 4):9-14, 1986.

Loprinzi CL et al: Phase III evaluation of four doses of megestrol acetate as therapy for patients with cancer anorexia and/or cachexia, *J Clin Oncol* 11:762-767, 1993.

Von Rhoenn JH et al: Megestrol acetate for treatment of cachexia associated with human immunodeficiency virus (HIV) infection, *Ann Intern Med* 109:840-841, 1988.

MELPHALAN

Other Names
Alkeran, Alkeran IV, L-PAM, L-phenylalanine mustard, L-sarcolysin, NSC-8806.

Indications
FDA approved for the treatment of multiple myeloma and nonresectable epithelial carcinoma of the ovary. Melphalan may also be a useful treatment for cancers of the breast, thyroid, and testes. The injectable formulation is approved for use when oral therapy is not indicated. The injectable formulation has been used in isolated limb perfusion (for melanoma) and as a part of induction regimens before bone marrow transplantation.

Classification
Alkylating agent.

Pharmacokinetics
Melphalan is erratically absorbed (25% to 90%) from the gastrointestinal tract and reaches peak plasma levels approximately 2 hours after dosing. Approximately 30% of the drug is bound to plasma proteins. Melphalan undergoes spontaneous hydrolysis in the bloodstream, and approximately 10% to 15% is eliminated in the urine as unchanged drug. Melphalan has an elimination half-life of 1.5 to 4 hours. Melphalan is not hemodialyzable.

Dose
The usual oral dose for patients with multiple myeloma is 0.25 mg/kg/day (in combination with prednisone 2 mg/kg/day) for 4 days repeated every 6 weeks. Other regimens have been given, including 0.1 to 0.15 mg/kg/day for 7 days every 4 weeks, 6 to 7 mg/m^2/day for 5 days every 6 weeks, and 0.1 to 0.15 mg/kg/day for 2 to 3 weeks followed by a maintenance dose of 2 to 4 mg daily when the bone marrow has recovered. A dose of 0.2 mg/kg/day for 5 days repeated every 4 weeks has been administered to patients with ovarian carcinoma. In bone marrow transplantation regimens, melphalan has been administered in doses of 50 to 60 mg/m^2/day for 3 days. Melphalan has also been given at a dose of 16 mg/m^2 intravenously every 2 weeks for 4 doses, then every 4 weeks. For isolated limb perfusion, doses of 10 mg/L of limb volume or 0.45 mg/kg (upper extremity) and 0.9 mg/kg (lower extremity) have been given. A 50% dose reduction of IV melphalan has been advocated for patients with a serum BUN of 30 mg/dL or higher.

Administration
Melphalan may be administered orally or intravenously as a solution of no greater than 0.45 mg/mL in normal saline over a period of 15 to 30 minutes. Infusion durations longer than 60 minutes are not recommended because of drug instability. The drug has also been given intraperitoneally or via isolated limb perfusion.

Toxicity

Hematological. Leukopenia and thrombocytopenia are expected and may be cumulative. Recovery may be prolonged for 6 to 8 weeks. If myelosuppression is not observed after oral dosing, poor oral absorption should be suspected. Hemolytic anemia rarely occurs.

Gastrointestinal. Nausea and vomiting occur infrequently after oral dosing, but may be severe after IV administration of larger doses. Mucositis, diarrhea, and oral ulcers occur infrequently.

Dermatological. Rash, pruritus, dermatitis, alopecia (uncommon).

Pulmonary. Pulmonary fibrosis and interstitial pneumonitis are rare.

Hypersensitivity. Urticaria, pruritus, exanthema, rash, anaphylaxis (rare).

Other. Amenorrhea and oligospermia are relatively common toxicities. Cataracts, vasculitis, and second malignancies are rare.

Storage and Stability

Tablets and vials are stored at room temperature. Melphalan solution, diluted to a final concentration of 2 mg/mL in normal saline, is stable for 1 hour. The manufacturer recommends that solutions of melphalan not be dispensed in glass containers. The reconstituted solution should not be refrigerated because the drug may precipitate.

Preparation

Reconstitute the 50-mg vial with 10 mL of the provided diluent to yield a 5 mg/mL solution. Further dilute the solution to a concentration no greater than 0.45 mg/mL in normal saline in a glass container.

Availability

Melphalan is commercially available as a 2-mg tablet and a 50-mg vial provided with a 10-mL vial of diluent.

Selected Readings

Hafstrom L et al: Regional hyperthermic perfusion with melphalan after surgery for recurrent malignant melanoma of the extremities, *J Clin Oncol* 9:2091-2094, 1991.

Samuels BL, Bitran JD: High-dose intravenous melphalan: a review, *J Clin Oncol* 13:1786-1799, 1995.

Sarosy G et al: The systemic administration of intravenous melphalan, *J Clin Oncol* 6:1768-1782, 1988.

MERCAPTOPURINE

Other Names

Purinethol, 6-mercaptopurine, 6-MP, NSC-755.

Indications

The oral formulation is FDA approved for remission induction and maintenance therapy of acute lymphatic leukemia and acute nonlymphocytic leukemia. Mercaptopurine (6-MP) may be a useful treatment for chronic myelogenous leukemia, non-Hodgkin's lymphoma, polycythemia vera, inflammatory bowel disease, and severe psoriatic arthritis. The injectable formulation is investigational.

Classification
Purine antimetabolite.

Pharmacokinetics
6-MP is well absorbed by mouth but undergoes extensive first-pass metabolism in the liver by xanthine oxidase. Thus approximately 10% to 20% of an oral dose reaches the bloodstream and achieves peak concentrations 2 hours after dosing. Because of xanthine oxidase inhibition, the oral bioavailability of 6-MP increases to 60% when allopurinol is administered. Approximately 20% of a dose is bound to plasma proteins and 10% to 40% is excreted in the urine as unchanged drug. 6-MP has an elimination half-life of 6 to 10 hours. 6-MP is dialyzable.

Dose
A common oral dose is 70 to 100 mg/m^2/day. Reduce the oral dose by 75% if allopurinol is coadministered. A common IV dose is 500 to 1000 mg/m^2/day for 2 to 3 days. Dose adjustment of the 6-MP administered by IV is not necessary with concomitant administration of allopurinol.

Administration
Oral or by IV infusion (as a 1 to 2 mg/mL solution) in normal saline or 5% dextrose over a period of 1 hour or longer.

Toxicity
Hematological. Leukopenia, thrombocytopenia, anemia. All are common, with leukopenia the most frequent dose-limiting toxicity.

Gastrointestinal. Occasionally, nausea, vomiting, anorexia, abdominal pain, diarrhea, and mucositis.

Dermatological. Hyperpigmentation, rash, and pruritus are rare. Extravasation of the IV formulation may cause tissue necrosis.

Hepatic. Jaundice, elevated hepatic transaminase levels, cholestasis, ascites, hepatic encephalopathy associated with hepatic necrosis and severe fibrosis. The onset is variable, usually occurring in 1 to 2 months. Deaths have occurred, most frequently associated with doses greater than 2.5 mg/kg/day.

Neurological. Headache.

Other. Hyperuricemia, weakness, fever, pancreatitis.

Storage and Stability
Tablets and the injectable formulation are stored at room temperature. Reconstituted vials are stable for 21 days at room or refrigeration temperature. Further dilution to 1 to 2 mg/mL with normal saline or 5% dextrose is stable for 3 days at room or refrigeration temperature.

Preparation
Add 49.8 mL of sterile water to the 500-mg vial to yield a concentration of 10 mg/mL. This is further diluted to 1 to 2 mg/mL in normal saline or 5% dextrose before administration.

Compatibilities
Mercaptopurine and methotrexate are compatible in solution.

Availability
Commercially available in 50-mg tablets. Vials containing 500-mg and 10-mg tablets are investigational and may be obtained from the NCI.

Selected Reading
Lennard L, Lilleyman JS: Are children with lymphoblastic leukemia given enough 6-mercaptopurine? *Lancet* 2:785-787, 1987.

MESNA
Other Names
Mesnex, Uromitexan, mesnum, sodium-2-mercaptoethanesulphonate, NSC-113891.

Indications
FDA approved for the prevention of ifosfamide-induced hemorrhagic cystitis. Also useful for preventing cyclophosphamide-induced hemorrhagic cystitis.

Classification and Mechanisms of Action
Mesna is a prophylactic agent used to prevent hemorrhagic cystitis induced by the oxasophosphorines (ifosfamide, cyclophosphamide). It has no intrinsic cytotoxicity and no antagonistic effects on radiotherapy or chemotherapy. Mesna binds with acrolein, the urotoxic metabolite produced by the oxasophosphorines, to produce a nontoxic thioether and slows the rate of acrolein formation by combining with the 4-hydroxy metabolites of the oxasophosphorines.

Pharmacokinetics
After IV administration, mesna is rapidly oxidized in the blood to the inactive compound dimesna, which is completely cleared from the body through the kidneys. Dimesna is reabsorbed through kidney tubules and is converted to mesna, which combines with acrolein to produce a nontoxic thioether. Approximately 50% of an oral dose of mesna is absorbed by mouth and reaches peak plasma concentrations 1 to 1.5 hours after administration (absorption half-life, 0.34 hours). Mesna and dimesna have elimination half-lives of approximately 0.5 and 1.2 hours, respectively.

Dose
The usual dose of mesna is 20% of the ifosfamide dose, given just before and 4 and 8 hours after ifosfamide (total mesna dose is 60% of

the ifosfamide dose). Mesna has also been given as a continuous infusion concurrently with ifosfamide; a total dose of mesna equal to the total dose of ifosfamide is given, preceded by a loading dose of 6% to 10% of the total ifosfamide dose.

Administration

Mesna is often given as an IV injection in 50 mL or more of 5% dextrose or normal saline over a period of 5 minutes or longer. Mesna has also been given as a continuous IV infusion and orally (as the injection mixed in tomato juice, orange juice, or carbonated beverage).

Toxicity

At the doses used for uroprotection, mesna is virtually nontoxic. However, the following adverse effects may be attributable to mesna:

Gastrointestinal. Nausea, vomiting, diarrhea, abdominal pain, and altered taste.

Dermatological. Rash, urticaria.

Other. Lethargy, headache, joint or limb pain, hypotension, fatigue, false-positive test for urinary ketones.

Storage and Stability

Intact ampules and vials are stored at room temperature. The multidose vial may be stored and reused for up to 8 days. Open ampules should not be reused because mesna reacts with oxygen to form dimesna. Diluted solutions (1 to 20 mg/mL) are stable for at least 24 hours under room or refrigeration temperatures. Mesna is chemically stable in the following solutions at room temperature: 5% dextrose in water, 48 hours (20 mg/mL) or 24 hours (1 mg/mL); 5% dextrose and 0.45% NaCl, 48 hours (20 mg/mL) or 72 hours (1 mg/mL); normal saline, 24 hours (1 mg/mL); lactated Ringer's solution, 24 hours (1 mg/mL).

Preparation

Mesna is available as an injectable solution. Mesna may be further diluted in 5% dextrose, 5% dextrose and 0.2% NaCl, 5% dextrose and 0.33% NaCl, 5% dextrose and 0.45% NaCl, normal saline, or lactated Ringer's solution to a final concentration of 1 to 20 mg/mL.

Incompatibilities

Mesna is incompatible in solution with cisplatin.

Compatibilities

Ifosfamide and mesna are compatible for continuous infusion in PVC bags containing 5% dextrose or normal saline. Mesna is reported to be compatible in solution with cyclophosphamide, etoposide, lorazepam, potassium chloride, bleomycin, and dexamethasone. A pharmacist should be consulted for additional information.

Availability
Commercially available in 2-mL ampules and 10-mL vials containing 100 mg/mL.

Selected Readings
Dechant KL et al: Ifosfamide/mesna: a review of its antineoplastic activity, pharmacokinetic properties and therapeutic efficacy in cancer, *Drugs* 42:428-467, 1991.
Schoenike SE, Dana WJ: Ifosfamide and mesna, *Clin Pharm* 9:179-191, 1990.

METHOTREXATE
Other Names
Methotrexate LPF, methotrexate sodium, MTX, Mexate, Mexate-AQ, Folex, Folex-Pfs, Abitrexate, Rheumatrex, amethopterin, NSC-740.

Indications
FDA approved for the treatment of choriocarcinoma, hydatidiform mole, acute lymphocytic leukemia; prophylaxis and treatment of meningeal lymphocytic leukemia, breast cancer, epidermal tumors of the head and neck, lung cancer, non-Hodgkin's lymphoma, cutaneous T-cell lymphoma, osteosarcoma, psoriasis, and rheumatoid arthritis (second- or third-line treatment). Methotrexate may be a useful treatment for acute nonlymphocytic leukemia, multiple myeloma, rhabdomyosarcoma, and cancers of the bladder, brain, cervix, esophagus, kidney, ovary, prostate, stomach, and testes.

Classification
Antimetabolite (antifol).

Pharmacokinetics
Doses up to 40 mg/m^2 are well-absorbed (75% to 95%) from the gastrointestinal tract. Higher oral doses are less absorbed. Peak plasma levels occur 0.5 to 2 hours after oral dosing. Methotrexate is distributed to body water and into breast milk. Patients with significant ascites or effusions will eliminate the drug more slowly than patients without these conditions. Approximately 10% of methotrexate is metabolized to 7-hydroxymethotrexate, a less water-soluble, potentially nephrotoxic metabolite. Approximately 90% of methotrexate is eliminated from the body in the urine as unchanged drug. The patient must have relatively normal kidney function to excrete the drug adequately and avoid excessive toxicity. The BUN and creatinine levels should be followed routinely. A 24-hour creatinine clearance before initiation of methotrexate therapy is often desirable. Methotrexate has an elimination half-life of approximately 3 hours. Patients with severe renal function impairment should not receive methotrexate. Patients with lesser degrees of renal impairment should receive an attenuated dose of methotrexate with leucovorin rescue. Methotrexate is not dialyzable, but charcoal hemoperfusion may lower serum levels. Methotrexate will inhibit DNA synthesis in bone marrow at

concentrations of 1×10^{-8} M, and will inhibit the growth of gastrointestinal epithelium at plasma concentrations as low as 5×10^{-9} M.

NOTE: Methotrexate 1×10^{-7} is equal to 0.1 μg/mL.

Dose

Parenteral doses vary from 20 to 40 mg/m² every 1 to 2 weeks (for the treatment of solid tumors) to 200 to 500 mg/m² every 2 to 4 weeks (for leukemias and lymphomas). As adjuvant treatment for osteosarcoma, doses of 12,000 to 15,000 mg/m² have been given with leucovorin rescue. The usual adult intrathecal dose is 10 to 15 mg in 7 to 15 mL of preservative-free saline (3 mL if given via an Ommaya reservoir). Doses greater than 80 mg/week should be accompanied by leucovorin rescue. See Table 3-2 for leucovorin dosing instructions.

Administration

"Small" doses (≤100 mg) are usually administered by IV bolus (without further dilution). Larger doses are usually given by IV infusion in 50 mL or more of 5% dextrose or normal saline over a 30-minute period or longer. Methotrexate has also been given intrathecally, intramuscularly, orally, intraarterially, intraperitoneally, and by intravesical instillation.

Toxicity

Hematological. Leukopenia and thrombocytopenia are dose related and more common (and more severe) with prolonged drug exposure. Nadir white blood cell and platelet counts occur 7 to 10 days after dosing and recovery occurs approximately 7 days later. Anemia occurs less frequently.

Gastrointestinal. Nausea and vomiting are uncommon with conventional doses and usually mild. Stomatitis is common (more common with high doses and longer infusion durations). Diarrhea, anorexia, hematemesis, and melena are uncommon. Gastrointestinal ulceration, enteritis, and/or intestinal perforation have been reported.

Dermatological. Skin erythema and/or rash, pruritus, urticaria, alopecia (rare), photosensitivity, furunculosis, depigmentation or hyperpigmentation, acne, telangiectasia, skin desquamation (exfoliative dermatitis), bullae formation, folliculitis.

Hepatic. Mild and transient increases of hepatic transaminase levels occur occasionally. Hepatic fibrosis and cirrhosis rarely occur and are more likely to occur in patients receiving long-term continuous or daily treatment.

Neurological. Encephalopathy, more commonly with multiple intrathecal doses and in patients who have received cranial irradiation; tiredness, weakness, confusion, ataxia, tremors, irritability, seizures, and coma have also been reported. Acute side effects of intrathecal methotrexate may include dizziness, blurred vision, headache, back pain, nuchal rigidity, seizures, paralysis, and hemiparesis.

Pulmonary. Pneumonitis, pulmonary fibrosis, cough, and dyspnea are rare.

Renal. Renal dysfunction is dose related and more likely to occur in patients with compromised renal function or dehydration, or in those receiving other nephrotoxic drugs. Renal function impairment is manifested by increased serum creatinine levels and hematuria. The patient's serum creatinine should be routinely monitored before therapy and intermittently during treatment with higher doses (e.g., ≥200 mg). Methotrexate levels (24 hours after dosing) should also be monitored.

Ocular. Conjunctivitis, excessive lacrimation, cataracts, photophobia, cortical blindness (high doses).

Other. Malaise, osteoporosis (aseptic necrosis of the femoral head), hyperuricemia, reversible oligospermia, allergic reactions (e.g., fever, chills, rash, urticaria, anaphylaxis), vasculitis, flank pain (associated with rapid IV infusion).

Storage and Stability
Store at room temperature protected from light. Reconstituted solutions are stable at room temperature for at least 4 weeks. Dilute solutions (2 to 25 mg/mL) are chemically stable for at least 3 months in the refrigerator. Solutions of 50 mg/100 mL in PVC bags of 5% dextrose may be frozen at −20° C for at least 30 days when thawed in 2 minutes by microwave radiation. There is no loss of potency after five freeze-thaw cycles.

Preparation
Lyophilized 20-, 50-, 100-, and 250-mg vials are reconstituted with sterile water, normal saline, or 5% dextrose to a concentration no greater than 25 mg/mL. The 1000-mg vials are reconstituted with 19.4 mL to provide a concentration of 50 mg/mL. Higher doses (>100 mg) are often further diluted with 50 mL or more of 0.45% NaCl, normal saline, or 5% dextrose.

Compatibilities
Compatible with sodium bicarbonate, cytarabine, cephalothin, fluorouracil, mercaptopurine, vincristine sulfate, hydrocortisone, dacarbazine, leucovorin, furosemide, and amino acids. At the "Y-site," methotrexate is compatible with fluorouracil, cisplatin, and heparin. A pharmacist should be consulted for additional information.

Incompatibilities
Incompatible in solution with bleomycin, doxorubicin, idarubicin, prednisolone sodium phosphate, droperidol, metoclopramide, and ranitidine. Aspirin, probenecid, and nonsteroidal antiinflammatory drugs may prolong methotrexate clearance and increase toxicity. These drugs should not be given to patients receiving larger doses of methotrexate (for 48 hours after a dose). Asparaginase and leucovorin abrogate the effects of methotrexate.

Availability
Commercially available as a lyophilized powder for injection (20-, 50-, 100-, 250-, and 1000-mg/vial); as a 25 mg/mL preservative-free, isotonic solution for injection (50-, 100-, 200- and 250-mg/vial); as a 25 mg/mL

(50- and 250-mg vials) preparation containing preservative, isotonic solution for injection, and as a 2.5 mg tablet.

Selected Reading

Anonymous: *Methotrexate*, Pearl River, NY, 1987, Lederle Laboratories, Professional Services, American Cyanamide Co.

MITOMYCIN

Other Names

Mutamycin, mitomycin-C, NSC-26980.

Indications

FDA approved for the treatment of disseminated adenocarcinoma of the stomach or pancreas (in combination with other drugs). Mitomycin may be a useful treatment for chronic myelogenous leukemia and cancers of the bladder, breast, cervix, colon, esophagus, gallbladder, head and neck, lung, and rectum.

Classification

Antitumor antibiotic.

Pharmacokinetics

Mitomycin is poorly absorbed by mouth. After IV administration the drug rapidly distributes to body tissues, excluding the brain. Mitomycin is inactivated by microsomal enzymes in the liver and is also metabolized in the spleen and kidneys. The presence of ascites does not affect the elimination of mitomycin even though the drug penetrates into ascitic fluid (40% of plasma concentrations). After intraarterial administration to the liver, approximately 25% is metabolized on first pass. Approximately 10% to 30% of the drug is eliminated unchanged in the urine. Renal dysfunction does not significantly alter mitomycin elimination. Mitomycin has an elimination half-life of 0.5 to 1 hour, and the drug is not hemodialyzable.

Dose

The usual IV dose range is 10 to 20 mg/m^2 once every 6 to 8 weeks. It has been recommended that total cumulative doses not exceed 50 mg/m^2 to avoid excessive toxicity. For instillation into the bladder, 20 to 40 mg mitomycin (mixed with 20 to 40 mL of water or saline) is given weekly for 8 weeks.

Administration

Using extravasation precautions, administer into a free-flowing IV line over a span of 2 to 5 minutes. Mitomycin has been given intravesically, intraperitoneally, and intraarterially. After intravesical instillation, patients are asked to retain the drug in the bladder for 2 to 3 hours before voiding.

Toxicity

Hematological. Leukopenia and thrombocytopenia are expected, occur late (nadir 4 to 5 weeks; recovery 2 to 3 weeks later), and are cumulative and dose limiting. Anemia and hemolytic-uremic syndrome (renal failure, profound thrombocytopenia, pulmonary edema, and hypotension) are uncommon. Hemolytic-uremic syndrome is associated with a high mortality rate (>50%) and may be more common in patients who have received a cumulative mitomycin dose in excess of 60 mg/m².

Gastrointestinal. Mild nausea and vomiting are common but usually prevented by antiemetic therapy. Symptoms usually begin 1 to 2 hours after IV administration and may persist for 3 to 4 hours. Nausea occasionally persists for a few days. Anorexia is common. Stomatitis and diarrhea are uncommon.

Dermatological. Alopecia (4%), dermatitis, photosensitivity, skin rash, and pruritus (4%) are uncommon toxicities. Tissue necrosis, ulceration, and cellulitis will occur if mitomycin extravasates. Skin erythema and ulceration can occur weeks to months after administration and may appear at a site that is distant from the site of injection.

Hepatic. Venoocclusive disease of the liver, manifested as abdominal pain, hepatomegaly, and liver failure in patients receiving mitomycin and autologous bone marrow transplantation.

Neurological. Paresthesias, lethargy, headache.

Renal. Nephrotoxicity (2% incidence overall). Frequency increases when doses exceed 50 mg/m² and is manifested as increased serum creatinine and BUN concentrations.

Pulmonary. Interstitial pneumonitis (with cough, dyspnea, hemoptysis, and/or pneumonia) is an infrequent toxicity and can be severe. Acute bronchospasm has been reported to occur in some patients receiving vinblastine or vindesine and mitomycin. Some advocate the administration of dexamethasone, 20 mg intravenously, before each dose of mitomycin to prevent this uncommon toxicity. Pulmonary fibrosis has been reported to occur in some patients after mitomycin-containing therapy.

Other. Fatigue (common), pain on injection, phlebitis, fever (rare), weakness, blurred vision (rare).

Storage and Stability
Unreconstituted vials are stored at room temperature. At a concentration of 0.5 mg/mL the drug is chemically stable for at least 7 days at room temperature and 14 days in the refrigerator. Further diluted to 0.2 to 0.4 mg/mL, mitomycin is stable for 3 hours in 5% dextrose, 12 hours in normal saline, and 24 hours in lactated Ringer's solution.

Preparation
Mitomycin is reconstituted with 10 (5-mg vial), 40 (20-mg vial), or 80 mL (40-mg vial) of sterile water to result in a solution containing 0.5 mg/mL.

Incompatibilities
Bleomycin (20 to 30 units/L) loses 20% to 52% of its potency over 7 days when combined with mitomycin (10 to 50 mg/L in normal saline).

Compatibilities

Mitomycin (5 to 15 mg) is compatible with heparin (1000 to 10,000 units) in 30 mL of normal saline for 48 hours at room temperature.

Availability

Commercially available as a lyophilized powder in 5-, 20-, and 40-mg vials.

Selected Readings

Cantrell JE, Phillips TM, Schein PS: Carcinoma-associated hemolytic-uremic syndrome: a complication of mitomycin C chemotherapy, *J Clin Oncol* 3:723-734, 1985.

Doll DC, Weiss RB, Issell BF: Mitomycin: ten years after approval for marketing, *J Clin Oncol* 3:276-286, 1985.

Dorr RT: New findings in the pharmacokinetic, metabolic, and drug-resistance aspects of mitomycin-C, *Semin Oncol* 15(suppl 3):32-41, 1988.

MITOTANE

Other Names

Lysodren, *o,p*'DDD, NSC-38721.

Indications

FDA approved for the treatment of adrenocortical cancer. Mitotane may also be useful in the treatment of Cushing's syndrome.

Classification and Mechanisms of Action

Mitotane is an adrenal cytotoxic agent; its exact mechanism of action is unknown. Mitotane may exert cytotoxic effects by damaging the mitochondria of adrenocortical cells. Mitotane modifies extraadrenal metabolism of exogenous and endogenous steroids and suppresses adrenocortical neoplasms by a cytotoxic effect.

Pharmacokinetics

Approximately 35% to 40% of an oral dose is absorbed and reaches peak serum concentrations 3 to 5 hours after dosing. Inhibition of adrenal function occurs after 2 to 4 weeks of continuous treatment. Serum concentrations of mitotane are not believed to correlate with antitumor effect. Mitotane is distributed to all body tissues with adipose tissue being a primary storage site. Mitotane is metabolized by the liver and eliminated in the bile (1% to 17%) and urine (10% to 25%). The drug has an elimination half-life of 18 to 160 days.

Dose

For the treatment of adrenocortical carcinoma the usual initial adult dose is 1000 to 6000 mg/day in 3 to 4 divided doses. The dose is usually increased to 9000 to 10,000 mg/day, the usual adult dose. The maximum tolerable dose is 2000 to 16,000 mg/day. For Cushing's syndrome, initial treatment is usually 3000 to 6000 mg/day in divided doses followed by smaller maintenance doses administered daily or a few times each week.

Administration
Oral.

Toxicity
Hematological. Thrombocytopenia and leukopenia are rare.

Gastrointestinal. Anorexia, nausea, and vomiting are reported in about 80% of patients and can be dose limiting. Diarrhea occurs in approximately 20% of the patients.

Dermatological. Maculopapular rash occurs in about 15% of patients; hyperpigmentation, chloasma, urticaria, erythema multiforme, periorbital or facial swelling, and perinasal scaling rarely occur.

Hepatic. Elevation of hepatic transaminase levels and hyperbilirubinemia.

Neurological. Depression, manifested as sedation, lethargy, and dizziness or vertigo occurs in 40% of patients. Irritability, confusion, headache, weakness, fatigue, and/or tremors occur less frequently. Functional impairment and brain damage may result from prolonged use of high doses. Serum concentrations ≥20 µg/mL are often associated with adverse central nervous system effects.

Cardiovascular. Flushing, orthostatic hypotension, hypertension are infrequent toxicities.

Pulmonary. Shortness of breath and wheezing are infrequent toxicities.

Endocrine. Most patients develop adrenocortical insufficiency. Glucocorticoid and mineralocorticoid replacement therapy may be necessary.

Metabolic. Hypercholesterolemia and hypouricemia frequently occur.

Ocular. Visual disturbances, blurred vision, diplopia, papilledema, lens opacity, cataracts, and retinopathy are rare.

Other. Fever, hematuria, hemorrhagic cystitis, and albuminuria are rare.

Storage and Stability
Mitotane is stored at room temperature. Containers bear expiration dates.

Incompatibilities
Spironolactone may antagonize the effects of mitotane.

Availability
Commercially available as a 500-mg scored tablet.

Selected Readings
Hague RV: Hepatic microsomal enzyme induction and adrenal crisis due to o,p'DDD therapy for metastatic adrenocortical carcinoma, *Clin Endocrinol* 53:51-57, 1989.
Luton JP: Clinical features of adrenocortical carcinoma, prognostic factors, and the effect of mitotane therapy, *N Engl J Med* 322:1195-1201, 1990.

MITOXANTRONE

Other Names
Novantrone, mitoxantrone hydrochloride, dihydroxyanthracenedione, DHAD, DHAQ, NSC-301739.

Indications
FDA approved for the treatment of acute nonlymphocytic leukemia. Mitoxantrone may be useful in the treatment of non-Hodgkin's lymphoma, breast and prostate cancers, and hepatocellular carcinoma.

Classification and Mechanisms of Action
Antitumor antibiotic (anthracenedione derivative).

Pharmacokinetics
Mitoxantrone is poorly absorbed by mouth. After IV administration, it is widely distributed throughout the body, metabolized by the liver, and excreted in the bile (30% unchanged) and urine (<10% unchanged). Approximately 80% of the drug is bound to plasma proteins. Elimination of the drug in patients with serum bilirubin concentrations of 1.3 to 3.4 mg/dL is similar to that observed in patients with normal bilirubin levels. Mitoxantrone has an elimination half-life of 2.3 to 13 days. Mitoxantrone is probably not removed by dialysis because of its extensive tissue binding.

M

Dose
A commonly used regimen for induction of acute nonlymphocytic leukemia is 12 mg/m^2/day for 3 days combined with cytarabine, 100 mg/m^2/day, as a 7-day continuous IV infusion. Subsequent treatments to maintain a complete remission in patients with acute leukemia utilize the same doses of mitoxantrone and cytarabine administered over 2 and 5 days, respectively. Mitoxantrone has also been administered at doses of 10 to 12 mg/m^2/day for 5 days as a treatment for patients with acute leukemia. For other malignancies a common dose is 12 mg/m^2 every 3 to 4 weeks.

Administration
Mitoxantrone has been given as an IV bolus (over a 3-minute or longer period), but it is recommended that the drug be administered by slow IV infusion (in 50 mL or more of 5% dextrose or normal saline) over a 15- to 30-minute or longer period. The drug has also been given as a continuous IV infusion, intramuscularly, intraperitoneally, and by intravesical instillation.

Toxicity
Hematological. Leukopenia is expected and dose limiting. Thrombocytopenia and anemia occur less frequently.

Gastrointestinal. Nausea and vomiting (usually preventable), diarrhea, mucositis (common), abdominal pain.

Dermatological. Alopecia is common but usually mild. Pruritus and dry skin have been reported.

Hepatic. Transient elevation of hepatic transaminase levels occur occasionally, jaundice (rare), hyperbilirubinemia is uncommon.

Neurological. Headache, seizures (rare).

Cardiovascular. Cumulative cardiomyopathy (congestive heart failure) can occur. Mitoxantrone is less cardiotoxic than doxorubicin and daunorubicin. However, monitoring left ventricular ejection fraction (LVEF) is recommended (see doxorubicin section). In patients without any risk factors for developing cardiomyopathy the risk of this toxicity appears to increase when cumulative doses exceed 140 mg/m^2. Arrhythmias, tachycardia, and chest pain occur infrequently.

Pulmonary. Cough and/or dyspnea are uncommon and may be associated with congestive heart failure.

Allergic. Hypotension, urticaria, and rash are uncommon toxicities.

Other. Blue discoloration of sclerae, blue-green discoloration of the urine that may persist for 24 to 48 hours after treatment. Fever, conjunctivitis, phlebitis, amenorrhea, tissue ulceration and necrosis on extravasation (rare).

Storage and Stability
Intact vials are stored at room temperature. Storage under refrigeration may cause formation of a precipitate that redissolves upon warming to room temperature. When diluted to 0.02 to 0.5 mg/mL in normal saline or 5% dextrose, the drug is chemically stable for at least 7 days at room temperature.

Preparation
Dilute in at least 50 mL normal saline or 5% dextrose before administration.

Incompatibilities
Heparin (1 to 10 units/mL with mitoxantrone, 50 to 200 µg/mL) causes an immediate precipitate. Hydrocortisone sodium phosphate (2 mg/mL with mitoxantrone, 50 µg/mL) causes an immediate precipitate.

Compatibilities
Hydrocortisone sodium succinate (0.1 to 2 mg/mL with mitoxantrone, 0.05 to 0.2 µg/mL in normal saline or 5% dextrose) is compatible for at least 24 hours at room temperature.

Availability
Commercially available as a 2 mg/mL solution (20-, 25-, and 30-mg vials).

Selected Readings
Anonymous: *Mitoxantrone*, Pearl River, NY, 1988, Lederle Laboratories, Professional Services, American Cyanamide Co.

Faulds D et al: Mitoxantrone: a review of its pharmacodynamic and pharmacokinetic properties, and therapeutic potential in the chemotherapy of cancer, *Drugs* 41:400-449, 1991.

Hiddemann W et al: High dose cytosine arabinoside and mitoxantrone: a highly effective regimen in refractory acute myeloid leukemia, *Blood* 69:744-749, 1987.

Larson RA et al: A clinical and pharmacokinetic study of mitoxantrone in acute non-lymphocytic leukemia, *J Clin Oncol* 5:391-397, 1987.

OCTREOTIDE

Other Names

Sandostatin, L-cysteinamide, SMS 201-995. Long-acting formulations: octreotide pamoate (SMS 201-995 pa LAR), SMS 201-995 LAR (octreotide acetate)

Indications

FDA approved for the control of symptoms in patients with carcinoid and vasoactive intestinal peptide–secreting tumors (VIPomas). Octreotide may be a useful treatment for pancreatic cancer and AIDS-associated diarrhea. Long-acting formulations of octreotide are undergoing evaluation in patients with cancers of the pancreas and breast.

Classification and Mechanisms of Action

Octreotide is a long-acting analogue of the natural hormone somatostatin that inhibits the secretion of serotonin, vasoactive intestinal peptide, gastrin, motilin, insulin, glucagon, secretin, and pancreatic polypeptide.

Pharmacokinetics

Octreotide is rapidly and completely absorbed after subcutaneous injection. The drug is widely distributed throughout the body, and approximately 65% is protein bound (primarily to lipoproteins). Octreotide has an elimination half-life of 1.5 hours, and its duration of action is around 12 hours. Approximately 30% of the drug is eliminated unchanged in the urine.

Dose

For the treatment of carcinoid tumors, the usual daily dose is 100 to 600 μg in two to four divided doses. For the treatment of tumors secreting vasoactive intestinal peptide, the usual daily dose is 200 to 300 μg in two to four divided doses. Doses greater than 450 μg/day are not usually necessary. Long-acting formulations of octreotide have been administered in doses of 80 to 160 mg every 4 weeks.

Administration

Usually administered subcutaneously. Rotation of the injection site is recommended. Octreotide has also been administered as a bolus IV injection (over a 3-minute period) and as a continuous infusion. The long-acting formulations of octreotide are administered intramuscularly.

Toxicity

Gastrointestinal. The most frequent side effects are abdominal pain or discomfort, loose stools, anorexia, and vomiting. Fat malabsorption occurs in

1% to 3% of patients. Rarely, gastrointestinal bleeding, heartburn, swollen stomach, and cholelithiasis may occur.

Dermatological. Pain at the injection site, flushing, edema, wheal and erythema at the injection site, hair loss, thinning of skin, skin flaking, bruising, bleeding from superficial wounds, rash, and/or pruritus may occur.

Hepatic. Hepatitis, jaundice, slight elevation of liver enzyme levels.

Neurological. Headache (2%), dizziness, light-headedness, fatigue, anxiety, depression, convulsions, drowsiness, vertigo.

Cardiovascular. Hypertension, shortness of breath, thrombophlebitis, ischemia, congestive heart failure, palpitations, orthostatic hypotension, chest pain.

Metabolic. Hypoglycemia, hyperglycemia, urine hyperosmolarity.

Other. Rhinorrhea, dry mouth, numbness, oliguria, prostatitis, hyperhidrosis, visual disturbance, chills, fever, throat discomfort, elevated creatine phosphokinase levels.

Storage and Stability
Ampules and vials of octreotide are stored in the refrigerator. Octreotide can be stored at room temperature for at least 14 days if protected from light. At concentrations of 5-, 50-, or 100 µg/mL in normal saline, octreotide is stable for at least 96 hours at room temperature.

Preparation
Octreotide injection may be further diluted in normal saline or 5% dextrose to concentrations of 5 to 100 µg/mL.

Incompatibilities
Octreotide is incompatible with 10% fat emulsion.

Compatibilities
Octreotide is compatible with heparin and certain total parenteral nutrition (TPN) solutions. However, the manufacturer does not recommend mixing of octreotide with TPN solutions. A pharmacist should be consulted for additional information.

Availability
Commercially available in 1-mL ampules containing 0.05, 0.1, and 0.5mg/mL. Octreotide is also available in a 5-mL multidose vial containing 0.2 and 1 mg/mL. The long-acting formulations of octreotide are investigational and are available in vials containing 40 mg/mL.

Selected Readings
Battershill PE: Octreotide: a review of its pharmacodynamic and pharmacokinetic properties, and therapeutic potential in conditions associated with excessive peptide secretion, *Drugs* 38:658-702, 1989.

Burch PA et al: A phase III evaluation of octreotide (Sandostatin) versus chemotherapy with 5-FU or 5-FU/leucovorin in advanced exocrine pancreatic cancer, *Proc Am Soc Clin Oncol* 14:203, 1995.

Katz MD: Octreotide: a new somatostatin analogue, *Clin Pharm* 8:255-273, 1989.

Maton PN: The use of the long-acting somatostatin analogue, octreotide acetate, in patients with islet cell tumors, *Gastroenterol Clin North Am* 18:897-922, 1989.

PACLITAXEL

Other Names
Taxol, NSC-125973.

Indications
FDA approved for the treatment of advanced ovarian and breast cancers. Paclitaxel may be useful for the treatment of cancers of the head and neck, lung, prostate, and stomach.

Classification
Plant alkaloid (antimicrotubule agent).

Pharmacokinetics
Paclitaxel is 95% to 98% protein bound and is metabolized to 7-epitaxol. Approximately 5% to 12% is excreted unchanged in the urine. The drug has an elimination half-life of approximately 5 hours, although some have reported half-lives in the range of 13 to 56 hours. Paclitaxel distributes to ascitic fluid, achieving concentrations around 40% of plasma levels. Elimination of paclitaxel is reduced by one third when the drug is administered immediately after administration of cisplatin.

Dose
The originally approved doses for patients with ovarian and breast cancer are 135 and 175 mg/m^2, respectively, every 3 weeks. In minimally pre-treated patients, many recommend higher doses in the range of 200 to 250 mg/m^2 every 3 weeks. A variety of doses and schedules have been used. The maximum tolerated dose is 30 mg/m^2/day for 5 days every 3 weeks. When combined with cisplatin (75 mg/m^2), paclitaxel is given at 135 mg/m^2 *followed by* cisplatin because there is an increased incidence of severe neutropenia when cisplatin is given before paclitaxel. When administered with cisplatin (75 mg/m^2) and filgrastim (G-CSF) the dose of paclitaxel can be increased in some patients to 250 mg/m^2. Doses of paclitaxel, 200 to 225 mg/m^2, have been combined with carboplatin (dose based on an AUC value of 6 to 7).

Administration
IV infusion (as a 0.3 to 1.2 mg/mL solution in 5% dextrose or normal saline) over 3 to 24 hours has been administered. Use of an in-line 0.2 µm filter is recommended when administering paclitaxel. Information is available demonstrating that paclitaxel can be administered over 1 hour. Premedication is recommended to reduce the incidence of hypersensitivity reactions: dexamethasone 20 mg orally, 6 and 12 hours before paclitaxel plus diphenhydramine 50 mg intravenously, and ranitidine 50 mg intravenously (or cimetidine 300 mg intravenously, or famotidine 20

mg intravenously) 30 to 60 minutes before administration of paclitaxel. If patients forget to take the oral doses of dexamethasone before paclitaxel, then an IV dose of dexamethasone 20 mg is administered 30 minutes before administration of paclitaxel. Some clinicians give this IV dexamethasone dose 30 minutes before paclitaxel, regardless of whether the two oral doses were taken, just to be cautious. Paclitaxel has also been given as a 96-hour continuous IV infusion and intraperitoneally (maximum tolerated dose, 175 mg/m^2).

Toxicity

Hematological. Neutropenia is dose limiting and does not appear to be cumulative; it occurs more often when a 24-hour (versus 3-hour) infusion of paclitaxel is administered. Nadir counts occur by day 8 to 11 and are often severe, with recovery occurring by day 21. Thrombocytopenia is usually not severe. Myelosuppression is most severe in patients who have received extensive prior treatment and in patients who receive cisplatin just before paclitaxel. Mild anemia is seen in approximately 20% of patients.

Gastrointestinal. Mucositis is dose related and cumulative (3% have greater than Grade I mucositis), occurs within 3 to 7 days and resolves 5 to 7 days thereafter. Nausea and vomiting are infrequent (4% incidence), as are diarrhea, taste changes, typhlitis (neutropenic enterocolitis), ischemic colitis, and pancreatitis.

Dermatological. Alopecia is universal, complete, and often sudden. Hair loss usually occurs 14 to 21 days after treatment and often affects all body hair (i.e., eyebrows, pubic hair). Many patients experience regrowth of hair after five to seven cycles of treatment. Injection site reactions (erythema, induration, tenderness, skin discoloration), infiltration (phlebitis, cellulitis, ulceration, and necrosis, rare), nail changes (e.g., discoloration, separation from the nail bed), radiation recall reactions, and rashes occur infrequently.

Hepatic. Minor elevation of hepatic transaminase levels, hyperbilirubinemia, hepatic failure, and hepatic necrosis have been reported.

Neurological. Peripheral neuropathy, more frequent with longer infusions, with doses over 170 mg/m^2, and in patients with a history of substantial alcohol use, diabetes, or diabetic neuropathy. Grade 2 peripheral neuropathies have been seen after 9 of 281 courses and appear to be cumulative. Transient myalgias and arthralgias begin within 2 to 3 days after treatment, occasionally resolve within 2 to 4 days, are amenable to treatment with nonsteroidal antiinflammatory drugs, and occur more often after higher doses. Mood alterations, light-headedness, neuroencephalopathy, hepatic encephalopathy, motor neuropathy, autonomic neuropathy, paralytic ileus, generalized weakness, and seizures are rare.

Cardiovascular. Bradycardia (40 to 60 bpm) is common, usually transient, and usually asymptomatic. Ventricular tachycardia (usually asymptomatic but potentially serious) and atypical chest pain occur less frequently. In patients with no prior history of cardiac problems and taking no cardiac medications, routine cardiac monitoring is not recommended. Syncope, hypotension, ventricular tachycardia, bigeminy, complete heart block requiring a pacemaker, and myocardial infarction have been reported rarely. Hypertension, possibly related to concomitant administration of dexamethasone, has been reported.

Pulmonary. Interstitial pneumonitis has been reported in some patients.

Hypersensitivity. Manifested as cutaneous flushing, hypotension, dyspnea with bronchospasm and bradycardia (40 to 60 bpm). Urticaria, abdominal and extremity pain, angioedema, and diaphoresis have also occurred. Half of the reported reactions occurred within 2 to 3 minutes of initiation of treatment (78% within 20 minutes), 50% occur after the first dose, and 40% after the second dose. In one series 11 reactions were observed in 32 patients receiving paclitaxel as a continuous infusion. Hypersensitivity reactions are of the same frequency for 24- and 3-hour infusions. Premedication, described on p. 170, is recommended.

Other. Fatigue, headache, minor elevations in serum creatinine and triglyceride levels, light-headedness, myopathy, sensation of flashing lights, and blurred vision.

Storage and Stability
The intact vials may be stored at room temperature. Refrigeration and freezing do not affect the potency of paclitaxel. Solutions diluted to a concentration of 0.3 to 1.2 mg/mL in normal saline or 5% dextrose are stable for at least 27 hours at room temperature.

Preparation
The concentrated solution must be diluted before use in normal saline, 5% dextrose, or 5% dextrose in Ringer's solution to a concentration of 0.3 to 1.2 mg/mL. Solutions exhibit a slight haze, common to all products containing nonionic surfactants. Glass, polypropylene, or polyolefin containers and non–PVC-containing (nitroglycerin) infusion sets should be used.

Incompatibilities
Avoid the use of PVC bags and infusion sets because of leaching of di-(2-ethylhexyl)phthalate (DEHP) (plasticizer).

Availability
Paclitaxel is commercially available as a 6 mg/mL solution in 30- and 100-mg vials.

Selected Readings
Chabner BA: Taxol. In DeVita Jr, Hellman S, Rosenberg SA, eds: *Principles and practice of oncology, PPO updates,* 5:1-10, 1991.

Gregory RE, DeLisa AF: Paclitaxel: a new antineoplastic agent for refractory ovarian cancer, *Clin Pharm* 12:401-415, 1993.

Pazdur R et al: The taxoids: paclitaxel (Taxol) and docetaxel (Taxotere), *Cancer Treat Rev* 19:351-386, 1993.

Rowinsky EK, Casenave LA, Donehower RC: Taxol: a novel investigational microtubule agent, *J Natl Cancer Inst* 82:1247-1259, 1990.

Rowinsky EK et al: Clinical toxicities encountered with paclitaxel, *Semin Oncol* 20:1-15, 1993.

PALA

Other Names
Sparfosate sodium, phosphonacetyl-L-aspartic acid, PALA disodium, NSC-224131.

Indications
PALA is an investigational agent that is being studied as a biochemical modifier of 5-fluorouracil (5-FU) cytotoxicity.

Classification
Antimetabolite (pyrimidine antagonist).

Pharmacokinetics
PALA is poorly absorbed by mouth. After IV administration, PALA is distributed widely throughout the body. Cerebrospinal fluid concentrations are approximately 18% to 40% of concurrent plasma levels 8 hours after administration. The majority (85%) of PALA is excreted unchanged in the urine. The drug has an elimination half-life of around 5 hours.

Dose
A commonly used dose regimen is 250 mg/m^2 (in combination with 5-FU) every week. As a single agent, PALA has been given in weekly doses of 3750 to 4000 mg/m^2.

Administration
PALA is usually given by IV push, but it may be administered by IV infusion (as a 1 mg/mL solution), over a 30-minute or longer period.

Toxicity
The adverse effects of PALA, used as a single agent, are described below. Used in combination with 5-FU or other drugs, additional side effects may occur as PALA may enhance the effects of other drugs.

Hematological. Leukopenia, thrombocytopenia, and anemia are usually mild and rarely dose limiting.

Gastrointestinal. Nausea (mild), vomiting (preventable), diarrhea (mild), mucositis (mild and transient), anorexia (uncommon).

Dermatological. Skin rash (erythematous, maculopapular) often involves the chest, face, back and skin-fold surfaces; cutaneous "flare reactions" may occur in previously irradiated sites.

Neurological. Paresthesias, lethargy, somnolence, ataxia (rare), seizures (rare).

Other. Keratoconjunctivitis, corneal ulceration, phlebitis, fever.

Storage and Stability
PALA is stable for at least 5 years at refrigeration and room temperatures. Diluted to a concentration of 1 mg/mL in 5% dextrose or normal saline, PALA is chemically stable for at least 14 days at room temperature.

Preparation

The desired dose of PALA may be further diluted to a concentration of 1 mg/mL in normal saline or 5% dextrose.

Availability

PALA is an investigational drug that is available from the NCI as a 100 mg/mL solution (500 mg/vial).

Selected Readings

Grem JL et al: Biochemistry and clinical activity of N-(phosphonacetyl)-L-aspartate: a review, *Cancer Res* 48:4441-4454, 1988.

Kemeny N et al: Biochemical modulation of bolus fluorouracil by PALA in patients with advanced colorectal cancer, *J Clin Oncol* 10:747-752, 1992.

PAMIDRONATE

Other Names

Aredia, pamidronate disodium, aminohydroxypropylidene biphosphonate, APD.

Indications

FDA approved for the treatment of hypercalcemia of malignancy and multiple myeloma. Pamidronate may also be useful for treatment of patients with osteolytic bone metastases (e.g., breast cancer), Paget's disease, and other bone-resorptive diseases.

Classification and Mechanisms of Action

Pamidronate is a biphosphonate that inhibits bone resorption. The drug exerts its actions through its effects on osteoclast precursors, possibly by adsorption of the drug to hydroxyapatite crystals in bone. The drug also inhibits parathyroid hormone–induced bone resorption.

Pharmacokinetics

Pamidronate is poorly absorbed (1% to 5%) by mouth. In animals the drug is widely distributed throughout the body, primarily to bone, spleen, and liver. Pamidronate has an elimination half-life of 27 hours, and approximately 50% is eliminated unchanged in the urine.

In conjunction with vigorous saline hydration for the treatment of hypercalcemia, pamidronate is given in a dose of 60 to 90 mg. Retreatment is not necessary in most patients. If retreatment is necessary, it is recommended that at least 7 days elapse from the time of the initial dose. The manufacturer recommends a dose of 60 to 90 mg for moderate hypercalcemia (serum calcium corrected for albumin, 12 to 13.5 mg/dL) and a starting dose of 90 mg for severe hypercalcemia (serum calcium corrected for albumin, >13.5 mg/dL). (Corrected serum calcium = serum calcium in mg/dL + 0.8[4.0 − serum albumin in g/dL].) For the treatment of osteolytic bone lesions associated with multiple myeloma, a dose of 90 mg is recommended. For the treatment of Paget's disease, the recommended dose is 30 mg/day for 3 days.

Administration

The manufacturer recommends that pamidronate be administered by IV infusion, in 1000 mL of 5% dextrose, normal saline, or 0.45% NaCl over a 4- (60-mg dose) to 24-hour (90-mg dose) period. Others have recommended that pamidronate (90 mg/500 mL maximum concentration) be administered at a rate no greater than 15 mg/hour. The drug has been given over a 1- to 4-hour period (60 mg/hr maximum).

Toxicity

Hematological. Anemia (6%), leukopenia (4%).

Gastrointestinal. Nausea (18% with 90-mg dose, 0% to 4% with 60-mg dose), vomiting (0% to 15%), abdominal pain (2%), anorexia (1% to 12%), constipation (up to 6%), gastrointestinal hemorrhage (up to 6%).

Neurological. Insomnia (1% to 2%), somnolence (1% to 6%), abnormal vision (2%), psychosis (0% to 4%).

Cardiovascular. Atrial fibrillation, hypertension, syncope, and tachycardia have been reported in up to 6% of the patients treated with pamidronate, 90 mg.

Pulmonary. Upper respiratory infection (2%), rales (up to 6%).

Electrolyte. Hypocalcemia (2% to 12%), hypokalemia (4% to 18%), hypomagnesemia (4% to 12%), hypophosphatemia (9% to 18%).

Other. Fatigue (12% with 90-mg dose), fever (18% to 50%), infusion site reaction (4% to 18%), hypothyroidism (6% with 90-mg dose), generalized pain (15%), bone pain (15%).

Storage and Stability

Pamidronate is stored at room temperature. Vials bear expiration dates. Reconstituted solutions (30 mg/10 mL) are stable for at least 24 hours in the refrigerator. Further diluted (30 to 90 mg in 1000 mL of 5% dextrose, normal saline or 0.45% NaCl), pamidronate is stable for at least 24 hours at room or refrigeration temperatures.

Preparation

Add 10 mL of sterile water to the 30-, 60-, or 90-mg vial to yield concentrations of 3, 6, or 9 mg/mL, respectively.

Incompatibilities

Pamidronate is incompatible with calcium-containing solutions, such as Ringer's solution. Concomitant use of vitamin D may antagonize the effects of pamidronate and should be avoided.

Availability

Pamidronate is commercially available as a lyophilized powder in 30-, 60-, and 90-mg vials.

Selected Readings
Berenson JR et al: Efficacy of pamidronate in reducing skeletal events in patients with advanced multiple myeloma, *N Engl J Med* 334:488-493, 1996.

Fitton A, McTavish D: Pamidronate: a review of its pharmacological properties and therapeutic efficacy in resorptive bone disease, *Drugs* 41:289-318, 1991.

Gucalp R et al: Comparative study of pamidronate disodium and etidronate disodium in the treatment of cancer-related hypercalcemia, *J Clin Oncol* 10:134-142, 1992.

van Holten-Verzantvoort ATM et al: Palliative pamidronate treatment in patients with bone metastasis from breast cancer, *J Clin Oncol* 11:491-498, 1993.

PENTOSTATIN

Other Names
Nipent, 2'-deoxycoformycin, dCF, co-vidarabine, NSC-218321.

Indications
FDA approved for the treatment of hairy cell leukemia in patients whose disease is no longer controlled by interferon alfa. Pentostatin may also be useful in the treatment of non-Hodgkin's lymphoma and cutaneous T-cell lymphoma.

Classification
Antimetabolite (adenosine deaminase inhibitor).

Pharmacokinetics
Approximately 4% of pentostatin is bound to plasma proteins. The majority of pentostatin is excreted unchanged in the urine. The plasma elimination half-life of pentostatin in patients with normal renal function (i.e., creatinine clearance of 60 mL/min or more) ranges from 5 to 6 hours. In patients with impaired renal function (i.e., creatinine clearance less than 50 mL/min) the elimination half-life may exceed 18 hours. High levels of deoxyadenosine can accumulate in the blood and brain. Urinary deoxyadenosine may exceed solubility in patients with sensitive neoplasms, such as acute lymphoblastic leukemia, unless a forced diuresis is arranged.

Dose
A common regimen is 4 mg/m^2 every 2 weeks.

Administration
Pentostatin is usually administered by IV bolus (usually in 25 to 50 mL of 5% dextrose or normal saline) or as an IV infusion over a 20-minute or longer period. It is recommended that 1000 to 2000 mL of hydration be given with each treatment.

Toxicity
Hematological. Severe leukopenia and lymphopenia occur commonly and can lead to serious infection. Thrombocytopenia and anemia are common (32% to 35%).

Gastrointestinal. Nausea (22% to 53%) and vomiting are not usually severe. Stomatitis (3% to 10%), diarrhea (15%), anorexia (16%), and altered taste are infrequent toxicities.

Dermatological. Skin rashes occur in up to 26% of the patients, may be severe, and worsen with continued therapy. Other dermatological toxicities include dry skin (3% to 17%), diaphoresis (3% to 10%), pruritus, skin discoloration, seborrhea, and eczema.

Hepatic. Elevated hepatic transaminase levels (19%), hepatitis (rare), hyperbilirubinemia.

Neurological. In phase I studies, neurological toxicities were often dose limiting. Neurological toxicities observed in these studies included lassitude, confusion, headache, fatigue, insomnia, expressive aphasia, slurred speech, depression, hallucinations, agitation, cerebral edema, seizures, and coma. The more severe toxicities rarely occur with conventional doses (i.e., 4 mg/m^2 every 2 weeks).

Pulmonary. Cough (17%), shortness of breath, respiratory insufficiency, and/or pulmonary infiltrates on chest radiographs are rare. Combined treatment of pentostatin and fludarabine is not recommended because of the increased risk of fatal pulmonary toxicity.

Renal. Elevated serum creatinine, acute tubular necrosis, hematuria, dysuria, and renal failure are uncommon.

Other. Keratoconjunctivitis, photophobia, fever (42%), chills (11%), arthralgia, myalgia (11%).

Storage and Stability
Unreconstituted drug vials are stored in the refrigerator. Reconstituted solutions (2 mg/mL) are chemically stable for 72 and 96 hours at room and refrigeration temperatures, respectively. Dilute solutions (10 mg/500 mL) are chemically stable at room temperature for 24 hours in 5% dextrose and 48 hours in normal saline or lactated Ringer's solution.

Preparation
The 10-mg vial is reconstituted with 5 mL of sterile water or normal saline to result in a 2 mg/mL solution. The desired dose is further diluted to concentrations of 1 mg/mL or less in normal saline, lactated Ringer's solution, or 5% dextrose.

Availability
Pentostatin, 10 mg/vial, is commercially available as a lyophilized powder.

Selected Readings
Grever MR et al: Low-dose deoxycoformycin in lymphoid malignancy, *J Clin Oncol* 3:1196-1201, 1985.

Grever M et al: Randomized comparison of pentostatin versus interferon alfa-2a in previously untreated patients with hairy cell leukemia: an intergroup study, *J Clin Oncol* 13:974-982, 1995.

Johnston JB et al: Efficacy of 2-deoxycoformycin 2' in hairy-cell leukemia: a study of the National Cancer Institute of Canada Clinical Trials Group, *J Natl Cancer Inst* 80:765-769, 1988.

Spiers ASD et al: Remissions in hairy-cell leukemia with pentostatin (2'-deoxycoformycin), *N Engl J Med* 316:825-830, 1987.

P

PIPOBROMAN
Other Names
Vercyte, A-8103, 8103-Abbott, NSC-25154.

Indications
Chronic granulocytic leukemia and polycythemia vera.

Classification
Alkylating agent.

Dose
In the treatment of chronic granulocytic leukemia, initially 1.5 to 2.5 mg/kg/day is used. The maintenance dose is 0.1 to 0.2 mg/kg/day to desired response. In the treatment of polycythemia vera, 1 mg/kg/day is the usual initial dose, followed by 0.1 mg/kg/day to the best response.

Administration
Oral.

Toxicity
Hematological. Bone marrow suppression is dose dependent. Leukopenia and thrombocytopenia are common. If anemia develops rapidly with reticulocytosis, a hemolytic process should be suspected, and treatment should be stopped.

Gastrointestinal. Nausea, vomiting, abdominal cramps, and diarrhea.

Dermatological. Skin rash.

Storage and Stability
Pipobroman is stored at room temperature. Containers bear expiration dates.

Availability
Pipobroman is commercially available in 25-mg scored tablets.

Selected Readings
Bernard J et al: The treatment of polycythemia vera by pipobroman: results in 63 patients treated between 1969 and 1977, *Nouv Presse Med* 7:3527-3530, 1978.
Monto RW et al: A-8103 in polycythemia vera, *JAMA* 190:833-836, 1964.

PLICAMYCIN
Other Names
Mithracin, mithramycin, NSC-24559.

Indications
FDA approved for the treatment of malignant tumors of the testis and hypercalcemia and hypercalcuria associated with a variety of advanced neoplasms.

Plicamycin may be useful in the treatment of chronic myelogenous leukemia in blast crisis.

Classification
Antitumor antibiotic.

Pharmacokinetics
Plicamycin is not well absorbed by mouth. After IV administration the drug predominately distributes to the liver, kidney, bone, and cerebrospinal fluid. Plicamycin is metabolized by the liver, and approximately 25% to 40% is eliminated unchanged in the urine. Plicamycin has an elimination half-life of around 2 hours.

Dose
For the treatment of testicular cancer, doses of 25 to 30 µg/kg/day for 8 to 10 days have been given. For the treatment of hypercalcemia of malignancy, doses of 25 to 30 µg/kg may be administered 1 to 3 times a week.

Administration
Plicamycin is administered by slow IV infusion (in 100 to 500 mL of normal saline or 5% dextrose) over a 30- to 60-minute or longer period (usually over a span of 4 to 6 hours).

Toxicity
Hematological. Leukopenia and anemia occur infrequently. Thrombocytopenia and hemorrhage occur more frequently and are dose related. Bleeding episodes occur approximately 12% of the time and are fatal in up to 6% of the patients who receive doses greater than 30 µg/kg/day and/or receive more than 10 doses. Facial flushing, epistaxis, and prolonged prothrombin time are frequent signs of this toxicity. Treatment should be held if any of these signs are present. An alternate-day schedule instead of daily dosing reduces the incidence of bleeding problems.

Gastrointestinal. Nausea and vomiting (more common with rapid IV infusion), anorexia, stomatitis, diarrhea.

Dermatological. Skin and soft-tissue damage (cellulitis, phlebitis) if extravasated, hyperpigmentation, toxic epidermal necrolysis, acneiform skin rash.

Hepatic. Elevated hepatic transaminase levels, hyperbilirubinemia.

Neurological. Headache, depression, dizziness, nervousness, drowsiness.

Renal. Proteinuria, azotemia, elevated serum creatinine levels.

Electrolyte. Hypocalcemia, hypophosphatemia, hypokalemia, hypomagnesemia, rebound hypercalcemia on discontinuation of treatment.

Other. Fever, weakness, fatigue, lethargy, periorbital pallor.

Storage and Stability
Unreconstituted drug should be stored in the refrigerator. Unreconstituted plicamycin is stable for 3 months at room temperature. At a concentration

of 500 µg/mL, the drug is chemically stable for at least 24 and 48 hours at room and refrigeration temperatures, respectively. After dilution in 5% dextrose or normal saline to a concentration of 24 µg/mL, plicamycin is stable for at least 24 hours at room temperature.

Preparation
The 2500-µg (2.5-mg) vial is reconstituted with 4.9 mL of sterile water to result in a 500 µg/mL solution. The desired dose of plicamycin is usually further diluted in 100 to 500 mL of normal saline or 5% dextrose.

Incompatibilities
Cellulose ester filters, iron, trace element solutions.

Availability
Plicamycin is commercially available as a lyophilized powder in 2500-µg (2.5 mg) vials.

Selected Readings
Schaiff RA, Hall TG, Bar RS: Medical treatment of hypercalcemia, *Clin Pharm* 8:108-121, 1989.
Shevrin DH et al: Treatment of cancer-associated hypercalcemia with mithramycin and oral etidronate disodium, *Clin Pharm* 4:204-205, 1985.

PORFIMER SODIUM
Other Names
Photofrin.

Indications
FDA approved for use with photodynamic therapy in the treatment of esophageal cancer.

Classification and Mechanisms of Action
Porphyrin compound with photosensitizing properties. Porfimer sodium within cells reacts with laser light to produce a photochemical reaction that results in the release of cytotoxic elements (e.g., singlet oxygen, superoxide and hydroxyl radicals).

Pharmacokinetics
Approximately 90% of porfimer sodium is protein bound. The drug is cleared from most tissues over 40 to 72 hours but some tissues (e.g., tumors, spleen, liver) retain the drug for a longer period of time. The elimination half-life of the drug is approximately 10 days.

Dose
Porfimer sodium is administered at a dose of 2 mg/kg 40 to 50 hours before illumination of the target tissue with laser light. Illumination of the target tissue with laser light is repeated 96 to 120 hours after administration of porfimer sodium.

Administration
Slow IV infusion over 3 to 5 minutes using extravasation precautions.

Toxicity
The toxicities listed are those that have been observed in patients receiving porfimer sodium in combination with laser light treatment for esophageal carcinoma.

Hematological. Anemia (32%).

Gastrointestinal. Constipation (24%), nausea (24%), vomiting (17%), abdominal pain (20%), dysphagia (10%), esophageal edema and/or bleeding (8%), esophagitis (5%), esophageal stricture (6%), hematemesis (8%), melena (5%), dyspepsia (6%), diarrhea (5%), anorexia (8%).

Dermatological. Photosensitivity reactions (e.g., erythema, edema, blistering) have been reported in approximately 20% of the patients. It is recommended that a test for residual photosensitivity be conducted before exposing any area of the body to direct sunlight. A small area of the skin should be exposed to sunlight for approximately 10 minutes. If a photosensitivity reaction occurs within 24 hours of the test, all areas of the skin should be protected for 2 weeks before repeating the test. If a photosensitivity reaction does not occur within 24 hours of the test, gradual resumption of outdoor activities may commence. *Ultraviolet light sunscreens will not prevent photosensitivity reactions.* Concomitant administration of other photosensitizing drugs (e.g., tetracyclines, sulfonylureas, thiazides, phenothiazines, griseofulvin) should be avoided.

Neurological. Insomnia (14%), anxiety (7%), confusion (8%).

Cardiovascular. Hypotension and hypertension have been reported in 6% to 7% of the patients. Atrial fibrillation, tachycardia, peripheral edema, and cardiac failure have been reported in approximately 6% to 10% of the patients.

Pulmonary. Pleural effusion (32%), dyspnea (20%), pneumonia (18%), pharyngitis (11%), cough (7%), tracheoesophageal fistula (6%).

Other. Fever (31%), chest pain (22%), pain (22%), back pain (11%), dehydration (7%), weight loss (9%), asthenia (6%).

Storage and Stability
Vials of porfimer sodium are stored at room temperature. Reconstituted solutions should be protected from bright light and used immediately.

Preparation
Add 31.8 mL of 5% dextrose or normal saline to the vial to result in a 2.5 mg/mL solution. The drug may be administered without further dilution.

Incompatibilities
Porfimer sodium is contraindicated in patients with porphyria.

Availability
Commercially available as a lyophilized powder in 75-mg vials.

PREDNIMUSTINE
Other Names
Sterecyt, Mostarinia, Leo 1031, NSC-134087.

Indications
Prednimustine is an investigational drug that may be useful in the treatment of chronic lymphocytic leukemia, non-Hodgkin's lymphoma, and cancers of the ovary, breast, and prostate.

Classification
Alkylating agent.

Pharmacokinetics
Prednimustine is poorly absorbed by mouth. The drug is metabolized by the liver, and up to 50% is excreted unchanged in the feces.

Dose
Various dose regimens have been studied. Continuous daily doses of 20 to 30 mg or intermittent dosing with 100 to 160 mg/m²/day for 3 to 5 days are most commonly used.

Administration
Oral, usually in two divided doses.

Toxicity
Hematological. Leukopenia and thrombocytopenia are common and often dose limiting.

Gastrointestinal. Mild nausea and vomiting occur infrequently. Diarrhea and gastritis have been reported.

Dermatological. Alopecia and skin rashes are uncommon toxicities.

Neurological. Confusion, euphoria.

Cardiovascular. Hypertension.

Other. Fever, urticaria, edema.

Storage and Stability
Prednimustine tablets are stored at room temperature.

Availability
Prednimustine is an orphan drug that is available as a 20-mg tablet.

Selected Readings
Boesen E, Mouridsen HT: Prednimustine in combination with methotrexate and 5-FU (PMF): a pilot study, *Cancer Treat Rep* 66:2081-2083, 1982.

Yarbro JW, Bornstein RS, Mastrangelo MJ, eds: Prednimustine, *Semin Oncol* 13(suppl 1):1-14, 1986.

PREDNISONE

Other Names

Deltasone, Orasone, Meticorten, Panasol-S, Liquid Pred, and others.

Indications

FDA approved for the treatment of endocrine disorders (adrenocortical insufficiency, hypercalcemia of malignancy, nonsuppurative thyroiditis), rheumatic disorders (rheumatoid arthritis, psoriatic arthritis, ankylosing spondylitis, bursitis, gouty arthritis, osteoarthritis, epicondylitis), collagen diseases (lupus, polymyositis), dermatological diseases (pemphigus, erythema multiforme, mycosis fungoides, psoriasis, seborrheic dermatitis), ophthalmic diseases (severe acute and chronic allergic and inflammatory processes), respiratory diseases (sarcoidosis, Löeffler's syndrome, berylliosis, aspiration pneumonitis), hematological disorders (idiopathic thrombocytopenic purpura [ITP] in adults, secondary thrombocytopenia in adults, hemolytic anemia, erythroblastopenia, congenital hypoplastic anemia), neoplastic diseases (leukemias and lymphomas in adults, acute leukemia of childhood), edematous states, gastrointestinal disorders (ulcerative colitis, regional enteritis), acute exacerbations of multiple sclerosis, tuberculous meningitis, and trichinosis with neurological or myocardial involvement.

Classification and Mechanisms of Action

Prednisone is a potent synthetic glucocorticoid that affects almost every body system. It has antiinflammatory, immunosuppressant, and minimal mineralocorticoid activity and antineoplastic properties. As an antineoplastic agent, prednisone may bind to specific proteins (receptors) within the cell, forming a steroid-receptor complex. Binding of the receptor-steroid complex with nuclear chromatin alters mRNA and protein synthesis within the cell.

Pharmacokinetics

Approximately 80% of a dose is absorbed by mouth, and 75% of the drug is bound to plasma proteins. Prednisone is metabolized by the liver and has an elimination half-life of 3.5 hours.

Dose

Common regimens include 40 mg/m²/day for 14 days, repeated every 28 days; 20 mg/m²/day for 7 days; and 100 mg/m²/day for 5 days, repeated every 3 to 4 weeks.

Administration

Oral.

Toxicity

Hematological. Leukocytosis, thrombocytosis.

Gastrointestinal. Nausea, vomiting, anorexia, increased appetite, weight gain, pancreatitis, aggravation of peptic ulcers, peptic ulceration.

Dermatological. Rash, skin atrophy, hirsutism, acne, facial erythema, ecchymoses, poor wound healing.

Neurological. Insomnia, muscle weakness, euphoria, psychosis, depression, headache, vertigo, seizures.

Cardiovascular. Fluid retention and edema, hypertension, thromboembolism.

Genitourinary. Menstrual changes (amenorrhea, menstrual irregularities).

Ocular. Cataracts, increased intraocular pressure, exophthalmos.

Metabolic. Hyperglycemia, decreased glucose tolerance, aggravation or precipitation of diabetes mellitus, adrenal suppression (with Cushingoid features), hypokalemia.

Other. Osteoporosis (and resulting back pain), serious infections (including herpes zoster, varicella zoster, fungal infections, *Pneumocystis carinii* pneumonia, tuberculosis), muscle wasting, aseptic necrosis of femoral head, suppression of reactions to skin tests.

Storage and Stability
Prednisone is stored at room temperature; bottles bear expiration dates.

Availability
Commercially available in 1-, 2.5-, 5-, 10-, 20-, 25-, and 50-mg tablets. Also available as a 1 mg/mL oral solution or syrup and as a 5 mg/mL oral solution.

Selected Readings
The Boston Collaborative Drug Surveillance Program: Acute reactions to prednisone in relation to dosage, *J Clin Pharmacol* 13:694-698, 1972.

Ling MHM, Perry PJ, Tsuang MT: Side effects of corticosteroid therapy: psychiatric aspects, *Arch Gen Psychiatry* 38:471-477, 1981.

PROCARBAZINE
Other Names
Matulane, Natulan, ibenzmethyzin, N-methylhydrazine, NSC-77213.

Indications
FDA approved for the treatment of Hodgkin's disease (stages III and IV) as a part of the Mustargen-Oncovin-procarbazine-prednisone (MOPP) regimen. Procarbazine may also be useful in the treatment of non-Hodgkin's lymphoma, multiple myeloma, melanoma, brain tumors, lung cancer, and polycythemia vera.

Classification
Alkylating agent.

Pharmacokinetics
Procarbazine is almost completely absorbed after oral administration and reaches peak plasma concentrations in 1 hour. Procarbazine penetrates

into the cerebrospinal fluid, it is metabolized by the liver, and less than 5% is eliminated in the urine as unchanged drug. Procarbazine has an elimination half-life of approximately 1 hour.

Dose

As a part of the MOPP and C-MOPP (cyclophosphamide-Oncovin-procarbazine-prednisone) regimens, procarbazine is given in a dose of 100 mg/m^2/day for 14 days and repeated every 4 weeks.

Administration

Oral.

Toxicity

Hematological. Leukopenia and thrombocytopenia occur frequently, usually 2 to 3 weeks after cessation of therapy. Anemia occurs less frequently.

Gastrointestinal. Nausea and vomiting occur commonly and may be dose limiting. Antiemetic drugs may be necessary. Anorexia, diarrhea (uncommon), stomatitis (uncommon), xerostomia, dysphagia, and constipation have been reported.

Dermatological. Skin rash, photosensitivity, urticaria, dermatitis, flushing, alopecia.

Neurological. Paresthesias, lethargy, weakness, dizziness, somnolence, nightmares, depression, insomnia, headache, visual disturbances, hallucinations, ataxia, nystagmus, seizures. Concomitant use with tricyclic antidepressants, opiate analgesics, or benzodiazepines may lead to enhanced central nervous system toxicities.

Cardiovascular. Hypotension, tachycardia, syncope. Concomitant use with sympathomimetics or foods with high tyramine content may lead to a sudden increase in blood pressure and hypertensive crisis.

Ocular. Photophobia, diplopia, papilledema, and retinal hemorrhage have been reported.

Other. Urinary frequency, hematuria, nocturia, gynecomastia, sterility, menstrual irregularities, fever, myalgia, arthralgia, second malignancy, allergic pneumonitis.

Drug interactions. Concurrent use of drugs and/or foods listed below *may* result in adverse effects such as headache, tremor, excitation, cardiac arrhythmia, nausea, vomiting, and visual disturbances. Procarbazine is a weak monoamine oxidase inhibitor, and this is the basis for some of the drug interactions listed.

Drugs. Ethanol, sympathomimetics (e.g., ephedrine, pseudoephedrine, isoproterenol, epinephrine), tricyclic antidepressants (e.g., imipramine, nortriptyline, amitriptyline, desipramine), monoamine oxidase inhibitors (e.g., pargyline), opiate analgesics (especially meperidine), antihistamines, phenothiazines, antihypertensive agents, and barbiturates.

Foods. Tyramine-rich foods (imported beer, fermented cheese, some wines), chocolate, fava beans.

Storage and Stability
Procarbazine is stored at room temperature; containers bear expiration dates.

Availability
Procarbazine is commercially available in 50-mg capsules.

Selected Readings
Anonymous: Foods interacting with MAO inhibitors, *Med Lett* 31:11-12, 1989.
Maxwell MB: Reexamining the dietary restrictions with procarbazine (an MAOI), *Cancer Nurs* 3:451-457, 1980.

PSC-833
Other Names
SDZ PSC 833.

Classification and Mechanisms of Action
Cyclosporine derivative, modulator of multidrug resistance. PSC-833 is a nonimmunosuppressive analogue of cyclosporine that is 5 to 20 times more potent than cyclosporine in its ability to modulate multidrug resistance in vitro. PSC-833 competitively inhibits the activity of the transmembrane protein P-glycoprotein. As a result, intracellular retention of doxorubicin, vinblastine, or other drugs in multidrug-resistant cells is enhanced.

Pharmacokinetics
Approximately 50% of PSC-833 reaches the bloodstream after oral administration. When the drug is administered by continuous IV infusion, doses of 6.6 mg/kg/day or more have been shown to result in plasma levels above 1000 ng/mL. Combined with etoposide, PSC-833 has been shown to decrease the elimination of etoposide by 41%, increase the elimination half-life by 39%, and increase the plasma AUC of etoposide by an average of 76% (range, 1% to 171%).

Dose
The optimal dose of PSC-833 has not been determined. The drug has been given 4 hours after administration of chemotherapy as a 2 mg/kg loading dose administered intravenously over a span of 4 hours concurrent with a continuous IV infusion of 10 mg/kg/day for 5 days. The loading dose and the continuous IV infusion are begun at the same time. The drug has also been given as an oral dose of 5 mg/kg 4 times daily for 5 days.

Administration
Oral (capsules or solution) or by IV infusion in a glass container over a period of 2 hours or longer. Normal saline, 100 mL, has been used to administer 2-hour infusions, and 500 mL of 5% dextrose have been used to administer the drug over a period of 24 hours. Polyvinylchloride-containing

containers and infusion sets should not be used to administer the parenteral formulation of PSC-833.

Toxicities

PSC-833 is a modulator of multidrug resistance that is used in combination with antineoplastic drugs.

Hematological. PSC-833 may enhance the myelosuppressive effects of antineoplastic drugs (e.g., etoposide).

Gastrointestinal. Nausea, vomiting (infrequent), constipation.

Hepatic. Transient elevation of hepatic transaminase levels. Hyperbilirubinemia occurs frequently and is usually asymptomatic.

Neurological. Cerebellar dysfunction (ataxia, incoordination, unsteadiness, difficulty in walking) are dose limiting. In some studies, symptoms appeared within 1 to 3 hours of IV administration and generally disappeared within 12 hours of discontinuation of the IV infusion. When PSC-833 was given as a continuous IV infusion, symptoms appeared 36 to 48 hours after initiation of treatment and resolved slowly over a period of 3 to 5 weeks. Dizziness, diplopia, paresthesias, and headache have also been reported.

Cardiovascular. Orthostatic hypotension occasionally occurs; hypertension has been reported.

Pulmonary. Moderate feeling of suffocation with sternal pressure and an urge to cough has been reported after IV administration.

Other. Anaphylactoid reactions possibly caused by the Cremophor EL diluent; mild hyperglycemia has been reported.

Storage and Stability

The parenteral formulation of PSC-833 is stored in the refrigerator and protected from light. Freezing of PSC-833 should be avoided. After dilution in dextrose 5% or normal saline, PSC-833 solution is stable for 24 hours. Capsules of PSC-833 are stored at room temperature.

Preparation

The parenteral formulation is diluted to a 1:20 to 1:50 volume in 5% dextrose or normal saline (in a glass bottle).

Incompatibilities

Polyvinylchloride containers and IV infusion sets.

Availability

PSC-833 is an investigational drug that is currently available from Novardis Pharmaceutical Corporation as a parenteral formulation (50 mg/mL), a solution for oral administration (100 mg/mL, 50 mL/bottle), and capsules (50 mg and 100 mg).

Selected Readings

Boesch D et al: In vivo circumvention of P-glycoprotein–mediated multidrug resistance of tumor cells with SDZ PSC 833, *Cancer Res* 51;4226-4233, 1991.

Boote DJ et al: Phase I study of etoposide with SDZ PSC 833 as a modulator of multidrug resistance in patients with cancer, *J Clin Oncol* 14:610-618, 1996.

Twentyman PR, Bleehen NM: Resistance modification by PSC-833, a novel non-immunosuppressive cyclosporin A, *Eur J Cancer* 27:1639-1642, 1991.

STREPTOZOCIN

Other Names
Zanosar, streptozotocin, NSC-85998.

Indications
FDA approved for the treatment of metastatic islet cell carcinoma of the pancreas. Streptozocin may be a useful treatment for carcinoid tumors, Hodgkin's disease, and pancreatic carcinoma.

Classification
Alkylating agent.

Pharmacokinetics
Streptozocin is poorly absorbed by mouth. After IV administration, the drug is primarily distributed in the kidneys, pancreas, and liver. Metabolites of streptozocin penetrate the cerebrospinal fluid (CSF), and drug levels in the plasma and CSF are equivalent 2 hours after administration. Streptozocin is extensively metabolized, and 10% to 20% is eliminated in the urine as unchanged drug. Streptozocin has an elimination half-life of 35 to 40 minutes; metabolites of the drug have half-lives around 40 hours.

Dose
Streptozocin is commonly given every 4 to 6 weeks at a dose of 500 to 1000 mg/m^2/day for 5 days. Doses of 1000 to 1500 mg/m^2/week have also been used. A single daily dose of 1500 mg/m^2 should not be exceeded because this may increase the likelihood of severe nephrotoxicity.

Administration
Streptozocin has been given by IV bolus, but is usually administered by slow IV infusion (in 100 mL or more of normal saline or 5% dextrose), usually over a period of 30 to 60 minutes. The drug has been given as a 5-day continuous IV infusion.

Toxicity
Hematological. Leukopenia and thrombocytopenia are rarely dose limiting. However, cumulative myelosuppression has been reported. Anemia and eosinophilia occur infrequently.

Gastrointestinal. Nausea and vomiting are common, often severe, and require antiemetic pretreatment. Symptoms begin 1 to 4 hours after administration of the drug. Anorexia, diarrhea, and abdominal cramps occur less frequently.

Hepatic. Mild, transient increases in hepatic enzyme levels occur in approximately 25% of the patients. Hypoalbuminemia has also been reported.

Neurological. Confusion, depression, and lethargy are rare and tend to occur most often in patients receiving streptozocin as a continuous 5-day IV infusion.

Renal. Nephrotoxicity is common, dose related, and sometimes irreversible. Early signs include hypophosphatemia, aminoaciduria, and/or proteinuria. Other manifestations may include renal tubular acidosis, Fanconi syndrome, azotemia, acetonuria, acute tubular necrosis, hyperchloremia, decreased creatinine clearance, and nephrogenic diabetes insipidus (rare).

Metabolic. Mild to moderate hyperglycemia, severe hypoglycemia, and insulin shock have been rarely reported in patients with insulinoma.

Other. Fever (rare), vein irritation during administration, second malignancy.

Storage and Stability
When streptozocin is stored in the refrigerator (2° C to 8° C) and protected from light, it is stable for 3 years. Streptozocin is stable at room temperature for at least 1 year after the date of manufacture. After reconstitution to a concentration of 100 mg/mL and after dilution to a concentration of 2 mg/mL in 5% dextrose or normal saline, the drug is chemically stable for at least 48 hours at room temperature and 96 hours under refrigeration.

Preparation
The 1000-mg vial is reconstituted with 9.5 mL of 5% dextrose or normal saline to yield a 100 mg/mL solution. The desired dose may be further diluted in 5% dextrose, normal saline, or 5% dextrose and normal saline.

Availability
Streptozocin, in a 1000 mg/vial, is commercially available as a lyophilized powder.

Selected Readings
Weiss RB: Streptozocin: a review of its pharmacology, efficacy and toxicity, *Cancer Treat Rep* 66:427-438, 1982.
Wiggans RG et al: Phase II trial of streptozocin, mitomycin-C, and 5-fluorouracil (SMF) in the treatment of advanced pancreatic cancer, *Cancer* 41:397-401, 1978.

S

SURAMIN
Other Names
Suramin sodium, Antrypol, Bayer 205, Germanin, Moranyl, Naganin, Naphuride, Naganol, Fourneau 309, NSC-34936.

Indications
Suramin is an investigational drug that has been shown to have activity against prostate cancer. Suramin may be a useful treatment for patients with adrenal carcinoma.

Classification and Mechanisms of Action

Suramin is a glycosaminoglycan (GAG) agonist-antagonist and a potent antitrypanosomal agent that may inhibit malignant cell growth by binding to growth factors, such as platelet-derived growth factor (PDGF), epidermal growth factor (EGF), transforming growth factor beta (TGF beta), and basic fibroblast growth factor (bFGF). Suramin may also exert antitumor activity by other mechanisms, including inhibition of growth regulatory proteins (such as transferrin), inhibition of glycosaminoglycan catabolism, and inhibition of DNA polymerases.

Pharmacokinetics

After IV administration suramin (>99%) is tightly bound to plasma proteins, primarily albumin. Suramin distributes primarily to the kidneys; 2% is eliminated unchanged in the bile, and the remainder is eliminated in the urine by renal excretion. Suramin has an elimination half-life of 40 to 50 days.

Dose

Suramin has been given as a continuous IV infusion, 350 mg/m^2/day, until the plasma suramin level reaches 250 to 300 µg/mL. Drug administration is usually stopped for a period of 2 months and treatment repeated if indicated. Several other dosing regimens have been evaluated, including 1440 mg/m^2 on day 1 followed by 720 mg/m^2 on days 2 and 8, and 576 mg/m^2 on day 9 repeated every 28 days for three courses.

Administration

Suramin has been given by IV bolus and by IV infusion over a period of 1 hour or longer. The drug has also been administered as a continuous IV infusion until the plasma suramin level reaches 250 to 300 µg/mL.

Toxicity

The most significant toxicities (e.g., neurotoxicity) are dose dependent. Life-threatening toxicities can be avoided in most cases by keeping the plasma concentration below 300 µg/mL.

Hematological. Leukopenia (usually mild); thrombocytopenia (may be dose limiting); elevated thrombin, prothrombin, and partial thromboplastin times; hemorrhage; anemia.

Gastrointestinal. Nausea, vomiting, metallic or salty taste in the mouth, constipation.

Dermatological. Erythematous rash (usually transient), urticaria, pruritus.

Hepatic. Elevated hepatic enzyme levels and hyperbilirubinemia.

Neurological. Paresthesias (distal end of the extremity and perioral); polyradiculoneuropathy (muscle weakness progressing to generalized flaccid paralysis), with maximum plasma level >386 µg/mL or more.

Renal. Proteinuria, decreased creatinine clearance, elevated serum creatinine levels, hypophosphatemia, hypomagnesemia, hematuria.

Adrenal. Adrenocortical insufficiency (increased adrenocorticotropin [ACTH] and plasma renin concentrations, decreased serum cortisol level, lack of response to ACTH stimulation).

Ocular. Vortex keratopathy, with lacrimation, photophobia, and blurred vision.

Other. Fever, malaise, and lethargy (often severe); hypocalcemia, pericardial effusion (rare).

Storage and Stability
Unreconstituted drug is stored at room temperature. At concentrations of 2, 10, and 20 mg/mL in sterile or normal saline (PVC containers), the drug is chemically stable for at least 21 days at room temperature. At a concentration of 8 mg/mL in 5% dextrose in Deltec cassette reservoirs, suramin is stable for 3 weeks at 4° C and −20° C.

Preparation
The 1000-mg vial is reconstituted with 10 mL of sterile water to yield a 100 mg/mL solution. The desired dose is further diluted to concentrations of 2 to 10 mg/mL in normal saline or 5% dextrose.

Availability
Suramin is an investigational drug that is available as a lyophilized powder from the NCI in 1000-mg vials.

Selected Readings
Eisenberger MA et al: Suramin, an active drug for prostate cancer: interim observation in a phase I trial, *J Natl Cancer Inst* 85:611-621, 1993.

Eisenberger MA et al: Phase I and clinical evaluation of a pharmacologically guided regimen of suramin in patients with hormone-refractory prostate cancer, *J Clin Oncol* 13:2174-2186, 1995.

Meyers C et al: Suramin: a novel growth factor antagonist with activity in hormone-refractory metastatic prostate cancer, *J Clin Oncol* 10:881-889, 1992.

Stein CA, LaRocca R, Myers C: Suramin: an old compound with new biology. In DeVita VT Jr, Hellman S, Rosenberg SA, eds: *Principles and practice of oncology, PPO updates,* 4:1-12, 1990.

T

TAMOXIFEN

Other Names
Nolvadex, tamoxifen citrate, Alpha-Tamoxifen, Med Tamoxifen, Nolvadex-D, Novo-Tamoxifen, Tamofen, Tamone, Tamoplex, NSC-180973.

Indications
FDA approved for the treatment of breast cancer in an adjuvant setting after initial surgical and/or radiation treatment. Tamoxifen is also approved for the treatment of metastatic breast cancer. The drug may be a useful treatment for mastalgia, gynecomastia, malignant melanoma, and cancers of the pancreas, endometrium, and liver. Tamoxifen may also be

a useful preventive treatment for patients with a very high risk of developing breast cancer.

Classification and Mechanisms of Action

Tamoxifen is a hormone antagonist (antiestrogen). Tamoxifen and its metabolites possess antiestrogenic activity as a result of their ability to compete with estradiol for binding to receptors in the cells of tumors that contain high amounts of estrogen receptors (such as breast cancer). The tamoxifen-estrogen receptor complex is translocated from the cytoplasm of cancer cells to the nucleus, where it reduces DNA synthesis and cellular responses to estrogen. Tamoxifen also has weak estrogenic properties.

Pharmacokinetics

Tamoxifen is well absorbed by mouth, reaching peak serum concentrations 3 to 6 hours after dosing. Tamoxifen is metabolized by the liver to several metabolites—the major one is N-desmethyltamoxifen. With continued dosing, serum concentrations of N-desmethyltamoxifen often exceed those of tamoxifen by twofold. Negligible amounts of N-desmethyltamoxifen and unchanged tamoxifen are excreted in the bile or urine. Tamoxifen and N-desmethyltamoxifen have elimination half-lives of approximately 7 and 14 days, respectively.

Dose

The usual dose regimen is 10 mg twice daily. Once-daily doses (20 mg) may also be used. Loading-dose regimens (100 mg twice daily for 5 to 7 days) have been used in the past to rapidly attain steady-state serum concentrations.

Administration

Oral.

Toxicity

Hematological. Thrombocytopenia is usually mild and transient. Leukopenia and anemia are infrequent (5% to 10%).

Gastrointestinal. Nausea (5% to 25%), vomiting, and anorexia occur occasionally and are rarely dose limiting. Diarrhea or constipation occur infrequently.

Dermatological. Rash and erythema are uncommon. Mild hair loss has been reported.

Hepatic. Increased hepatic enzyme levels and cholestasis are rare. A few cases of severe hepatotoxicity (fatty liver, hepatitis, cholestasis, hepatic necrosis) have been reported.

Neurological. Depression, dizziness, light-headedness, headache, confusion, lassitude, and/or syncope are uncommon.

Cardiovascular. Hot flashes are the most common side effect (25% to 32% incidence). Although not proven to be beneficial, clonidine, 25 to 75 μg twice daily (or by patch delivery system), has been used to lessen the severity of this toxicity. Thrombophlebitis, thromboembolism, pulmonary embolism, fluid retention, and edema are infrequent toxicities.

Genitourinary. Vaginal bleeding or discharge, amenorrhea (16%), menstrual irregularities (12%), pruritus vulvae, and endometriosis are infrequent toxicities.

Ocular. Retinopathy, decreased visual acuity, cataracts, optic neuritis, and/or corneal opacity are rare with conventional doses.

Other. Tumor "flare" may occur in the first month of therapy, manifested as an increase in tumor-related symptoms, such as bone pain (sometimes accompanied with hypercalcemia), increase in tumor size, and/or erythema. This reaction subsides quickly. Increased thyroxine concentrations occur rarely. The long-term use of tamoxifen may increase the risk of developing endometrial cancer.

Storage and Stability
Tamoxifen is stored at room temperature; containers bear expiration dates.

Incompatibilities
Phenobarbital may decrease and bromocriptine may increase serum concentrations of tamoxifen. Tamoxifen may potentiate the anticoagulant effects of warfarin.

Availability
Tamoxifen is commercially available in 10- and 20-mg tablets.

Selected Readings
Fisher B et al: A randomized clinical trial evaluating tamoxifen in the treatment of patients with node-negative breast cancer who have estrogen-receptor–positive tumors, *N Engl J Med* 320:479-484, 1989.

Fisher B et al: Endometrial cancer in tamoxifen-treated breast cancer patients: findings from the National Surgical Adjuvant Breast and Bowel Project (NSABP) B-14, *J Natl Cancer Inst* 86:527-537, 1994.

Nayfield SG et al: Potential role of tamoxifen in prevention of breast cancer, *J Natl Cancer Inst* 83:1450-1459, 1991.

T

TEGAFUR
Other Names
Ftorafur, UFT (combined with uracil).

Indications
UFT is an investigational agent that may be a useful treatment for colorectal carcinoma and other cancers for which fluorinated pyrimidines are a useful treatment.

Classification
Pyrimidine antimetabolite.

Pharmacokinetics
Tegafur is metabolized to 5-fluorouracil after administration. Peak serum levels of 5-fluorouracil occur approximately one hour after oral administration of tegafur.

Dose
UFT has been administered at a dose of 300 mg/m^2/day for 28 days followed by 7 days of rest. This 5-week cycle is repeated until the patient no longer benefits from the therapy. Daily doses are calculated, rounded up or down to the nearest 100 mg, and each daily dose is divided into three equal parts taken approximately every 8 hours. UFT is most often administered with oral leucovorin, 15 to 150 mg/day, in three divided doses.

Administration
Oral.

Toxicity
Hematological. Leukopenia and thrombocytopenia are uncommon (less than 3% incidence of severe myelosuppression). Anemia has been reported to occur rarely in studies conducted in Japan.

Gastrointestinal. Diarrhea (10%) and abdominal cramps (3%) are dose related and are the most common adverse effects. Nausea, vomiting (5%), and anorexia occasionally occur. Hemorrhagic enteritis, mucositis, and pancreatitis have been reported.

Dermatological. Rash or itching occur infrequently; urticaria (rare).

Hepatic. With prolonged use, elevations of liver enzyme levels may occur and be dose limiting. Fulminant hepatitis has rarely been reported.

Neurological. Headache, malaise, or vertigo (rare). Leukoencephalopathy has been reported in patients receiving UFT in Japan.

Pulmonary. Interstitial pneumonia has been rarely observed in patients receiving UFT in Japan.

Renal. Proteinuria or hematuria (rare).

Other. Fatigue (5%); fever, arthralgia, or glycosuria (rare).

Storage and Stability

Capsules are stored at room temperature; containers bear expiration dates.

Incompatibilities
Tegafur and other fluorinated pyrimidines adversely interact with halogenated antiviral agents (e.g., sorivudine, netivudine). The catabolism of the fluorinated pyrimidine is inhibited, and life-threatening myelosuppression may occur. Deaths have been reported when tegafur or 5-fluorouracil has been administered to patients receiving sorivudine or netivudine.

Availability

UFT is an investigational drug that is available in capsules for oral administration from Taiho Pharmaceutical Co., Ltd. (Tokyo). Each capsule contains 100 mg of tegafur and 224 mg of uracil.

Selected Readings

Pazdur R et al: Phase II trial of uracil and tegafur plus oral leucovorin: an effective oral regimen in the treatment of metastatic colorectal carcinoma, *J Clin Oncol* 12:2296-2300, 1994.

Pazdur R et al: Comparative steady state pharmacokinetics of oral UFT versus protracted intravenous 5-fluorouracil (FU), *Proc Am Soc Clin Oncol* 15:1498, 1996.

Peck R et al: Inhibition of dihydropyrimidine dehydrogenase by 5-propynyluracil, a metabolite of the anti-varicella zoster virus agent netivudine, *Clin Pharmacol Ther* 59:22-31, 1996.

Saltz LB et al: A fixed-ratio combination of uracil and ftorafur (UFT) with low dose leucovorin, *Cancer* 75:782-785, 1995.

TEMOZOLOMIDE

Other Names

CCRG 81045, SCH 52365, NSC-362856.

Indications

Temozolomide is an investigational drug that is being evaluated as a treatment for patients with brain tumors, melanoma, and other malignancies.

Classification and Mechanisms of Action

An imidazotetrazine derivative of mitozolomide, also related to dacarbazine (DTIC). Temozolomide is an alkylating agent. It is a pro-drug whose active metabolite—monomethyl triazenoimidazole carboxamide (MTIC)—is formed by chemical degradation at physiological pH.

Dose

The initial dose is 150 mg/m^2/day for 5 consecutive days (total dose of 750 mg/m^2) for patients who have received previous chemotherapy. For patients who have not previously received chemotherapy, the initial dose is 200 mg/m^2/day for 5 consecutive days (total dose of 1000 mg/m^2). Doses need to be rounded to the nearest 20 mg to accommodate for capsule strength. Treatment cycles have been repeated every 28 days.

T

Administration

Oral, on an empty stomach. It has been recommended that patients refrain from eating 4 hours before and 2 hours after each dose. The capsules should not be crushed or dissolved.

Toxicity

Hematological. Leukopenia, lymphopenia, thrombocytopenia, and anemia usually occur 2 to 8 weeks after the start of treatment.

Gastrointestinal. Nausea; vomiting is usually preventable and limited to the first day of treatment. Constipation, anorexia, diarrhea, and stomatitis have been reported.

Dermatological. Alopecia (usually mild to moderate), skin rash, pruritus.

Hepatic. Elevation of hepatic enzyme levels is uncommon and usually mild.

Neurological. Headache, lethargy.

Other. Hyperglycemia, impaired renal function, fever.

Storage and Stability
Temozolomide capsules should be stored at room temperature in original packaging and should be protected from moisture. Medication should be dispensed to patients in amber plastic containers.

Availability
Temozolomide is investigational and available from the NCI in 20- and 100-mg capsules.

Selected Readings
Bleehen NM et al: Cancer research campaign phase II trial of temozolomide in metastatic melanoma, *J Clin Oncol* 13:910-913, 1995.
Newlands ES et al: Phase I trial of temozolomide, *Cancer* 65:287-291, 1992.

TENIPOSIDE
Other Names
Vumon, VM-26, PTG, thenylidene-lignan-P, NSC-122819.

Indications
FDA approved for the treatment of children with relapsed or refractory acute lymphoblastic leukemia (in combination with cytarabine). Teniposide has been found to have activity in other neoplasms, including adult leukemias and small-cell lung cancer.

Classification
Plant alkaloid (topoisomerase II inhibitor).

Pharmacokinetics
After IV administration, teniposide is extensively (99%) bound to plasma albumin. The drug is metabolized by the liver, and 4% to 14% is eliminated unchanged in the urine. Teniposide has a terminal half-life of approximately 5 hours. The clearance of teniposide is increased significantly in patients receiving anticonvulsant medications (e.g., phenobarbital, phenytoin, carbamazepine).

Dose
Teniposide is administered in a dose of 165 mg/m^2 in combination with cytarabine 300 mg/m^2 intravenously, twice weekly for 8 to 9 doses, for the

treatment of acute lymphocytic leukemia. Occasionally, maintenance doses of teniposide, 250 mg/m^2/week, are given for a period of 4 to 8 weeks. Several other regimens have been used, including 100 mg/m^2 once or twice weekly, 20 to 60 mg/m^2/day for 5 days, and 250 mg/m^2/week for a period of 4 to 8 weeks. As a single agent in the treatment of small-cell lung cancer, a dose of 80 to 90 mg/m^2/day for 5 days has been used.

Administration

Teniposide for injection is administered by slow IV infusion (as a 0.1 to 0.4 mg/mL solution in 5% dextrose or normal saline) over *at least 30 minutes*. The drug has also been given as a continuous IV infusion and intraperitoneally.

Toxicity

Hematological. Leukopenia is expected and dose limiting (nadir 10 to 14 days). Thrombocytopenia and anemia occur less frequently.

Gastrointestinal. Nausea and vomiting occur occasionally (29%) and are usually preventable with antiemetic drugs. Anorexia, diarrhea (33%), stomatitis (76%), and abdominal pain (with intraperitoneal administration) may also occur. Abdominal pain may be dose limiting when teniposide is administered intraperitoneally.

Dermatological. Alopecia occurs in 10% to 30% of patients and is generally mild. Skin rashes have been reported in 3% of the patients.

Hepatic. Elevated hepatic transaminase levels, hyperbilirubinemia.

Neurological. Fatigue, seizures, paresthesias (all rare). Somnolence and hypotension have been reported in children receiving sedative antiemetics (e.g., promazine and diphenhydramine) in combination with teniposide and cytarabine.

Cardiovascular. Hypotension is associated with rapid IV administration.

Hypersensitivity. Anaphylaxis (rare); reactions may include blood pressure changes, bronchospasm, tachycardia, urticaria, facial flushing, diaphoresis, periorbital edema, vomiting, and/or fever.

Other. Fever (rare); elevated levels of BUN and serum creatinine (rare); local IV site phlebitis, secondary malignancy (acute nonlymphocytic leukemia).

Storage and Stability

The manufacturer recommends that teniposide be stored at refrigeration temperature and protected from light. Freezing does not adversely affect the stability of teniposide. After dilution in normal saline or 5% dextrose to concentrations of 0.1 to 0.4 mg/mL, the drug is chemically stable for at least 24 hours at room or refrigeration temperatures in glass containers. In plastic containers, 0.1 mg/mL of teniposide in normal saline is stable for 8 hours at room and refrigeration temperatures. *Teniposide exhibits poor stability in plastic containers when mixed with 5% dextrose and precipitation may occur within 4 hours.*

Preparation
Teniposide is often diluted in glass containers to a concentration of 0.4 mg/mL or less in normal saline or 5% dextrose. Teniposide has also been diluted to a concentration 1.0 mg/mL in normal saline or 5% dextrose. Plastic containers may be used if normal saline is the diluent and the drug is used within 8 hours.

Incompatibilities
Teniposide and heparin are incompatible; precipitation of teniposide may occur.

Availability
Teniposide is commercially available 50-mg (10 mg/mL) ampules.

Selected Readings

Grem JL et al: Teniposide in the treatment of leukemia: a case study of conflicting priorities in the development of drugs for fatal diseases, *J Clin Oncol* 6:351-379, 1988.

O'Dwyer PJ et al: Teniposide: a review of 12 years of experience, *Cancer Treat Rep* 68:1455-1466, 1984.

Pui C-H et al: Acute myeloid leukemia in children treated with epipodophyllotoxins for acute lymphoblastic leukemia, *N Engl J Med* 325:682-687, 1991.

THIOGUANINE

Other Names
6-Thioguanine, 6-TG, Lanvis, Thioguanine Tabloid, aminopurine-6-thiol-hemihydrate, NSC-752.

Indications
Oral thioguanine is FDA approved for remission induction, consolidation, and maintenance therapy of acute nonlymphocytic leukemia. Thioguanine may be a useful treatment for acute lymphocytic leukemia and chronic myelogenous leukemia. The injectable formulation of thioguanine is investigational.

Classification
Purine antimetabolite.

Pharmacokinetics
Thioguanine is incompletely (14% to 46%) and slowly absorbed by mouth and reaches maximum plasma concentrations approximately 8 hours after dosing. Thioguanine is extensively metabolized by the liver to several metabolites. Negligible amounts of thioguanine are eliminated unchanged in the urine. The elimination half-life of the drug is reported to range from 1.5 to 11 hours.

Dose
Range of 2 to 3 mg/kg/day orally for both children and adults. Combined with daunorubicin and cytarabine in the treatment of acute nonlymphocytic

leukemia, thioguanine has been given at a dose of 100 mg/m^2 every 12 hours for a 14-day period. The IV formulation of thioguanine has been evaluated in patients with solid tumors at a dose of 55 mg/m^2/day for 5 days, repeated every 4 weeks.

Administration

Thioguanine is taken orally, between meals if possible. The drug may also be given by IV infusion in 250 to 500 mL of 5% dextrose or normal saline over a period of *at least 30 minutes or longer*. Rapid IV infusion may induce bronchospasm and cardiovascular collapse.

Toxicity

Hematological. Leukopenia and thrombocytopenia, with nadirs occurring 10 to 14 days after administration. Anemia occurs occasionally.

Gastrointestinal. Nausea (infrequent), vomiting (infrequent), anorexia, stomatitis, diarrhea.

Dermatological. Rash, dermatitis.

Hepatic. Elevated hepatic transaminase levels, hyperbilirubinemia, jaundice, venoocclusive disease.

Neurological. Loss of vibratory sensation, unsteady gait.

Cardiovascular. Bronchospasm and cardiovascular collapse may be associated with rapid IV infusion (i.e., infusion over a period of less than 30 minutes).

Renal. Elevated BUN and serum creatinine concentrations, hyperuricemia (caused by tumor cell lysis).

Storage and Stability

Tablets are stored at room temperature; containers bear expiration dates. Unreconstituted vials are stable for at least 4 years under refrigeration and 3 years at room temperature. At a concentration of 15 mg/mL the drug is chemically stable for at least 24 hours at refrigeration temperatures. After further dilution in 500 mL of 5% dextrose or normal saline, thioguanine is chemically stable for at least 24 hours at room and refrigeration temperatures.

Preparation

The 75-mg vial is reconstituted with 5 mL of normal saline to result in a 15 mg/mL solution. The desired dose may be further diluted with 500 mL of 5% dextrose or normal saline. An oral suspension of thioguanine can be made from the tablets. A pharmacist should be consulted for additional information.

Compatibilities

A 1 mg/mL solution containing 0.5 mEq of sodium bicarbonate for every 75 mg of thioguanine is stable for 8 hours in 5% dextrose or normal saline.

Availability

Thioguanine 40-mg tablets are commercially available. The injectable formulation, 75 mg/vial, is investigational and is available as a lyophilized powder from the NCI.

Selected Readings

Brox LW, Birkett L, Belch A: Clinical pharmacology of oral thioguanine in acute myelogenous leukemia, *Cancer Chemother Pharmacol* 6:35-38, 1981.

Kovach JS et al: Phase I trial of parenteral 6-thioguanine given on 5 consecutive days, *Cancer Res* 46:5959-5962, 1986.

THIOTEPA

Other Names

Thioplex; triethylenephosphoramide; N,N',N"-triethylene-thiophosphoramide; tris(1-aziridinyl)phosphine sulfide; TESPA; TSPA; NSC-6396.

Indications

FDA approved for the treatment of adenocarcinoma of the breast, adenocarcinoma of the ovary, intracavitary effusions, superficial papillary bladder cancer, and Hodgkin's and non-Hodgkin's lymphomas. Thiotepa may be useful in bone marrow transplantation treatment programs and as a treatment for lung cancer.

Classification

Alkylating agent.

Pharmacokinetics

Thiotepa is poorly absorbed from the gastrointestinal tract. Between 10% and 100% is absorbed through bladder mucosa after intravesical instillation. Thiotepa is extensively metabolized by the liver, its major metabolite (TEPA) has cytotoxic activity, and only trace amounts of thiotepa and TEPA appear in the urine. Thiotepa has an elimination half-life of 2 to 3 hours (from plasma) and 8 hours (from cerebrospinal fluid after intrathecal administration). TEPA has an elimination half-life of 15 to 18 hours.

Dose

Nontransplant doses: 12 to 16 mg/m^2 every 1 to 4 weeks.
Transplant doses: up to 900 mg/m^2.
Intravesical instillation: 30 to 60 mg every week for 4 weeks.
Intrathecal doses: 1 to 10 mg/m^2 once or twice weekly.

Administration

Thiotepa has been given by IV push, but it may be administered by IV infusion in 50 mL or more of 5% dextrose or normal saline, over a 10-minute period or longer. Thiotepa has also been administered as an ophthalmic instillation, intrathecally, as an intravesical instillation, intraarterially (i.e., regional perfusion), intratumorally, intrapleurally, intraperitoneally, intrapericardially, and intramuscularly.

Toxicity

Systemic effects may occur after intravesical instillation or intracavitary administration.

Hematological. Leukopenia is expected and often dose limiting (nadir, 10 to 14 days after administration). Thrombocytopenia and anemia occur less frequently. Myelosuppression may be cumulative.

Gastrointestinal. Nausea and vomiting are uncommon with nontransplantation doses. Anorexia, diarrhea, and abdominal pain are uncommon. Stomatitis may be severe with bone marrow transplantation doses.

Dermatological. Alopecia (rare with conventional doses), hives, rash, pruritus, contact dermatitis, fingernail changes; bronzing, erythema and desquamation of the skin in patients receiving >900 mg/m^2 before bone marrow transplantation.

Hepatic. Elevated hepatic transaminase levels occur and are usually mild and transient.

Neurological. Headache, dizziness, weakness of lower extremities, paresthesias (with intrathecal injection). Cognitive impairment (e.g., stupor, coma) is the dose-limiting toxicity of high-dose thiotepa (first observed at 1125 mg/m^2 and increasing in severity at higher doses).

Pulmonary. Apnea (in patients receiving succinylcholine).

Urinary (in patients receiving thiotepa by intravesical instillation). Abdominal pain, hematuria, hemorrhagic cystitis (rare), dysuria, frequency, urgency, ureteral obstruction, and impairment of renal function (rare).

Ocular (after ophthalmic instillation). Irritation, skin pigmentation in the periorbital region, blurred vision, conjunctivitis.

Other. Second malignancy (i.e., leukemia), pain at site of injection (rare), impaired fertility (i.e., azoospermia, amenorrhea), fever (rare), angioedema (rare), hypersensitivity reactions (e.g., rash, urticaria, laryngeal edema, wheezing).

Storage and Stability

Thiotepa is stored in the refrigerator. At a concentration of 10 mg/mL the drug is stable for at least 24 hours at room temperature and 5 days in the refrigerator. After dilution in normal saline to concentrations of 1 or 3 mg/mL in polyvinylchloride containers, thiotepa is stable for at least 48 hours in the refrigerator and 24 hours at room temperature. At a concentration of 5 mg/mL the drug is stable for at least 24 hours at room and refrigeration temperatures. Solutions of thiotepa, 0.5 mg/mL, are unstable at 24 hours and should be used immediately.

Preparation

The 15-mg vial is reconstituted with 1.5 mL of sterile water to result in a 10 mg/mL solution. The desired dose is further diluted with normal saline. The reconstituted solution should be filtered using a 0.22 μm filter.

Solutions that remain opaque or that have particulate matter after filtration should not be used.

Compatibilities

Thiotepa is compatible with 2% procaine hydrochloride and/or epinephrine 1:1000.

Availability

Thiotepa, 15 mg/vial, is commercially available as a lyophilized powder.

Selected Readings

Anonymous: *Thiotepa: alkylating agent for cancer chemotherapy*, Pearl River, NY, 1986, Lederle Laboratories, Professional Services Department.

Herzig RH et al: Phase I-II studies with high-dose thiotepa and autologous marrow transplantation in patients with refractory malignancies. In *Advances in cancer chemotherapy: high-dose thiotepa and autologous marrow transplantation*, Proceedings of a symposium held October 25, 1986 in Dallas, Texas. Herzig GP (symposium chairman), Park Row Publishers, 1987.

Zincke H et al: Intravesical thio-tepa and mitomycin C treatment immediately after transurethral resection and later for superficial bladder cancer: a prospective, randomized, stratified study with crossover design, *J Urol* 134:1110-1114, 1985.

TOMUDEX

Other Names

ZD 1694, N-(5-[N-(3,4-dihydro-2-methyl-4-oxoquinazolin-6-ylmethyl)-N-methylamino]-2-thenoyl)-L-GLUTAMIC ACID, NSC-639186.

Indications

Tomudex is an investigational drug that appears to be a useful treatment for patients with colorectal carcinoma.

Classification and Mechanisms of Action

Thymidylate synthase inhibitor. Thymidylate synthase is a key enzyme in the synthesis of thymidine triphosphate, a nucleotide required for DNA synthesis.

Pharmacokinetics

Tomudex exhibits a triexponential pattern of elimination after IV administration. The beta half-life ranges from approximately 1 to 3 hours; the elimination half-life varies widely, from 8 to 105 hours. When doses greater than 0.6 mg/m^2 are administered the drug is routinely assayed at the beginning of the subsequent course of therapy (3 weeks later). The drug does not appear to accumulate with repeated administration.

Dose

A dose of 3 mg/m^2 repeated every 3 weeks is undergoing evaluation in phase II and phase III studies. A dose of 3.4 mg/m^2 every 3 weeks was shown to be dose limiting in a recent phase I study.

Administration

IV infusion over a 15-minute period or longer.

Toxicity

Hematological. Leukopenia is dose limiting and has occurred in approximately 60% of the patients receiving a dose of 3 mg/m^2 every 3 weeks. In one third of these patients the nadir white blood cell count was Grade III or Grade IV. The nadir leukocyte count occurs around day 8 (range, days 7 to 21) with recovery occurring approximately 10 days later. Thrombocytopenia has been reported to occur in 25% of the patients and be clinically significant in a small percentage of these patients. Thrombocytopenia leading to fatal pulmonary hemorrhage has been reported in one patient who received 3.5 mg/m^2.

Gastrointestinal. Gastrointestinal toxicities have been reported to be dose related and diarrhea has been dose limiting in some patients. At a dose of 3 mg/m^2, diarrhea has been reported to occur in 60% of the patients, with 26% of the patients experiencing severe or life-threatening diarrhea. Severe diarrhea generally occurs 1 week after the second dose. Nausea and vomiting have been observed in approximately 50% of the patients who have received doses of 1.6 mg/m^2 or greater. The onset of these symptoms generally occurred 2 or 3 days after administration of the drug. Grade II mucositis has been observed in 48% of the patients who received Tomudex at a dose of 3 mg/m^2.

Dermatological. Rash (35%).

Hepatic. Reversible elevations of hepatic transaminase levels, occasionally severe. Hyperbilirubinemia has also been observed.

Other. Dose-limiting malaise, which was prolonged in some patients, was observed at a dose of 3.5 mg/m^2 every 3 weeks. Accompanying the malaise were symptoms of asthenia, nausea, anorexia, fatigue, and resulting decreases in performance status. Fever and flulike symptoms occur occasionally.

Storage and Stability

Initial results for the 0.1% strength formulation supports an 18-month shelf life when stored at 4° C, protected from light. The formulation has also been shown to be adequately stable in normal saline and 5% dextrose, within a concentration range of 2 μg/mL to 200 μg/mL for at least 12 hours if protected from light.

Preparation

Reconstitute with 4 mL of sterile water for injection to produce an isotonic solution containing 0.5 mg/mL. The drug may be diluted with 5% dextrose or normal saline. The maximum concentration of the final solution must not be less than 2 μg/mL or exceed 200 μg/mL. At these concentrations the drug should be protected from light and used within 12 hours.

Availability
Tomudex is available as an investigational drug in 2-mg vials of lyophilized powder and 10-mL vials containing a 1 mg/mL solution.

Selected Readings
Clarke SJ et al: Phase I trial of ZD1694, a new folate-based thymidylate synthase inhibitor, in patients with solid tumors, *J Clin Oncol* 14:1495-1503, 1996.

Cunningham D et al: 'Tomudex' (ZD1694): results of a randomised trial in advanced colorectal cancer demonstrate efficacy and reduced mucositis and leucopenia, *Eur J Cancer* 31A:1945-1954, 1995.

Zalcberg JR et al: ZD1694: A novel thymidylate synthase inhibitor with substantial activity in the treatment of patients with advanced colorectal cancer, *J Clin Oncol* 14:716-721, 1996.

TOPOTECAN
Other Names
Hycamptin, topotecan hydrochloride, topotecan AC/AF, hycamptamine, SKF 104864-A, NSC-609699.

Indications
FDA approved for the treatment for patients with metastatic ovarian carcinoma after failure of initial or second-line therapy.

Classification
Topoisomerase I inhibitor.

Pharmacokinetics
Approximately 22% to 48% of a dose of topotecan is eliminated unchanged in the urine. Topotecan has an elimination half-life of approximately 2 to 3 hours. There does not appear to be a strong correlation with AUC (area under the plasma concentration time curve) and ANC (absolute neutrophil count). Approximately 35% of topotecan is bound to plasma proteins. Elimination of topotecan is delayed in patients with compromised renal function. Patients with hyperbilirubinemia appears to eliminate the drug slower than patients with normal serum bilirubin levels, but clinically significant differences in toxicity between the two groups have not been observed.

Dose
The approved dose of topotecan is 1.5 mg/m^2/day for 5 days by IV infusion over a 30-minute period for the first four courses of treatment. Subsequent treatments should be administered at a dose of 1.25 mg/m^2/day for 5 days. It is recommended that the daily dose be reduced to 0.75 mg/m^2 for patients with moderate renal impairment (creatinine clearance 20 to 40 mL/min). Dose adjustments are not necessary for patients with hyperbilirubinemia (e.g., bilirubin 1.7 to 15 mg/dL). Topotecan has been evaluated investigationally in other doses and schedules in patients with solid tumors and leukemias. Listed on p. 205 are some of the regimens that have been evaluated in adult patients with solid tumors.

Single dose of 1.3 to 1.6 mg/m^2 by IV infusion over a 0.5-, 2-, and 24-hour period and repeated every 3 to 4 weeks.

Weekly dose of 1.5 to 1.75 mg/m^2/day by IV infusion over a 24-hour period.

Continuous infusion over a 72-, 96-, or 120-hour period at a dose of 0.65 to 2.0 mg/m^2/day and repeated every 3 to 4 weeks.

Administration

Topotecan is administered intravenously, usually in 100 mL or more of normal saline or 5% dextrose over a 30-minute period or longer.

Toxicity

Hematological. Dose-limiting leukopenia is the major toxicity of topotecan (nadir, days 10 to 12; recovery by days 15 to 21 after daily × 5 regimens). With the doses recommended for the treatment of women with ovarian cancer, neutropenia (500 cells/mm3 or less) is reported to occur in 81% of the patients. Thrombocytopenia occurs frequently but is rarely dose limiting. Anemia is common (i.e., >2% decline in hematocrit in 80%, >4% decline in 30% to 50%) and occasionally (14%) precipitous. Approximately 50% of the patients have required red blood cell transfusions during treatment with topotecan. Myelosuppression induced by topotecan (1.25 mg/m^2/day for 5 days) is more severe if combined with cisplatin (50 mg/m^2 on day 1).

Gastrointestinal. Severe (Grades 3 and 4) nausea and vomiting are reported to occur in approximately 10% of the patients. Diarrhea is common (25% to 42%) but is severe in approximately 5% of the patients. Diarrhea usually begins during or shortly after infusion of topotecan and lasts 2 to 3 days. Anorexia, constipation, abdominal pain, mucositis, and xerostomia are rarely dose limiting.

Dermatological. Total alopecia is common (42%). Skin rash (mild) occurs infrequently and on occasion may be accompanied by pruritus and/or urticaria. Acne and fever blisters have been reported.

Hepatic. Elevated hepatic enzyme levels and hyperbilirubinemia are uncommon toxicities.

Neurological. Headache occurs frequently. Dizziness, light-headedness, peripheral neuropathy, and Horner's syndrome have been reported.

Cardiovascular. Hypertension and tachycardia have been reported infrequently.

Pulmonary. Dyspnea has been reported to occur in 20% of the patients, severe (Grades 3 and 4) in 4% to 6%.

Renal. Elevated serum creatinine concentrations and hematuria rarely occur.

Other. Fever, fatigue (severe in 8%), malaise (severe in 2%), arthralgia (severe in 1%), asthenia (severe in 5%), myalgia, and weight loss have been reported.

Storage and Stability

Topotecan is stored at room temperature. After reconstitution to concentrations from 10 µg/mL to 500 µg/mL, the solution is chemically stable for 21 days at room and refrigeration temperatures. Dilution to concentrations of 20 µg/mL and 100 µg/mL in plastic containers of 5% dextrose or normal saline are stable for at least 48 hours at room temperature.

Preparation

Add 4 mL of sterile water to the 4-mg vial to yield a concentration of 1 mg/mL.

Availability

Topotecan (4 mg/vial) is commercially available.

Selected Readings

Kudelka AP et al: Phase II study of intravenous topotecan as a 5-day infusion for refractory epithelial ovarian carcinoma, *J Clin Oncol* 14:1552-1557, 1996.

Rowinsky EK et al: Phase I and pharmacologic study of topotecan: a novel topoisomerase I inhibitor, *J Clin Oncol* 10:647-656, 1992.

TOREMIFENE

Other Names

Fareston, toremifene citrate, toremifenum, FC-1157a.

Indications

FDA approved for the treatment of advanced breast cancer.

Classification and Mechanisms of Action

Toremifene has a high affinity for estrogen receptors. Thus part of its mechanism of action may involve binding to estrogenic receptors that become translocated in the nucleus where DNA synthesis is inhibited. However, toremifene has also been shown to have cytostatic effects in estrogen receptor–negative cells.

Pharmacokinetics

Toremifene is rapidly absorbed after oral administration and reaches peak serum concentrations within 3 to 4 hours of dosing. Toremifene is almost totally bound to serum proteins (92% to albumin). Toremifene exhibits a biphasic elimination pattern with a distribution half-life of approximately 4 to 4.5 hours and an elimination half-life of approximately 5 to 6 days. Toremifene is metabolized in the liver to at least two metabolites (i.e., N-desmethyl-toremifene, 4-hydroxy-toremifene) that have equivalent antiestrogenic activity.

Dose

Phase I studies evaluated doses ranging from 20 to 400 mg/day for 8 weeks. Phase II studies have employed doses of 60 and 200 mg/day. Toremifene 68 mg/day has equivalent antiestrogenic activity as tamoxifen, 60 mg/day.

Administration
Oral, once daily.

Toxicity
Hematological. Marked decline in erythrocyte sedimentation rate (common).

Gastrointestinal. Nausea (6% to 31%), upper abdominal pain (4% to 10%), vomiting (0% to 12%), anorexia (0% to 9%), diarrhea (4%), constipation (3%), increased appetite (2%).

Dermatological. Urticaria (rare).

Neurological. Dizziness or vertigo (10%), lethargy/fatigue (10%), headache (9%), insomnia, tremulousness.

Ocular. Dryness and cataracts have been reported in a few patients.

Pulmonary. Pulmonary embolism (rare).

Other. Hot flashes (10% to 30%), sweating (13%), hypercalcemia (rare), vaginal discharge (8%), vaginal bleeding (3%), mildly reduced levels of antithrombin III (58%).

Storage and Stability
Toremifene tablets are stored at room temperature and are stable for at least 3 years from the date of manufacture.

Availability
Toremifene is commercially available as 60-mg tablets.

Selected Readings
Hamm JT et al: Phase I study of toremifene in patients with advanced cancer, *J Clin Oncol* 9:2036-2041, 1991.

Hayes DF et al: Randomized comparison of tamoxifen and two separate doses of toremifene in postmenopausal patients with metastatic breast cancer, *J Clin Oncol* 13:2556-2566, 1995.

Vogel CL et al: Multicenter phase II efficacy trial of toremifene in tamoxifen-refractory patients with advanced breast cancer, *J Clin Oncol* 11:345-350, 1993.

TRETINOIN

Other Names
Vesanoid, all-trans-retinoic acid, TRA, ATRA, vitamin A acid, NSC-122758.

Indications
FDA approved for the treatment of acute promyelocytic leukemia.

Classification and Mechanisms of Action
Tretinoin is a derivative of vitamin A. The drug binds to a cellular protein that facilitates the transfer of tretinoin from cellular cytoplasm into the nucleus. Within the nucleus, tretinoin binds to a chromosomal receptor that is near the chromosomal lesion that is associated with acute

promyelocytic leukemia (APL). Differentiation of APL cells occurs after administration of tretinoin.

Pharmacokinetics

Tretinoin is a natural retinoic acid metabolite (basal concentrations, 3 to 4 ng/mL). After oral administration peak plasma levels (e.g., 1 μM after an 80 mg dose) occur in 1 to 4 hours. The drug rapidly disappears from the systemic circulation (elimination half-life, 40 minutes), does not penetrate into the cerebrospinal fluid, and is almost totally metabolized (<1% eliminated unchanged in the urine). Patients on low-fat diets may not absorb retinoic acid adequately. Ketoconazole may inhibit the metabolism of tretinoin.

With continued treatment, plasma levels decline and increased urinary excretion of metabolites occurs, indicating increased metabolism of the drug, which often coincides with relapse of acute promyelocytic leukemia (APL).

Dose

For the treatment of APL: 45 mg/m²/day (rounded up to the nearest 10 mg) for 30 days. If a partial response is obtained, treatment is continued until a complete response is achieved or there is progression of disease. If a complete response is attained, treatment is continued for another 60 days (minimum, 90 total days of treatment). Doses of 175 mg/m²/day have been evaluated in the treatment of other malignancies. In a study evaluating tretinoin in patients with brain tumors, each 8-week course of tretinoin consisted of daily administration for 6 weeks followed by a 2-week period of no treatment.

Administration

Oral, once daily in the morning. The daily dose has also been administered in two divided fractions.

Toxicity

Hematological. Leukocytosis (40%). A rapid increase in white blood cell count has resulted in leukostasis and hemorrhage in a few patients. Leukocyte counts tend to reach peak levels within 6 to 16 days after initiation of treatment. Less common toxicities include anemia, increased erythrocyte sedimentation rate, and thrombocytosis.

Gastrointestinal. Nausea, vomiting, and anorexia are uncommon. Xerostomia occurs occasionally, and pancreatitis is rare.

Dermatological. Dry skin and mild exfoliation occur in most patients. Rash, cheilitis, cracked lips, inflamed lips, pruritus, and photosensitivity are also common side effects. Alopecia (mild thinning) is an infrequent toxicity.

Hepatic. Transient elevation of hepatic enzyme levels and hyperbilirubinemia occur occasionally but may persist for weeks after treatment is discontinued.

Neurological. Headache is common, occurs several hours after dosing, and is managed with mild analgesics. Lethargy, fatigue, pseudotumor cerebri (dose limiting in children), and mental depression occur infrequently.

Cardiopulmonary. "Retinoic acid syndrome" occurs in 10% to 25% of patients, occurs within 2 days to 3 weeks after initiation of treatment, and can be fatal. High fever, respiratory distress, pulmonary infiltrates, and pericardial and/or pleural effusion may be accompanied by heart failure and hypotension. Some patients have required intubation and mechanical ventilation. Initiation of treatment with corticosteroids at the first sign of dyspnea has been recommended.

Ocular. Dryness, corneal erosion, blurred vision, papilledema, corneal opacities, night blindness, conjunctivitis, xerophthalmia.

Other. *Tretinoin is teratogenic. Fetal abnormalities (e.g., thymic aplasia, craniofacial malformation) are likely if in utero exposure to tretinoin occurs.* Nasal congestion, bone pain (10% to 25%), myalgia and arthralgia (common), muscle weakness, osteophyte formation, elevated cholesterol and triglyceride levels (common), fever, and xanthomas (rare) have been reported in patients receiving tretinoin. Hyperhistaminemia (100 times normal) resulting in shock and severe gastric and duodenal ulceration has been reported.

Storage and Stability
Tretinoin capsules are stored at room temperature protected from light. Each bottle bears an expiration date.

Incompatibilities
It is suggested that topical tretinoin (Retin-A) be avoided. Tretinoin is contraindicated in patients allergic to parabens or vitamin A.

Availability
Tretinoin is commercially available as a 10-mg capsule.

Selected Readings
Atiba JO et al: All-transretinoic acid (atRA): a new and effective salvage agent for recurrent high grade malignant glioma (RHGMG), *J Clin Oncol* 14:1746, 1996.
Koike T et al: Brief report: severe symptoms of hyperhistaminemia after the treatment of acute promyelocytic leukemia with tretinoin (all-trans-retinoic acid), *N Engl J Med* 327:385-387, 1992.
Levien TL, Baker DE: Reviews of tramadol and tretinoin, *Hosp Pharm* 31:54-73, 1996.
Smith MA et al: Retinoids in cancer therapy, *J Clin Oncol* 10:839-864, 1992.

TRIMETREXATE
Other Names
Neutrexin, TMQ, TMTX, NSC-352122.

Indications
FDA approved for the treatment of patients with *Pneumocystis carinii* infection who are intolerant of or refractory to trimethoprim-sulfamethoxazole therapy. Trimetrexate may also be a useful treatment for cancers of the lung, head and neck, and colon.

Classification
Antimetabolite (antifol).

Pharmacokinetics

Trimetrexate is rapidly absorbed (19% to 67%) after oral administration, reaching peak plasma concentrations in 1 hour. After IV administration the drug distributes throughout the body but does not appear to accumulate in pleural or ascitic fluid. Trimetrexate is metabolized by the liver, with 6% to 25% appearing in the urine as unchanged drug. Trimetrexate has an elimination half-life of 11 to 16 hours. However, trimetrexate clearance is decreased and toxicity is increased in patients with hypoalbuminemia (serum albumin level less than 3.5 g/dL).

Dose

The recommended dose for the treatment of *Pneumocystis carinii* infection is 45 mg/m²/day for 21 days with *concomitant* leucovorin. Leucovorin must be administered for 3 days after cessation of treatment with trimetrexate. Leucovorin may be administered orally or by IV infusion at a dose of 20 mg/m² every 6 hours for 24 days. For the treatment of patients with cancer, doses of 8 to 12 mg/m²/day for a 5-day period repeated every 3 to 4 weeks have been evaluated. When followed by leucovorin rescue, trimetrexate (110 mg/m²) has been administered in combination with fluorouracil (500 mg/m²) on a weekly basis for a 6-week period followed by 2 weeks of no treatment.

Administration

Trimetrexate has been given by IV push, but it is usually administered by IV infusion, in 50 mL or more of *5% dextrose only* over a 60- to 90-minute period. Trimetrexate has also been given by shorter IV infusions and as a continuous IV infusion.

Toxicity

Patients with hypoalbuminemia (less than 3.5 g/dL) are more likely to experience severe or life-threatening anemia, mucositis, and thrombocytopenia.

Hematological. Myelosuppression (leukopenia, thrombocytopenia, anemia) is dose related and occasionally dose limiting. Concomitant leucovorin significantly reduces the incidence of these toxicities.

Gastrointestinal. Mucositis can be dose limiting and severe. Nausea, vomiting, anorexia, and diarrhea occur infrequently.

Dermatological. Maculopapular skin rash (occasionally with erythroderma), pruritus, hyperpigmentation, partial alopecia, radiation recall reactions (rare).

Hepatic. Transient elevations of liver enzyme levels (17%).

Renal. Transient elevation of serum creatinine level (4% to 8%).

Other. Fever (40%), shaking chills, malaise (12%).

Storage and Stability

Unreconstituted vials are stored at room temperature. At a concentration of 12.5 mg/mL, trimetrexate is stable for at least 7 days at room and refrigeration temperatures. After dilution in 5% dextrose to a concentration of 0.25 to 2 mg/mL, the drug is chemically stable for at least 24 hours at room and refrigeration temperatures.

Preparation

The 25-mg vial is reconstituted with 2 mL of sterile water to result in a 12.5 mg/mL solution. The desired dose may be further diluted in 5% dextrose. *Do not use chloride-containing solutions to reconstitute or dilute trimetrexate, or a black precipitate will form.*

Incompatibilities

Trimetrexate is incompatible with chloride- or anion-containing solutions.

Availability

Trimetrexate is commercially available as a lyophilized powder in 25-mg vials.

Selected Readings

Bertino JR et al: Clinical pharmacology and metabolism of trimetrexate, *Semin Oncol* 15(suppl 2):10-16, 1988.

Conti JA et al: Trial of sequential trimetrexate, fluorouracil, and high-dose leucovorin in previously treated patients with gastrointestinal carcinoma, *J Clin Oncol* 12:695-700, 1994.

Eisenhauer EA et al: Trimetrexate: predictors of severe or life-threatening toxic effects, *J Natl Cancer Inst* 80:1318-1322, 1988.

Grem JL et al: Correlates of severe or life-threatening toxic effects from trimetrexate, *J Natl Cancer Inst* 80: 1313-1318, 1988.

URACIL MUSTARD

Other Names

Uramustine, NSC-34462.

Indications

FDA approved for the treatment of chronic lymphocytic leukemia, chronic myelocytic leukemia, non-Hodgkin's lymphoma, cutaneous T-cell lymphoma, thrombocytosis, and polycythemia vera. Uracil mustard may be a useful treatment for patients with ovarian carcinoma.

Classification

Alkylating agent.

U

Pharmacokinetics

Uracil mustard is absorbed by mouth, and less than 1% is detected in the urine.

Dose

Single weekly dose: 0.15 mg/kg (adults) or 0.3 mg/kg (children) for 4 doses. Treatment is repeated if a therapeutic response is observed. Other regimens: 1 to 2 mg/day until the desired hematological response is obtained or 3 to 5 mg/day for 7 days followed by 1 mg/day until the desired response is obtained. Each of these regimens may be followed by a 1 mg/day maintenance dose.

Administration
Oral.

Toxicity
Hematological. Myelosuppression is dose related. Leukopenia and thrombocytopenia occur most often, with nadir counts 2 to 4 weeks after beginning treatment. Anemia occurs less frequently.

Gastrointestinal. Nausea, vomiting, anorexia, and/or diarrhea.

Dermatological. Alopecia, dermatitis, pruritus, and abnormal skin pigmentation.

Neurological. Nervousness, irritability, depression, mental confusion.

Allergic. Capsules of uracil mustard contain tartrazine. Patients with aspirin hypersensitivity may develop reactions, including bronchial asthma.

Other. Hepatotoxicity, azoospermia, amenorrhea.

Storage and Stability
Capsules of uracil mustard are stored at room temperature. Containers bear an expiration date.

Availability
Uracil mustard is commercially available as a 1-mg capsule.

Selected Readings
Gold GL et al: The use of mechlorethamine, cyclophosphamide, and uracil mustard in neoplastic disease: a cooperative study, *J Clin Pharmacol* 10:110-120, 1970.
Shamasunder HK, Gregory SA, Knospe WH: Uracil mustard in the treatment of thrombocytosis, *JAMA* 244:1454-1455, 1980.

VINBLASTINE
Other Names
Velban, Velsar, Alkaban AQ, Velbe, vinblastine sulfate, vincaleukoblastine, VLB, NSC-49842.

Indications
FDA approved for the treatment of Hodgkin's disease, non-Hodgkin's lymphoma, cutaneous T-cell lymphoma (advanced stages), carcinoma of the testis, Kaposi's sarcoma, histiocytosis X, choriocarcinoma, and breast cancer. Vinblastine may be useful in the treatment of chronic myelogenous leukemia, melanoma, neuroblastoma, and cancers of the kidney, bladder, cervix, head and neck, ovary, and lung.

Classification
Plant alkaloid (tubulin inhibitor).

Pharmacokinetics

Vinblastine is poorly absorbed by mouth. The drug is metabolized by the liver to desacetylvinblastine, which is active, and nonactive metabolites. Less than 1% of vinblastine or desacetylvinblastine is eliminated unchanged in the urine. Vinblastine is not hemodialyzable and has an elimination half-life of approximately 20 hours.

Dose

Commonly used doses range from 6 to 10 mg/m^2 every 2 to 4 weeks in combination with other drugs. Vinblastine has also been given weekly and as a continuous infusion in a dose of 1.7 to 2.0 mg/m^2/day over a 96-hour period.

Administration

Vinblastine is most commonly given by IV push using extravasation precautions. The drug has been administered by continuous IV infusion in 50 mL or more of 5% dextrose or normal saline over a 96-hour period.

Toxicity

Hematological. Leukopenia is dose limiting. Thrombocytopenia and anemia occur less frequently.

Gastrointestinal. Nausea and vomiting are infrequent toxicities, and constipation occurs occasionally (see neurological side effects). Abdominal pain (cramps), anorexia, diarrhea, mucositis, and gastrointestinal hemorrhage are rare.

Dermatological. Alopecia (uncommon), epilation, skin and soft-tissue damage if extravasated (the manufacturer recommends subcutaneous injection of hyaluronidase and application of heat to help disperse the drug), rash, photosensitivity.

Neurological. Neurological adverse effects are dose related and occur infrequently with conventional doses. Toxicities may include peripheral neuropathy (loss of deep tendon reflexes, paresthesias, paralysis), autonomic neuropathy (constipation, paralytic ileus, urinary retention, orthostasis), vocal cord paralysis, myalgias, Raynaud's phenomenon, headache, seizures, depression, dizziness, and malaise.

Pulmonary. Bronchospasm and acute dyspnea are uncommon and more commonly occur when vinblastine and mitomycin are administered in combination. Pulmonary edema has been rarely reported.

Other. Severe pain in the jaw, pharynx, bones, back, or limbs after injection; syndrome of inappropriate antidiuretic hormone (SIADH), fever, and ischemic cardiotoxicity.

V

Storage and Stability

Vials are stored in the refrigerator. Vinblastine, reconstituted to a concentration of 1 mg/mL, is stable for 14 and 30 days at room and refrigeration temperatures, respectively. Further diluted to a concentration of 0.01 mg/mL in normal saline or 5% dextrose, vinblastine is stable for at least 5 days at room temperature.

Preparation
The 10-mg vial of lyophilized powder is reconstituted with 10 mL of bacteriostatic normal saline to yield a concentration of 1 mg/mL. Doses for continuous infusion may be further diluted with 50 mL or more of normal saline or 5% dextrose in water.

Incompatibilities
Furosemide, heparin, Infusaid pumps.

Compatibilities
Vinblastine is physically stable in normal saline solutions for at least 5 days, alone or mixed with doxorubicin, at room or refrigeration temperatures. Vinblastine is also compatible in solution with metoclopramide, dacarbazine, or bleomycin. A pharmacist should be consulted for additional information.

Availability
Vinblastine is commercially available in 10-mg vials, as a lyophilized powder and as a 1 mg/mL solution.

Selected Readings
Fraschini G et al: Five-day continuous-infusion vinblastine in the treatment of breast cancer, *Cancer* 56:225-229, 1985.

Kris MG et al: Dyspnea after vinblastine or vindesine administration in patients receiving mitomycin plus vinca alkaloid combination therapy, *Cancer Treat Rep* 68:1029-1031, 1984.

VINCRISTINE
Other Names
Oncovin, Vincasar Pfs, Vincrex, vincristine sulfate, VCR, leucocristine, NSC-67574.

Indications
FDA approved for the treatment of acute leukemia, Hodgkin's disease, non-Hodgkin's lymphoma, rhabdomyosarcoma, neuroblastoma, Ewing's sarcoma, and Wilm's tumor. Vincristine may be useful in the treatment of chronic leukemias, Kaposi's sarcoma, soft-tissue sarcomas, osteosarcoma, multiple myeloma, trophoblastic neoplasms, malignant melanoma, and cancers of the colon, rectum, brain, breast, cervix, head and neck, ovary, lung, and thyroid.

Classification
Plant alkaloid (tubulin inhibitor).

Pharmacokinetics
Vincristine is poorly absorbed by mouth. After IV dosing the drug is widely distributed throughout the body (excluding the cerebrospinal fluid). Vincristine is metabolized by the liver and 40% to 70% is excreted

in the bile. Less than 1% is excreted unchanged in the urine. Vincristine is not hemodialyzable and has an elimination half-life of approximately 85 hours.

Dose
Commonly used doses range from 0.5 to 1.4 mg/m² every 1 to 4 weeks. Limiting a total individual dose to 2 mg is advocated by many but may not be necessary. Continuous infusion regimens of 0.5 mg/day to 0.5 mg/m²/day for 4 days have also been used.

Administration
Usually given through a free-flowing IV line using extravasation precautions. Occasionally it is administered by continuous IV infusion in 50 mL or more of 5% dextrose or normal saline over a 96-hour period.

Toxicity
Hematological. Leukopenia (mild and rare), thrombocytopenia (rare), anemia.

Gastrointestinal. Nausea and vomiting are rare, constipation (see neurological side effects), abdominal pain (cramps), anorexia, diarrhea.

Dermatological. Alopecia (12% to 45%), skin and soft-tissue damage if extravasated (the manufacturer recommends subcutaneous injection of hyaluronidase and application of heat to help disperse the drug), rash (uncommon).

Hepatic. Elevations of hepatic transaminase levels are usually mild and transient.

Neurological. Peripheral neuropathy (loss of deep tendon reflexes, paresthesias, paralysis), autonomic neuropathy (constipation, paralytic ileus, urinary retention, orthostasis), ataxia, hoarseness, myalgia, cortical blindness, headache, seizures. Fatal ascending paralysis follows intrathecal administration. Foot pain with severe motor weakness has been observed after treatment with vincristine and filgrastim (granulocyte colony-stimulating factor [G-CSF]).

Pulmonary. Bronchospasm and acute dyspnea have been reported and appear to occur more frequently when vincristine is administered with mitomycin.

Ocular. Diplopia, ptosis, photophobia, cortical blindness (see neurological toxicity), optic atrophy, ophthalmoplegia, corneal hypesthesia.

Other. Severe pain in the jaw, pharynx, bones, back, and limbs after injection, syndrome of inappropriate antidiuretic hormone (SIADH), fever, pancreatitis (rare).

Storage and Stability
Vincristine is stored in the refrigerator. The drug is stable for at least 30 days at room temperature. Vincristine is chemically stable when further diluted in normal saline or 5% dextrose for at least 4 days at room

temperature (7 days in the refrigerator), alone or mixed with doxorubicin in glass or PVC containers.

Preparation
Doses for continuous infusion are further diluted with 50 mL or more of normal saline or 5% dextrose.

Incompatibilities
Furosemide, idarubicin, some in-line filters, polysiloxane containers used in portable delivery devices.

Compatibilities
Vincristine is compatible with doxorubicin, bleomycin, cytarabine, fluorouracil, methotrexate, and metoclopramide. A pharmacist should be consulted for additional information.

Availability
Vincristine is commercially available as a solution in a concentration of 1 mg/mL in 1-, 2-, and 5-mL vials and 1- and 2-mg syringes (Hyporet).

Selected Readings
Chauncey TR, Shanel JL, Fox JH: Vincristine neurotoxicity, *JAMA* 254:507, 1985.
Jackson DV et al: Single agent vincristine by infusion in refractory multiple myeloma, *J Clin Oncol* 3:1508-1512, 1985.
Weintraub M et al: Severe atypical neuropathy associated with colony-stimulating factors and vincristine, *J Clin Oncol* 14:935-940, 1996.

VINORELBINE
Other Names
Navelbine, vinorelbine tartrate, 5'-noranhydrovinblastine, NVB.

Indications
FDA approved for the treatment of non–small-cell lung cancer as a single agent or in combination with cisplatin. Vinorelbine may also be useful in the treatment of breast cancer.

Classification
Vinca alkaloid (tubulin inhibitor).

Pharmacokinetics
Approximately 26% of vinorelbine is bioavailable after oral administration. The drug is metabolized in the liver and has an elimination half-life of approximately 23 hours.

Dose
The usual IV dose, as a single agent or in combination with cisplatin, is 30 mg/m^2/week. Vinorelbine has been evaluated in oral doses of 50 to 80 mg/m^2/week.

Administration

Vinorelbine is a moderate vesicant and can produce phlebitis. The drug is most often administered intravenously (using extravasation precautions) over a 5- to 10-minute period. Adequate flushing of the vein with 100 to 200 mL of 5% dextrose or normal saline after administration is recommended to decrease the risk of phlebitis. The orally-administered drug is generally taken on an empty stomach as a single dose.

Toxicity

Hematological. Leukopenia and neutropenia are the most frequent dose-limiting toxicities. Leukopenia generally begins 1 week after administration with recovery 8 to 10 days thereafter. Mild to moderate anemia is infrequent. Thrombocytopenia rarely occurs. Hematological toxicity does not appear to be cumulative.

Gastrointestinal. Nausea and vomiting after IV administration are generally mild and controllable with standard antiemetic drugs. Severe nausea and vomiting have been reported more frequently after oral administration. Mild to moderate constipation, anorexia, stomatitis, diarrhea, and abdominal pain have been reported in approximately 18% to 38% of the patients.

Dermatological. Significant alopecia is uncommon and appears to be related to the duration of the treatment. Phlebitis, characterized by erythema, vein discoloration, and tenderness extending over the length of the infused vein, is an occasional toxicity. Vinorelbine is a moderate vesicant, similar to vincristine and vinblastine.

Hepatic. Transient and mild elevations of hepatic enzyme levels have been reported.

Neurological. Fatigue has been reported in 27% of the patients treated with vinorelbine and tended to worsen with continued treatment. Severe peripheral neuropathy is rare and may appear as decreased deep tendon reflexes, constipation, paresthesias, and/or hypesthesia. Loss of deep tendon reflexes may be cumulative. Tumor pain and jaw pain are infrequent, but may be severe.

Cardiovascular. Chest pain, with or without ECG changes, has been reported in several patients treated with vinorelbine. Many of the patients experiencing chest pain had either a history of cardiovascular disease or a tumor within the chest. The precise cause of the chest pain has not been determined. Myocardial infarction has also been reported in a few patients; all of these patients had a prior history of severe cardiovascular disease.

Pulmonary. Acute reversible dyspnea after IV administration has been reported and may be an allergic phenomenon, as with other vinca alkaloids. Hypoxemia and interstitial pneumonitis have been reported infrequently. Treatment with corticosteroids may be beneficial in patients who develop pulmonary toxicities.

Other. Mild to moderate asthenia is common. Syndrome of inappropriate secretion of antidiuretic hormone (SIADH), fatigue, and hemorrhagic cystitis have been rarely reported after administration of vinorelbine.

V

Storage and Stability

Intact vials are stored in the refrigerator (2° C to 8° C) and protected from light. The parenteral formulation is stable at room temperature for at least 72 hours. Vials should not be frozen. Vinorelbine, diluted in 50 to 100 mL of 5% dextrose or normal saline, is stable for at least 24 hours at room and refrigeration temperatures.

Preparation

Vinorelbine must be diluted before administration. Concentrations of 1.5 or 3.0 mg/mL have been diluted with 5% dextrose or normal saline and administered with a syringe. For administration in an IV container, vinorelbine may be diluted in 5% dextrose, normal saline, 0.45% NaCl, 5% dextrose and 0.45% NaCl, Ringer's solution, or lactated Ringer's solution to a concentration of 0.5 to 2.0 mg/mL.

Availability

Commercially available as a 10 mg/mL solution in 1-mL ampules and 5-mL vials. Oral capsules in 10- and 40-mg units are investigational.

Selected Readings

LeChevalier T et al: Randomized study of vinorelbine and cisplatin versus vindesine and cisplatin versus vinorelbine alone in advanced non–small-cell lung cancer: results of a European multicenter trial including 612 patients, *J Clin Oncol* 12:360-367, 1994.

Toso C, Lindley C: Vinorelbine: a novel vinca alkaloid, *Am J Health-Sys Pharm* 52:1287-1304, 1995.

Weber BL et al: Intravenous vinorelbine as first-line and second-line therapy in advanced breast cancer, *J Clin Oncol* 13:2722-2730, 1995.

GENERAL REFERENCES

American Medical Association: *AMA drug evaluations*, Chicago, 1996, The Association.

Chabner BA, Collins JM, eds: *Cancer chemotherapy: principles and practice*, Philadelphia, 1990, JB Lippincott.

Chabner BA, Longo DL: *Cancer chemotherapy and biotherapy: principles and practice*, ed 2, Philadelphia, 1996, Lippincott-Raven.

DeVita VT Jr, Hellman S, Rosenberg SA, eds: *Cancer: principles and practice of oncology*, ed 5, Philadelphia, 1997, Lippincott-Raven.

Durivage HJ, Burnham NL: Prevention and management of toxicities associated with antineoplastic drugs, *J Pharm Pract* 4:27-48, 1991.

McEvoy JK, ed: *AHFS drug information*, Washington, DC, 1996, American Society of Health-System Pharmacists.

National Cancer Institute: *NCI investigational drugs: pharmaceutical data–1994*, Bethesda, Md, 1994, National Institutes of Health.

Olin BR, Hebel SK, Hagemann RC, eds: Antineoplastic agents. In *Facts and comparisons: drug information*, St. Louis, 1996, Facts and Comparisons, pp 642-689h.

Perry MC, editor: Toxicity of chemotherapy, *Semin Oncol* 19:453-609, 1992.

Physician's desk reference, ed 51, Montvale, NJ, 1997, Medical Economics Co.

Reynolds JEF, ed: *Martindale: the extra pharmacopoeia*, ed 29, London, 1989, The Pharmaceutical Press.

United States Pharmacopeial Convention: *USP drug information*, Rockville, Md, 1996, The Convention.

4

Biological Response Modifiers

The immune system is responsible for protecting the body from harmful substances such as bacteria, viruses, and cancer. External defenses, such as the skin, mucous membranes, and gastric acid, prevent the absorption of harmful substances. Internal defenses, such as the lymphoid organs, tissues, and cells, rid the body of substances that have penetrated our external defenses. Internal defenses can be either nonspecific (e.g., neutrophils, macrophages) or specific (e.g., T-lymphocytes).

The immune system is responsible for recognizing foreign substances (antigens), eliminating them, and remembering that they were once present. Re-exposure to the antigen produces an immune response. Many investigators believe the immune system is responsible for the elimination of malignant cells. In a patient with a rapidly progressive malignancy, the immune system has failed to function properly.

Early work with nonspecific stimulators of the immune system, such as bacillus Calmette-Guérin (BCG), methanol-extracted residue of BCG (MER-BCG), *Corynebacterium parvum (C. parvum),* and levamisole yielded few successes. Most studies, with the exception of levamisole plus 5-fluorouracil as adjuvant treatment for Duke's C colon cancer and intravesical BCG for bladder cancer, failed to demonstrate any benefit when these agents were used alone as systemic therapy for advanced disease or as an adjuvant to surgery for "localized" malignancies.

More recent investigations of immunological responses and approaches for the treatment of cancer followed these early disappointments. These studies have increased our knowledge of tumor immunology and coupled with recombinant DNA technology have led to the development of many of the biological response modifiers that are available for the treatment of patients with cancer.

In this chapter is a brief discussion of tumor immunology and general classes of available biological response modifiers. For an extensive review of tumor immunology, see the general references provided at the end of this chapter.

ANTITUMOR IMMUNITY

When the immune system responds to the presence of a foreign substance, or antigen, it does so in two possible ways. In the humoral response, B-lymphocytes recognize and attach to the antigen. Plasma cells are then formed that produce antibodies against the antigen. In the cell-mediated response, T-lymphocytes (T-helper cells or cytotoxic T-lymphocytes) recognize the foreign substance and either directly kill the invader or elicit the production of antibody from plasma cells. Regulation of T-lymphocyte proliferation and activity is largely mediated by cytokines such as interleukin-1 (IL-1), interleukin-2 (IL-2), and tumor necrosis factor (TNF).

The concept known as *natural immunity* or *immune surveillance* implies that the immune system is capable of recognizing all tumor cells as foreign. Natural killer (NK) cells (another type of lymphocyte) and macrophages confer this type of immunity. However, views are divided on the concept of immune surveillance because not all human tumors elicit an immune response or they are not particularly sensitive to the effects of NK cells. Although it is not precisely known how NK cells, macrophages, and certain lymphocytes recognize and kill tumor cells, studies with these cell types have resulted in antitumor therapies. These cells can be removed from the body, can be induced by cytokines (such as IL-2), and later can be reinfused to the patient as a form of treatment. As will be discussed in this chapter, many of the cytokines that are a natural part of the immune system are presently available for the treatment of cancer or will be in the future.

CLINICAL DEVELOPMENT OF THE BIOLOGICAL RESPONSE MODIFIERS

The target cells of the biological response modifiers are the host effector cells, such as the T-helper lymphocytes, not the cancer cells. As a result, classical dose-response relationships that exist for antineoplastic drugs may not exist for agents that are intended to augment the immune system. Administration of a biological response modifier at its maximally tolerated dose may not be the optimal dose for modulation of the immune system. In some cases, the maximally tolerated dose may be inferior to a lower dose. Alternatively, the higher dose may increase the severity of adverse effects without a concomitant increase in the desired biological effect. The clinical development and early human testing of biological response modifiers are designed to determine the optimal biologic dose (OBD), the relationship between the OBD and the optimal therapeutic effect and, if necessary, the maximally tolerated dose (MTD). Unfortunately, it is often unclear which of the many effector cell functions are directly related to tumor response.

HEMATOPOIETIC GROWTH FACTORS

Hematopoietic growth factors are glycoproteins that bind to specific cell surface receptors and stimulate the proliferation, differentiation, and activation of blood cells from different lineages. They were discovered and are defined by their ability to support colony formation in vitro, hence the name *colony-stimulating factor*. Blood cell formation involves a complex network of cytokines. In hematology and oncology the goal of therapy with hematopoietic growth factors is to increase the number of functional white blood cells so that host defense mechanisms can be maintained, to increase the number of platelets so that bleeding problems can be avoided, and/or to increase the number of red blood cells so that red blood cell transfusions can be avoided. Success of treatment with growth factors will be measured in terms of decreased neutropenia, infection, use of antibiotics, transfusion requirements, hospital admissions for fever, decreased length of stay, and reduced treatment costs. Other applications will be to examine the efficacy of increasing dose intensity of chemotherapy using growth factors to avoid myelosuppression. The success of these studies will be measured by increases in tumor response, disease-free interval, and survival.

INTERFERONS

The phenomenon known as *viral interference* (i.e., prevention of viral infection after initial exposure) has been known for many years. In 1957 Issacs and Lindenmann, while studying viral interference in vitro, reported the discovery of a substance that was able to induce cellular resistance to viral challenge. They called this substance *interferon*. In 1969 the interferons were shown to have antitumor effects. In 1973 methods were developed that permitted the isolation of interferons from human blood. Interferons are a family of species-specific proteins that, among other functions, induce antiviral resistance in cells. They are naturally secreted by human cells after viral challenge. The interferons were originally described according to their cell of origin, later according to physical-chemical properties, and now according to their antigenic type. Experimental studies in man in the 1970s and early 1980s were performed with interferon prepared from human leukocytes exposed to the Sendai virus. Interferon was isolated from leukocytes that were collected primarily by the Finnish Red Cross. These preparations contained approximately 0.5% pure interferon and at least 16 other species of interferon alfa. Since then, recombinant DNA technology has provided a way to produce massive amounts of pure interferon of a single species. Interferons are available for use in the treatment of patients with cancer and other disease as a mixture of alfa interferons (interferon alfa-n3: Alferon, interferon alfa-n1: Wellferon) or as single recombinant proteins (interferon alfa-2a: Roferon, interferon alfa-2b: Intron-a, or interferon gamma-1b: Actimmune).

Although the interferons are described in the following sections as single agents for the treatment of malignant and other conditions, some studies suggest that they may be useful when combined with antineoplastic drugs or other biological agents, such as tumor necrosis factor and gamma interferon.

INTERLEUKINS

The interleukins are lymphokines, substances secreted by T cells, mono-cytes, macrophages, and other cells and are important mediators of many immune responses. The recent advances in genetic engineering have enabled researchers to identify and evaluate the biological activities of several different interleukins. Not all of the interleukins that have been identified have been evaluated in humans. Others have undergone extensive study and are no longer being pursued as potential treatments for patients with cancer. The interleukins included in this chapter are those that have been approved for the treatment of cancer (IL-2, aldesleukin) and a few others currently undergoing clinical evaluation.

PREVENTION AND MANAGEMENT OF TOXICITIES

Most biological response modifiers (BRMs) produce similar side effects, although a few unique toxicities have been observed. As outlined for interferon, treatment with a BRM produces predictable acute and chronic constitutional symptoms. The flulike syndrome of fevers, chills, rigors, and myalgias is the most common acute side effect for most of the BRMs. Exceptions include granulocyte colony-stimulating factor (G-CSF), lev-amisole, and BCG. Fatigue and neurological side effects are common chronic side effects. Less predictable, except for high-dose IL-2 therapy, is the broad range of potential organ system toxicities (Table 4-1). Most side effects that are observed, however, are dependent on dose, dura-tion of treatment, schedule, route of administration, or a combination of these variables.

Patients need to be aware of the side effects that are likely to occur, and they must be informed about what they can do to prevent or mini-mize the severity of these side effects. They also need to know that virtu-ally all of the side effects are reversible, most subsiding within a few days after stopping treatment.

The severity (or perceived severity) of symptoms varies from patient to patient. The lack of acute side effects is not usually predictive of adverse effects that may occur after weeks to months of treatment. Many of the side effects are subjective (i.e., fatigue, bone pain) and accurate documen-tation requires frequent communication and the cooperation of the patient and health care provider.

Neurological side effects, such as mood or behavior changes, may be subtle. Family members and friends are a valuable source of information regarding these types of side effects.

Health care providers must be aware of the full range of possible tox-icities associated with BRM treatment (Table 4-1). Factors that may inten-sify a particular toxicity or mask its detection must be eliminated before treatment is begun and avoided during therapy. Premedication and other preventative measures must be instituted at the onset of treatment and adjusted accordingly as therapy progresses.

Several biological agents are discussed in this revision, including a few that were not included in the previous edition. Reviews have also been updated. The format for the listing of biological agents is the same as that

TABLE 4-1

Prevention and Treatment of Adverse Reactions Associated With BRM Therapies

Major adverse events	Causative BRM	Prevention and management
Flulike symptoms (fever, chills, rigors)	Interferons, interleukins, TNF, GM-CSF	Dose at bedtimes; premedicate with acetaminophen, 650 mg every 4 hours ± indomethacin 50 to 75 mg every 8 hours; begin therapy 8 hours before interleukin or TFN therapy; use meperidine, 50 mg IV, if necessary to manage rigors; maintain adequate hydration
Constitutional systems (fatigue, myalgias, arthralgias, headache)	Interferons, interleukins, TNF	Analgesics for pain; supportive care for fatigue; tell patient to arrange most important activities when energy levels are highest (e.g., in the morning) and allow for frequent rest periods
Hematological (anemia, thrombocytopenia)	IL-2, interferons	Monitor complete blood count and platelets daily during treatment; teach patient to watch for signs and symptoms associated with neutropenia, thrombocytopenia, and anemia
Gastrointestinal (anorexia, nausea, vomiting, diarrhea, GI bleeding)	Interleukins, TNF	Premedicate with antiemetic(s), administer antidiarrheal drugs if necessary; instruct patient on ways to increase caloric intake; teach patient about signs of GI bleeding; obtain a stool hemoccult daily
Hepatic (hyperbilirubinemia, elevated transaminase levels)	IL-2, interferons	Exclude patients with significant liver disease; monitor liver function tests daily during treatment; avoid concurrent administration of hepatoxic drugs; teach patient to report signs of hepatic toxicity (darkened urine, generalized itching, yellowing of skin or sclera)

BRM, biological response modifiers; *TNF,* tumor necrosis factor; *G-CSF,* granulocyte colony-stimulating factor; GM-CSF, granulocyte-macrophage colony-stimulating factor; *IL-2,* interleukin 2; *BUN,* blood urea nitrogen; *BCG,* bacillus Calmette-Guérin.

Continued

TABLE 4-1
Prevention and Treatment of Adverse Reactions Associated With BRM Therapies—cont'd

Major adverse events	Causative BRM	Prevention and management
Renal (oliguria, elevated serum creatinine levels)	IL-2	Exclude patients with serum creatinine ≥1.6 mg/dL; monitor intake and output every 4 to 8 hours and serum creatinine, BUN, and electrolytes daily; administer fluids and dopamine if necessary
Urinary (dysuria, hematuria, frequency)	BCG	Forewarn patients; monitor urinalysis for blood; administer analgesics if necessary
Cardiopulmonary (capillary leak: hypotension pulmonary edema, weight gain)	IL-2, TNF, GM-CSF (in excessive doses)	Require normal cardiac stress test and pulmonary function before treatment; monitor vital signs every 4 hours, weight every day, intake and output every 8 hours; administer vasopressors and fluids if necessary; teach patient to report irregular pulse, palpitations, chest pain, or shortness of breath
Neurological (Depression: mental status changes, disorientation, somnolence, impaired memory)	IL-2, interferons in high doses	Avoid sedative medications and alcohol if possible; teach family and friends about potential adverse events to help monitor subtle changes; mental status examination every 8 hours; discontinue therapy at first signs of toxicity
(Excitation: dizziness, agitation, confusion)	Levamisole	Monitor signs and symptoms; teach family and friends about potential adverse events to help monitor subtle changes
Musculoskeletal (bone pain)	G-CSF, GM-CSF, IL-3	Medicate with acetaminophen 650 mg every 6 hours *or* more potent analgesic if necessary
Dermatological (erythema, rash, pruritus)	IL-2, TNF, levamisole	Routine assessment of symptoms, administer antipruritic medications and/or lotions if necessary

in Chapter 3. The general guidelines enumerated in Chapter 3 also apply to the reviews of the biological agents.

ALDESLEUKIN

Other Names
Proleukin, interleukin-2, IL-2, rIL-2, T-cell growth factor, T-cell replacing factor, TRF, NSC-373364.

Indications
FDA approved for the treatment of metastatic renal cell carcinoma in adults. IL-2 may be a useful treatment for patients with malignant melanoma, Kaposi's sarcoma (combined with zidovudine [AZT]), and non-Hodgkin's lymphoma.

Mechanisms of Action
IL-2 is a glycoprotein produced and released during an immune response by stimulated T-helper cells. IL-2 has been called *T-cell growth factor* because of its role in regulating the maturation and replication of T-lymphocytes. Recombinant IL-2 differs from natural IL-2 by two amino acids. There are no known differences in the biological activity and pharmacological profile between the two products. IL-2 activity is measured in units. One "Cetus unit" is equivalent to 6 international units (IU). In each mg of protein there are 18×10^6 IU (or 3×10^6 Cetus units). In the body, IL-2 mediates the expansion of reactive T-lymphocytes (cells that possess IL-2 receptors) after they contact an antigen. All four subsets of T-lymphocytes (i.e., T-helper cells, cytolytic T-cells, suppressor T-cells, and memory T-cells) as well as monocytes and B-lymphocytes are influenced by IL-2. Natural killer T-lymphocytes incubated with IL-2 are called *lymphokine-activated killer* (LAK) cells. Cytolytic T-lymphocytes incubated with IL-2 are called *tumor-infiltrating lymphocytes* (TIL).

Pharmacokinetics
IL-2 is not absorbed after oral administration. After IV administration, IL-2 rapidly distributes throughout the body, including the cerebrospinal fluid. IL-2 is metabolized in the kidneys and has an elimination half-life of 30 to 90 minutes. Elimination of IL-2 occurs via glomerular filtration and tubular secretion. The elimination of IL-2 is not dramatically affected in patients with reduced creatinine clearance because of tubular secretion.

Dose
For the treatment of renal cell carcinoma the recommended dose is 600,000 IU/kg every 8 hours for a total of 14 doses over 5 consecutive days. After a 9-day period of no treatment, IL-2 at the same dose and schedule is repeated. Of the 28 doses intended, an average of eight doses are withheld because of toxicity. In patients who appear to be obtaining benefit from the first course of treatment, a second course may be administered. It is recommended that the second course be initiated 7 weeks after the date the patient was discharged from the hospital.

It is recommended that therapy be permanently discontinued if any of the following toxicities are observed: sustained ventricular tachycardia, unresponsive or uncontrolled cardiac arrhythmia, recurrent chest pain with ECG changes, documented angina or myocardial infarction, pericardial tamponade, intubation required for more than 72 hours, renal dysfunction requiring greater than 72 hours of dialysis, coma or toxic psychosis lasting more than 48 hours, uncontrolled seizures, bowel ischemia, bowel perforation, or gastrointestinal bleeding requiring surgery.

Administration
IL-2 is administered intravenously, usually in 50 mL or more of 5% dextrose and water over a period of 20 to 30 minutes. IL-2 has also been administered by continuous IV (more toxic by this route), subcutaneously, intramuscularly, intraperitoneally, via intrahepatic intraarterial infusion, and by isolated limb perfusion.

Toxicity
High-dose IL-2 also causes capillary leak and suppression of hematopoiesis, leading to anemia, thrombocytopenia, and neutropenia. High-dose IL-2 is an intensive therapy that causes many adverse effects. IL-2 affects the endothelium, causing increased capillary permeability and emigration of lymphoid cells and proteinaceous fluids from the peripheral blood into the interstitium of many organs. Most of the serious toxicities caused by IL-2 are a result of capillary leak.

Hematological. Eosinophilia >40,000/mm^3 (21% to 30%), thrombocytopenia <25,000/mm^3 (16%), platelet transfusion required in 36%, anemia requiring transfusion (62% required ≥4 units packed red blood cells [PRBC], 43% required ≥8 units PRBC), lymphocytosis (75%), leukopenia, transient neutropenia <500/mm^3 (0% to 3%), lymphocytopenia, mildly elevated prothrombin time.

Gastrointestinal. Nausea or vomiting (81%), dyspepsia, diarrhea (67% to 84%), abdominal distention, mucositis (32%), xerostomia, anorexia (27%), gastrointestinal necrosis and perforation (1% to 2%), gastrointestinal bleeding requiring surgery (13%), pancreatitis (rare).

Dermatological. Erythema (41%), rash (26%), pruritus (20% to 48%), dry skin (15%), exfoliative dermatitis (14%), alopecia, vitiligo, injection site reactions after subcutaneous administration. Skin rash (cutaneous macular erythema) usually begins 2 to 3 days after the onset of treatment and is most prominent on the head and neck but may involve the entire body. Within 72 hours after treatment is discontinued the erythema resolves and desquamation follows. Although pruritus may persist for 3 to 6 weeks, normal-appearing skin is usually present within 2 to 3 weeks.

Hepatic. Reversible cholestasis. Hyperbilirubinemia occurs commonly and generally returns to baseline 5 to 6 days after stopping IL-2 therapy. Transient elevation of hepatic enzyme levels (56%). Jaundice has been reported in 11% of patients receiving IL-2.

Neurological. Changes in mental status (73%), impaired memory, irritability, aphasia, headache (12%), somnolence (5% to 13%), disorientation (13% to 35%), stupor, coma (2% to 8%), dizziness (17%), sleep disorders, vivid dreams, paranoia, emotional lability, light-headedness, motor neurological disorders, abnormalities of special senses. Rare neurological toxicities include transient ischemic attack, leukoencephalopathy, peripheral neuropathy, carpal tunnel syndrome, brachial plexopathy, and seizure.

Cardiovascular. Arrhythmias (6% to 17%), hypotension requiring vasopressors (50% to 70%), tachycardia (70%), severe peripheral edema (3%), weight gain $\geq$10% of body weight (32%), angina/ischemic attacks (1% to 3%), myocardial injury (0.5% to 2%). Rare reports of thrombosis, pericardial effusion, stroke, myocarditis, and congestive heart failure. Hypotension begins within a few hours of beginning treatment and returns to baseline within 24 to 48 hours of discontinuing IL-2 therapy.

Pulmonary. Dyspnea (52%), respiratory distress (3% to 23%), intubation required (1% to 6%), pulmonary edema (10%), pleural effusion (3% to 7%), wheezing (6%), tachypnea (8%). Rare reports of apnea, pneumothorax, and hemoptysis.

Renal. Transient increase in serum creatinine levels (61% to 83%) and oliguria begin within 24 to 48 hours after starting IL-2 treatment (29% to 44%). Renal function returns to normal in 7 days (64%), 14 days (84%), and 30 days (95%). In earlier studies, approximately 2% of patients have required dialysis. With current treatment guidelines the need for dialysis is rare.

Metabolic. Hypomagnesemia (16%), acidosis (16%), hypocalcemia (15%), hypophosphatemia (11%), hypokalemia (9%), hyperuricemia (9%), hypoalbuminemia (8%), hyponatremia (7%), adrenal insufficiency (rare), hypothyroidism (may persist for months).

Other. Fatigue and malaise (53%), fever and chills (41% to 89%), myalgia (6%), 10% or greater increase in weight (32%), nasal congestion, central line sepsis (69%), malignant hyperthermia (rare).

Storage and Stability

Intact vials are stored in the refrigerator. Once reconstituted, IL-2 is stable for 48 hours at refrigerated and room temperature when further diluted in 5% dextrose.

Preparation

IL-2 is provided as a lyophilized powder containing 22 million IU/vial. Vials are reconstituted with 1.1 mL sterile water to yield an 18-million IU/mL solution. Direct the diluent down the side of the vial to avoid foaming. The diluted solution is to be added to 50 mL of 5% dextrose in a polyvinylchloride container.

Incompatibilities

IL-2 is incompatible with normal saline (results in a precipitate) and bacteriostatic solutions. The manufacturer has indicated that dilution of IL-2 with albumin should be avoided.

Availability

IL-2 is commercially available as a lyophilized powder in vials containing 22-million IU (1.3 mg).

Selected Readings

Belldegrun A et al: Effects of interleukin-2 on renal function in patients receiving immunotherapy for advanced cancer, *Ann Intern Med* 107:817-822, 1987.

Gaspari AA et al: Dermatologic changes associated with interleukin-2 administration, *JAMA* 258:1624-1629, 1987.

Kintzel PE, Calis KA: Recombinant interleukin-2: a biological response modifier, *Clin Pharm* 10:110-128, 1991.

Lee RE et al: Cardiorespiratory effects of immunotherapy with interleukin-2, *J Clin Oncol* 7:7-20, 1989.

Schwartzentruber DJ: Biologic therapy with interleukin-2: clinical applications: principles of administration and management of side effects. In DeVita VT Jr, Hellman S, Rosenberg SA, eds: *Biologic therapy of cancer*, ed 2, Philadelphia, 1995, JB Lippincott, pp 235-249.

Sznol M: Biologic therapy with interleukin-2: clinical applications, other cancers. In DeVita VT Jr, Hellman S, Rosenberg SA, eds: *Biologic therapy of cancer*, ed 2, Philadelphia, 1995, JB Lippincott, pp 269-278.

Thompson JA et al: Influence of dose and duration of infusion of interleukin-2 on toxicity and immunomodulation, *J Clin Oncol* 6:669-678, 1988.

Williams TM, Fox KR, Kant JA: Interleukin-2: basic biology and therapeutic use, *Hematol Pathol* 5:45-55, 1991.

Yang JC: Biologic therapy with interleukin-2: clinical applications, renal cell cancer. In DeVita VT Jr, Hellman S, Rosenberg SA, eds: *Biologic therapy of cancer,* ed 2, Philadelphia, 1995, JB Lippincott, pp 262-269.

BACILLUS CALMETTE-GUÉRIN

Other Names

Theracys, ImmuCyst, Tice BCG, BCG.

Indications

FDA approved for the treatment of primary and relapsed carcinoma in situ of the urinary bladder. Theracys is approved to eliminate residual tumor cells and reduce the frequency of recurrence. Tice BCG is approved as first- or second-line treatment for patients who cannot undergo radical surgery. BCG is not approved for the treatment of papillary tumors occurring in the absence of carcinoma in situ. Other forms of BCG are approved for immunization against tuberculosis and are not discussed.

Mechanisms of Action

It is unclear whether the effects of BCG are the result of an immune reaction to the bacillus that extends to tumor antigens on the surface of the neoplastic cell or to a nonspecific inflammatory reaction. It has been proposed that the antitumor effects of BCG are mediated by release of tumor necrosis factor (TNF) from activated macrophages.

Dose

When administered by intravesical instillation, BCG is administered in 50 to 53 mL of normal saline. Patients are told to avoid urinating for 2 hours after BCG has been given. Treatment is usually repeated weekly for 6 weeks. The usual dose of Tice BCG is one ampule (i.e., 50 mg). The usual weekly dose of BCG live (Theracys, ImmuCyst) is three vials (each containing 27 mg). Six-week courses of treatment with Theracys may be repeated at 3, 6, 12, 18, and 24 months after the initial treatment, and 6-week courses of Tice BCG may be repeated monthly for 6 to 12 months.

Administration

BCG is administered intravesically for the treatment of in situ bladder cancer. Treatment is usually initiated within 1 to 2 weeks after biopsy or resection. Other routes of administration (i.e., intradermal, percutaneous, intralesional, intrapleural) have been evaluated in the treatment of other malignancies. It is not recommended that BCG be administered if the patient has hematuria or an active urinary tract infection because these conditions increase the risk of developing posttreatment systemic tuberculosis.

Toxicity

Hematological. Anemia and leukopenia, rarely severe, have been reported. Aplastic anemia has been reported.

Gastrointestinal. Nausea and vomiting have been reported in 3% to 16% of the patients, anorexia in 2% to 10%, diarrhea in 1% to 6%, and mild abdominal pain in 1.5% to 3%.

Dermatological. Skin rash (erythema nodosum). When administered percutaneously or intradermally, the expected reaction is a small red papule that scales, ulcerates, and dries, leaving a small pink or bluish scar after about 3 months. More severe ulceration, abscesses, and granulomas may occur and are worse with larger doses. Generalized rashes, lymphadenitis, or lymphangitis can also occur.

Genitourinary. Intravesical administration is frequently associated with dysuria (62%, severe in 3% to 10%), hematuria (40%, severe in 7% to 17%), urinary frequency (40%, severe in 2% to 7%), and cystitis (6% to 30%, severe in 2%), which may require interruption or discontinuation of therapy. Bladder irritation usually occurs 2 to 4 hours after instillation and may last 1 to 2 days. Other genitourinary toxicities are rarely severe and may include urinary urgency (6% to 18%), urinary incontinence (2% to 6%), pain (4% to 6%), nocturia (0% to 4%), and urethritis (0% to 1%).

Other. Almost all patients will develop positive conversion of the tuberculin skin test. This usually occurs after 3 to 12 weeks of intravesicular therapy and is not permanent. Fever, chills, lethargy, and malaise are common (41%). Osteomyelitis, tuberculous meningitis, anaphylaxis, and Guillain-Barré syndrome have occurred rarely. Disseminated BCG infection occasionally occurs and may be fatal. The likelihood of developing a systemic BCG infection may be increased if treatment is administered when the patient has a urinary tract infection.

Storage and Stability

The intact ampules and vials are stored in the refrigerator. After reconstitution, BCG preparations are to be used within 2 hours. It is recommended that BCG preparations be protected from light (i.e., sunlight and artificial light).

Preparation
Care should be taken by those handling BCG to avoid contact with the product. Contact with BCG may cause conversion to tuberculin reactivity. BCG live (Theracys) is reconstituted with the provided diluent, 1 mL/vial. Three vials are further diluted with 50 mL of normal saline (53 mL total/dose). Tice BCG is reconstituted with 1 mL of sterile water per ampule. One ampule is further diluted with 49 mL of normal saline.

Disposal
Containers that have come in contact with BCG preparations are to be considered as infectious waste. The NCI recommends that containers, syringes, and other equipment used for handling the vaccine be sterilized before disposal.

Availability
Tice BCG contains 100 to 800 million colony-forming units (approximately 50 mg) of BCG bacillus as a freeze-dried suspension for reconstitution, in 2-mL ampules. Each 1-mL vial of BCG live (Theracys) contains 340 ± 300 million colony-forming units (approximately 27 mg) of BCG bacillus as a freeze-dried suspension for reconstitution.

Selected Readings
Batts CN: Adjuvant intravesical therapy for superficial bladder cancer, *DICP Ann Pharmacother* 26:1270-1276, 1992.

Herr HW: Local therapy with biologic agents, instillation therapy for bladder cancer. In DeVita VT Jr, Hellman S, Rosenberg SA, eds: *Biologic therapy of cancer,* ed 2, Philadelphia, 1995, JB Lippincott, pp 705-711.

Herr HW et al: Intravesical bacillus Calmette-Guérin therapy prevents tumor progression and death from superficial bladder cancer: ten-year follow-up of a prospective randomized trial, *J Clin Oncol* 13:1404-1408, 1995.

Lamm DL et al: A randomized trial of intravesical doxorubicin and immunotherapy with Bacille Calmette-Guérin for transitional-cell carcinoma of the bladder, *N Engl J Med* 325:1205-1209, 1991.

Orihuela E et al: Toxicity of intravesical BCG and its management in patients with superficial bladder tumors, *Cancer* 60:326-333, 1987.

BROPIRIMINE
Other Names
Remisar, 2-amino-5-bromo-6-phenyl-4(3H)-pyrimidone, ABPP, 5-bromo-6-phenylisocytosine.

Indications
Bropirimine is an investigational drug that has been shown to be useful in the treatment of patients with in situ carcinoma of the bladder. Objective responses have been observed in patients with melanoma and low-grade non-Hodgkin's lymphoma. Topically administered bropirimine has been shown to be a useful treatment for genital herpes simplex virus infections.

Classification and Mechanisms of Action

Bropirimine is a biological response modifier. The mechanisms by which bropirimine exerts its antitumor effects may be due to its immunomodulatory (i.e., increased natural killer cell) activity and interferon-inducing activity. Bropirimine may be synergistic when combined with antineoplastic drugs or other biological response modifiers.

Pharmacokinetics

Bropirimine is well absorbed (at least 45%) after oral administration. Peak plasma levels of bropirimine occur approximately 1 to 4 hours after administration. Studies in animals indicate that the absorption of bropirimine may be increased if the drug is administered in conjunction with food. Bropirimine is highly protein bound (greater than 90%) and metabolized in the liver to at least two glucuronic metabolites. After oral administration of 250 to 1000 mg, approximately 45% to 60% of the drug is excreted in the urine as bropirimine and its metabolites within 24 hours. Less of the drug is detected in the urine when higher doses are administered, which may be indicative of reduced oral absorption at doses greater than 1000 mg. Bropirimine has a terminal half-life of 2.5 to 4.5 hours.

Dose

In the treatment of bladder carcinoma in situ, bropirimine has been administered in doses of 3000 mg/day for 3 consecutive days each week. Each daily dose is divided into three fractions (1000 mg/dose) and taken with food at 2-hour intervals. Current studies are evaluating up to 1 year of treatment.

Administration

Oral or topical.

Toxicity

Gastrointestinal.   Nausea (15% to 30%); vomiting (5% to 10%); diarrhea, constipation, abdominal pain, and anorexia are infrequent toxicities.

Dermatological.   Rash, pruritus, diaphoresis.

Hepatic.   Elevation of hepatic enzyme levels (rare).

Neurological.   Fatigue (30% to 40%), headache (15% to 30%), dizziness (uncommon), transient paresthesias (rare).

Cardiovascular.   Tachycardia (infrequent), palpitations (rare).

Genitourinary.   Increased frequency and hematuria (rare).

Other.   Asthenia (15%), fever (14%), chills, flulike symptoms (17%), hypersensitivity reaction (hives, dyspnea), myalgia, arthralgia.

Storage and Stability

Bropirimine tablets and ointment are stored at room temperature and protected from light. The drug is chemically stable for at least 5 years from the date of manufacture.

Availability
Bropirimine is an investigational drug that is currently available in 250-mg tablets and as a 20 mg/mL ointment.

Selected Readings
Merritt J et al: Phase I/II trial of oral bropirimine (BROP) in superficial bladder cancer, *Proc Am Soc Clin Oncol* 9:143, 1990.
Sarosdy MF et al: Phase I trial of oral bropirimine in superficial bladder cancer, *J Urol* 147:31-33, 1992.

EPOETIN ALFA
Other Names
Epogen, Procrit, erythropoietin, EPO, erythropoietin alfa.

Indications
FDA approved for the treatment of anemia associated with chronic renal failure, zidovudine (AZT) therapy in patients with HIV infection, and cancer chemotherapy for nonmyeloid malignancies.

Mechanisms of Action
Epoetin alfa (EPO) is a lineage-specific inducer of erythrocyte production. EPO stimulates the division and differentiation of erythrocyte progenitor cells within the bone marrow. EPO does not have any effects on leukocytes, platelets, or their progenitors. Reticulocyte counts begin to rise within 10 days of initiating treatment. Elevation of hematocrit, hemoglobin, and red blood cell levels usually occurs within 2 to 6 weeks of treatment onset. The rate of the elevation of red blood cell levels, hemoglobin, and hematocrit is dose dependent.

Pharmacokinetics
After subcutaneous administration, peak serum levels of EPO occur within 5 to 24 hours. EPO has an elimination half-life of 4 to 13 hours. The elimination half-life does not appear to be affected by renal function, although the half-life of EPO is approximately 20% shorter in normal volunteers.

Dose
For patients with anemia caused by cancer chemotherapy, EPO is not recommended if erythropoietin levels are greater than 200 mU/mL. The recommended starting dose for patients with anemia caused by cancer chemotherapy is 150 units/kg, 3 times each week. If anemia is not corrected after 8 weeks of treatment, the dose may be increased to 300 units/kg 3 times weekly. Doses are adjusted to maintain the desired hematocrit level (i.e., around 36%).

Administration
EPO is administered by subcutaneous injection.

Toxicity
The adverse events described are those reported after the use of EPO in patients receiving cancer chemotherapy.

Gastrointestinal. Diarrhea (21%), nausea (17%), vomiting (17%).

Dermatological. Pain at site of injection, rash.

Cardiovascular. Edema (17%), hypertension (rare).

Neurological. Paresthesia (11%), dizziness (5%).

Other. Fever (29%), asthenia (13%), fatigue (13%), shortness of breath (13%).

Storage and Stability

EPO is stored in the refrigerator. The 1-mL vials do not contain a preservative, and it is recommended that one vial be used per dose. The 2-mL (20,000-unit) vial contains a preservative and may be stored in the refrigerator for at least 21 days. EPO should not be frozen.

Preparation

EPO is administered without further dilution. Do not shake the vial because this may adversely affect potency.

Compatibilities

EPO is compatible with bacteriostatic normal saline.

Availability

EPO is commercially available as an injectable solution in 1-mL vials containing 2000, 3000, 4000, and 10,000 units and a 2-mL vial containing 20,000 units (10,000 units/mL).

Selected Readings

Graber SE, Krantz SB: Erythropoietin: biology and clinical use, *Hematol Oncol Clin North Am* 3:369-400, 1989.

Means RT Jr: Erythrocte-stimulating factors. In DeVita VT Jr, Hellman S, Rosenberg SA, eds: *Biologic therapy of cancer,* Philadelphia, 1995, JB Lippincott, pp 190-201.

Miller CM et al: Phase I-II trial of erythropoietin in the treatment of cisplatin-associated anemia, *J Natl Cancer Inst* 84:98-103, 1992.

Platanias LC et al: Treatment of chemotherapy-induced anemia with recombinant human erythropoietin in cancer patients, *J Clin Oncol* 9:2021-2026, 1991.

FILGRASTIM

Other Names

Neupogen, Granulocyte Colony-Stimulating Factor, G-CSF, rG-CSF recombinant-methionyl human granulocyte-colony stimulating factor, r-met HuG-CSF, NSC-614629.

Indications

FDA approved to decrease the incidence of infection in patients with nonmyeloid tumors receiving myelosuppressive chemotherapy and to reduce the duration of neutropenia in patients receiving bone marrow transplantation. G-CSF may also be useful as a rescue treatment for febrile neutropenic patients; as a treatment for aplastic anemia, cyclic neutropenia, congenital neutropenia, and myelodysplastic disorders; and to augment peripheral stem cell collection.

Mechanisms of Action

G-CSF is produced by monocytes, fibroblasts, and endothelial cells of the bone marrow. G-CSF supports the proliferation, differentiation, and activation of committed progenitor cells of the granulocyte series. G-CSF also enhances neutrophil chemotaxis and phagocytosis. After a single subcutaneous dose of G-CSF the absolute neutrophil count (ANC) decreases 50% to 75% for the first 30 minutes before rising to a maximum 8 to 10 hours later. If G-CSF is not administered again, the ANC will normalize within 24 to 48 hours. The level of neutrophilia observed is dose-related.

Pharmacokinetics

G-CSF is not absorbed by mouth. G-CSF can be detected in the serum within 5 minutes of a subcutaneous injection; peak serum concentrations occur within 2 to 8 hours. G-CSF is metabolized in the liver and kidneys. It has an elimination half-life of 3 to 5 hours.

Dose

The recommended starting dose is 5 µg/kg/day for up to 14 days beginning 24 hours after completion of chemotherapy. Higher doses of G-CSF may be administered in subsequent cycles according to the duration and severity of myelosuppression. In general, G-CSF may be discontinued when the ANC is greater than 10,000/mm^3 *after* the expected chemotherapy-induced nadir. G-CSF has also been administered as a 5-day course of treatment at a dose of 5 µg/kg/day on days 15 through 19 of a 3-week chemotherapy regimen. Within 2 to 4 hours of bone marrow transplantation, G-CSF is administered at a dose of 5 µg/kg/day for 21 days. To reduce wastage and cost, daily doses are often rounded off to the nearest vial size (300 or 480 µg). Doses of 100 µg/kg/day or greater have been administered without the occurrence of dose-limiting toxicities.

Administration

Subcutaneous injection is the preferred route of administration. G-CSF may also be administered intravenously, usually as an infusion over at least 30 minutes. Continuous infusions, by either the intravenous or subcutaneous route, have also been used.

Toxicity

Hematological. Initial decrease in ANC (within 5 minutes, may last up to 1 hour). Transient decreases in platelet counts have been reported in patients receiving "high doses." Progression of myelodysplastic syndromes (especially in patients with "excess blasts") may occur.

Gastrointestinal. Nausea (rare), vomiting (rare), diarrhea (rare), anorexia (rare).

Dermatological. Local inflammation at the injection site, skin rash (rare), cutaneous vasculitis (rare), flare in psoriasis, mild alopecia with long-term administration (rare), Sweet's syndrome (acute febrile neutrophilic dermatosis).

Hepatic. Mild elevation of lactic dehydrogenase, alkaline phosphatase, and transaminase levels.

Cardiovascular. Fluid retention; pericardial effusion (rare).

Neurological. Severe motor weakness and foot pain have been observed after the use of G-CSF in combination with chemotherapy regimens containing vincristine.

Musculoskeletal. Transient bone pain (15% to 39% incidence), usually mild to moderate in severity. The pain has been described as a pulsating deep pain in the lower back, pelvis, or sternum. The pain usually begins after initiation of treatment and just before the onset of neutrophil recovery. Resolution usually occurs without stopping treatment and always resolves within a few hours after discontinuation.

Other. Fatigue, elevated uric acid levels, flushing (rare), mild headache, and chest tightness. Splenomegaly is relatively common in patients receiving chronic therapy with G-CSF, but it is rarely of clinical significance.

Storage and Stability

G-CSF should be refrigerated and not allowed to freeze. It is stable for at least 10 months when refrigerated. There is significant loss of activity when the product is stored above or below 2° C to 8° C. G-CSF is stable in plastic syringes for at least 24 hours or 7 days at room and refrigeration temperatures, respectively. At a concentration of 5 µg/mL or greater in 5% dextrose, G-CSF is stable for 7 days at room or refrigerator temperatures. At dilutions from 2 to 15 µg/mL, albumin in a final concentration of 2 mg/mL should be added to protect against adsorption. Addition of albumin is unnecessary when the drug is diluted to a concentration greater than or equal to 15 µg/mL in 5% dextrose. Concentrations of less than 2 µg/mL should not be used. Dilutions of G-CSF in 5% dextrose are stable in glass bottles, polyvinylchloride, polyolefin, or polypropylene bags and IV sets, and Travenol infusors.

Preparation

Draw appropriate dose into a syringe for subcutaneous injection. If G-CSF is further diluted for IV administration, use only 5% dextrose.

Incompatibilities

Normal saline.

Availability

G-CSF is supplied as a 300 µg/mL solution in vials containing 1 mL (300 µg/vial) and 1.6 mL (480 µg/vial).

Selected Readings

American Society of Clinical Oncology: Update of recommendations for the use of hematopoietic colony-stimulating factors: evidence-based clinical practice guidelines, *J Clin Oncol* 14:1957-1960, 1996.

ASCO Ad Hoc Colony-Stimulating Factor Guidelines Expert Panel: American Society of Clinical Oncology recommendations for the use of hematopoietic colony-stimulating factors: evidence-based, clinical practice guidelines, *J Clin Oncol* 12:2471-2508, 1994.

Bensinger TR et al: Transplantation of allogeneic peripheral blood stem cells mobilized by recombinant human granulocyte colony-stimulating factor, *Blood* 85:1655-1658, 1995.

Geller RB: Use of cytokines in the treatment of acute myelocytic leukemia: a critical review, *J Clin Oncol* 14:1371-1382, 1996.

Hollingshead LM, Goa KL: Recombinant granulocyte colony stimulating factor (rG-CSF): a review of its pharmacological properties and prospective role in neutropenic conditions, *Drugs* 42:300-330, 1991.

Klumpp TR et al: Granulocyte colony-stimulating factor accelerates neutrophil engraftment following peripheral-blood stem-cell transplantation: a prospective, randomized trial, *J Clin Oncol* 13:1323-1327, 1995.

Lieschke GJ, Burgess AW: Granulocyte colony-stimulating factor and granulocyte-macrophage colony-stimulating factor, *N Engl J Med* 327:28-35, 99-106, 1992.

Miller LL, Nagler CH: Colony-stimulating factors: clinical applications. In DeVita VT Jr, Hellman S, Rosenberg SA, eds: *Biologic therapy of cancer,* Philadelphia, 1995, JB Lippincott, pp 141-182.

Ohno R et al: Effect of granulocyte colony-stimulating factor after intensive induction therapy in relapsed or refractory acute leukemia, *N Engl J Med* 323:871-877, 1990.

Peters WP, Rosner G, Ross M: Comparative effects of granulocyte-macrophage colony-stimulating factor (GM-CSF) and granulocyte colony-stimulating factor (G-CSF) on priming peripheral blood progenitor cells for use with autologous bone marrow after high-dose chemotherapy, *Blood* 81:1709-1719, 1993.

Ribas A et al: Five-day course of granulocyte colony-stimulating factor in patients with prolonged neutropenia after adjuvant chemotherapy for breast cancer is a safe and cost-effective schedule to maintain dose-intensity, *J Clin Oncol* 14:1573-1580, 1996.

INTERFERONS

Interferon is a glycoprotein with a molecular weight of 20,000 composed of approximately 150 amino acids. It consists of multiple species. Interferons are available as a mixture of alfa interferons (interferon alfa-n3: Alferon, interferon alfa-n1: Wellferon) or as single recombinant proteins (interferon alfa-2a: Roferon, interferon alfa-2b: Intron-a, or interferon gamma-1b: Actimmune).

ALPHA INTERFERONS

Other Names

Interferon alfa-2a, IFN alfa-2a, Roferon, NSC-367982.
Interferon alfa-2b, IFN alfa-2b, Intron-A, NSC-377523.
Interferon alfa-n1, IFN alfa-n1, Wellferon.
Interferon alfa-n3, IFN alfa-n3, Alferon.

Indications

The FDA-approved indications are listed in Table 4-2. In addition to these indications, the alfa interferons may be useful in the treatment of multiple myeloma, chronic myelogenous leukemia, bladder carcinoma

TABLE 4-2

Approved Indications for Biological Agents Used in the Treatment of Patients With Cancer

Biological agent	Indications*
Aldesleukin	Renal cell cancer *Malignant melanoma, Kaposi's sarcoma, non-Hodgkin's lymphoma*
BCG	Carcinoma in situ of the bladder
Bropirimine	Investigational (carcinoma in situ of the bladder)
Epoetin alfa	Anemia associated with cancer chemotherapy, zidovudine (AZT) therapy in patients with HIV infection, and chronic renal failure
Filgrastim (G-CSF)	Neutropenia caused by cancer chemotherapy, reducing the duration of neutropenia in patients receiving bone marrow transplantation *Rescue treatment for febrile neutropenia, aplastic anemia, cyclic neutropenia, congenital neutropenia, myelodysplastic disorders, augmentation of autologous peripheral stem cell collection*
Interferon alfa-n1	Investigational
Interferon alfa-n3	Condylomata acuminata
Interferon alfa-2a	Hairy cell leukemia, Kaposi's sarcoma of AIDS *Adjuvant treatment of malignant melanoma, chronic hepatitis B, chronic hepatitis non-A non-B/C, condylomata acuminata, multiple myeloma, chronic myelogenous leukemia, bladder carcinoma (intravesical instillation), low grade non-Hodgkin's lymphoma, cutaneous T-cell lymphoma, essential thrombocythemia, renal cell carcinoma*
Interferon alfa-2b	Hairy cell leukemia, adjuvant treatment of malignant melanoma, Kaposi's sarcoma of AIDS, chronic hepatitis B, chronic hepatitis non-A non-B/C, condylomata acuminata *Multiple myeloma, chronic myelogenous leukemia, bladder carcinoma (intravesical instillation), low-grade non-Hodgkin's lymphoma, cutaneous T-cell lymphoma, essential thrombocythemia, renal cell carcinoma*

*Roman typeface designates FDA-approved indications; italics represent compendia-based indications from the Association of Community Cancer Centers (ACCC) Compendia-Based Drug Bulletin, 5(2), 1996 and the three federally recognized compendia. To obtain additional information contact the ACCC, 11600 Nebel St. Suite 201, Rockville, MD 20852. The three compendia are (1) *United States Pharmacopeia, Drug Information (USP-DI),* The US Pharmacopeial Convention, Inc., 12601 Twinbrook Parkway, Bethesda, MD, 20852; (2) *AMA Drug Evaluations,* American Medical Association, Division of Drugs and Toxicology, 535 N. Dearborn St., Chicago, IL 60610; and (3) *American Society of Hospital Pharmacists (AHFS) Drug Information,* American Society of Hospital Pharmacists, Inc., 4630 Montgomery Ave., Bethesda, MD 20814.

Continued

TABLE 4-2
Approved Indications for Biological Agents Used in the Treatment of Patients With Cancer—cont'd

Biological agent	Indications*
Interferon alfa-2c	Investigational
Interferon beta-1b	Multiple sclerosis (ambulatory patients with relapsing-remitting disease)
	AIDS-related Kaposi's sarcoma, renal cell carcinoma, melanoma, cutaneous T-cell lymphoma, acute non-A non-B/C hepatitis
Interferon gamma-1b	Infections associated with chronic granulomatous disease
	Ovarian carcinoma
Interleukin-3	Investigational (thrombocytopenia)
Interleukin-4	Investigational (regional perfusion, melanoma, sarcoma)
Interleukin-6	Investigational
Interleukin-11	Investigational
Levamisole	Adjuvant treatment of colon cancer in combination with fluorouracil
	Melanoma
MGDF	Investigational (reversal and prevention of thrombocytopenia)
Sargramostim (GM-CSF)	Reducing the duration of neutropenia caused by bone marrow transplantation and treatment of myelogenous leukemia in adults
	Myelosuppression associated with chemotherapy, rescue treatment for febrile neutropenia, aplastic anemia, cyclic neutropenia, congenital neutropenia, myelodysplastic disorders, augmentation autologous peripheral stem cell collection
Thrombopoietin	Investigational (reversal and prevention of thrombocytopenia)
Tumor necrosis factor	Investigational (regional perfusion, melanoma, sarcoma)

(intravesical instillation), low-grade non-Hodgkin's lymphoma, cutaneous T-cell lymphoma, essential thrombocythemia, and renal cell carcinoma. In patients with chronic myelogenous leukemia, cytogenetic conversion to Ph1 chromosome negativity occurs in approximately 40% of patients after a median of 9 months of treatment, and 90% of responding patients maintain their remission with continued therapy.

Classification and Mechanisms of Action
The interferons induce antiviral proteins in cells without directly influencing the virus. Interferons also inhibit tumor growth via an interaction with 2'5'-oligoadenylate synthetase and other means, namely by increasing tumor antigenicity, down regulation of oncogenes (e.g., c-*myc*, c-*fos*),

inducing differentiation, affecting antibody production, and regulating cytotoxic effector cells. Its direct antiproliferative properties (e.g., inhibition of cell growth) may explain its activity in certain malignancies. Interferons also inhibit P450 enzymes. This phenomenon may result in reduced hepatic metabolism of aminophylline, barbiturates, carmustine, and other drugs.

Pharmacokinetics

Interferons are not absorbed by mouth; they must be administered parenterally. Maximum serum levels of IFN alfa-2b occur approximately 3 to 12 hours after intramuscular administration. Interferons are metabolized almost totally by renal tubules. Very little interferon is reabsorbed into the circulation from the kidneys. There is no need to reduce the dose of interferon in patients with reduced creatinine clearance. Although the interferons have a short elimination half-life (i.e., approximately 2 to 3 hours for IFN alfa-2b), their antiviral and other effects persist for up to 72 hours after a single dose.

Dose

Hairy cell leukemia. 2 million IU/m^2 subcutaneously, 3 times weekly (IFN alfa-2b), or 3 million IU subcutaneously daily for a period of 16 to 24 weeks, then 3 times weekly (IFN alfa-2a). Administration of the dose at bedtime may reduce the severity of some side effects. Treatment is usually administered for 1 year.

Kaposi's sarcoma of AIDS. 30 million IU/m^2 subcutaneously, 3 times weekly (IFN alfa-2b), or 36 million IU subcutaneously daily for a period of 10 to 12 weeks, then 36 million IU 3 times weekly (IFN alfa-2a). The dose needs to be reduced in patients also receiving zidovudine (AZT). Dose-limiting toxicity is seen in most of the patients taking AZT, 100 to 200 mg every 4 hours with IFN alfa-2a, 9 million IU/day.

Condylomata acuminata. 1 million IU, injected into each lesion 3 times weekly for 3 weeks (repeat the 3-week treatment in 12 to 16 weeks if necessary) (IFN alfa-2b), or 250,000 IU injected into each lesion twice weekly for a period up to 8 weeks (IFN alfa-n3).

Chronic hepatitis non-A, non-B/C. 3 million IU subcutaneously 3 times weekly for a 16-week period (IFN alfa-2b).

Chronic hepatitis B. 5 million IU/day subcutaneously or 10 million IU 3 times weekly (30 to 35 million IU/week) for a 16-week period (IFN alfa-2b).

Adjuvant treatment for malignant melanoma. 20 million IU/m^2/day for 5 days, repeated weekly for 4 weeks, followed by 10 million IU/m^2 3 times each week for 48 weeks (IFN alfa-2b).

Chronic myelogenous leukemia. 5 million IU/m^2/day.

Multiple myeloma. 2 million IU/m^2 3 times weekly as maintenance therapy in patients who attain a response to induction chemotherapy.

Other malignancies. Various doses (i.e., 3 to 10 million IU/m^2) and schedules (i.e., daily, daily for 5 days repeated every 3 to 4 weeks, or every other day) have been used.

Administration

The preferred route of administration is subcutaneous. Interferons have also been given intramuscularly, intravenously, intralesionally, intravesically, intraperitoneally, and topically. When interferon is administered intravenously, it is often mixed in 50 to 100 mL of normal saline and given over a period of 10 to 15 minutes. Alfa interferons have also been administered as a continuous IV or subcutaneous infusion.

Toxicity

Hematological. Mild leukopenia (50%), thrombocytopenia (35%), and anemia (27%) are not usually dose limiting.

Gastrointestinal. Mild nausea (30% to 50%), vomiting (10% to 17%), diarrhea (30% to 40%), anorexia (45% to 65%), aberrant taste, flatulence, constipation, and gastric distress have been reported. These side effects occasionally occur and are rarely severe.

Dermatological. Mild alopecia is observed in some patients after 4 months of therapy. Skin rash and injection site reactions occur in 21% to 25% of patients. Other uncommon side effects include dry skin, flushing, increased eye lash growth, and urticaria.

Hepatic. Mild elevations of hepatic transaminase levels occur in approximately 25% to 46% of patients with hairy cell leukemia. Hyperbilirubinemia and hepatitis rarely occur.

Neurological. Somnolence and mild paresthesias occur in about 25% of the patients. Dizziness has been reported in 21% to 41% of the patients. Depression, visual and sleep disturbances, tremor, seizures, acute paranoid reactions, aphasia, agitation, anxiety, and dizziness have occurred with high doses (i.e., > 20 million units/m^2).

Cardiovascular. Cough (27%), dyspnea (11%), hypotension (5%), edema (3% to 9%), chest pain (4%), hypertension. Arrhythmias (atrial or ventricular), tachycardia, and myocardial infarction have been rarely reported.

Renal. Proteinuria and elevations of serum creatinine levels occur in less than 2% of the patients; elevation of BUN levels have been reported to occur in 4% of the patients.

Flulike symptoms. Fever, chills, diaphoresis, and rigors occur universally regardless of dose, route, or schedule. The usual onset occurs 1 to 2 hours after a dose, peaks within 4 to 8 hours, and may persist for 18 hours. These effects tend to lessen with continued dosing. Prophylactic treatment with acetaminophen blunts the severity of these side effects.

Constitutional symptoms. Fatigue (90%), myalgias (70%), arthralgias (5% to 24%), and headaches (70%) may be dose limiting. These symptoms usually occur during the first or second week of treatment. Chronic fatigue is dose limiting when doses are greater than 3 to 4 million units 3 times weekly. In patient's with Kaposi's sarcoma of AIDS, an 84% incidence of chronic fatigue has been reported.

Other. Weight loss (14% to 25%), impotence (6%), night sweats (8%), rhinorrhea (4%), sinusitis (0% to 3%). Rarely reported toxicities include hypothyroidism, conjunctivitis, injection site inflammation, broncho-spasm, tachypnea, cyanosis, earache, eye irritation, and rhinitis.

Storage and Stability

The intact vials of IFN alfa-2a, IFN alfa-2b, and IFN alfa-n3 are stored in the refrigerator. At the time of this writing, IFN alfa-n1 must be stored in the freezer before use. All containers bear expiration dates.

Reconstituted solutions of IFN alfa-2a are stable for 2 weeks at room temperature and 1 month in the refrigerator. IFN-alfa 2a is stable for 48 hours in 5% dextrose at a concentration of 60,000 IU/mL and in normal saline at a concentration of 40,000 IU/mL.

Reconstituted solutions of IFN alfa-2b are stable for 1 month at refrigeration temperatures and for 2 weeks at room temperature when mixed as directed by the manufacturer.

Preparation

IFN alfa-2a powder for injection: add 3 mL of accompanying diluent to the vial containing 18 million IU to yield 6 million IU/mL.

IFN alfa-2b powder for injection

Vial strength (million IU)	Diluent (mL)	Final concentration (million IU/mL)
3	1	3
5	1	5
10*	1	10
18	1	18
25	5	5
50†	1	50

*For condylomata acuminata.
†For Kaposi's sarcoma of AIDS.

For IV injection, it is recommended that IFN alfa-2b be administered as a 100,000 IU/mL solution to minimize adsorption of the drug to glass and plastic containers. The manufacturer does not recommend use of the 10, 18, or 25 million IU vials for IV administration.

Incompatibilities

IFN alfa-2b is incompatible with 5% dextrose solution and with a component of the Travenol infusor. Interferon has been shown to inhibit the metabolism of aminophylline by as much as 33% to 81%.

Compatibilities

IFN alfa-2b is compatible in normal saline, Ringer's injection, lactated Ringer's solution, and 5% sodium bicarbonate injection.

Availability

IFN alfa-2a is commercially available as an injectable solution (3, 6, 9, 18, and 36 million IU/mL) and as a lyophilized powder (6- and 18-million IU/vial).

IFN alfa-2b is commercially available as a lyophilized powder in vials containing 3, 5, 10, 18, 25, and 50 million IU and as an injectable solution in vials containing 10 million IU/2 mL, 22.8 million IU/3.8 mL (6 million IU/mL), and 25 million IU/5 mL.

IFN alfa-n3 is commercially available as an injectable solution in 1-mL vials containing 5 million IU/mL.

IFN alfa-n1 (Wellferon) is investigational and has been provided by the NCI or the manufacturer in 1-mL vials containing 8 to 12 million IU/mL.

Selected Readings

Browman GP et al: Randomized trial of interferon maintenance in multiple myeloma: a study of the National Cancer Institute of Canada Clinical Trials Group, *J Clin Oncol* 13:2354-2360, 1995.

Foon KA: Biologic therapy with interferon-alfa and beta: clinical applications, hairy cell leukemia, chronic myelogenous leukemia, and myeloproliferative disorders. In DeVita VT Jr, Hellman S, Rosenberg SA, eds: *Biologic therapy of cancer*, ed 2, Philadelphia, 1995, JB Lippincott, pp 365-373.

Golomb HM, Jacobs A et al: Alpha-2 interferon therapy of hairy-cell leukemia: a multicenter study of 64 patients, *J Clin Oncol* 4:900-905, 1986.

Hoofnagle JH et al: Treatment of chronic non-A, non-B hepatitis with recombinant human alpha interferon, *N Engl J Med* 315:1575-1578, 1986.

Kirkwood JM: Biologic therapy with interferon-alfa and beta: clinical applications, melanoma. In DeVita VT Jr, Hellman S, Rosenberg SA, eds: *Biologic therapy of cancer*, ed 2, Philadelphia, 1995, JB Lippincott, pp 388-411.

Kirkwood JM et al: Interferon alfa-2b adjuvant therapy of high-risk resected cutaneous melanoma: the Eastern Cooperative Oncology Group Trial EST 1684, *J Clin Oncol* 14:7-17, 1996.

Krown SE: Biologic therapy with interferon-alfa and beta: clinical applications, Kaposi's sarcoma. In DeVita VT Jr, Hellman S, Rosenberg SA, eds: *Biologic therapy of cancer*, ed 2, Philadelphia, 1995, JB Lippincott, pp 411-419.

Krown SE et al: Interferon-alfa with zidovudine: safety, tolerance, and clinical and virologic effects in patients with Kaposi sarcoma associated with acquired immunodeficiency syndrome, *Ann Intern Med* 112:812-821, 1990.

Mandelli F et al: Maintenance treatment with recombinant interferon alfa-2b in patients with multiple myeloma responding to conventional induction chemotherapy, *N Engl J Med* 322:1430-1434, 1990.

Perrillo RP et al: A randomized, controlled trial of interferon alfa-2b alone and after prednisone withdrawal for the treatment of chronic hepatitis B, *N Engl J Med* 323:295-301, 1990.

Salmon SE: Biologic therapy with interferon-alfa and beta: clinical applications, multiple myeloma. In DeVita VT Jr, Hellman S, Rosenberg SA, eds: *Biologic therapy of cancer*, ed 2, Philadelphia, 1995, JB Lippincott, pp 420-426.

Williams RD: Intravesical interferon alfa in the treatment of superficial bladder cancer, *Semin Oncol* 5:10-13, 1988.

INTERFERON BETA-1B

Other Names

Betaseron, interferon beta, IFN-beta, recombinant beta interferon, rIFN-B, IFN-Bser, NSC-373361.

Indications

FDA approved for use in ambulatory patients with relapsing-remitting multiple sclerosis. IFN-beta may also be useful in the treatment of

AIDS-related Kaposi's sarcoma, renal cell carcinoma, melanoma, cutaneous T-cell lymphoma, non small-cell cancer of the lung, and acute non-A, non-B hepatitis.

Classification and Mechanisms of Action

IFN-beta binds to the same cellular receptor sites as the alpha interferons. IFN-beta has antiviral, antiproliferative (cytostatic), and immunomodulatory properties. Its direct antiproliferative properties (e.g., inhibition of cell growth and differentiation) may account for its activity in certain malignancies. The mechanisms by which IFN-beta exerts its effects on multiple sclerosis are not known.

Pharmacokinetics

Peak serum concentrations of IFN-beta occur within 1 to 8 hours after subcutaneous injection. The apparent bioavailability of IFN-beta after subcutaneous administration is 50%. The elimination half-life has been calculated as 8 minutes to 4.3 hours.

Dose

For the treatment of multiple sclerosis, the recommended dose is 0.25 mg (8 million IU) subcutaneously every other day. Various doses have been evaluated in the treatment of malignancies, including 90 million IU/day for 10 days, repeated every 21 days; and 180 million IU 3 times a week.

Administration

IFN-beta has been administered subcutaneously, intramuscularly, intranasally, intravesically, intraperitoneally, intrathecally, topically, and intravenously, usually as an infusion over a 10- to 15-minute period.

Toxicity

Hematological. Neutropenia (18% may have an absolute neutrophil count less than 1500/mm^3), lymphopenia (84% will have a lymphocyte count less than 1500/mm^3), thrombocytopenia (uncommon), anemia (rare).

Gastrointestinal. Mild nausea, vomiting (21%), mild diarrhea (35%), constipation (24%).

Dermatological. Rash, alopecia (4%), injection site reaction (85%), diaphoresis (23%), photosensitivity (rare).

Hepatic. Significant elevation of hepatic transaminase levels has been reported to occur in 5% to 19% of the patients.

Neurological. Somnolence (6%), confusion (at high doses), paresthesia, tremor, seizures (rare), paranoia (rare), aphasia (3%), agitation (2%), anxiety, dizziness, transient visual disturbances (7%).

Cardiovascular. Tachycardia (6%), palpitations (8%), generalized edema (8%), hypertension (7%), arrhythmias, myocardial infarction (rare).

Flulike symptoms. Flulike symptoms occur in at least 54% of the patients. Fever, chills, diaphoresis, and rigors occur regardless of dose, route, or schedule. The usual onset occurs 1 to 2 hours after a dose, peaks within 4 to 8 hours, and may persist for 18 hours. These effects tend to lessen with continued dosing. Prophylactic treatment with acetaminophen blunts the severity of these side effects.

Constitutional symptoms. Fatigue (common), myalgias (44%), arthralgias, and headaches (84%) may be dose limiting. These symptoms usually occur during the first or second week of treatment. Chronic fatigue is dose limiting with higher doses.

Other. Asthenia (49%), abdominal pain (32%), sinusitis (36%), dyspnea (8%), laryngitis (6%), hypoglycemia (15%), proteinuria (6%), weight gain (4%), weight loss (4%), conjunctivitis (12%), menstrual abnormalities (17%), cystitis (15%).

Storage and Stability
Unreconstituted vials are stored at refrigeration temperatures. The manufacturer recommends that reconstituted solutions of IFN-beta be used within 3 hours.

Preparation
The lyophilized product is reconstituted by adding 1.2 mL of the provided diluent to the 0.3-mg vial (9.6 million IU) to result in a concentration of 0.25 mg/mL (8 million IU/mL). For intravenous injection the IFN-beta may be further diluted with 5% dextrose or normal saline.

Availability
IFN-beta is commercially available as a lyophilized powder in 0.3-mg (9.6 million IU) vials.

Selected Readings
Foon KA: Biologic therapy with interferon-alfa and beta: clinical applications, hairy cell leukemia, chronic myelogenous leukemia, and myeloproliferative disorders. In DeVita VT Jr, Hellman S, Rosenberg SA, eds: *Biologic therapy of cancer*, ed 2, Philadelphia, 1995, JB Lippincott, pp 365-373.

Schiller J et al: Randomized phase II-III trial of combination beta and gamma interferons and etoposide and cisplatin in inoperable non small-cell cancer of the lung, *J Natl Cancer Inst* 81:1739-1743, 1989.

INTERFERON GAMMA
Other Names
Actimmune, interferon gamma-1b, IFN-gamma.

Indications
FDA approved to decrease the severity and frequency of serious infections associated with chronic granulomatous disease. Interferon gamma may be a useful treatment for patients with ovarian carcinoma or combined with melphalan and tumor necrosis factor (TNF) given by isolated limb perfusion for patients with melanoma of the extremity.

Pharmacokinetics

Interferon gamma is not absorbed by mouth. Approximately 90% of the drug is absorbed after subcutaneous administration. Peak plasma concentrations occur 4 and 7 hours after administration by intramuscular and subcutaneous routes, respectively. The elimination half-life is approximately 6 hours after subcutaneous administration, 40 minutes after intravenous administration, and 3 hours after intramuscular dosing. The maximum serum concentration occurs 7 hours after subcutaneous injection.

Dose

For patients with a body surface area greater than 0.5 m^2: 50 $\mu g/m^2$/dose (1.5 million IU/m^2/dose). For patients with a body surface area less than or equal to 0.5 m^2: 1.5 $\mu g/kg$/dose (3 million IU/m^2/dose). One dose is administered 3 times each week (usually on a Monday, Wednesday, and Friday of each week). For patients with ovarian carcinoma, interferon gamma has been administered intraperitoneally at a dose of 20 million IU/m^2 twice weekly for a period of 3 to 4 months. Combined with melphalan and tumor necrosis factor (TNF) administered by isolated limb perfusion (ILP), interferon gamma has been administered subcutaneously at a dose of 200 μg/day on the 2 days preceding ILP. Interferon gamma, 200 μg, was also added to the perfusate containing TNF and melphalan.

Administration

Subcutaneous injection is the preferred route of administration. Interferon gamma has also been given intramuscularly, intravenously over a 1-minute or longer period, intraperitoneally, and by isolated limb perfusion. When administered into the peritoneal cavity, interferon gamma has been diluted in 250 mL of normal saline and infused over a 2-hour period.

Toxicity

Hematological. Leukopenia occurs frequently but is rarely of clinical significance. Decreased hemoglobin and hematocrit (uncommon), thrombocytopenia, prolonged PT and PTT, and hemolysis (rare). Deep venous thrombosis and pulmonary embolism have been reported. After intraperitoneal administration, Grade 3 neutropenia and anemia were observed in 4% and 3% of the patients, respectively.

Gastrointestinal. Diarrhea (14%), nausea (10%), vomiting (13%), abdominal pain (8% after IV use, 13% after intraperitoneal use), anorexia (3%), weight loss, stomatitis, pancreatitis, gastrointestinal bleeding in patients with a prior history (rare).

Dermatological. Rash, injection site reactions.

Hepatic. Increased hepatic transaminase levels occur after intravenous and intraperitoneal administration.

Neurological. Headache (33% after IV administration, 9% after intraperitoneal administration), decreased alertness, confusion, dizziness, parkinson-like symptoms, disorientation, hallucinations, transient ischemic attack, and seizures. Paresthesias have been reported in 6% of the patients receiving interferon gamma via the intraperitoneal route.

Cardiovascular. Hypotension, primary atrioventricular block, peripheral vasoconstriction, syncope, tachyrhythmia, myocardial infarction.

Pulmonary. Tachypnea, interstitial pneumonitis, bronchospasm.

Renal. Elevated BUN or creatinine levels, acute renal failure.

Constitutional symptoms. Fever commonly occurs after all routes of administration; chills (14%), myalgias (6%), fatigue (14%), night sweats.

Other. Hyponatremia, hyperglycemia, increased triglyceride levels.

Preparation
Available as sterile liquid.

Storage and Stability
Interferon gamma-1b is stored in the refrigerator. It is stable for 12 hours at room temperature. The manufacturer recommends discarding any unused portion of a vial after withdrawing the desired dose.

Availability
Commercially available as 100 μg (3 million units) per 0.5-mL vial.

Selected Readings
Ijzermans JNM, Marquet RL: Interferon-gamma: a review, *Immunobiology* 179:456-473, 1989.

Kurzrock R et al: Pharmacokinetics, single-dose tolerance and biological activity of recombinant gamma-interferon in cancer patients, *Cancer Res* 45:2866-2872, 1985.

Pujade-Lauraine E et al: Intraperitoneal recombinant interferon gamma in ovarian cancer patients with residual disease at second-look laparotomy, *J Clin Oncol* 14:343-350, 1996.

Quesada JR: Biologic therapy with interferon-gamma. In DeVita VT Jr, Hellman S, Rosenberg SA, eds: *Biologic therapy of cancer*, ed 2, Philadelphia, 1995, JB Lippincott, pp 435-442.

INTERLEUKIN-3
Other Names
IL-3, recombinant IL-3, hematopoietic cell growth factor, HCGF, mast cell growth factor, MCGF, multi-potential colony-stimulating factor, multi-CSF.

Indications
IL-3 may be useful, in combination with G-CSF or GM-CSF, as an adjunctive treatment to high-dose chemotherapy or bone marrow transplantation because of its ability to stimulate the production of platelets.

Mechanisms of Action
IL-3 is produced by T cells. IL-3 supports the proliferation of early hematopoietic progenitors (myeloid, erythroid, and megakaryocytes) as well as mature eosinophils, monocytes, and mast cells. IL-3 has been shown to induce acute nonlymphocytic leukemia blasts to proliferate.

IL-3 produces a dose-dependent increase in white blood cell (WBC) counts (up to a threefold increase at 500 µg/m²), eosinophils (up to a 50-fold increase at 500 µg/m²), and platelets (a 1.5- to 1.8-fold increase at 250 to 500 µg/m²). Increases in reticulocyte counts and hemoglobin levels have also been reported in a minority of the patients treated with IL-3. The effects of IL-3 are delayed; it may take 10 to 14 days of treatment to achieve a positive response. The effects of IL-3 are long lasting; leukocyte and platelet levels may remain elevated for several days after treatment has been stopped.

Pharmacokinetics

IL-3 is not absorbed by mouth. It has an elimination half-life of 18 to 68 minutes. A dose of 250 µg/m² routinely results in serum concentrations 10 to 20 ng/mL. The maximum serum concentration occurs 2 to 4 hours after a subcutaneous dose.

Dose

Most studies have utilized doses of 8 to 10 µg/kg (320 to 400 µg/m²) daily for 14 to 28 days. Doses up to 1000 µg/m2 have been administered. IL-3, at a dose of 7.5 µg/kg/day, has been combined with GM-CSF, 3 µg/kg/day. Sequential administration of IL-3 and GM-CSF has been shown to produce significant improvement in platelet recovery compared with IL-3 and GM-CSF given concurrently or GM-CSF given alone.

Administration

IL-3 may be given as a subcutaneous injection or as an IV infusion over a period of 4 hours or longer.

Toxicity

Hematological. An increase in bone marrow blast cells has been reported in a patient with refractory anemia with excess blasts. IL-3 was discontinued and the marrow blast cell count returned to "normal" within 1 week.

Gastrointestinal. Nausea (14% to 25%), diarrhea.

Dermatological. Urticaria, rash, pruritus, inflammation at the injection site (erythema and edema 50% in some studies).

Hepatic. Elevated hepatic transaminase levels.

Cardiovascular. Hypotension.

Flulike symptoms. Fever and chills are common. Approximately 5 hours after administration of a subcutaneous dose, a maximum temperature of 39.5° C will occur in 80% of the patients. The fever typically lasts 3 to 4 hours. When IL-3 is given intravenously, the fever begins with the infusion and abates within 2 hours.

Musculoskeletal. Bone pain, usually mild. At doses greater than 500 µg/m², bone pain is observed in 50% of the patients. Myalgia may accompany bone pain.

Other. Headache, often requiring treatment with acetaminophen or codeine, is dose related. All patients who receive 1000 µg/m²/day experience headaches. Exacerbation of asthma, fatigue, dyspnea, malaise, and polyserositis have been reported after treatment with IL-3.

Storage and Stability
The unreconstituted drug is stable for at least 6 months in the refrigerator. Reconstituted IL-3 is stable for 30 hours at room temperature.

Preparation
Add 2 mL sterile water to the 150-µg vial of IL-3 to yield an isotonic solution with a concentration of 75 µg/mL. Add 1 ml of sterile water to the 300-µg vial to yield an isotonic solution with a concentration of 300 µg/mL. IL-3 may be further diluted in normal saline.

Availability
IL-3 is investigational and is available as a lyophilized powder in 150- and 300-µg vials.

Selected Readings
Biesma B et al: Effects of interleukin-3 after chemotherapy for ovarian cancer, *Blood* 80:1141-1148, 1992.

Ganser A et al: Effects of recombinant human interleukin-3 in patients with myelodysplastic syndromes, *Blood* 76:455-462, 1990.

Ganser A et al: Clinical effects of recombinant human interleukin-3, *Am J Clin Oncol*14(suppl 1):51-63, 1991.

Hoelzer D, Siepelt G, Ganser A: Interleukin-3 alone and in combination with GM-CSF in the treatment of patients with neoplastic disease, *Semin Hematol* 28(2 suppl 2):17-24, 1991.

Kurzrock R et al: Phase I study of recombinant human interleukin-3 in patients with bone marrow failure, *J Clin Oncol* 9:1241-1250, 1991.

Lindemann A et al: Biological effects of recombinant human interleukin-3 in vivo, *J Clin Oncol* 9:2120-2127, 1991.

INTERLEUKIN-4
Other Names
IL-4, recombinant human IL-4, rhuIL-4, B-cell growth factor, BCGF, B-cell stimulating factor, BSF, T-cell growth factor II, TCGF-II, NSC-618085.

Indications
IL-4 is an investigational agent that may be useful in the treatment of patients with malignant melanoma.

Mechanisms of Action
IL-4 has immunomodulatory and antiproliferative properties. It is capable of stimulating the proliferation of activated B and T cells and the differentiation and functional activity of cells of myelomonocytic origin (e.g., induces MHC class II antigens on B cells, increases immunoglobulin secretion by B cells).

Pharmacokinetics

After subcutaneous injection, IL-4 can be detected in the serum 8 to 12 hours later. After IV intravenous administration, IL-4 rapidly distributes throughout the body. IL-4 has an elimination half-life of less than 1 hour.

Dose

The maximum tolerated dose is 5 µg/kg/day when administered subcutaneously. The maximum tolerated dose of IL-4, given intravenously in three equally divided doses, is approximately 15 to 20 µg/kg/dose.

Administration

Administered by subcutaneous injection, IV bolus injection, and continuous IV infusion. Administration of IL-4 by intraarterial and intratumoral injection is being evaluated.

Toxicity

Hematological. Elevated white blood cell and platelet counts, reductions in lymphocyte and monocyte counts, thrombocytopenia, prolonged prothrombin and partial thromboplastin times.

Gastrointestinal. Mucositis, gastritis, gastrointestinal ulceration, gastrointestinal hemorrhage, nausea, vomiting, anorexia, diarrhea (dose limiting in some studies).

Dermatological. Diffuse erythematous/papular rash, sweating, injection site reactions after subcutaneous injection.

Hepatic. Elevated hepatic enzyme levels occur frequently and are often associated with the subcutaneous route of administration. Hepatic encephalopathy is rare.

Neurological. Visual hallucinations, photophobia, disorientation, paranoid reactions, confusion, somnolence, Bell's palsy.

Cardiovascular. Cardiac arrhythmias (usually with doses greater than 600 µg/m^2), pericarditis, chest pain, syncope, hypotension (which may require vasopressors), myocardial infarction, cardiomegaly, congestive heart failure, generalized edema, and vascular leak syndrome.

Pulmonary. Dyspnea, bronchospasm, pleural effusion.

Musculoskeletal. Back pain, myalgia, arthralgia, lethargy, rhabdomyolysis.

Flulike symptoms. Headache (occasionally dose limiting), fever, chills, and rigors, usually subsiding after 24 hours; fatigue, malaise, and arthralgia.

Other. Anaphylaxis and acute hypersensitivity reactions, mild to moderate elevation of serum creatinine levels, hyponatremia, hypoglycemia, nasal/sinus congestion.

Storage and Stability

Vials are stored in the refrigerator. After reconstitution, the solution is stable for 24 hours at refrigeration temperatures.

Preparation

Each vial is reconstituted with 1.2 mL sterile water to yield a solution containing 25, 100, 200, or 400 µg/mL. An overfill of 0.2 mL is provided to compensate for residual volume in the vial and in the syringe/needle hub during withdrawal.

Availability

IL-4 is available from the NCI as a lyophilized powder in 25-, 100-, 200-, and 400-µg vials.

Selected Readings

Margolin K et al: Phase II studies of recombinant human interleukin-4 in advanced renal cancer and malignant melanoma, *J Immunother* 15:147-153, 1994.

Okabe M, Saike I, Miyazaki T: Inhibitory anti-tumor effects of interleukin-4 on Philadelphia chromosome positive acute lymphocytic leukemia and other hematologic malignancies, *Leuk Lymphoma* 8:57-63, 1992.

Puri RK, Siegel JP: Interleukin-4 and cancer therapy, *Cancer Invest* 1194:473-486, 1993.

Truitt RL, Borden EC, Keever CA: Role of IL-4, IL-6 and IL-12 in cancer therapy. In DeVita VT Jr., Hellman S, Rosenberg SA, eds: *Biologic therapy of cancer*, ed 2, Philadelphia, 1995, JB Lippincott, pp 279-293.

LEVAMISOLE

Other Names

Ergamisol, Termizole, Ketrax, NSC-177023.

Mechanisms of Action

Levamisole is an antihelmintic drug. It is also believed that levamisole stimulates the immune system, particularly macrophages and T-lymphocytes. However, the exact mechanism of action for its antitumor activity is unknown. Levamisole does not have cytotoxic effects.

Indications

FDA approved as adjuvant treatment in combination with fluorouracil after surgical resection in patients with Duke's C colon cancer. Levamisole may also be a useful treatment for patients with malignant melanoma.

Pharmacokinetics

Levamisole is rapidly absorbed by mouth, reaching peak serum concentrations within 1.5 to 2 hours. It is extensively metabolized by the liver. Approximately 5% of the drug is excreted into the urine as unchanged drug. Levamisole has an elimination half-life of 3 to 4 hours; its metabolites have half-lives around 16 hours.

Dose

Levamisole is given in combination with 5-fluorouracil at a dose of 50 mg every 8 hours for 3 consecutive days. Treatment is repeated every 2 weeks and continued for 1 year (26 total treatments). Studies are in progress to determine whether 6 months of therapy (13 total treatments) will give equivalent results, but the data are not yet conclusive enough to provide an answer.

Administration
Oral.

Toxicity

Hematological. Leukopenia and thrombocytopenia occur infrequently and are not believed to be a result of impairment of bone marrow function. Leukopenia and thrombocytopenia are not associated with agranulocytosis. Agranulocytosis is rare and may occur suddenly, with recovery usually occurring within 1 to 2 weeks after discontinuing treatment.

Gastrointestinal. Nausea, occasional vomiting, diarrhea, anorexia, constipation, bitter or metallic taste, stomatitis.

Dermatological. Rash, pruritus, exfoliative dermatitis (0.5%), alopecia (rare).

Hepatic. Elevated hepatic transaminase levels. Significant elevation of transaminase levels has been reported in approximately 2% to 3% of patients receiving fluorouracil and levamisole. Symptoms are rarely associated with this toxicity and transaminase levels return to normal after discontinuation of therapy.

Neurological. Insomnia, euphoria, sensory stimulation, headache, fatigue, dizziness, parkinsonian reactions, tardive dyskinesia, agitation, confusion, nightmares, hallucinations, paranoia, coma, paresthesias, tremor, ataxia, spasms, headache, jitters, and cerebral demyelinization. Cerebral demyelinization occurs rarely and may be manifest as ataxia, confusion, mental status changes, focal neurological findings, and/or seizures.

Other. Flulike syndrome (fever, chills, myalgias, arthralgias), proximal muscle weakness, arthritis, edema and swelling of extremities, hypertension, hypotension, fluid retention, conjunctivitis (rare), proteinuria (rare), syndrome of inappropriate antidiuretic hormone (rare).

Storage and Stability
The drug is stable for many years when stored at room temperature and protected from light. The container lists the expiration date.

Incompatibilities
Drug interactions: Increased levels of phenytoin (Dilantin) may result after initiation of treatment with levamisole. Increased levels of warfarin and prolonged prothrombin time may be caused by the addition of levamisole. Alcohol may cause a disulfiram reaction.

Availability
Commercially available in 50-mg tablets.

Selected Readings
Hamilton JM, Friedman MA: 5-FU/levamisole update. In DeVita VT Jr, Hellman S, Rosenberg SA, eds: *Principles and practice of oncology, PPO updates,* 8(11):1-7, 1994.

Moertel CG et al: Levamisole and fluorouracil for adjuvant therapy of resected colon cancer, *N Engl J Med* 322:352-358, 1990.

Moertel CG et al: Intergroup study of fluorouracil plus levamisole as adjuvant therapy for stage II/Duke's B2 colon cancer, *J Clin Oncol* 13:2936-2943, 1995.

Parkinson DR: Levamisole. In DeVita VT Jr, Hellman S, Rosenberg SA, eds: *Biologic therapy of cancer*, ed 2, Philadelphia, 1995, JB Lippincott, pp 795-801.

Van Wauwe J, Janssen PAJ: On the biochemical mode of action of levamisole: an update, *Int J Immunopharmacol* 13:3-9, 1991.

MEGAKARYOCYTE GROWTH AND DEVELOPMENT FACTOR

Other Names

MGDF, rHuMGDF.

Indications

MGDF may be useful as an adjunctive treatment to high-dose chemotherapy or conditioning regimens for bone marrow transplantation because of its ability to stimulate the production of platelets.

Mechanisms of Action

MGDF is a lineage-specific inducer of platelet production. MGDF has no effects on systemic leukocyte or hemoglobin levels. Peak platelet counts occur approximately 2 weeks after a 10-day course of treatment.

Dose

The optimal dose and schedule have not been determined. MGDF has been administered daily for 10 days before and for 17 days after chemotherapy. Doses of 0.03 to 1 μg/kg/day have been administered.

Administration

MGDF is administered by subcutaneous injection.

Toxicity

Dermatological. Rash.

Cardiovascular. Deep venous thrombosis, pulmonary embolism, thrombophlebitis.

Availability

MGDF is investigationally available from Amgen.

Selected Readings

Begley G et al: Randomized, double-blind, placebo-controlled phase I trial of pegylated megakaryocyte growth and development factor administered to patients with advanced cancer after chemotherapy, *Proc Am Soc Clin Oncol* 15:271, 1996.

Fanucchi M et al: Safety and biologic effects of pegylated megakaryocyte growth and development factor in lung cancer patients receiving carboplatin and paclitaxel: randomized, placebo-controlled phase I study, *Proc Am Soc Clin Oncol* 15:271, 1996.

SARGRAMOSTIM

Other Names
Leukine, Prokine, granulocyte-macrophage colony-stimulating factor, GM-CSF, rGM-CSF, NSC-617589.

Sargramostim is derived from yeast.

Indications
Sargramostim (GM-CSF) is FDA approved for myeloid reconstitution after autologous bone marrow transplantation (ABMT) and to abrogate myelosuppression associated with chemotherapy, including patients with acute leukemia. *Use of GM-CSF is contraindicated in patients whose bone marrow or peripheral leukemic myeloid blast cell counts are greater than or equal to 10%.* GM-CSF may also be useful as a rescue treatment for febrile neutropenic patients; as a treatment for aplastic anemia, cyclic neutropenia, congenital neutropenia, or myelodysplastic disorders; to augment autologous peripheral stem cell collection; and to reduce the severity of mucositis after chemotherapy.

Mechanisms of Action
GM-CSF supports the production of granulocyte and monocyte precursors. GM-CSF is produced by T cells, fibroblasts, and endothelial cells of the bone marrow. GM-CSF supports the production, differentiation, and activation of granulocyte and monocyte precursors. In "high" doses, GM-CSF may increase the production of red blood cell and platelet precursors.

Pharmacokinetics
GM-CSF is not absorbed by mouth and is degraded by the liver and kidneys. GM-CSF can be detected in the serum within 5 minutes of a subcutaneous injection; peak serum concentrations occur within 2 hours. GM-CSF is metabolized in the liver and kidneys. GM-CSF has an elimination half-life of approximately 2 to 3 hours and remains detectable in the serum for up to 6 hours after subcutaneous injection.

Dose
Phase I studies have demonstrated that the maximum tolerated dose of GM-CSF is approximately 30 µg/kg/day. In addition, the dose and peak serum level have been shown to correlate with adverse side effects. In the treatment of neutropenia after ABMT, sargramostim is given at a dose of 250 µg/m^2/day for 21 consecutive days. Treatment with GM-CSF is begun 2 to 4 hours after infusion of the bone marrow. The manufacturer recommends stopping GM-CSF if the absolute neutrophil count (ANC) exceeds 20,000/mm^3. GM-CSF has been given at a dose of 5 µg/kg/day for 10 to 14 days beginning 24 hours after completion of chemotherapy. Higher doses of GM-CSF have been administered in subsequent cycles according to the duration and severity of myelosuppression. To reduce wastage and cost, doses are often rounded off to the nearest vial size.

Administration

GM-CSF is usually mixed in 50 mL of normal saline and administered to bone marrow transplant patients as a 2- to 4-hour intravenous infusion. GM-CSF has also been given by subcutaneous injection and as a continuous IV infusion.

Toxicity

The adverse effects of GM-CSF are dose related. Doses of 30 µg/kg/day or greater may induce capillary leak and a host of related adverse effects. Lower doses (e.g., 5 µg/kg/day or 250 µg/m²/day) produce side effects that are similar to those caused by G-CSF.

First-dose effect. Flushing sensation, hypotension (58%), hypertension (21%), tachycardia, dyspnea, hypoxia, nausea, vomiting, fever, rigor, syncope, and leg spasms. The symptoms usually begin 1 to 2 hours after injection, and are more common when GM-CSF is administered intravenously.

Hematological. Initial decrease in ANC for 4 to 24 hours. Transient, sometimes significant decrease in platelet counts with high doses. Thrombosis at the catheter tip has occurred in patients receiving doses above 30 µg/kg/day. Progression of myelodysplastic syndromes (especially in patients with "excess blasts") may occur.

Gastrointestinal. Anorexia, nausea, vomiting, abnormal taste.

Dermatological. Local erythema, skin rash, injection site reactions.

Hepatic. Mild elevation of hepatic enzyme levels, abnormal clotting times, and hypoalbuminemia have been reported.

Neurological. Headache, confusion, neuropathies.

Cardiovascular. Dose-related. Fluid retention, pericardial effusion, thrombophlebitis, pericarditis, cardiac arrhythmias, atrial fibrillation.

Pulmonary. At high doses: dyspnea (caused by fluid retention and capillary leak syndrome), pleuritis.

Musculoskeletal. Transient bone pain, usually mild to moderate in severity. The pain has been described as a pulsating deep pain in the lower back, pelvis, or sternum. The pain usually resolves without stopping treatment and always resolves within a few hours after discontinuation.

Other. Fever, flulike syndrome (chills, rigors, myalgias), fatigue, arthralgias, hypersensitivity reactions.

Storage and Stability

Intact vials should be kept refrigerated. Solutions of GM-CSF that have been reconstituted with 1 mL sterile water or 1 mL bacteriostatic sterile water are stable in the vial or in a polypropylene syringe for at least 30 days at room or refrigeration temperatures. Dilute solutions (2.5, 8, or 12 µg/mL) are stable in PVC containers for at least 48 hours at room or refrigeration temperatures. Solutions diluted to a concentration less than 10 µg/mL require the addition of albumin at a concentration of 1 mg/mL to minimize adsorption of GM-CSF to the container and IV tubing.

Preparation

When mixing GM-CSF, care must be taken to keep the product from foaming and to avoid excess agitation. The diluent should be injected against the side of the vial. Do not shake the vial. Add 1 mL of sterile water for injection to the 250- or 500- µg vial to achieve final concentrations of 250 or 500 µg/mL. GM-CSF may be further diluted with normal saline to a concentration of no less than 10 µg/mL. Solutions containing less than 10 µg/mL may require the addition of albumin (at a final concentration of 0.1%) to prevent GM-CSF from adhering to glass or plastic containers.

Availability

GM-CSF is commercially available as a lyophilized powder in vials containing 250 and 500 µg, and as a 500 µg/ml solution in a 1-mL vial.

Selected Readings

Advani R et al: Granulocyte-macrophage colony-stimulating factor (GM-CSF) as adjunct to autologous stem cell transplantation for lymphoma, *Ann Intern Med* 116:183-189, 1992.

Bregni M et al: Comparative effects of granulocyte-macrophage colony-stimulating factor in patients with chemotherapy-related febrile neutropenia, *J Clin Oncol* 14:628-635, 1996.

Chi K-H et al: Effect of granulocyte-macrophage colony-stimulating factor on oral mucositis in head and neck cancer patients after cisplatin, fluorouracil and leucovorin chemotherapy, *J Clin Oncol* 13:2620-2628, 1995.

Eaton VE: *Breakthroughs in biotechnology: a pharmacist's guide to GM-CSF,* Philadelphia, 1991, Office of Professional Programs, Philadelphia College of Pharmacy and Science, pp 1-14.

Gulati SC, Bennett CL: Granulocyte-macrophage colony-stimulating factor (GM-CSF) as adjunct therapy in relapsed Hodgkin's disease, *Ann Intern Med* 116:177-182, 1992.

Hermann F et al: Hematopoietic responses in patients with advanced malignancy treated with recombinant human granulocyte-macrophage colony-stimulating factor, *J Clin Oncol* 7:159-167, 1989.

Miller LL, Nagler CH: Colony-stimulating factors: clinical applications. In DeVita VT Jr, Hellman S, Rosenberg SA, eds: *Biologic therapy of cancer,* ed 2, Philadelphia, 1995, JB Lippincott, pp 141-182.

Rowe JM et al: A randomized placebo-controlled phase III study of granulocyte macrophage colony-stimulating factor in adult patients (>55 to 70 years of age) with acute myelogenous leukemia: a study of the Eastern Cooperative Oncology Group (E1490), *Blood* 86:457-462, 1995.

Ruef C, Coleman DL: Granulocyte-macrophage colony-stimulating factor: pleiotropic cytokine with potential clinical usefulness, *Rev Infect Dis* 12:41-62, 1990.

THROMBOPOIETIN

Other Names

TPO, recombinant human thrombopoietin, rhTPO.

Indications

Thrombopoietin (TPO) may be useful as an adjunctive treatment to high-dose chemotherapy or conditioning regimens for bone marrow transplantation because of its ability to stimulate the production of platelets.

Mechanisms of Action

TPO is a lineage-specific inducer of platelet production. TPO has no effects on systemic leukocyte or hemoglobin levels. Maximum platelet counts have been observed within 1 to 2 weeks after a single dose. Examination of bone marrow after administration of TPO has demonstrated increased levels of all CD14+ and CD34+ cell subsets.

Pharmacokinetics

The elimination half-life of TPO is approximately 20 hours and increases with increasing doses. TPO has been detected in the blood 5 days after administration of a single dose.

Dose

The optimal dose and schedule have not been determined. A single dose, administered 1 to 4 days after chemotherapy has been evaluated. Single doses of 0.3 µg/kg have little effect on platelet counts, whereas a dose of 2.4 µg/kg has been shown to elevate baseline platelet counts by over 200%.

Administration

TPO may be given as an IV bolus injection.

Toxicity

Neurological. Mild transient headache occurs occasionally.

Availability

TPO is an investigational compound that is available from Genentech.

Selected Readings

Vadhan-Raj S et al: Single-dose therapy with recombinant human thrombopoietin (rhTPO) in patients receiving cytotoxic chemotherapy, *J Clin Oncol* 14:1747, 1996.

Weber JS, Gordon MS: Platelet-stimulating factors. In DeVita VT Jr, Hellman S, Rosenberg SA, eds: *Biologic therapy of cancer*, ed 2, Philadelphia, 1995, JB Lippincott, pp 183-189.

TUMOR NECROSIS FACTOR

Other Names

rTNF-alpha, TNF-alpha, cachectin.

Indications

Tumor necrosis factor (TNF) has not been shown to be a useful antitumor agent when administered by intravenous or intramuscular injection. Some activity is observed against Kaposi's sarcoma after intralesional injection. TNF has been shown to be very active against malignant melanoma when the TNF is administered by isolated limb perfusion in combination with interferon gamma and melphalan.

Mechanisms of Action

TNF is a naturally occurring protein that is secreted by macrophages in response to infection. In combination with IL-1 and IL-6, TNF is an important factor in the acute phase reaction to an infection. TNF is a polypeptide cytokine that mediates inflammation and immune effector cell regulation. The direct cytotoxic effects of TNF appear to be cell-cycle dependent with prolonged exposure yielding greater cell kill in vitro. Other actions may account for some of the antitumor activity of TNF, such as endothelial cell effects and procoagulation (hemorrhagic necrosis), enhanced macrophage cytotoxicity, activation of NK cells, or as a part of an inflammatory reaction. Synergism with TNF and gamma interferon has been demonstrated.

Pharmacokinetics

Peak levels of TNF occur 30 minutes after IV injection and 2 to 3 hours after initiation of a continuous IV infusion. Despite continued infusion, levels of TNF are undetectable within 6 to 12 hours. TNF has an elimination half-life of 10 to 16 minutes after systemic administration of 25 to 100 $\mu g/m^2$. The half-life after administration of higher doses (e.g., 150 to 727 $\mu g/m^2$) is 40 to 80 minutes.

Dose

Systemically administered TNF has been utilized on varied regimens, including daily for 5 days, twice daily for 5 days, and 3 times weekly. The maximum tolerated dose is approximately 200 to 300 $\mu g/m^2$/day. Intralesional injections are usually given at a dose of 25 to 300 $\mu g/m^2$ 3 times weekly. When given by isolated limb perfusion, 3 to 6 mg is added to the perfusate of crystalloid (700 mL) and packed red blood cells (1 unit). Intraperitoneal and intravesical doses ranging from 50 to 1800 $\mu g/m^2$ have been evaluated.

Administration

TNF has been given by isolated limb and organ perfusion, IV bolus, IV infusion over 24 hours or longer, intraperitoneally, and by subcutaneous, intramuscular, intraarterial, intravesical, and intralesional injection.

Toxicity

The toxicities seen after administration with TNF are dependent on dose and schedule of administration, although similar toxicities are seen in patients receiving TNF by IV bolus or continuous infusion.

Hematological. Mild leukopenia (after high doses or repeated IV administration); thrombocytopenia is not common or severe; eosinophilia; transient leukocytosis is dose related and lasts approximately 24 hours after a single dose; immune thrombocytopenia in patients also receiving IL-2 has been reported. Disseminated intravascular coagulation has been reported in patients receiving systemic TNF.

Dermatological. Tenderness, erythema, induration, and inflammation at the site of subcutaneous or intramuscular injection.

Gastrointestinal. Abdominal pain, dose-related nausea and vomiting, anorexia, diarrhea. Abdominal pain and peritonitis are dose limiting when TNF is administered intraperitoneally.

Hepatic. The following effects are usually mild and transient: hyperbilirubinemia, elevated hepatic transaminase levels (40%), and elevated alkaline phosphatase levels.

Neurological. Headache, confusion, speech disorders, somnolence, lethargy, hallucinations, seizures.

Cardiovascular. Hypotension occurs frequently and has been dose limiting in most phase I studies. Hypotension usually occurs within 12 or 24 hours after initiation of a continuous IV infusion. Intravenous vasopressors are necessary in some patients. Hypotension also occurs when TNF is administered by isolated limb perfusion. In one study, 4 to 6 mg of TNF was administered by isolated limb perfusion. The incidence of Grade 3 or 4 hypotension was 39%. Other cardiovascular adverse effects include fluid retention, tachycardia, and hypertension (often related to a febrile episode).

Pulmonary. Dyspnea (rare), wheezing, pulmonary edema.

Renal. Mild elevation of serum creatinine and BUN levels.

Other. Fever occurs in all patients regardless of the route of administration or dose and generally resolves within a few hours; chills, rigor, myalgia, fatigue, malaise, phlebitis, hypophosphatemia. Regional toxicities after isolated limb perfusion include mild chronic edema (56%), muscle tenderness with atrophy (8%), blistering (50%), paresthesia (40%), and arterial occlusion requiring amputation in one patient.

Storage and Stability
Vials are shipped frozen on dry ice and must be stored in the refrigerator. If TNF is received thawed, do not use. Small perturbations in storage temperature are tolerable (e.g., several hours at 25° C). Small colorless particles of protein may be visible, are not unusual, and do not alter the potency of TNF. Vigorous handling results in aggregation of the protein and may create cloudy solutions that should not be used.

Preparation
Before use the vial should be gently swirled to ensure uniform mixing of the contents. TNF is sensitive to shear-induced stress; do not shake vials. TNF is diluted only in normal saline. Adsorption of TNF to glassware, plastic IV sets, and syringes occurs when delivered intravenously or diluted to concentrations <10 µg/mL. To prevent adsorption, it is recommended that human albumin be added at a final concentration of 2 mg/mL. Human albumin effectively reduces adsorption at TNF concentrations as low as 0.1 µg/mL.

Availability
TNF-alfa, 0.5-mg/vial, is available from the NCI.

Selected Readings
Creagan ET, Kovach TS, Moertel CG: Phase I clinical trial of recombinant human tumor necrosis factor, *Cancer* 62:2467-2471, 1988.

Fraker DL, Alexander HR, Pass HI: Biologic therapy with TNF: systemic administration and isolation-perfusion. In DeVita VT Jr, Hellman S, Rosenberg SA, eds: *Biologic therapy of cancer,* ed 2, Philadelphia, 1995, JB Lippincott, pp 329-345.

Fraker DL et al: Treatment of patients with melanoma of the extremity using hyperthermic isolated limb perfusion with melphalan, tumor necrosis factor, and interferon gamma: results of a tumor necrosis factor dose-escalation study, *J Clin Oncol* 14:479-489, 1996.

Jakubowski AA et al: Phase I trial of intramuscularly administered tumor necrosis factor in patients with advanced malignancy, *J Clin Oncol* 7:298-303, 1989.

Lienard D et al: High-dose recombinant tumor necrosis factor alpha in combination with interferon gamma and melphalan in isolation perfusion of the limbs for melanoma and sarcoma, *J Clin Oncol* 10:52-60, 1992.

Spriggs DR et al: Recombinant human tumor necrosis factor administered as a 24-hour infusion, *J Natl Cancer Inst* 80:1039-1044, 1988.

REFERENCES

Atkins MB, Trehu EG, Mier JW: Combination cytokine therapy. In DeVita VT Jr, Hellman S, Rosenberg SA, eds: *Biologic therapy of cancer,* ed 2, Philadelphia, 1995, JB Lippincott, pp 443-466.

Bregman MD, Meyskens FL: Human recombinant alpha- and gamma-interferons enhance the cytotoxic properties of tumor necrosis factor on human melanoma, *J Biol Response Mod* 7:384-389, 1988.

Geller RB: The use of cytokines in the treatment of acute myelocytic leukemia: a critical review, *J Clin Oncol* 14:1371-1382, 1996.

Irwin MM: Patients receiving biological response modifiers: an overview of nursing care, *Oncol Nurs Forum* 14:32-37, 1987.

Issacs A, Lindenmann J: Viral interference: the interferon, *Proc R Soc Lond (Biol)* 147:258-267, 1957.

Miller LL, Nagler CH: Colony-stimulating factors: clinical applications. In DeVita VT Jr, Hellman S, Rosenberg SA, eds: *Biologic therapy of cancer,* ed 2, Philadelphia, 1995, JB Lippincott, pp 141-182.

Miller RG, Tannock IF: Immunology and immunotherapy of cancer. In Tannock IF, Hill RP, eds: *The basic science of oncology,* ed 2, New York, 1992, McGraw-Hill, pp 232-255.

Morstyn G, Foote MA, Mazanet R: Haematopoietic growth factors in cancer chemotherapy, *Exp Opin Invest Drugs* 4:515-523, 1995.

Restifo NP, Wunderlich JR: Biology of cellular immune responses. In DeVita VT Jr, Hellman S, Rosenberg SA, eds: *Biologic therapy of cancer,* ed 2, Philadelphia, 1995, JB Lippincott, pp 3-37.

Rosenberg SA: The immunotherapy and gene therapy of cancer, *J Clin Oncol* 10:180-199, 1992.

Sandstrom SK: Nursing management of patients receiving biologic therapy, *Semin Oncol Nurs* 12:152-162, 1996.

Siegel JP et al: Development of biological therapeutics for oncologic use. In DeVita VT Jr, Hellman S, Rosenberg SA, eds: *Biologic therapy of cancer,* ed 2, Philadelphia, 1995, JB Lippincott, pp 879-890.

Vose JM, Armitage JO: Clinical applications of the hematopoietic growth factors, *J Clin Oncol* 13:1023-1035, 1995.

Weber JS, Gordon MS: Platelet-stimulating factors. In DeVita VT Jr, Hellman S, Rosenberg SA, eds: *Biologic therapy of cancer,* ed 2, Philadelphia, 1995, JB Lippincott, pp 183-189.

5

Cancer Chemotherapy Administration

Technology and cancer treatment are dynamic factors in oncology that influence the way we deliver care, the setting, and the needs of the patient and family for information, support, and resources. Advances in therapeutic strategies, supportive care, and new technology present a constant challenge to the oncology health professional.

The majority of systemic cancer therapy is administered in the outpatient setting, either in physician offices, clinics, day hospitals, or the home. The profile of patients and types of treatments in these settings has changed dramatically in the past decade. Higher patient volume and acuity levels, combined with increasingly complex and more intensive therapy, have significantly challenged our resources and those of the patient and family. The changing health care environment has eliminated participation in care as a decision choice for patients. Patients and their identified caregivers must be adequately prepared with the knowledge and skill required to fulfill their designated roles in cancer care. The oncology health care provider maintains the responsibility for education and evaluation of care delivery by patients and their designated caregivers. The scope and labor intensity of this teaching responsibility varies tremendously and is dependent on major variables of staff resources, patient status, caregiver resources, and complexity of therapeutic approaches.

This chapter provides information and guidelines for nursing, physician, and pharmacy staff in the delivery of cancer chemotherapy across various settings. The first and most important factor for safe drug delivery and optimal patient care is knowledge. Comprehensive knowledge, from the initial drug indications through predicted side effects, and supportive care provide the basis for patient teaching, safe drug administration, prevention of complications, and interventions for side effects.

Oncology physicians, nurses, and pharmacists represent the health care team primarily responsible for safe chemotherapy drug delivery. Each team member is responsible for standards unique to their discipline and for collaboration as a multidisciplinary team in their setting for the prescription, admixture, administration, and disposal of drugs, as well as care of the patient receiving chemotherapy. National standards and guidelines for controlling exposure to antineoplastic agents have been provided by the Occupational Safety and Health Administration (OSHA) of the United States (1995). Standards for nursing education, practice, and administration of therapy are provided by the Oncology Nursing Society (1996). Guidelines for handling of chemotherapy drugs by pharmacy personnel are provided by the American Society of Hospital Pharmacists (1990). National recommendations provide a framework for multidisciplinary teams at the institutional level to design policies and procedures for safe delivery of antineoplastic drugs. Most institutions have educational programs that certify nurses and pharmacy personnel for the handling and delivery of cancer chemotherapy drugs and policies for writing orders, verification, and dose modifications (Fischer et al, 1996). Implementation of policies, adherence to institutional guidelines, and routine evaluation are critical components of the multidisciplinary team's responsibility for quality control of cancer chemotherapy.

CONTROLLING EXPOSURE TO ANTINEOPLASTIC DRUGS

Risk of exposure to potential adverse effects of cytotoxic drugs is based on the known mutagenic, carcinogenic, and teratogenic properties of selected drugs and information that is derived from experimental animal data and human data with drugs given at therapeutic levels. In addition, there are reported studies that have attempted to identify biological absorption in nurses and pharmacists who handle chemotherapy drugs, suggesting that there is some risk to low-level, long-term exposure. Results of these studies are inconsistent but should be heeded because the actual occupational risk remains unknown.

Inhalation, absorption, and ingestion are the three major sources of exposure to antineoplastics. The first solid evidence that biological absorption may occur as a result of low-level exposure was reported by Hirst et al (1983). Urine samples were analyzed from nurses administering large doses of cyclophosphamide. Most urine sample results were negative for the presence of the drug, but cyclophosphamide was detected in a few urine samples, confirmed by gas chromatography and mass spectrometry.

Other investigators have used urine mutagenicity and chromosome aberrations in circulating lymphocytes as indicators of exposure to cytotoxic drugs. Increased mutagenic activity and increased levels of urinary thioethers in the urine of nurses exposed to chemotherapeutic drugs have been reported (Falck et al, 1979; Bos et al, 1982; Anderson et al, 1982; Rogers and Emmett, 1987; Caudell et al, 1988; Karakaya, Burgaz, and Bayan, 1989). Yet a similar number of investigations has failed to show any difference between nurses who were or were not exposed to these drugs (Venitt et al, 1984; Staiano et al, 1981; Hoffman, 1983; Cloak et al, 1985). Factors such as cigarette smoking, alcohol, diet, and medications are known to affect the outcome of such testing (Burgaz, Ozdamar, and Karakaya, 1988), and not all studies control for these variables. Stucker et al (1986) reported significant increases in urine mutagenicity in nurses handling cytotoxic drugs but failed to detect any cytogenetic abnormalities.

Reproductive risks have been raised with reports of an increase in the number of spontaneous abortions among nurses working with antineoplastics compared with controls (Selevan et al, 1985; Rogers and Emmett, 1987). Lack of information on specific levels of exposure, a retrospective approach to the studies, and lack of identification of maternal risk factors for fetal loss such as alcohol intake, cigarette smoking, and prior fetal loss suggest caution in interpretation of the results. Nonetheless, exposure of pregnant workers, especially in the first trimester (or men trying to procreate), is a valid concern based on the known effects of exposure to these drugs at therapeutic dose levels.

Long-term effects of handling hazardous drugs remain unknown, but guidelines to limit exposure are essential. In 1995 OSHA revised the recommendations for hazardous drug handling of antineoplastics and expanded the scope of the recommendations by including other hazardous drugs such as ganciclovir and pentamidine. The recommendations provided in this informational guidance document (OSHA, 1995) apply to all settings (i.e., hospitals, physician offices, home care) where employees are exposed to hazardous drugs.

The first step to prevent employee exposure is education of all personnel about occupational exposure, potential risk of exposure to hazardous drugs, explanation and rationale for measures to reduce exposure, and plans for monitoring and assessing the effectiveness of protective measures. The environment in which the employee works, tasks performed (preparation, administration, or both), the average number of drug exposures per week, the number of consecutive days worked with drug exposure, the type of protective measures offered by the employer, the percentage of reported accidental skin contacts, and adherence to recommended protective measures are important factors for the individuals at risk.

Work-practice guidelines to reduce exposure are no longer optional, and the employer is responsible for education, implementation, assessment, and periodic reevaluation. Individual health protection is the responsibility of the employee, who should be well informed and adhere to protective guidelines and institutional policies. Results of studies that assessed practice related to the 1986 OSHA guidelines for handling cytotoxic drugs reported varying rates of compliance, especially for the use of protective equipment (Valanis et al, 1992; Mahon et al, 1994). Some recommendations, such as the use of gowns during drug administration, have been associated with lower compliance rates than other protective guidelines. The actual degree of risk associated with administration and concern about patient reactions have been cited for these lower rates of compliance. Each institution must integrate the OSHA recommendations together with the available scientific evidence into its policies to minimize any occupational hazardous drug risk. A policy for the protection of employees is critical but requires institutional support to implement it in all sites and must include available resources, education, and routine surveillance. The current OSHA (1995) recommendations are presented in Table 5-1.

TABLE 5-1
Prevention of Employee Exposure to Hazardous Drugs (OSHA, 1995)

Recommendation	Comment
1. Hazardous drug safety and health plan	
Develop a plan according to the ASHP (1990) criteria that is available and accessible to all employees. Designate personnel responsible for implementation of the plan and review effectiveness at least annually.	To protect employees from health hazards associated with handling hazardous drugs and to minimize exposure.
2. Drug preparation precautions	
Work area: A restricted, preferably centralized area is recommended for preparation of hazardous drugs. Eating, drinking, smoking, chewing gum, applying cosmetics, and storing food prohibited.	Minimizes exposure. Minimizes ingestion exposure.
Biological Safety Cabinets (BSC): Class II or III are recommended because they vent to the outside. The blower should be on at all times; if turned off, the BSC should be decontaminated and covered until airflow is resumed. The BSC should be serviced and certified by a qualified technician every 6 months or any time the BSC is moved or repaired.	Until a BSC is installed; a NIOSH-approved respirator must be worn; usage must comply with OSHA's respiratory protection standard. Permanent respirator use is *not* recommended.
Protective equipment: Wear protective gloves, latex preferable. For latex allergy, consider the use of vinyl or nitrile gloves or glove liners. Change gloves hourly or immediately if torn, punctured, or contaminated with a spill. Wash hands before gloves are put on and after removal.	Thickness of gloves provides best protection against permeability, which is the rationale for latex recommendation. All gloves are permeable to some extent, and permeability increases with time.

ASHP, American Society of Hospital Pharmacists; *NIOSH,* National Institute of Occupational Safety and Health.

Continued

TABLE 5-1
Prevention of Employee Exposure to Hazardous Drugs (OSHA, 1995)—cont'd

Recommendation	Comment
2. Drug preparation precautions (cont'd)	
Wear disposable, lint-free, low permeability fabric gown with closed front, long sleeves, and elastic or knot-closed cuffs.	Gowns provide an additional barrier to potential skin contact (direct or aerosol). No ideal material has been identified, but some gowns have reinforced sleeves to minimize permeability in the most exposure-prone areas.
Face and eye protection must be provided whenever splashes, sprays, or aerosols from hazardous drugs may be generated.	To prevent or minimize eye, nose, or mouth contamination.
Work equipment: Place absorbent plastic-backed paper liner on work surface; use Luer lock fittings; have covered disposable container to contain excess solution and have hazardous drug–labeled plastic bags for disposal of used protective equipment and any contaminated materials.	Change liner every shift (hospital) or at the end of the day (ambulatory).
Work practices: Use aseptic technique for drug preparation; put on protective equipment before working in the BSC; label all drugs according to standard pharmacy labeling practices and for identification as a hazardous drug.	Minimizes exposure.
Whenever possible, prime drug administration sets in the BSC before addition of the drug.	If priming must occur outside the BSC, prime with non-drug-containing fluid or use a back-flow closed system (ASHP, 1990).
Avoid positive and negative pressures in medication vials. Use of venting devices is recommended, along with appropriate employee education. An alternative to venting devices is adding diluent slowly in small amounts, allowing displaced air to escape into the syringe.	Reduces aerosol exposure.

For ampules, wrap a sterile gauze around ampule neck before breaking; if diluent is needed, inject slowly down the side wall of the ampule.

Prevents cuts, aerosolization, and skin contamination.

Tablets that may produce dust or potential exposure to the handler should be counted in the BSC.

3. Drug administration

Wash hands before and after; wear protective gloves and gown; discard gloves after each use.

Minimizes direct skin exposure.

Infusion sets should have Luer lock fittings; use plastic-back absorbent pad under tubing during administration; use sterile gauze at injection sites.

Minimizes exposure through skin contact by potential drug leakage.

Do not clip needles or syringes; place in puncture-resistant container. Dispose of administration sets intact.

Minimizes possible contamination from needle sticks or aerosol exposure.

Have spill kit available and accessible.

Administration of aerosolized hazardous drugs requires special engineering controls for employee protection.

4. Caring for patients receiving hazardous drugs

Observe universal precautions to prevent contact with blood or other potentially infectious material. Wear protective gloves and gowns when dealing with excreta, specifically urine, of patients who have received hazardous drugs within the past 48 hours.

Minimizes exposure to all personnel.

Linen contaminated by hazardous drugs or excreta from patients (as above) is a potential source of exposure; use gloves during handling and place in marked laundry bags. Contents should be prewashed and then added to other laundry for a second wash.

Continued

TABLE 5-1
Prevention of Employee Exposure to Hazardous Drugs (OSHA, 1995)—cont'd

5. Waste disposal

Use thick, leak-proof, labeled plastic bags for discarded protective equipment and materials. Keep waste bag inside a covered waste container labeled *HD Waste Only*; have one receptacle located in each area of drug preparation and administration; do nor move from one area to another.

Hazardous drug–related wastes should be handled separately from other trash and disposed of according to appropriate regulations for hazardous waste. Check current regulations and institutional policy.

6. Spills

Personal contamination: Immediately remove protective clothing and wash affected skin with soap and water. If eye exposure has occurred, flush with water or isotonic eyewash for 5 minutes; seek prompt medical attention; document exposure in the employee's record.

Small spills (<5 mL): Immediately clean up spill while wearing protective gowns, gloves, and splash goggles. Wipe liquids with absorbent gauze pads and solids with wet absorbent gauze; clean spill area three times with detergent solution followed by clean water; pick up broken glass with a small scoop.
    Isolates and contains contaminated materials.

Large spills: Isolate area and avoid aerosol generation. Limit liquid spread by covering with absorbent sheets or spill-control pads.
    Reduces absorption exposure risk.

Spills in the BSC: If greater than 150 mL or the contents of one vial, decontamination of the interior BSC is recommended after spill cleanup.

7. Medical surveillance

Workers with potential exposure to hazardous drugs should be monitored in a systematic program, such as preplacement, periodic, and exit medical examinations; postexposure evaluation, and maintenance of exposure records for all employees.

Reproductive toxicity of hazardous drugs should be explained to all employees with potential exposure. Although the data on reproductive risks are inconclusive, the facility should have a policy for worker exposure in male and female employees.

Employees need to be informed so that they can understand the carcinogenic potential of the drugs and reproductive risks.

8. Hazard communication

Employers are responsible for developing, implementing, and maintaining a written hazard communication program, which should include all drugs that represent a health hazard to employees.

9. Information dissemination

All employees must be informed of drugs that may present a hazard, and knowledge and competence of those workers should be evaluated on a regular basis; updated information should be provided as it evolves.

10. Record keeping

Workplace exposure records associated with handling hazardous drugs are to be kept and made available for the duration of employment plus 30 years; training records should be maintained for 3 years from the date of training.

DRUG ADMINISTRATION

A comprehensive physical and psychosocial assessment of the patient (Table 5-2) is indicated before initiation of therapy to establish baseline information, determine appropriateness of the treatment and setting, evaluate venous access, and identify patient and family resources and needs. Adequate preparation of the patient and staff for treatment decreases the risk of unpredictable problems and unnecessary time delays, reduces potential protocol violations, minimizes emotional distress, and enhances the patient–caregiver relationship.

Administration of chemotherapeutic drugs requires knowledge and, in most cases, skill. Cancer chemotherapy treatment follows the five basic pharmacological principles: right patient, right drug, right dose, right route, and right time. Orders should always be verified and drug doses recalculated and checked against the order (ONS, 1996). A written policy defining verification (e.g., knowledge of the protocol regimen and correct drugs for day in the cycle of the drug regimen) and personnel responsibility for order writing and verification is strongly recommended. Assessment should also include evaluating appropriate laboratory values, checking the need for pretreatment medications or supportive therapy such as hydration, and ensuring the patient's understanding and readiness for the therapy.

Dose Calculation

Drug doses are most often calculated according to the patient's body surface area (meter squared, or m^2) and occasionally by weight (kilograms). One exception to using BSA for drug calculation is carboplatin dosing, for which the Calvert formula (Calvert et al 1989; Calvert, Newell, and Gore,

TABLE 5-2
Pretreatment Assessment Checklist

History physical	Social	Psychological	Sexual
Extent of disease	Role responsibilities	Emotional status	Sexual preference
Comorbid conditions	Financial resources	Handling of past crises	Significant other
Current medications	Health insurance coverage	Informational needs	Sexual activity
Allergies	Employment	Available support	Reproductive status
Prior cancer treatment	Family structure/ relationship	Body image	Birth control
System review (physiological and functional)	Cultural factors	Role of religion	
Cardiovascular			
Integumentary			
Respiratory			
Genitourinary			
Gastrointestinal			
Neurological			
Hematopoietic			

1992) is recommended. The formula uses the creatinine clearance level, and the calculation is based on glomerular filtration rate and plasma concentration (see Appendix A, Table A-6).

The patient's body surface area is most commonly determined by height and weight nomograms (see Appendix A, Tables A-1 and A-2), although formulas can also be used (see Appendix A, Table A-1). The proper dose for obese patients is controversial. Some clinicians suggest that the dose should be calculated on the basis of the patient's ideal weight; therefore information is included based on height and ideal weight (see Appendix A, Table A-3). Other clinicians perceive ideal weight as an overcorrection. On the basis of an analysis of doses (actual compared with ideal weight) in 3732 protocol patients, it has been suggested that actual body weight be used with only two exceptions: in clinical trials using very high doses of drugs and in clinically obese patients, defined as those weighing 30% or more over ideal body weight. If actual weight had been used for dose calculations, 48% of patients would have had a 10% increase in drug dose, and only 8% would have received a 25% increase (Gelman et al, 1987). It was concluded that using actual weight may provide greater consistency of drug dosing among different protocols and institutions. It was also noted that hematological toxicity may be greater with dose increases of 10% or more but would remain within acceptable levels.

Hypersensitivity Reactions

There are four classes of hypersensitivity reactions to drugs. Type I class represents immediate hypersensitivity reactions that occur with chemotherapy drugs. Regardless of the specific nature of the reaction (anaphylactic or anaphylactoid), there is a rapid release of various mediators of the reaction (histamine, prostaglandins, leukotrienes, platelet-activating factor, slow-reacting substance of anaphylaxis, and eosinophil chemotactic factor) that are responsible for the subsequent clinical manifestations (Craig and Capizzi, 1985). Most anaphylactic reactions occur unexpectedly; however, identification of drugs with known risks, prophylactic treatment when indicated, a careful pretreatment assessment (including allergy history), availability of emergency drugs and equipment, and rapid assessment of the extent and severity of the reaction will greatly minimize any untoward outcome (Bochner and Lichtenstein, 1991; ONS, 1996). A variety of chemotherapy drugs has been associated with immediate hypersensitivity reactions (Table 5-3), although L-asparaginase and paclitaxel are associated with a higher, more predictable risk. Guidelines to prevent or minimize risk from a reaction from L-asparaginase include consideration of pretreatment with intravenous diphenhydramine, available intravenous access, and use of the subcutaneous or intramuscular route for injection (Weiss, 1992). For paclitaxel, premedication is recommended with dexamethasone 20 mg administered orally 12 and 6 hours before the paclitaxel, and diphenhydramine 50 mg and cimetidine 300 mg (or ranitidine 50 mg) administered intravenously 30 to 60 minutes before the paclitaxel. For all chemotherapy drugs with a known potential risk of immediate hypersensitivity reactions, the following clinical guidelines are recommended (Bochner and Lichtenstein, 1991; ONS, 1996).

- Carefully assess patients for clinical signs and symptoms (Table 5-4), and have emergency drugs available and accessible.

TABLE 5-3

Immediate Hypersensitivity Reactions: Predicted Risk of Chemotherapy Drugs

High risk	Low to moderate risk	Rare risk
L-Asparaginase*	Anthracylines	Cytarabine
Paclitaxel	Bleomycin	Cyclophosphamide
	Carboplatin	Chlorambucil
	Cisplatin	Dacarbazine
	Cyclosporine	5-Fluorouracil
	Docetaxel	Ifosfamide
	Etoposide	Mi271toxantrone
	Melphalan IV	
	Methotrexate	
	Procarbazine	
	Teniposide	

*Significantly increased risk with IV route.

TABLE 5-4

Clinical Signs and Symptoms of Immediate Hypersensitivity

Organ system	Subjective complaints	Objective findings
Respiratory	Dyspnea, inability to speak, tightness in chest	Stridor, bronchospasm, decreased air movement
Skin	Pruritus, urticaria	Cyanosis, urticaria, angioedema
Cardiovascular	Chest pain, increased heart rate	Tachycardia, hypotension, arrhythmias
CNS	Dizziness, agitation, anxiety	Decreased sensorium, loss of consciousness
Gastrointestinal	Abdominal pain, nausea	Increased bowel sounds, diarrhea, vomiting

From Craig JB, Capizzi RL: The prevention and treatment of immediate hypersensitivity reactions from cancer chemotherapy, *Semin Oncol Nurs* 1:285-291, 1985.
CNS, Central nervous system.

- Once a reaction occurs, immediately stop the chemotherapy infusion. Notify the physician or emergency team.
- Maintain intravenous access; administer emergency drugs per standing order or physician order; closely monitor the patient's vital signs; maintain adequate oxygenation, cardiac output, airway, and tissue perfusion; have quick access to life-support therapies in case of failure to respond to initial pharmacological interventions (Table 5-5).
- Document the reaction, treatment, and patient responses.

TABLE 5-5
Pharmacological Treatment of Systemic Anaphylaxis in Adults*

Agents	Indications	Dosages	Goals	Complications
AIRWAY OR CUTANEOUS REACTIONS				
Initial therapy				
Epinephrine	Bronchospasm, laryngeal edema, urticaria, angioedema	0.3-0.5 mL of 1:1000 dilution (0.3-0.5 mg) subcutaneously every 10-20 min	Maintain airway patency, reduce fluid extravasation and pruritus	Arrhythmias, hypertension, nervousness, tremor
Oxygen	Hypoxemia	40%-100%	Maintain $PO_2 \geq 60$ mm Hg	None
Metaproterenol[†]	Bronchospasm	0.3 mL (5% solution) in 2.5 mL of saline, inhaled through nebulizer	Maintain airway patency	Same as for epinephrine
Secondary therapy[‡]				
Aminophylline	Bronchospasm	Loading dose if necessary (6 mg/kg intravenously over a 30-min period); 0.3-0.9 mg/kg/hr intravenously as maintenance dose[§]	Maintain airway patency	Arrhythmias, nausea, vomiting, seizures

From Bochner BS, Lichtenstein LM: Anaphylaxis, *N Engl J Med* 324:1785-1790, 1991.
*Dosages, choice of specific agents, efficacy, and safety must be individualized. PO_2 denotes partial pressure of oxygen, and D_5W 5% aqueous dextrose solution.
[†]Albuterol (0.5 mL of the 0.5% solution in 2.5 mL of saline) or isoetharine (0.5 mL of the 1% solution in 2 mL of saline) can also be used.
[‡]These agents have little or no efficacy during the acute anaphylactic reaction; they may reduce or prevent recurrent or prolonged reactions.

Continued

TABLE 5-5
Pharmacological Treatment of Systemic Anaphylaxis in Adults—cont'd

Agents	Indications	Dosages	Goals	Complications
AIRWAY OR CUTANEOUS REACTIONS (cont'd)				
Corticosteroids	Bronchospasm	250 mg of hydrocortisone or 50 mg of methylprednisolone intravenously every 6 hr for 2-4 doses	Block or reduce prolonged or late-phase reactions	Hyperglycemia, fluid retention
Antihistamines	Urticaria	25-50 mg of hydroxyzine or diphenhydramine intramuscularly or orally every 6-8 hr as needed	Reduce pruritus, antagonize H_1 effects of histamine	Drowsiness, dry mouth, urinary retention
		300 mg of cimetidine intravenously or orally every 6 hr	Antagonize H_2 effects of histamine	
CARDIOVASCULAR REACTIONS				
Initial therapy				
Intravenous fluids (saline, colloid)	Hypotension	1 liter every 20-30 min as needed	Maintain systolic blood pressure $\geq$80-100 mm Hg	Congestive heart failure, pulmonary edema

Epinephrine	Hypotension	Same as for intravenous fluids	1 mL of 1:1000 dilution in 500 mL of D_5W intravenously at a rate of 0.5-5 μg (0.25-2.5 mL)/min	Arrhythmias, hypertension, nervousness, tremor
Secondary therapy				
Norepinephrine	Hypotension	Same as for intravenous fluids	4 mg in 1 liter of D_5W intravenously at a rate of 2-12 μg (0.5-3 mL)/min	Same as for epinephrine
Antihistamines	Hypotension	Antagonize H_1 and H_2 effects of histamine on myocardium and peripheral vasculature	25-50 mg of hydroxyzine or diphenhydramine intramuscularly or orally every 6-8 hr as needed; 300 mg of cimetidine intravenously or orally every 6 hr	Drowsiness, dry mouth, urinary retention
Glucagon[||]	Refractory hypotension	Increase heart rate and cardiac output	1 mg in 1 liter of D_5W intravenously at a rate of 5-15 μg (5-15 mL)/min	Nausea

[§]Lower rates are suggested for older patients, those taking medications that reduce metabolism, those with hepatic dysfunction, and those with congestive heart failure; higher rates should be used in younger persons or cigarette smokers.

[||]May be particularly useful in patients taking β-adrenergic blockers, since its ability to stimulate both inotropic and chronotropic cardiac function may be unaltered by β-adrenergic blockade.

Most immediate hypersensitivity reactions to chemotherapy will resolve with administration of epinephrine, with or without antihistamines, corticosteroids, and fluids. The duration of monitoring after such a reaction is dependent on the patient status and the type and severity of the hypersensitivity reaction.

ROUTES OF DRUG ADMINISTRATION

The goal of therapy and the available form of the drug are primary factors dictating the route of drug administration. Once a therapy is recommended by the physician, the clinician (usually a certified oncology nurse) should be aware of the implications of each route of administration (Table 5-6). Specific assessment of the patient related to route of drug administration should be conducted to identify factors that may influence outcome, such as compliance with oral prescriptions of chemotherapy or ability and resources for administering supportive therapy (i.e., filgrastim [G-CSF] injections). The routes of chemotherapy drug administration include systemic (oral, subcutaneous, intramuscular, and intravenous) and regional approaches (intraperitoneal, intravesical, intrathecal, intraarterial, intrapleural, and topical). Systemic drug administration is the most common method of drug delivery. Many drugs are prescribed in the oral form alone or in combination with other drugs. Oral administration presents unique challenges to the oncology clinician. It is important to emphasize that oral drug delivery requires the same attentiveness to dose calculation, patient teaching, monitoring of side effects, follow-up, and compliance evaluation. Administration of chemotherapy by subcutaneous and intramuscular routes is relatively uncommon. In contrast, the administration of biologicals by the subcutaneous route is very common, requiring time to assess receptivity and resources of the patient and family or designated support person. Many written and audiovisual guides for use in teaching patients to perform subcutaneous injections are available, but these should not negate the importance of the role of the nurse in assessing learning and skill performance of the procedure.

INTRAVENOUS DRUG DELIVERY

Intravenous drug delivery is the predominate approach to systemic cancer therapy. Successful intravenous drug administration is dependent on patient factors and the knowledge and skill of the nurse or physician in vascular access and drug-administration procedures. Intravenous drug delivery is accomplished through peripheral insertion of a steel needle or plastic catheter or through a central venous access device.

Peripheral Venous Access
The patient should be well informed and comfortably positioned. The clinician should have easy access to both arms and minimize or avoid potential occupational exposure by following universal precautions and

TABLE 5-6
Routes of Administration of Antineoplastic Agents

Route	Advantages	Disadvantages	Potential complications	Nursing implications
Oral	Ease of administration	Inconsistency of absorption	Drug-specific complications	Evaluate compliance with medication schedule; teach patient handling techniques
Subcutaneous, intramuscular	Ease of administration Decreased side effects	Requires adequate muscle mass and tissue for absorption	Infection, bleeding	Evaluate platelet count (>50,000); use smallest gauge needle possible; prepare injection site with an antiseptic solution; assess injection site for signs and symptoms of infection
IV	Consistent absorption required for vesicants	Sclerosing of veins over time	Infection, phlebitis	Check for blood return before and after administration of drugs
Intraarterial*	Increased doses to tumor with decreased systemic toxic effects	Requires surgical procedure or special radiography equipment placement	Bleeding, embolism	Monitor for signs and symptoms of bleeding; monitor partial thromboplastin time, prothrombin time

From Oncology Nursing Society: *Cancer chemotherapy guidelines and recommendations for practice*, Pittsburgh, 1996, Oncology Nursing Press.
NOTE: Specialized nursing education may be required for certain administration methods. Refer to individual state nurse practice acts and agency policies and procedures.

Continued

TABLE 5-6
Routes of Administration of Antineoplastic Agents—cont'd

Route	Advantages	Disadvantages	Potential complications	Nursing implications
External pump	With intraarterial port, patient freedom increased	Patient lies flat for 3-7 days during drug infusion	Pump occlusion malfunction	Intense patient education needed for pump and catheter care
Internal (implanted) pump	Greater mobility	Cost effective only with long-term therapy (i.e., 3-6 months)	Pump occlusion malfunction	Specialized nursing education needed regarding arterial pumps and catheters
Intrathecal,* intraventricular	More consistent drug levels in cerebrospinal fluid	Requires lumbar puncture or surgical placement of reservoir or implanted pump for drug delivery	Headaches, confusion, lethargy, nausea and vomiting, seizures	Observe site for signs of infection; monitor functioning of reservoir or pump; assess patient for headache or signs of increased intracranial pressure
Intraperitoneal*	Direct exposure of intraabdominal metastases to drug	Requires placement of Tenckhoff catheter or intraperitoneal port	Abdominal pain, abdominal distention, bleeding, ileus, intestinal perforation, infection	Warm chemotherapy solution to body temperature; check patency of catheter or port; instill

Intrapleural	Sclerosing of pleural lining to prevent recurrence of effusions	Requires insertion of a thoracotomy tube	Pain, infection	solution according to protocol—infuse, dwell, and drain or continuous infusion Monitor for complete drainage from pleural cavity before instillation of drug; after instillation, clamp tubing and reposition patient every 10-15 minutes for 2 hours; attach tubing to suction for 18 hours; assess patient for pain or anxiety; provide analgesia and emotional support
Intravesicular	Direct exposure of bladder surfaces to drug	Requires insertion of Foley catheter	Urinary tract infections, cystitis, bladder contracture, urinary urgency, allergic drug reactions	Maintain sterile technique when inserting Foley catheter; instill solution, clamp catheter for 1 hour, and unclamp to drain

recommendations for handling of hazardous drugs. The following procedural guidelines are provided to optimize safe, effective drug delivery by peripheral venous access.

1. Thoroughly wash hands and put on protective gloves.
2. Exercise patience in vein selection; begin distally and work proximally. Avoid extremities with lymphedema, impaired circulation, edema, sites where venipuncture has been performed within the previous 24 hours, hematomas, axillary lymph node dissections, local infection, and phlebitis. To minimize potential patient morbidity from drugs capable of producing tissue necrosis, avoid the antecubital fossa, wrist, and dorsum of the hand. Warm soaks for 10 to 15 minutes may enhance detection of a potential site in patients with limited vascular access.
3. Choose a cannula based on the purpose, rate of flow, and duration of therapy; the size and availability of the patient's veins; and your own experience and success with each type of cannula. If a short-term infusion (<24 hours) is planned, either a steel needle or an appropriate plastic catheter can be used.
4. Prepare the skin with povidone-iodine solution. An alternative to iodine is 70% alcohol alone, rubbed vigorously for 1 minute.
5. Once the cannula is successfully placed, apply enough tape to secure it but not to obscure the end so that infiltration of fluid can be immediately detected, especially if a known vesicant is to be given.
6. Test patency of the cannula with 5% dextrose in water or normal saline, which should flow freely. If the flow is slow or intermittent, recheck the cannula, taping, and IV system (if used), and then recheck patency.
7. If venipuncture has been unsuccessful after two attempts, ask a colleague for assistance.
8. Drugs should be administered as ordered and according to protocol directions. For bolus injections and drugs infused through the side arm of IV tubing, infuse the drug slowly to prevent leakage around the needle and pressure on the wall of the vein. Blood return should be checked frequently.
9. The cannula and tubing should be flushed with solution between drugs and after completion of the last drug administered.
10. Heed any patient complaints. Stop drug administration for any complaints that might indicate extravasation (see Chapter 10). Evaluate with a saline flush. If there is any doubt, restart the infusion. Venous irritation or phlebitis, which may produce varying degrees of local pain, have been associated with several drugs: amsacrine, carmustine, cisplatin, dacarbazine, dactinomycin, daunorubicin, doxorubicin, etoposide, idarubicin, mechlorethamine, mitomycin, mitoxantrone, teniposide, vinblastine, vincristine, and vinorelbine tartrate. Ice applied above the IV site may alleviate the acute discomfort during drug administration for some of the drugs, such as dacarbazine, whereas for others, such as vinorelbine tartrate, adherence to the infusion time recommendations is the most important

intervention (Rittenberg, Gralla, and Rehmeyer, 1995). If discomfort persists from the venous irritation or phlebitis, warm soaks daily to the affected area may help; follow-up assessment, including careful evaluation of the level of discomfort and effectiveness of interventions, is warranted.

11. Record drug administered, dose, route of administration, type and volume of solution, and any adverse reactions.

Central Venous Access

Limited vascular access, intensive chemotherapy, parenteral nutrition, continuous drug delivery, and projected long-term need for venous access are the major indications for central venous catheters in cancer patients. The use of central catheters has escalated in cancer therapy as a result of broader therapeutic indications and improvements in the types and selection of devices. Technological advances in the plastics industry have diminished the incidence and severity of catheter complications with the introduction of polyurethane and silastic elastomer materials for catheter construction (Baranowski, 1993; Hadaway, 1995). Catheter materials are also radiopaque, which is a critically important feature in determining correct placement and evaluation of catheter malfunction. The cited improvements in catheter construction have diminished but not eliminated catheter-associated complications. Thrombosis and fibrin sheath formation producing partial or complete catheter occlusion are examples of persistent catheter problems faced daily by clinicians. Guidelines for catheter care in conjunction with algorithms for determining and managing catheter complications provide consistent approaches to maintaining patent functional catheters, thereby maximizing professional practice and minimizing patient stress and complication rates.

There are three major types of central venous access devices used in cancer therapy: nontunneled, tunneled, and implanted ports. Nontunneled catheters include short-term percutaneously inserted catheters, peripherally inserted catheters, and apheresis catheters (Table 5-7). The percutaneous short-term catheters are most frequently used in the acute care setting for immediate need for central venous access or high acuity patients who require multilumen infusional therapies. Exit site care and restriction of activities limit the utility of these catheters beyond the short-term or acute-care indications that have been cited. Midline catheters (Table 5-7) refer to peripherally inserted catheters that terminate in the upper arm at the axillary vein, not at the superior vena cava, which is the usual endpoint for a central venous catheter (Goodwin and Carlson, 1993). Similarly, catheters that terminate before or at the subclavian vein and not at the superior vena cava should be described as long-line catheters, not central catheters. Clarity of terms is critical to practice and care of patients with peripherally inserted venous access devices.

The peripherally inserted catheter, referred to as *PICC* or *PIC* catheter in the literature, offers an alternative to the existing short-term peripheral catheters and tunneled catheters. These catheters are peripherally inserted into the basilic or cephalic vein and advanced centrally, terminating at the

TABLE 5-7
Vascular Access Devices

	Midline	Peripherally inserted central catheters	Tunneled	Implanted ports	Apheresis catheters
Material used	Elastomeric hydrogel, silicone elastomer, polyurethane	Elastomeric hydrogel, silicone elastomer, polyurethane	Silicone elastomer	Silicone elastomer, polyurethane	Silicone elastomer, polyurethane
Available gauge, length	24 g to 16 g 3 to 8 inches	23 g (1.9F) to 16 g (4.8F) 15 to 27 inches	2.7F to 12.5F 29.5 to 42.7 inches	4F to 12F 19.7 to 34.5 inches	8.4F to 11.5F 5.4 to 18 inches
Double lumens available	Yes	Yes	Yes	Yes	Yes
Insertion site(s)	Basilic, cephalic, or median cubital veins of antecubital region	Basilic, cephalic, or median cubital veins of antecubital region	Enters vein at the proximal cephalic, axillary, or distal subclavian and exits lower chest wall at a lower, predetermined site	Enters vein at the antecubital or subclavian site with suture line closing port pocket close to this location; may be at numerous other anatomic locations, such as peritoneal, arterial, and epidural	Right internal jugular preferred; also subclavian and femoral

Tip location	Upper arm in axilla, distal to the shoulder; neonates and pediatric locations may be midthigh to upper thigh if lower extremity is used	SVC; innominate, subclavian, proximal axillary may also be chosen depending on patient condition and type of infusate; IVC in neonates or pediatrics when lower extremity insertion site is used	SVC or IVC if SVC cannot be cannulated	SVC or IVC if SVC cannot be cannulated	SVC
Method of insertion	Over-the-needle (Landmark only) or through-the-introducer with break-away needle or peel-away sheath	Through-the-introducer with break-away needle, peel-away sheath, or short over-the-needle catheter; Seldinger over-wire	Seldinger over-wire or cutdown with surgically created tunnel	Seldinger over-wire or cutdown with surgically created pocket for port	Seldinger over-wire or cutdown
Indications	IV solutions for replacement/hydration; most IV medications, admixture should be isoosmotic to decrease chemical vein irritation	SVC or IVC location—all types of fluids, medications, nutrition; if tip is in other veins, solution should be isoosmotic	All types of fluids, medications, and nutrition	All types of fluids, medications, and nutrition	Hemodialysis, apheresis

Continued

From Hadaway LC: Comparison of vascular access devices, *Semin Oncol Nurs* 11:154-166, 1995.
SVC, Superior vena cava; IVC, inferior vena cava; IV, intravenous.

TABLE 5-7
Vascular Access Devices—cont'd

	Midline	Peripherally inserted central catheters	Tunneled	Implanted ports	Apheresis catheters
Limitations of use	Solution with dextrose content more than 10% to 12.5%; continuously infused vesicants; lack of antecubital veins suitable for catheter insertion and advancement	Lack of antecubital veins suitable for catheter insertion and advancement; anomalies of central venous structure; thrombosis of veins	Anomalies of central venous structure; thrombosis of veins	Anomalies of central venous structure; thrombosis of veins	Anomalies of central venous structure; thrombosis of veins

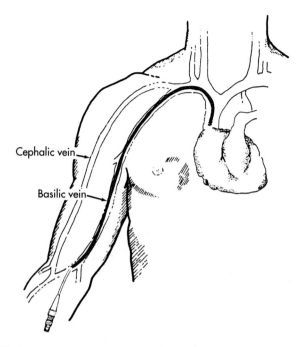

FIG. 5-1 Peripherally inserted catheter (PICC) placement. (From Reyman PW: Chemotherapy: principles of administration. In Groenwald S, Frogge M, Goodman M, Yarbo C: *Cancer nursing principles and practice*, ed 3, Boston, 1993, Jones & Bartlett, pp 314.)

superior vena cava (Fig. 5-1). Although some of these catheters have been used as long-line catheters, terminating in the subclavian or axillary vein, the optimal tip location is the superior vena cava, and radiologic examination is recommended after placement (James, Bledsoe, and Hadaway, 1993). Radiologic confirmation of correct tip position will also minimize or eliminate complications associated with tip malposition, especially in the asymptomatic patient (LaFortune, 1993). Educational programs have been designed to qualify clinicians—specifically, registered nurses—to insert and manage these catheter lines (Kyle and Myers, 1990).

The most common indication for a PICC line is antibiotics, but these lines are also used for parenteral nutrition, hydration, chemotherapy, pain control, and blood products. These catheters can be inserted at the bedside, are used for hospital or home infusion, are easily removed, are economical, are available with dual lumens, have been used successfully with immunosuppressed patients, and have been reported to remain in place up to several

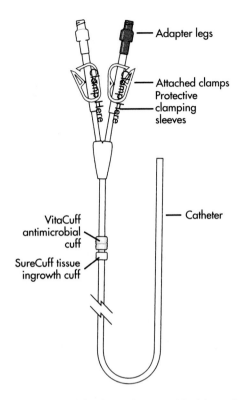

FIG. 5-2 Multilumen tunneled catheter. (Courtesy of Bard Access System, Salt Lake City, Utah.)

months (Goodwin and Carlson, 1993). A month or less is the most common duration of catheter dwelltime because completion of therapy is the reason for removal in the majority of patients. Disadvantages of PICC lines include daily to weekly care requirements, occlusive exit-site dressing, careful attention to prevent dislodgement (may be sutured), availability of a qualified nurse for insertion, difficulty or inability to draw blood, and body image concerns (Winslow, Trammell, and Camp-Sorrell, 1995). Complications are similar to other central lines and include occlusion, phlebitis, insertion malposition, dislodgement, infection, and breakage (James, Bledsoe, and Hadaway, 1993; Goodwin and Carlson, 1993).

Tunneled central venous catheters are available in single, double, or triple lumens with either a Dacron or collagen matrix cuff, which provides a mechanical barrier to organisms (Hadaway, 1995) (Fig. 5-2). These

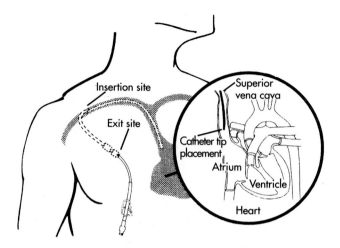

FIG. 5-3 Placement of tunneled central venous access catheter. (Courtesy of Bard Access Systems, Salt Lake City, Utah.)

catheters either are open at the end or are the Groshong type, with a closed distal tip with a three-way slit valve. The type of valve construction of the Groshong catheter is unique and eliminates the need for heparin flushes or external clamps because it restricts the backflow of blood (Winslow, Trammell, and Camp-Sorrell, 1995). Physicians insert tunneled central catheters under general or local anesthesia into one of the central veins, with the catheter tip resting in the right atrium. The catheter is tunneled for several inches through subcutaneous tissue to a separate incision, usually on the chest wall, allowing the catheter to exit at a site that is easy to see and care for and distanced from the entry point into the major vein (Fig. 5-3). After insertion, the type, length, size, length of external portion of the catheter, and confirmation of the catheter tip position should be documented. All catheters should flush easily and have adequate blood return immediately after insertion, and patients should be observed at the insertion, exit, and tunnel sites (Hadaway, 1995).

Scientific evidence is lacking for a definitive standard of catheter care and maintenance. The major components of care include exit site care, cap change, flushing, and dressing change (Table 5-8). Guidelines for care are based on available clinical literature and scientific principles related to skin integrity, risk of infection, and hemostasis (Winslow, Trammell, and Camp-Sorrell, 1995). Because of variations in catheter care and lack of definitive research, it is imperative to have institutional agreement on policies, procedures, and teaching for catheter care for continuity of both patients and staff in the hospital and ambulatory care settings. It is equally important to have a mechanism established for periodic review

TABLE 5-8
Clinical Parameters for Tunneled Catheter Care and Use

Care component	Procedure
Saline flush for Groshong-type catheters	Flush briskly with 5 mL before and after each use and weekly in-between use; use 10-20 mL after blood sampling or infusion of viscous fluids.
Flush for open-end catheters	Flush with 5-10 mL of normal saline before and after use, followed by a heparin flush of 3-5 mL of a 10-100 units/mL concentration. The concentration of 100 units/mL is more commonly supported in the literature (Winslow, Trammer, and Camp-Sorrell, 1995) but the heparin concentration of 10 units/mL appears to be a common practice trend. Maintain positive pressure at end of procedure to minimize reflux of blood. The frequency of heparin flush varies from daily to weekly.
Exit site care	Consider sterile technique initially after insertion until site is healed, generally 3-4 weeks, and in immunocompromised patients. Cleanse with a known effective antiseptic solution beginning with application of alcohol to remove skin oils and cells, followed by alcohol, iodophors, chlorhexidine gluconate, or tincture of iodine/70% alcohol (Baranowski, 1993). Hydrogen peroxide may be added to remove crusts.
Ointment at exit site	Efficacy is controversial; if used, change dressing every 48 hours (Winslow, Trammell, and Camp-Sorrell, 1995).

Dressing change	
Gauze, nonocclusive	Change every 48 hours.
Occlusive (gauze/tape or transparent)	Change every 5-7 days; consider more often for patients at higher risk for infection.
No dressing	Controversial, may consider for nonimmunosuppressed patient following complete healing of exit site.
Cap change	For infrequent access, change weekly (Winslow, Trammell, and Camp Sorrell, 1995). For routine use, change daily to 2-3 times per week. Change whenever there are signs of blood, precipitates, or leaks.
Clamping	Use for accessing and deaccessing open-ended catheters; if clamp is not available, have patient perform the Valsalva maneuver at the time the catheter is open to air; do *not* use clamps for Groshong catheters.
Blood sampling	Discard 5-10 mL of blood from catheter before your blood sample for laboratory analysis except for specimens for blood cultures. Coagulation values may be altered when drawn through a heparinized catheter (Pinto, 1994); other factors, such as specific drug levels, may alter laboratory results drawn from a central catheter, which may indicate a repeat test (Baranowski, 1993).

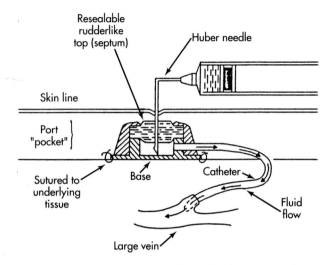

FIG. 5-4 Port design. (From Camp-Sorrell D: Implantable ports: everything you always wanted to know, *J Intrav Nurs* 15(5), 264, 1992.)

and revision of policies to incorporate changes as new information evolves from practice and research.

Implanted Ports

An infusion port is a subcutaneous device that consists of a portal body, septum, reservoir, and catheter (Fig. 5-4). Ports can be placed for venous, intraarterial, intraperitoneal, intrapleural, or epidural access (Fig. 5-5) and are available from multiple manufacturers. The portal body is made from stainless steel, titanium, plastic, or polysulfone, with heights of 9.8 mm to 17 mm, diameters of 16.5 mm to 40 mm, internal body volumes of 0.2 mL to 1.47 mL, and weights ranging from 2.1 g to 28.8 g. Within the portal body is a self-sealing silicone septum that requires a noncoring needle for access (Camp-Sorrell, 1992). Ports are manufactured with attachable or preattached catheters made of silicone or polyurethane; multiple lumens are available, and the ports are available in pediatric and low-profile styles (Reymann, 1993). The catheter size and tip depend on the type of access for which the port system was designed. Venous ports have either an open end or a Groshong-type closed tip end with slit valve; peritoneal catheters have several slits at the lower end of the catheter, similar to peritoneal dialysis catheters; epidural catheters are open-ended, and arterial catheters either are open-ended or have a one-way valve at the distal end to prevent blood backflow (Camp-Sorrell, 1992). New types of ports continue to be designed and tested for additional access sites, such as intraosseous access or for improvements in function, such as altered

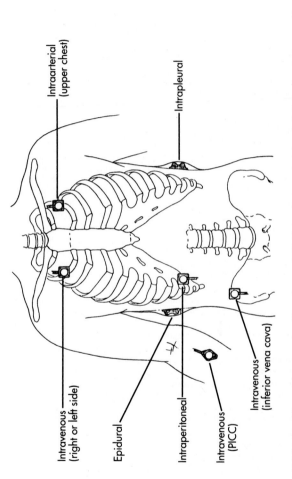

Intraarterial (upper chest)

Intrapleural

Intravenous (right or left side)

Epidural

Intraperitoneal

Intravenous (PICC)

Intravenous (inferior vena cava)

FIG. 5-5 Implantable port placement sites. (From Reyman PW: Chemotherapy: principles of administration. In Groenwald S, Frogge M, Goodman M, Yarbo C: *Cancer nursing principles and practice,* ed 3, Boston, 1993, Jones & Bartlett, pp 314.)

reservoir styles to improve flow and reduce dead space for collection of residues (Hadaway, 1995).

The venous infusion ports are the most commonly used port devices in practice. The port is placed under the skin with the incision above or below the septum of the device. For easy access and stability, ports are implanted between the chest midline and distal third of the clavicle. A needle can be inserted for access immediately if use is critical. If not, a 2- to 5-day delay is recommended to allow resolution of postoperative tenderness and edema.

Advantages of the implanted system include excellent patient acceptance, no dressing changes, heparinization monthly, no restriction on patient activity, less nursing time required for patient and family teaching, no exit site for potential infection, functional life of several years, appropriateness for intermittent or continuous therapy across a variety of settings, and association with a low maintenance cost. Disadvantages include needle puncture for access, high initial cost, surgical procedure required for placement and removal, risk of drug extravasation in the subcutaneous tissues of the pocket because of needle malposition or dislodgement, and risk of backtracking of the drug secondary to a clotted catheter or fibrin sheath.

The basic principles for access and maintenance are (1) using Huber needles for access, (2) flushing the system for patency, (3) maintaining positive pressure when withdrawing the needle, and (4) heparinizing once monthly and after each use. The Huber-point needles are designed with a deflected point that prevents coring of the septum and are available as a single needle that can be attached to a syringe or extension tubing or as a single device. A right-angle Huber needle is recommended if the needle is to remain in place (Baranowski, 1993) (Fig. 5-4). The extension tubing or single device (Huber needle with preattached tubing) offers a closed system, decreases the risk of compromising sterility, has a self-sealing rubber cap or Y site, and facilitates changing of syringes, blood drawing, and flushing.

Before a port is accessed, it is important to identify the type of device and characteristics of the specific product. Verification from the patient's record or confirmation from the surgeon is essential. If the patient is in a nonhospital setting, a policy to record the type of device should be established.

Guidelines for access procedures for ports generally adhere to aseptic technique, although clean technique has been suggested as an acceptable, safe, less costly, and less time-consuming method of preparation (Schulmeister, 1987; Long and Ovaska, 1992). The following guidelines are consistent with the generally accepted aseptic approach (ONS, 1996).

1. Assemble all necessary equipment.
2. Wash hands thoroughly.
3. Stabilize port with index finger and thumb of nondominant hand, and palpate septum of port with opposite hand.
4. Prepare skin over port with povidone-iodine or alcohol.
5. Using aseptic technique, fill the extension tubing and Huber needle with saline, expelling all air.
6. Stabilize port and access with Huber needle at a 90-degree angle (Fig. 5-4).

7. Flush with 5 to 10 mL of normal saline to check for patency.
8. If resistance is met, try to advance the needle farther into the septum until it hits the needle stop. If unsuccessful, try another needle and reenter port.
9. If withdrawal of blood is required, discard the first 5 mL to 10 mL, except for specimens for blood cultures (Moore et al, 1986). A syringe for withdrawing blood can be used, exerting very slow, steady pressure, or preferably, the Vacutainer blood-drawing method can be used. The latter is time-efficient and decreases the risk of blood exposure to the caregiver. After blood withdrawal or blood administration, flush the port with 20 mL of normal saline followed by a heparin flush (100 units/mL).
10. For long-term or continuous infusions, secure the needle hub with a small pad and sterile strips or tape, and secure with an occlusive, transparent dressing. The transparent dressing allows close observation of the site for any signs of erythema, irritation, or infiltration.
11. When therapy or access is completed, flush with 3 mL to 5 mL of 100 units/mL of heparin flush. When 0.5 mL is remaining, withdraw the needle, maintaining slight pressure to heparin lock the system. This will decrease the risk of backflow of blood into the catheter or reservoir.

Access of ports for other placement sites and routes of administration follows the same principles for venous access. Flushing recommendations vary by type of port and system accessed. For arterial ports, flush before with 5 mL of normal saline; after medication, flush with 20 mL of normal saline followed by a 5 mL heparin flush of 1000 units/mL, which should also be done weekly for nonaccessed ports. For peritoneal ports, flush before and after medication with 20 mL of compatible solution followed by 5 mL to 10 mL of normal saline flush. There is no maintenance flush for epidural ports (Camp-Sorrell, 1992).

Complications of Central Venous Catheters

Complications associated with central venous catheters include infection, occlusion, migration, venous thrombosis, malposition, air embolism, vessel perforation, breakage, and extravasation of medication. Nurses must be alert to signs and symptoms associated with potential catheter complications (Table 5-9).

Local and systemic infection is a common complication. Local infection may occur at the exit site, subcutaneous tunnel, or port pocket for implanted ports. Stringent site care and a 10- to 14-day course of oral or IV antibiotics is usually a successful strategy to eliminate local infection and preserve the function and utility of the catheter (Rumsey and Richardson, 1995). Catheter-related septicemia is a major risk. Determination of the catheter as the source of the septicemia is usually accepted on the basis of higher numbers of organisms recovered from blood cultures drawn from the catheter compared with those from the peripheral blood, and clinical symptoms suggesting systemic infection when there is no other apparent source (Baranowski, 1993). Initially, catheter-related

TABLE 5-9
Potential Complications of Central Venous Catheters

Complication	Frequency	Signs and symptoms
Infection	Common	
Local		Induration, erythema, exudate, tenderness
Systemic		Fever, chills, malaise, diaphoresis, tachycardia
Withdrawal occlusion	Common	Ability to flush catheter but unable to withdraw blood
Complete occlusion	Occasional	Inability to flush catheter or withdraw blood
Migration or malposition	Uncommon	Lack of blood return; flushing problems; swelling in ipsilateral extremity; dyspnea; discomfort with infusion
Extravasation	Uncommon	Swelling in the area of port pocket or subcutaneous tunnel; local symptom complaints, such as pain or burning; slow infusion rate
Separation of catheter from port	Rare	Lack of blood return; local swelling; change in ability to infuse fluids; patient complains of altered sensation in portal site
Venous perforation	Rare	Symptom related to site of perforation but shortness of breath most common (Baranowski, 1993)

Twiddler's syndrome: intentional or unintentional manipulation of port	Rare	A flipped portal body resulting in an inability to determine hub, port, or septal area
Pinch-off syndrome: anatomic, mechanical compression of the catheter at the costoclavicular space between the clavicle and first rib	Rare	Withdrawal occlusion, resistance to infusion; irregular flushing pattern with patient positioning; may lead to catheter fracture, which has been associated with cardiac arrhythmias and potential for drug extravasation (Ingle, 1995)
Venous thrombosis	Rare	Discomfort, pain, or swelling in chest wall, scapula, or shoulder area; pattern of venous distention in neck, shoulder, or chest wall; inability to flush device
Breakage: internal or external	Rare	Leakage; reflux of blood into catheter or extension tubing; unexplained drainage on dressing; air embolism (Ingle, 1995)
Dislodgment of needle in septum of port or inadequate needle length	Uncommon, rare	Inability to infuse; local swelling; inability to withdraw blood; potential for extravasation

sepsis should not dictate catheter removal until a trial of IV antibiotics is administered through the catheter. If the catheter is a double or triple lumen, administration of antibiotics should be alternated among each of the lumens. Removal of a catheter is generally indicated when associated symptoms of sepsis do not resolve after IV antibiotics are given through the catheter; the causative organism is fungi or bacilli, the patient experiences chills and hypotension after irrigation of the catheter, or there is evidence of endocarditis (Liepman, Jones, and Kauffman, 1984; Rumsey and Richardson, 1995).

Partial or complete catheter occlusion is a very common clinical problem. The causes include position of the catheter tip against the vessel wall, a fibrin sheath, thrombus in the lumen or at the catheter tip, fluid or drug precipitate, or malposition. Partial occlusions are often related to tip position, fibrin sheath formation, or a clot at the tip of the catheter, the latter two resulting in blood withdrawal occlusion ("one-way catheter"). Brisk irrigations with 10 mL to 30 mL of normal saline or changing the patient's position to reposition the catheter tip (turning side to side, leaning forward, elevating arms, coughing, deep breathing, lying supine) are often successful interventions. Prevention strategies include strict adherence to flushing procedures, low-dose oral anticoagulants, and prophylactic use of fibrinolytic agents (Baranowski, 1993). If blood withdrawal occlusion persists despite vigorous flushing, consult with the physician to consider a chest radiograph or dye study to confirm the position of the catheter (and/or document presence of a fibrin sheath) or instillation of a fibrinolytic agent.

Completely occluded catheters prevent administration of any fluids or withdrawal of blood. All possible causes should be evaluated to determine the most appropriate intervention. If the patient has an implanted port, the needle placement should be checked or changed. If complete occlusion persists, attempt a gentle flush/aspiration using a 10-mL syringe filled with 5 mL of saline. If unsuccessful and a clot is suspected, consult with the physician about instillation of a lytic agent (commonly urokinase 5000 IU/ml). Instill the lytic agent in an amount equal to the catheter and reservoir volume and leave for a duration of 5 to 30 minutes. The size of the syringe used to instill the lytic agent has been controversial. Historically, 1-mL tuberculin syringes were used, but in recognition of the pressure tolerance of the available catheters, use of 3- to 5-mL syringes is the current practice recommendation (Martin, Walker, and Goodman, 1996). For completely occluded catheters, a 10-mL syringe is recommended for instillation of the lytic agent. This is more difficult and requires patience, but the benefit is felt to outweigh the risks of exceeding the 25 to 40 pounds per square inch (PSI) that most catheters can tolerate (Baranowski, 1993). Attempt aspiration and if unsuccessful, repeat procedure. The length of time urokinase is left in the catheter on subsequent attempts varies from 1 to 24 hours, and the number of doses safely administered in a 24-hour period is largely dependent on the individual patient's status. For unresolved occlusions, alteplase (t-PA), a recombinant tissue plasminogen activator, has been successfully used in a small number of patients (Atkinson, Bagnall, and Gomperts, 1990); however, confirmation of its efficacy is required as well as evaluation of cost.

For suspected drug precipitate, catheter patency can be restored if the solubility of the fluid can be changed by altering the pH, resulting in returning the precipitate into solution. Instillation of 0.1 N hydrochloric acid (HCl) has been used successfully in restoring patency in catheters obstructed by precipitates such as lipids or calcium and phosphorous incompatibilities with TPN (Baranowski, 1993; Rumsey and Richardson, 1995).

REGIONAL DRUG DELIVERY

Infusion of chemotherapeutic drugs directly into the area of the tumor has theoretical advantages over the systemic route of administration. The most common approaches to regional drug perfusion include intraarterial, intraperitoneal, and intraventricular.

Intraarterial

The intraarterial route for regional drug delivery has been attempted in several malignancies such as head and neck tumors and limb perfusions for melanoma, but liver metastasis has been the primary target for intraarterial drug delivery. Arterial perfusion with chemotherapy can be delivered through an externally placed percutaneous catheter, an implanted port-catheter system, or implanted infusion pump. Percutaneous catheters are inserted under local anesthesia and placement is confirmed by angiography. Patients usually require hospitalization and bedrest with femoral artery access (Lynes, 1993). There is minimal use of these catheters in practice because of the high complication rate, especially for hepatic perfusion, and the availability of implanted devices.

Subcutaneously implanted ports are similar to the venous access ports. The most common indication is hepatic metastases, and catheters are usually placed in the common hepatic artery with the port body on either side of the rib cage. Access and use of this system require a noncoring needle, a 10 mL or larger syringe for flushing, aseptic technique, sterile occlusive dressing, a 5 mL flush of normal saline on access and a 20 mL flush of normal saline followed by 5000 units heparin at the completion of therapy, and 5000 units heparin weekly when catheter is not in use to maintain patency (Almadrones, Campana, and Dantis, 1995). Infusion pumps are used to deliver the therapy, and the patient can be at home. Totally implantable infusion pumps are available and permit safe, reliable, and prolonged delivery of chemotherapy.

Once a patient is determined to be eligible for hepatic artery perfusion, the pump is surgically implanted into a subcutaneous pocket in the abdominal wall. Infusaid introduced the first implantable pump, which now is available in several models (100, 200, 400, 500, and 1000). The Infusaid 400 model is the most widely used pump. It has a side port for bolus instillation of medication in addition to the continuous drug delivery and is available with single or dual catheters. The pump is disc-shaped, is about the size of a hockey puck, and has two chambers—an inner chamber for solution or drug and an outer chamber (vapor pressure) that provides the power source for drug delivery.

These pumps must be surgically implanted, with a typical hospitalization of 6 to 8 days. Complications include seroma, infection, catheter displacement, and occlusion. The pump causes a slight protuberance on the abdominal wall, and the drug or solution is injected subcutaneously through a self-sealing port located in the center of the pump. The pump has a 50-mL capacity, with an average set rate of 3 to 6 mL/day, requiring a refill approximately every 2 weeks. It is recommended that the daily flow rate be verified before chemotherapy treatment by emptying the pump and recharging it with saline or water and heparin (von Roemeling et al, 1986). The flow rate may be verified using the following formula:

$$\text{Flow rate (mL/day)} = \frac{\text{Initial volume (mL)} - \text{remaining volume (mL)}}{\text{Number of days since last refill}}$$

The pressure from the injection of a drug or solution activates the vapor pressure in the outer chamber of the pump to produce the power to deliver the solution. The procedure for filling the infused pump is described in Box 5-1.

Disadvantages of the Infusaid implantable pump are high cost (i.e, pump, surgeon fee, hospitalization), the inability to change the flow rate, inability to adjust the volume of solution, variations in flow rate caused by changes in body temperature and elevation, and restriction of the choice of drug because of concentration limits of the 50-mL capacity. Despite years of experience with intraarterial perfusion, indications for regional arterial therapy are limited and the risk to benefit profile remains controversial, especially for hepatic metastases.

Intraventricular

Prophylaxis or treatment of the central nervous system (CNS) can be performed via lumbar puncture, an implanted pump, or Ommaya reservoir. The Ommaya reservoir is the preferred device for obtaining cerebrospinal fluid (CSF) specimens and for delivering drugs into the CSF. The design of this device is a mushroom-shaped dome that has a reservoir attached to a ventricular catheter. There are several models with reservoir sizes of 1.5 cm and 2.5 cm, with either bottom burr hole inlet or flat bottom side inlet designs (Almadrones, Campana, and Dantis, 1995). An Ommaya reservoir is inserted by a neurosurgeon into the right frontal region under the scalp, and the catheter is positioned into the lateral ventricle through a burr hole. The reservoir can be used 48 hours after insertion, even though sutures remain until 7 to 10 days after surgical placement. Patients should be instructed to avoid trauma to the area, and hair is allowed to regrow except for a 2.5- to 3-cm area that will be shaved for access procedures (Esparza and Weyland, 1982). Infection, malfunction, catheter displacement, and spread of tumor cells by catheter placement are potential but uncommon complications.

Infection is an ongoing potential complication of reservoir usage. The patient should be routinely monitored for tenderness, erythema, drainage, fever, neck stiffness, and headache. Careful adherence to aseptic technique for access of the reservoir is the best preventive strategy against infection. Depending on institutional policy, physicians or nurses who have received specialized instruction may access the Ommaya reservoir.

BOX 5-1
Procedure for Filling the Infusaid Pump

EQUIPMENT

50-mL syringe (remove plunger)
50-mL syringe filled with chemotherapeutic agent or saline and heparin
(50,000 units) (total volume always equals 50 mL)
1½-in, 22-gauge Huber-point needle (curved) with connecting tubing or
1½-in, 22-gauge straight needle with a three-way stopcock
Povidone-iodine swabs (3)
Alcohol wipes (3)
Adhesive bandage
Sterile gloves

PROCEDURE

1. Prepare a sterile field containing sterile equipment.
2. Palpate pump; attempt to locate the septum.
3. Cleanse the area over the pump with alcohol and povidone-iodine
   swabs three times using a circular motion.
4. Put on sterile gloves. Place the Huber-point needle on a three-way stopcock and attach a 50-mL syringe. Turn the stopcock to off OR attach the
   needle to the tubing and attach a 50-mL syringe to the tubing. Clamp
   the tubing. Relocate the septum. Insert the needle perpendicular to the
   septum. The needle will puncture the septum and meet the needle stop.
   Open the stopcock or clamp and observe fluid rising in the syringe as the
   pump empties.
5. Once the fluid has stopped rising in the syringe, note the amount and
   disconnect the syringe from stopcock or tubing. The needle will be open
   to air, but air will not enter the pump because it is pressurized. Discard
   pump fluid properly as one would a chemotherapeutic agent.
6. Connect the syringe filled with chemotherapy or saline to the stopcock
   or tubing. While the needle is maintained in the pump, inject contents
   of the syringe.
7. Check for correct placement (fluid will rise in the syringe when pressure
   is released from the plunger).
8. Once completed, remove the syringe and needle while stabilizing the
   pump. Apply an adhesive bandage.
9. Calculate the rate of flow by subtracting the amount left in the syringe
   at the time of emptying from 50 mL and divide by the total number of
   days since the pump was filled. This will reveal the mL/day flow and
   ensure that the patient is receiving the appropriate dose of the drug as
   planned. Most pumps will infuse between 1.5 and 2.5 mL/day (consult
   individual manufacturer's insert). Temperature elevation and the use of
   less than 50,000 units of heparin and 50 mL of solution will increase the
   speed of the pump.

From Goodman M: Delivery of cancer chemotherapy. In Baird S, McCorkle R,
Grant M, eds: *Cancer nursing: a comprehensive textbook,* Philadelphia, 1991,
WB Saunders Co, pp 291-320.

PATIENT INFORMATION CARD

CARE OF YOUR OMMAYA RESERVOIR

Introduction:

An Ommaya reservoir is a small plastic dome-like device with a small tube. It is placed underneath the scalp and connects with a hollow section within the brain that contains cerebrospinal fluid. This device is put in place in the operating room. You will be given medications to prevent pain. The Ommaya is usually left in place permanently unless complications occur.

Purpose:

The purpose of an Ommaya reservoir is to provide a method for:

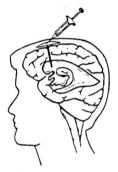

1. Giving medication directly into the fluid of the brain and spine without having to do a spinal tap.
2. Measuring the pressure of this fluid.
3. Obtaining specimens for examination.

Procedure for Using the Ommaya Reservoir:

1. Use of the reservoir is a sterile procedure so please do not touch the area once the procedure has begun.
2. Scalp hair over the Ommaya will be shaved when necessary before using the reservoir.
3. The area will be thoroughly scrubbed with a betadine solution. Please inform your doctor if you are allergic to iodine, in which case Phisohex will be used.
4. You may be asked to wear a mask during the procedure. The doctors and nurses may also be wearing masks.

A

FIG. 5-6 A, Patient teaching card for the Ommaya reservoir. (From Esparaza DM, Weyland JB: Nursing care of the patient with an Ommaya reservoir, *Oncol Nurs Forum* 9:17-20, 1982.

5. During the procedure your position may vary. The nurse will give you instructions.
6. You should not experience any pain during this procedure. There is no need to "numb" the area with a local anesthetic.
7. A small needle will be inserted into your reservoir and spinal fluid may first be removed. Then medication may be given.
8. The procedure will take a short period of time.
9. After the procedure you may be instructed to lie down for a short period. Then you may resume usual activities.
10. Possible problems you may have following the procedure are:
    a. Nausea and vomiting
    b. Headache
    c. Dizziness
    These effects will last a short time. If they continue, notify your doctor.

Special Instructions Regarding Your Ommaya:

1. The Ommaya does not require special care once the suture line has healed. The area should be kept dry until the sutures are removed. You should avoid injury to the area.
2. Do report these side effects to your doctor immediately because they may indicate problems (infection) with your Ommaya reservoir:
   a. Tenderness, redness or drainage from the site
   b. The site becomes unusually warm to the touch
   c. Fever of 101° or greater
   d. Neck stiffness
   e. Headache with or without vomiting

   If you are an outpatient, you can contact your nurse or doctor at the following numbers:

   8:00 a.m.-5:00 p.m. Call Station _____ Phone _____
   After 5:00 p.m. or on Weekends & Holidays call _____

B

FIG. 5-6 B, Reverse side of patient teaching card for the Ommaya reservoir.

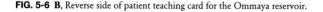

With maintenance of strict aseptic technique, the following procedural guidelines are recommended.

1. Educate the patient and obtain informed consent (Fig. 5-6).
2. Place the patient in a supine position.
3. With aseptic technique, prepare the skin over the area and puncture the reservoir obliquely with a 23- to 25-gauge scalp vein needle.
4. Remove fluid by gravity. Never forcefully aspirate. The amount of fluid removed must equal what is to be returned.
5. Inject medication slowly into the reservoir. Solution for the drug admixture should be normal saline without preservative.
6. To aid in drug dispersement, pump the reservoir (with a 2 × 2-in. gauze, gently place finger on top of the reservoir and push and release once or twice). This procedure can also be used to evaluate catheter function. If the reservoir does not refill or fills very slowly, a physician should be notified, and radiologic confirmation of placement may be indicated.
7. Dress the site with a sterile gauze.
8. The patient should remain in a supine position without a pillow for at least 30 minutes.

Intraperitoneal

Delivery of chemotherapy into the peritoneal cavity has been investigated in patients with malignant ascites and intraabdominal metastases primarily from carcinomas of the colon and ovary. The major advantage of intraperitoneal chemotherapy is pharmacological; that is, higher concentrations of some drugs can be delivered to the tumor than could be safely administered by other routes. Cytotoxicity is enhanced by direct drug contact with the cells in the peritoneal cavity and by very high drug concentrations.

Access can be achieved with a semipermanent Tenckoff catheter or a Tenckoff catheter attached to a subcutaneous implanted port. Instituting therapy involves surgical implantation of a catheter. Postoperative procedures vary from no flushing to intermittent dialysis exchanges through the catheter. Postoperative complications of catheter placement include intestinal perforation, bleeding, ileus, and incisional discomfort (Jenkins et al, 1982). The Tenckhoff catheter attached to a subcutaneously implanted port (Fig. 5-5) has become the device of choice for intraperitoneal drug delivery. The implanted port has eliminated exit site care, potential exit site infection, and restriction on patient activity. To access the implanted port, the same guidelines as described for intravenous port access should be followed with the exception of a larger volume flush (20-mL heparin flush of 100 units/mL).

Intraperitoneal drug delivery follows the same basic principles as peritoneal dialysis (Doane, Fisher, and McDonald, 1990). The solution should be allowed to reach room temperature or may be warmed to body temperature, and fluids run in and out by gravity. For chemotherapy, patency should be assessed by a 10- to 20-mL flush with normal saline before drug administration. The prescribed dose of chemotherapy is usually prepared in 2 L of solution. The fluid is instilled by gravity, and it usually takes at least 30 to 40 minutes with the implanted systems. Patients are instructed to change position periodically to permit optimal drug distribution in the abdominal cavity. Drainage is by gravity, but outflow problems are common. They may be caused by malposition of the catheter, a fibrin sheath at the tip of the catheter, or kinking of the catheter. Aspiration with a syringe, irrigation with normal saline, or changing the patient's position are often successful interventions used to institute outflow.

Outflow problems occur in one third to one half of patients and result in less than 50% recovery of fluid instilled (Hoff, 1987; Almadrones and Yerys, 1990). This does not present a significant clinical problem for most treatment patients because most drugs are removed via the portal circulation and metabolized by the liver before entering the systemic circulation and the fluid is absorbed over a few days. For patients with ascites, however, outflow obstruction may be a problem, and a percutaneous paracentesis may be needed. Other complications that occur much less frequently include bacterial or chemical phlebitis, leakage of the chemotherapeutic agent, and infection.

Symptoms associated with treatment include abdominal distention and drug-related side effects. The increase in abdominal pressure from fluid volume can produce a variety of clinical symptoms such as pain, nausea, anorexia, shortness of breath, diarrhea, constipation, and esophageal reflux (Swenson and Eriksson, 1986). Pain is the most common symptom. In a review of 137 patients who received intraperitoneal therapy, 25% reported mild discomfort (no analgesia required), 12% had moderate pain (analgesia given), and 11% reported severe pain during instillation that required narcotics and discontinuance of the procedure (Almadrones and Yerys, 1990). The mild discomfort was described as bloating or fullness and disappeared within 1 to 2 days after treatment.

Drug-related side effects are agent specific and similar to those observed with systemic intravenous therapy. It is important to remember that drugs are eliminated from the body by usual routes after absorption from the peritoneal cavity. Thus intraperitoneal cisplatin is associated with the same long-term and short-term toxicity as intravenous administration, although timing of onset may differ because of delayed absorption from the peritoneal cavity.

Intrapleural

Thoracentesis can be a therapeutic intervention for malignant pleural effusions, but efficacy is limited. Management of pleural effusions includes insertion of a chest tube, drainage of the fluid, and administration of a sclerosing agent. The goal of pleural sclerosis is pleurodesis, the fusion of the visceral and parietal pleurae, which prevents further accumulation of fluid (Little, 1994). The thoracostomy or chest tube remains in place until daily drainage is in the range of 100 to 250 mL to maximize the goal of pleural adherence. At this point, a chemical agent (a known pleural irritant) is instilled, which produces pleural inflammation. Pain during the procedure is common, but severity is dependent on the chemical irritant chosen for the procedure. Sedation, lidocaine administered through the chest tube, and systemic pain medication after the procedure are recommended to maintain

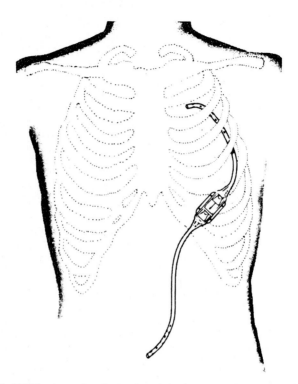

FIG. 5-7 Placement of a pleuroperitoneal shunt. (From Little AG: Malignant pleural effusion. In McKenna RJ, Murphy GP, eds: Cancer surgery, Philadelphia, 1994, JB Lippincott, p 354.)

patient comfort (Little, 1994). Management of specific drug-related side effects (i.e., nausea), assessment and monitoring of respiratory status, chest tube security, and level of patient comfort are other critical care components.

The use of pleuroperitoneal shunts for patients with malignant effusions is an alternative to the sclerosing procedures and has been associated with successful palliation (Little, 1994). The shunt consists of a double-valved pump chamber with connecting pleural and peritoneal catheters (Fig. 5-7). Success of this approach is dependent on the patient's ability and receptivity to use the pump portion of the shunt to transport the fluid against the pressure gradient from the pleural to peritoneal space. A potential serious disadvantage of this approach is dissemination of malignant cells, although this has not yet been reported (Little, 1994).

TABLE 5-10
Advantages and Disadvantages of Different Types of Ambulatory Infusion Pumps

Type of device	Advantages	Disadvantages
Syringe	Lightweight and portable Cost-effective Ease of patient use Excellent for antibiotics and pain management No dose calculations Little or no maintenance Visualize drug flow Alarms	Device can fracture and break if dropped Limited volumes Not for large-volume infusions Drug stability factor Requires adequate manual dexterity to work with syringe and tubing Free-flow risk
Elastomeric	Lightweight, portable, and concealable Ease of patient use Excellent for antibiotics No programming No maintenance Reservoir and tubing attached	Difficult to fill Admixture considerations Drug stability factor Calculate concentrations and volumes Limited infusion rates Not for large-volume infusions Reimbursement concerns Cost prohibitive in long-term therapies
Peristaltic	Provides intermittent and continuous infusions All types of infusion therapy Alarm systems Wide range of infusion rates and volumes	Requires programming Carrying pouch heavy when full Upstream occlusion Free-flow risk Labor intensive

From Rapsilber LM, Camp-Sorrell D: Ambulatory infusion pumps: application to oncology. *Semin Oncol Nurs* 11:213-220, 1995.

AMBULATORY INFUSION PUMPS FOR DRUG DELIVERY

External infusion pumps are used in oncology, most frequently for continuous intravenous chemotherapy treatments but also for regional drug delivery, pain control, hydration, and home antibiotic therapy.

Several factors must be considered for ambulatory drug delivery, including the type of drug, venous access (central access recommended), patient-family participation, cost, ability of the patient and family to learn and manage the mechanical devices, support services in the community, availability of staff to teach and problem solve, and the amount of teaching time required. The availability of home support services that have expertise with infusion devices has had a dramatic impact on the ability to deliver this type of therapy safely and efficiently. Technical skill, 24-hour coverage, drug preparation and equipment, educational instruction and reinforcement, and third-party reimbursement are available with many visiting nurse and home infusion agencies.

Infusion pumps can be classified by their mechanism of operation (peristaltic, syringe, elastomeric reservoir), mode of drug delivery (continuous, intermittent, bolus, single- or multiple-solution), and therapeutic application (patient-controlled analgesia or cancer treatment) (Kwan, 1991). The size, weight, accessories, cost, flow rate, fluid capacity, energy source, and alarm mechanisms vary by type and individual model of pump (Rapsilber and Camp-Sorrell, 1995).

The selection of an infusion pump should be based on the type of therapy and the advantages and disadvantages of each type of pump (Table 5-10). In addition, the health care professional must be knowledgeable and skilled in the use of ambulatory infusion pumps, and the patient and caregiver must be well educated and have a comfort level with the operation, alarm system, and potential complications (Rapsilber and Camp-Sorrell, 1995).

For updates on products and devices for intravenous therapy, the *Outpatient Intravenous Therapy (OPIT) Source Book* (Tice, 1996) will be available on the World Wide Web. To obtain the internet address for the OPIT Source Book, call (206) 627-1072, fax (206) 756-4999, or e-mail OPITSB@aol.com.

REFERENCES

Almadrones L, Campana P, Dantis EC: Arterial, peritoneal and intraventricular access devices, *Semin Oncol Nurs* 11:194-202, 1995.

Almadrones L, Yerys C: Problems associated with administration of intraperitoneal therapy using the Port-A-Cath system, *Oncol Nurs Forum* 17:75-80, 1990.

American Society of Hospital Pharmacists: Technical assistance bulletin on handling cytotoxic and hazardous drugs, *Am J Hosp Pharm* 47:1033-1049, 1990.

Anderson RW et al: Risk of handling injectable antineoplastic agents, *Am J Hosp Pharm* 39:1881-1887, 1982.

Atkinson JM, Bagnall HA, Gomperts E: Investigational use of tissue plasminogen activator (t-PA) for occluded central venous catheters, *J Parenter Enteral Nutr* 14: 310-311, 1990.

Baranowski L: Central venous access devices: current technologies, uses and management strategies, *J Intrav Nurs* 16: 167-194, 1993.

Bochner BS, Lichtenstein LM: Anaphylaxis, *N Engl J Med* 324:1785-1790, 1991.

Bos RP et al: Mutagenicity of urine from nurses handling cytostatic drugs: influence of smoking, *Int Arch Occup Environ Health* 50:359-369, 1982.

Burgaz S, Ozdamar YN, Karakaya AE: A signal assay for the detection of genotoxic compounds: the application on the urines of cancer patients on chemotherapy and nurses handling cytotoxic drugs, *Hum Toxicol* 7:557-560, 1988.

Calvert AH et al: Carboplatin dosage: prospective evaluation of a simple formula based on renal function, *J Clin Oncol* 7:1748-1756, 1989.

Calvert AH, Newell DR, Gore ME: Future directions with carboplatin: can theraputic monitoring, high dose administration and hematologic support with growth factors expand the spectrum compared with cisplatin? *Semin Oncol* 19:155-163, 1992.

Camp-Sorrell D: Implantable ports, *J Intrav Nurs* 15:262-272, 1992.

Caudell KA et al: Quantification of urinary mutagens in nurses during potential antineoplastic agent exposure: a pilot study with concurrent environmental and dietary control, *Cancer Nurs* 11:41-50, 1988.

Cloak M et al: Occupational exposure of nursing personnel to antineoplastic agents, *Oncol Nurs Forum* 12:33-39, 1985.

Craig JB, Capizzi RL: The prevention and treatment of immediate hypersentivity reactions from cancer chemotherapy, *Semin Oncol Nurs* 1:285-291, 1985.

Doane LS, Fisher LM, McDonald W: How to give peritoneal chemotherapy, *Am J Nurs* 4:58-66, 1990.

Esparza DM, Weyland JB: Nursing care of the patient with an Ommaya reservoir, *Oncol Nurs Forum* 9:17-20, 1982.

Falck K et al: Mutagenicity in urine of nurses handling cytotoxic drugs, *Lancet* 1:1250-1251, 1979.

Fischer DS et al: Improving the chemotherapy use process, *J Clin Oncol* 14:3148-3155, 1996.

Gelman RS et al: Actual versus ideal weight in the calculation of surface area effects on dose of 11 chemotherapy agents, *Cancer Treat Rep* 71:907-911, 1987.

Goodwin ML, Carlson I: The peripherally inserted central catheter, *J Intrav Nurs* 16:92-103, 1993.

Hadaway LC: Comparison of vascular access devices, *Semin Oncol Nurs* 11:154-166, 1995.

Hirst M et al: Caution on handling antineoplastic drugs, *N Engl J Med* 309:188-189, 1983.

Hoff ST: Concepts in intraperitoneal chemotherapy, *Semin Oncol Nurs* 3:112-117, 1987.

Hoffman DM: Lack of urine mutagenicity of nurses administering pharmacy prepared doses of antineoplastic agents, *Am J IV Ther Clin Nutr* 10:28-31, 1983.

Ingle RJ: Rare complications of vascular access devices, *Semin Oncol Nurs* 11:184-193, 1995.

James L, Bledsoe L, Hadaway LC: A retrospective look at tip location and complications of peripherally inserted central catheter lines, *J Intrav Nurs* 16:104-109, 1993.

Jenkins J et al: Technical considerations in the use of intraperitoneal chemotherapy administered by Tenckhoff catheter, *Surg Gynecol Obstet* 154:858-864, 1982.

Karakaya AE, Burgaz S, Bayan A: The significance of urinary thioesters as indicators of exposure to alkylating agents, *Arch Toxicol* 13(suppl):117-119, 1989.

Kwan JW: High technology i.v. infusion devices, *Am J Hosp Pharm* 48:S36-S51, 1991.

Kyle SK, Myers JS: Peripherally inserted central catheters: development of a hospital-based program, *J Intrav Nurs* 13:287-290, 1990.

LaFortune S: The use of confirming x-rays to verify tip position for peripherally inserted catheters, *J Intrav Nurs* 16:246-250, 1993.

Liepman MK, Jones PG, Kauffman CA: Endocarditis as a complication of indwelling right atrial catheters in leukemia patients, *Cancer* 54:804-807, 1984.

Little AG: Malignant pleural effusion. In McKenna RJ, Murphy GP, eds: *Cancer surgery,* Philadelphia, 1994, JB Lippincott, pp 351-356.

Long CM, Ovaska M: Comparative study of nursing protocols for venous access ports, *Cancer Nurs* 15:18-21, 1992.

Lynes AC: Percutaneous hepatic arterial chemotherapy and chemoembolization, *Cancer Nurs* 16:283-287, 1993.

Mahon SM et al: Safe handling practices of cytotoxic drugs: results of a chapter survey, *Oncol Nurs Forum* 21:1157-1165, 1994.

Martin VR, Walker FE, Goodman M: Delivery of cancer chemotherapy. In: McCorkle R et al, eds: *Cancer nursing: a comprehensive textbook*, Philadelphia, 1996, WB Saunders, pp 315-433.

Moore CL et al: Nursing care and management of venous access ports, *Oncol Nurs Forum* 13:35-39, 1986.

Occupational Safety and Health Administration: *Controlling occupational exposure to hazardous drugs* (OSHA Instruction CPL 2-2.20B), Washington, DC, 1995.

Oncology Nursing Society: *Cancer chemotherapy guidelines and recommendations for practice,* , Pittsburgh, 1996, Oncology Nursing Press.

Pinto KM: Accuracy of cogulation values obtained from a heparinized central venous catheter, *Oncol Nurs Forum* 21:573-575, 1994.

Rapsilber LM, Camp-Sorrell D: Ambulatory infusion pumps: application to oncology, *Semin Oncol Nurs* 11:213-220, 1995.

Reymann PE: Chemotherapy: principles of administration. In Groenwald S et al, eds: *Cancer nursing principles and practice*, Boston, 1993, Jones & Bartlett, pp 293-330.

Rittenberg CN, Gralla R, Rehmeyer TA: Assessing and managing venous irritation associated with vinorelbine tartrate (Navelbine), *Oncol Nurs Forum* 22:707-710, 1995.

Rogers B, Emmett EA: Handling antineoplastic agents: urine mutagenicity in nurses, *IMAGE* 19:108-113, 1987.

Rumsey KA, Richardson DK: Management of infection and occlusion associated with vascular access devices, *Semin Oncol Nurs* 11:174-183, 1995.

Selevan SG et al: A study of occupational exposure to antineoplastic drugs and fetal loss in nurses, *N Engl J Med* 313:1173-1178, 1985.

Staiano N et al: Lack of mutagenic activity in urine from hospital pharmacists admixing antitumor drugs, *Lancet* 1:615-616, 1981.

Stucker I et al: Urine mutagenicity, chromosomal abnormalities and sister chromatic exchanges in lymphocytes of nurses handling cytostatic drugs, *Int Arch Occup Environ Health* 57:195-205, 1986.

Swenson KK, Eriksson JH: Nursing management of intraperitoneal chemotherapy, *Oncol Nurs Forum* 13:33-39, 1986.

Tice AD, ed: *Outpatient intravenous therapy sourcebook*, Tacoma, Wash, 1996, Opit Source Book.

Valanis B et al: Antineoplastic drug handling protection after OSHA guidelines: comparison by profession, handling activity and work site, *J Occup Med* 34:149-155, 1992.

Venitt S et al: Monitoring exposure of nursing and pharmacy personnel to cytotoxic drugs: urinary mutation assays and urinary platinum as markers of absorption, *Lancet* 1:74-77, 1984.

von Roemeling R et al: Chemotherapy via implanted infusion pump: new perspectives for delivery of long term continuous treatment, *Oncol Nurs Forum* 13:17-24, 1986.

Weiss RB: Hypersensitivity reactions, *Semin Oncol* 19:458-477, 1992.

Winslow MN, Trammell L, Camp-Sorrell D: Selection of vascular access devices and nursing care, *Semin Oncol Nurs* 11:167-173, 1995.

6

Combination
Chemotherapy

During the 1950s, drugs were used mainly as single agents and yielded only a few complete responses with short durations. Choriocarcinoma was one of the few malignancies cured by single-agent chemotherapy (Berkowitz, Goldstein, and Bernstein, 1982). We can now add hairy cell leukemia to the list (Piro et al, 1990). The 1960s marked the beginning of the era of combination chemotherapy and was dominated by the cell kill hypothesis (Skipper et al, 1964). This hypothesis utilized kinetic, biochemical, and pharmacological principles in the design of combination chemotherapy regimens. Early combination successes include the Cooper regimen for advanced breast cancer (cyclophosphamide, methotrexate, 5-fluorouracil, vincristine, and prednisone) (Cooper, 1969) and MOPP chemotherapy (mechlorethamine, vincristine [Oncovin], procarbazine, and prednisone) for Hodgkin's disease (DeVita, Serpick, and Carbone, 1970). In contrast to single-agent chemotherapy, combination therapy often increases the number of complete responses and duration of the responses, and the cure rate is often higher with combinations even for patients with widespread disease (DeVita and Schein, 1973). Combination chemotherapy regimens have been designed on the basis of cell cycle specificity, drugs with different modes of action, varied toxicities, equal effectiveness of drugs, and synergy between drugs.

Literally hundreds of combination chemotherapy regimens have been developed. Many of them are listed in the on-line computer service *Physician's Data Query* (PDQ) system operated by the National Cancer Institute (NCI). As a quick reference for those who use combination chemotherapy, we have compiled a selection of completed studies with references to the original or follow-up report by the investigators. This is not meant as a "cookbook," but as a resource for oncology professionals who are familiar with the therapy. It is meant to provide references without having to go to the library or do a computer search. With this in mind, we have restricted inclusions to articles in English and in journals or proceedings more readily available to oncology professionals. Additional treatment options are to be found in oncology textbooks (see Appendix B, General Bibliography). When the compilation of chemotherapy protocols in this book is used as a guide, *it is imperative to consult the original or cited literature to verify dosage* (transcription or printing errors do occur), to check timing and sequencing, for suggested dose-reduction schedules, and to ascertain the need for ancillary support such as hydration or antiemetics or prophylaxis of allergic reactions. When we refer to repetition of a chemotherapy combination at a stated interval, we frequently use the terms *course* or *cycle* interchangeably, as they often are in the literature. If combined modality therapy is being used with radiation, dosage reduction is usually necessary and should be stated in the original report of combined-modality therapy. In addition, appropriate antiemetics, hydration, and colony-stimulating factors are occasionally mentioned in commenting on a particular regimen, but these would be too repetitive to list with every protocol. Clinicians should be familiar with these supportive measures, most of which are detailed in other relevant chapters.

The patient's quality of life is a central consideration in all therapy and is deservedly receiving more attention in the literature (Gelber, Goldhirsch, and Cavalli, 1991; Cella, 1995). Patients will generally accept more toxic side effects in an attempt to cure them or significantly prolong their lives but may be unwilling to tolerate much discomfort for palliation or a Phase I trial. That is a decision that belongs to the patient and should be made as part of an informed consent. Every patient is entitled to full information before agreeing to therapy, whether that therapy is considered "routine" or "standard" or is part of an investigational protocol approved by an Institutional Review Board (IRB) with a formalized consent form.

It will be noted that we have added a brief discussion to each tumor site to put it in perspective. We hope that this will be helpful. In addition, we have added sections on carcinoma of unknown primary, Kaposi's sarcoma, and renal cell carcinoma because combination therapy for those sites has become available. We have retained some regimens that are more than 25 years old because they are still being used or are frequently referred to in the current literature as points of comparison, and we have deleted others that are rarely used. We have tried to define acronyms where used. We have also compiled a list of drugs for which letters of the alphabet have been used to construct acronyms and to list the many drugs for which a single letter has been used (see Appendix A, Table A-10). Regimens for children's cancers (e.g., Wilms' tumor) have been deleted, and others are only occasionally listed because more than 80% of children with systemic cancer are treated on protocol (see Chapter 12).

New combinations are being developed every week and will require critical evaluation. We can expect biological response modifiers, radiation sensitizers, hormones, antihormones, and monoclonal antibodies to be used with chemotherapy in the future in many combinations and permutations. Although we have used many of the regimens listed, we do not endorse any as being necessarily superior, not even the ones developed or pioneered in our own institution. We have attempted to reflect the current literature as we see it. Others will see it slightly differently. Some combinations that were once regarded as "standard" or well established have since been shown to have toxicity disproportionate to their efficacy so that they have a negative therapeutic index for many patients. We have not included in this chapter any preparative high-dose chemotherapy regimens for use with bone marrow or peripheral blood stem cell transplantation. We have intentionally placed a new chapter, High-Dose Chemotherapy With Stem Cell Support, at some distance (see Chapter 9) to avoid confusion and potentially life-threatening errors.

We have commented on chemotherapy errors and resulting tragedies elsewhere (Fischer et al, 1996) and offered suggestions to minimize these errors. These suggestions included restriction of the ordering of chemotherapy to board-certified or eligible oncologists or to oncology fellows after a period of supervision and with continuing oversight, not accepting verbal orders except to reduce a dose, having patients on a dedicated oncology ward with a dedicated cadre of oncology nurses trained and certified to give cancer chemotherapy, and having a group of oncology trained and certified pharmacists dispensing cytotoxic chemotherapy drugs. Independent verification of all orders by each of those involved is mandatory. The orders should be checked against the IRB protocol, a copy of the original article, a textbook, or a handbook such as this. All orders should be written using generic or US Assigned Names for uniformity, for easy reference, and to prevent errors. If indicated, trade names or common abbreviations can be listed in parentheses if they will add clarity.

What therapeutic regimen should be used for the patient? Time, experience, and prospective randomized trials will eventually select the better regimens for the general patient population. Participation in good clinical trials should be encouraged when appropriate for the patient. Individual choices of single-agent therapy in cancer of the pancreas, stomach, thyroid, and brain may be just as efficacious as combination chemotherapy. For some cancers, such as renal cell carcinoma, there is no really useful chemotherapy, and biological response modifiers are being evaluated. Since our last edition, six major new drugs have become commercially available (paclitaxel, docetaxel, vinorelbine, irinotecan, topotecan, and gemcitabine) and are being evaluated in a multitude of combinations. The studies are early and will require more experience before their place in the chemotherapy armamentarium is clarified. However, a few are listed in combinations and more will be in the future. Overall, some of the listed combination therapies offer no survival advantage but some palliation, often at the price of considerable toxicity. Many of the regimens listed are "salvage regimens" to be used after failure of initial therapy for the patient who wants to "keep fighting." Many are second-line alternatives for the patient who has an organ disease that contraindicates the use of a superior regimen (e.g., cardiac disease with an abnormal ejection fraction or renal disease with an abnormal creatinine clearance). However, it is just as important for the oncologist to know when not to treat and when to stop treating as it is to know when and how to treat (see discussion of end-of-life decisions in Chapter 7). Determining what is best for a particular patient will always be the job of the experienced, conscientious clinician. When such a decision is impossible, as it will often be because not enough information is available, the patient should be entered in an appropriate research study to help develop the data to make future decisions.

REFERENCES

Berkowitz RA, Goldstein DP, Bernstein MR: Methotrexate with citrovorum factor rescue as primary therapy for gestational trophoblastic disease, *Cancer* 50:2024-2027, 1982.

Cella DF: Measuring quality of life in palliative care, *Semin Oncol* 22(2 suppl 3):73-81, 1995.

Cooper RE: Combination chemotherapy in hormone resistant breast cancer, *Proc Am Assoc Cancer Res* 10:15, 1969.

DeVita VT Jr, Schein PS: The use of drugs in combination for the treatment of cancer, *N Engl J Med* 288:998-1006, 1973.

DeVita VT Jr, Serpick AA, Carbone PP: Combination chemotherapy in the treatment of advanced Hodgkin's disease, *Ann Intern Med* 73:881-895, 1970.

Fischer DS et al: Improving the cancer chemotherapy use process, *J Clin Oncol* 14:3148-3155, 1996.

Gelber RD, Goldhirsch A, Cavalli F: Quality-of-life adjusted evaluation of adjuvant therapies for operable breast cancer, *Ann Intern Med* 114:621-628, 1991.

Piro LD et al: Lasting remissions in hairy-cell leukemia induced by a single infusion of 2-chlorodeoxyadenosine, *N Engl J Med* 322:1117-1121, 1990.

Skipper HE, Schabel FM, Wilcox WS: Experimental evaluation of potential anticancer agents. XII. On the criteria and kinetics associated with "curability" of experimental leukemia, *Cancer Chemother Rep* 35:1-111, 1964.

ADRENAL CORTICAL CARCINOMA

Adrenal cortical carcinoma is a rare tumor that is functional in about 10% of cases. When localized, it may be surgically curable. Recurrent or metastatic disease may be palliated with radiation or chemotherapy. There is no evidence that chemotherapy increases survival, but palliation may be achieved with single agent mitotane or doxorubicin or one of several combination chemotherapy regimens. Neither adjuvant radiation nor chemotherapy has been shown to improve survival. Functional tumors may sometimes be improved symptomatically with aminoglutethimide, metyrapone, or ketoconazole.

CAP–CYCLOPHOSPHAMIDE-DOXORUBICIN-CISPLATIN

Cyclophosphamide. 600 mg/m^2 intravenously on day 1.

Doxorubicin. 40 mg/m^2 intravenously on day 1.

Cisplatin. 50 mg/m^2 intravenously on day 1.

NOTE: Repeat the cycle every 21 days.

Selected Reading

van Slooten H, van Oosterom AT: CAP (cyclophosphamide, doxorubicin and cisplatin) regimen in adrenal cortical carcinoma, *Cancer Treat Rep* 67:377-379, 1983.

CE–CISPLATIN-ETOPOSIDE

Cisplatin. 40 mg/m^2 intravenously on days 1 to 3.

Etoposide. 100 mg/m^2 intravenously on days 1 to 3.

NOTE: Repeat the cycle every 3 weeks. Although the report is of two cases, the responses after failure of mitotane are impressive.

Selected Readings

Johnson DH, Greco FA: Treatment of metastatic adrenal cortical carcinoma with cisplatin and etoposide (VP-16), *Cancer* 58:2198-2202, 1986.

CE–CISPLATIN-MITOTANE

Cisplatin. 100 mg/m^2 (good risk) or 75 mg/m^2 (poor risk) intravenously every 3 weeks.

Mitotane. 1000 mg orally 4 times a day with escalation as tolerated.

Cortisone acetate. 25 mg twice a day.

Fludrocortisone acetate. 0.1 mg by mouth daily.

Selected Readings

Bukowski RM et al: Cisplatin (CDDP) and mitotane in metastatic adrenal carcinoma: a Southwest Oncology Group Study, *Proc Am Soc Clin Oncol* 9:136, 1990.

Bukowski FM et al: Phase II trial of mitotane and cisplatin in patients with adrenal carcinoma: a Southwestern Oncology Group study, *J Clin Oncol* 11:161-165, 1993.

FDC–FLUOROURACIL-DOXORUBICIN-CISPLATIN

5-Fluorouracil. 500 mg/m^2 by 1-hour IV infusion on days 1 to 3.

Doxorubicin. 60 mg/m^2 intravenously on day 2.

Cisplatin. 120 mg/m^2 intravenously on day 2.

NOTE: Hydration and mannitol diuresis are essential on day 2. Repeat every 4 weeks.

Selected Reading

Schlumberger M et al: 5-fluorouracil, doxorubicin, and cisplatin as treatment for adrenal cortical carcinoma, *Cancer* 67:2997-3000, 1991.

MS–MITOTANE-STREPTOZOCIN

Mitotane. 2000 to 4000 mg/day by mouth as individually tolerated.

Streptozocin. 1000 mg intravenously on days 1 to 5 and then 1500 to 2000 mg per month maintenance.

Selected Reading

Eriksson B et al: Treatment of hormone-producing adrenocortical cancer with *o,p'*DDD and streptozocin, *Cancer* 59:1398-1403, 1987.

ANAL CARCINOMA

Anal carcinoma is an uncommon but often curable disease. Traditionally, surgery was the treatment of choice and remains so in some cases. In an increasing percentage of cases, radiation therapy with fluorouracil and mitomycin has been proved to have an approximately comparable cure rate with preservation of a functioning anus and rectum. Studies are in progress to determine whether equivalent results can be obtained with radiation and fluorouracil and elimination of the added toxicity of mitomycin or the substitution of the less toxic porfiromycin.

FLUOROURACIL-MITOMYCIN

5-Fluorouracil. 1000 mg/m^2/day by continuous IV infusion for 4 days (maximum dose, 1500 mg/day).

Mitomycin. 10 mg/m^2 intravenously on day 1.

NOTE: Radiation may be delivered in a single course of 250 cGy/day 5 days a week for 4 weeks (5000 cGy) or in a split course with 2500 cGy in 2 weeks and an additional 2500 cGy beginning on day 43, in which case the above chemotherapy is repeated.

Selected Reading

Cummings BJ et al: Epidermoid anal cancer: treatment by radiation alone or by radiation and 5-fluorouracil with and without mitomycin, *Int J Radiat Oncol Biol Phys* 21:1115-1125, 1991.

MITOMYCIN-FLUOROURACIL

5-Fluorouracil. 1000 mg/m^2/day by continuous IV infusion on days 1 to 4 and 29 to 32.

Mitomycin. 15 mg/m^2 intravenously on day 1.

NOTE: Radiation therapy, 200 cGy/day, is administered for 5 days a week to a total dose of 3000 cGy.

Selected Reading

Leichman L et al: Cancer of the anal canal, *Am J Med* 78:211-215, 1985.

BLADDER (TRANSITIONAL CELL) CARCINOMA

Transitional cell carcinoma is the second most common tumor of the genitourinary tract, the fifth most common cancer, and the twelfth most frequent cause of cancer death. Treatment of superficial disease is by cautery and topical chemotherapy and biologicals. Invasive disease is treated with surgery with or without radiation and adjuvant chemotherapy. Metastatic disease is treated with palliative systemic cytotoxic combination chemotherapy. Active systemic single agents include methotrexate, cisplatin, vinblastine, doxorubicin, epirubicin, cyclophosphamide, mitoxantrone, carboplatin, gallium nitrate, ifosfamide, and paclitaxel. Combinations are more effective than single agents systemically. Active topical intravesical agents include BCG, doxorubicin, epirubicin, mitomycin, and thiotepa. Interferon-alfa and bropiramine, an oral interferon inducer, are being tested for treatment of superficial bladder cancer.

CISCA–CISPLATIN-CYCLOPHOSPHAMIDE-DOXORUBICIN

Cisplatin. 100 mg/m^2 intravenously on day 2.

Cyclophosphamide. 650 mg/m^2 intravenously on day 1.

Doxorubicin. 50 mg/m^2 intravenously on day 1.

NOTE: Hydration and mannitol for diuresis are very important. Repeat the cycle every 21 to 28 days.

Selected Reading
Sternberg JJ et al: Combination chemotherapy (CISCA) for advanced urinary tract carcinoma, *JAMA* 238:2282-2287, 1977.

CMV–CISPLATIN-METHOTREXATE-VINBLASTINE

Methotrexate. 30 mg/m^2 on days 1 and 8.

Vinblastine. 4 mg/m^2 intravenously on days 1 and 8.

Cisplatin. 100 mg/m^2 by IV infusion over a 4-hour period on day 2 after vigorous hydration.

NOTE: Repeat the cycle every 3 weeks as tolerated. Wei (Wei et al, 1996) uses methotrexate 40 mg/m^2 days 1 and 8, with acceptable toxicity.

Selected Readings
Harker WG et al: Cisplatin, methotrexate, and vinblastine (CMV): an effective chemotherapy regimen for metastatic transitional cell carcinoma of the urinary tract, *J Clin Oncol* 3:1463-1470, 1985.

Wei CH et al: Adjuvant methotrexate, vinblastine and cisplatin chemotherapy for invasive transitional cell carcinoma: Taiwan experience, *J Urol* 155:118-125, 1996.

MAC–METHOTREXATE-DOXORUBICIN-CYCLOPHOSPHAMIDE

Methotrexate. 30 mg/m^2 intravenously on days 1 and 8.

Doxorubicin. 30 mg/m^2 intravenously on day 1.

Cyclophosphamide. 300 mg/m^2 intravenously on day 1.

NOTE: Repeat the cycle every 21 days.

Selected Reading
Tanock IF, Gospodarowicz M, Evans WK: Chemotherapy for metastatic transitional carcinoma of the urinary tract: a prospective trial of methotrexate, adriamycin, and cyclophosphamide (MAC) with cisplatinum for failure, *Cancer* 51:216-219, 1983.

M-VAC–METHOTREXATE-VINBLASTINE-DOXORUBICIN-CISPLATIN

Methotrexate. 30 mg/m^2 intravenously on days 1, 15, and 22.

Vinblastine. 3 mg/m^2 intravenously on days 2, 15, and 22.

Doxorubicin. 30 mg/m² intravenously on day 2.

Cisplatin. 70 mg/m² intravenously on day 2 after vigorous hydration.

NOTE: On days 15 and 22, vinblastine (3 mg/m² intravenously) and methotrexate (30 mg/m² intravenously) are administered only if the white blood cell (WBC) count is greater than 2500 cells/µL and the platelet count is greater than 100,000 cells/µL. Cycles are repeated every 28 days even if an interim dose is withheld because of myelosuppression or mucositis. The dose of doxorubicin is reduced to 15 mg/m² in patients who have received more than 2000 cGy in 5 days to the pelvis. The use of granulocyte colony-stimulating factor (G-CSF) has allowed better adherence to the scheduled therapy with less neutropenia and its resulting toxicity.

Selected Readings

Gabrilove JL et al: Effect of granulocyte colony-stimulating factor on neutropenia and associated morbidity due to chemotherapy for transitional-cell carcinoma of the urothelium, *N Engl J Med* 318:1414-1422, 1988.

Loehrer PJ et al: A randomized comparison of cisplatin alone or in combination with methotrexate, vinblastine and doxorubicin in patients with metastatic urothelial carcinoma: a cooperative group study, *J Clin Oncol* 10:1066-1073, 1992.

Sternberg CN et al: Methotrexate, vinblastine, doxorubicin, and cisplatin for advanced transitional cell carcinoma of the urothelium, *Cancer* 64:2448-2458, 1989.

M-VAC: HIGH DOSE

Methotrexate. 30 mg/m² intravenously on days 1, 16, and 23.

Vinblastine. 4 mg/m² intravenously on days 2, 16, and 23.

Doxorubicin. 60 mg/m² intravenously on day 2.

Cisplatin. 100 mg/m² intravenously on day 2.

Sargramostim (rh GM-CSF). 250 µg/m² subcutaneously on days 3 to 13.

NOTE: May be repeated at 28-day intervals depending on toxicity and recovery, and amount of prior therapy (since this is a salvage regimen). Although molgramostim was used in the original study, sargramostim may be used in the same dosage or filgrastim (G-CSF) may be substituted at 5 µg/kg/day on days 3 to 13.

Selected Reading

Logothetis CJ et al: Escalated therapy for refractory urothelial tumors: methotrexate-vinblastine-doxorubicin-cisplatin plus unglycosylated recombinant colony-stimulating factor, *J Nat Cancer Inst* 82:667-672, 1990.

M-VEC—METHOTREXATE-EPIRUBICIN-VINBLASTINE-CISPLATIN

Methotrexate. 30 mg/m² intravenously on days 1, 15, and 22.

Vinblastine. 3 mg/m² intravenously on days 2, 15, and 22.

Epirubicin. 50 mg/m² intravenously on day 2.

Cisplatin. 70 mg/m² intravenously on day 2.

NOTE: M-VEC is a modification of M-VAC using epirubicin instead of doxorubicin to reduce cardiac toxicity. M-VECa is a further modification to reduce renal, gastroin-

testinal, and neural toxicity by substituting carboplatin 250 mg/m² on day 2 for cisplatin. The carboplatin regimen had the expected reduced toxicities and had increased hematological toxicity as anticipated but was significantly less effective in this trial. The study has been criticized for selecting a carboplatin dose that many regard as too low and not comparable to the cisplatin dose with which it was compared.

Selected Reading

Petrioli R et al: Comparison between a cisplatin-containing regimen and a carboplatin-containing regimen for recurrent or metastatic bladder cancer patients, *Cancer* 77:344-351, 1996.

MVNC—METHOTREXATE-VINBLASTINE-MITOXANTRONE-CARBOPLATIN

Methotrexate. 50 mg/m² intravenously on days 1 and 15.

Vinblastine. 3 mg/m² intravenously on day 1.

Mitoxantrone. 10 mg/m² intravenously on day 1.

Carboplatin. 200 mg/m² intravenously on day 1.

NOTE: Repeat every 4 weeks. Leucovorin 15 mg (total) is given orally 24 hours after each dose of methotrexate. Only four courses are administered until there is evidence of incomplete but continuing response, in which case additional courses may be cautiously given.

Selected Reading

Waxman J et al: New combination chemotherapy program for bladder cancer, *Br J Urol* 63:68-71, 1989.

VIG—VINBLASTINE-IFOSFAMIDE-GALLIUM NITRATE

Vinblastine. 0.11 mg/kg intravenously days 1 and 2.

Ifosfamide. 1200 mg/m² intravenously on days 1 to 5.

Mesna. 240 mg/m² intravenously 15 minutes before each dose of ifosfamide and 4 and 8 hours later, on days 1 to 5.

Gallium nitrate. 300 mg/m² by continuous 24-hour IV infusion.

Calcitrol. 0.5 µg/day orally starting 3 days before each course (except the first) and continuing through fifth and final day of each course.

Filgrastim. (G-CSF) 5 µg/kg/day on days 7 to 16 of each cycle.

NOTE: Repeat every 21 days. Reduce dose of ifosfamide and gallium nitrate by 25% if creatinine is >2 mg/dL; hold ifosfamide if urinary red blood cell count is >25/HPF on days 1 to 5; reduce VIG doses 20% for poor-risk patients (i.e., age >70 years, prior cisplatin therapy, prior nephrectomy or pelvic radiotherapy).

Selected Reading

Einhorn LH et al: Phase II trial of vinblastine, ifosfamide, and gallium combination chemotherapy in metastatic urothelial carcinoma, *J Clin Oncol* 12:2271-2276, 1994.

BRAIN TUMORS

Although the fifteenth most common cause of cancer and the tenth most frequent cause of cancer death, brain tumors are disproportionately devastating to the persona of the victim. They are treated surgically, when possible, with frequent radiation and/or chemotherapy postoperatively. The approach differs somewhat depending on whether the tumor is metastatic or primary and on its histology. Single-agent chemotherapy with carmustine (BCNU), lomustine (CCNU), high-dose methotrexate, or cisplatin may be as effective (or ineffective) as combination chemotherapy and is usually less toxic. Neoadjuvant therapy is being evaluated. Childhood brain tumors are almost always treated on cooperative group studies.

CARMUSTINE-CISPLATIN-RADIOTHERAPY

Carmustine. 40 mg/m^2/day intravenously on days 1 to 3.

Cisplatin. 40 mg/m^2/day intravenously on days 1 to 3.

NOTE: The drugs are given by continuous infusion, with the total dose of each being 120 mg/m^2 per cycle. If tolerated, cycles are repeated every 28 days for three cycles and then external beam radiation therapy is given in slightly different doses in the two reports.

Selected Readings

Gilbert MR et al: A phase II trial of continuous infusion chemotherapy, external beam radiotherapy, and local boost radiotherapy for malignant gliomas, *Proc Am Soc Clin Oncol* 12:176, 1993.

Grossman SA et al: BCNU/cisplatin followed by radiation in poor prognosis patients with high grade astrocytomas, *Proc Am Soc Clin Oncol* 11:149, 1992.

CYCLOPHOSPHAMIDE-VINCRISTINE

Cyclophosphamide. Up to 1000 mg/m^2 intravenously over a 1-hour period on days 1 and 2 with a goal of 1000 mg/m^2 each day.

Vincristine. 1.0 mg/m^2 (maximum, 2.0 mg) on day 1.

NOTE: Repeat every 3 or 4 weeks for 12 months or until progression.

Selected Reading

Longee DC et al: Treatment of patients with recurrent gliomas with cyclophosphamide and vincristine, *J Neurosurg* 72:583-588, 1990.

IFOSFAMIDE-CARMUSTINE-RADIOTHERAPY

Ifosfamide. 1200 mg/m^2 intravenously on days 1 to 5.

Carmustine. 30 mg/m^2 intravenously on days 1, 3, and 5.

NOTE: Concomitant with the start of chemotherapy, whole-brain irradiation is given in fractions with appropriate supporting care. After a therapy-free interval of approximately 5 weeks (depending on recovery of marrow depression), the concomitant radiotherapy and chemotherapy are repeated twice so that the whole brain receives 4500 cGy. Then the primary tumor is boosted to 5000 to 6000 cGy using smaller ports.

During radiotherapy courses, all patients receive oral dexamethasone 4 mg daily. The authors do not mention using mesna. We recommend giving mesna 400 mg/m² intravenously at 15 minutes, 4 hours, and 8 hours after starting ifosfamide on days 1 to 5.

Selected Reading
Lange OF, Haase K-D, Scheef W: Simultaneous radio- and chemotherapy of inoperable brain tumors, *Radiother Oncol* 8:309-314, 1987.

PCV PLUS RT–LOMUSTINE-VINCRISTINE-PROCARBAZINE

Whole-brain radiation.   180 to 200 cGy/day to a total of 6000 cGy.

Hydroxyurea.   400 mg/m² by mouth every other day of radiation therapy.

Within 14 days of completion of radiation therapy, give the following:

Lomustine.   110 mg/m² orally on day 1.

Procarbazine.   60 mg/m² orally on days 8 to 21.

Vincristine.   1.4 mg/m² intravenously on days 8 and 29.

NOTE: Repeat PCV every 6 to 8 weeks for 1 year or until tumor progression. This regimen apparently prolongs survival in astrocytoma but not in glioblastoma multiforme.

Selected Reading
Levin VA et al: Superiority of post-radiotherapy adjuvant chemotherapy with CCNU, procarbazine and vincristine (PCV) over BCNU for anaplastic gliomas: NCOG 6G61 final report, *Int J Radiat Oncol Biol Phys* 18:321-324, 1990.

BREAST CARCINOMA

Although it is now the second most common cause of cancer death in women, breast carcinoma remains the most frequent cancer in women. Initial therapy is usually surgical and often curative. Depending on stage, age, and receptor status, adjuvant therapy is frequently employed (i.e., radiation, hormonal, or cytotoxic chemotherapy or some combination thereof). Neoadjuvant therapy is being evaluated for large, bulky tumors. Recurrent or metastatic disease is often palliated with hormonal manipulation. This used to involve oophorectomy, hypophysectomy, or adrenalectomy in the premenopausal and estrogen therapy in the late postmenopausal patient. More recently, the antiestrogen tamoxifen has been the hormonal agent of first choice, with androgens (e.g., fluoxymesterone), progestins (e.g., megestrol acetate), or aromatase inhibitors (e.g., aminoglutethimide) used as secondary hormonal therapy. Several new hormonal agents have recently become available, including antiestrogens (e.g., toremifene), more specific aromatase inhibitors (e.g., arimidex), and luteinizing hormone–releasing hormone (LHRH) analogues (e.g., leuprolide and goserelin).

Many cytotoxic chemotherapeutic drugs have shown varying degrees of activity in the adjuvant or palliative treatment of breast cancer. For many years, the most widely used were cyclophosphamide, methotrexate, fluorouracil, doxorubicin, thiotepa, mitomycin, vinblastine, vincristine, and prednisone, alone or in various combinations, some of which are listed below. Activity has more recently been demonstrated for paclitaxel, epirubicin, mitoxantrone, ifosfamide, cisplatin, etoposide, docetaxel, vinorelbine, gemcitabine, and edatrexate. Some of these drugs are used as single agents. Various combinations of these agents have been and are being evaluated in clinical trials and some are in stage III trials with preliminary reports available. We list a few of the more well-studied regimens and a few of the early phase II trial combinations for salvage therapy with the caution that more experience with them is needed to establish their efficacy, dosage, and toxicity. Finally, there are high hopes for the curative potential of high-dose chemotherapy (HDC) with stem cell (bone marrow or peripheral blood stem cell) support. These are in various stages of evaluation in cancer centers and should be used only by those oncologists with special training in this area. To avoid the danger of inadvertently using HDC by error, we list those regimens in a separate HDC section in Chapter 9.

ADJUVANT METHOTREXATE-FLUOROURACIL

Methotrexate. 100 mg/m^2 intravenously on days 1 and 8.

Fluorouracil. 600 mg/m^2 intravenously 1 hour after methotrexate days 1 and 8.

Leucovorin. 10 mg/m^2 orally every 6 hours for six doses beginning 24 hours after methotrexate.

NOTE: A course is given every 28 days for 12 months.

Selected Readings

Fisher B et al: A randomized clinical trial evaluating sequential methotrexate and fluorouracil in the treatment of patients with node-negative breast cancer who have estrogen-receptor–negative tumors, *N Engl J Med* 320:473-478, 1989.

Fisher B et al: Sequential methotrexate and fluorouracil for the treatment of node-negative breast cancer patients with estrogen receptor–negative tumors: eight-year results from National Surgical Adjuvant Breast and Bowel Project (NSABP) B-13 and first report of findings from NSABP B-19 comparing methotrexate and fluorouracil with conventional cyclophosphamide, methotrexate, and fluorouracil, *J Clin Oncol* 14:1982-1992, 1996.

AC–DOXORUBICIN-CYCLOPHOSPHAMIDE

Doxorubicin. 60 mg/m^2 intravenously on day 1.

Cyclophosphamide. 600 mg/m^2 intravenously on day 1.

NOTE: Repeat the cycle every 21 days. Usual course is four cycles.

Selected Reading

Fisher B et al: Two months of doxorubicin-cyclophosphamide with and without interval reinduction therapy compared with six months of cyclophosphamide, methotrexate and fluorouracil in positive-node breast cancer patients with tamoxifen-nonresponsive tumors: results from the National Surgical Adjuvant Breast and Bowel Project B-15, *J Clin Oncol* 8:1483-1496, 1990.

ATC–DOXORUBICIN-PACLITAXEL-CYCLOPHOSPHAMIDE

Doxorubicin. 90 mg/m^2 intravenously on days 1, 15, and 29.

Paclitaxel. 250 mg/m^2 intravenously on days 43, 57, and 71 by 24-hour infusion.

Cyclophosphamide. 3000 mg/m^2 intravenously on days 85, 99, and 113.

NOTE: Each drug is repeated every 14 days for three courses, then the next drug for three courses, etc. For all nine cycles, support with 5 µg/kg G-CSF subcutaneously. To avoid hypersensitivity reactions with paclitaxel, premedicate with the usual three-drug regimen of dexamethasone, diphenhydramine, and cimetadine (or ranitidine).

Selected Reading

Hudis CA et al: Sequential adjuvant therapy with doxorubicin/paclitaxel/cyclophos-phamide for resectable breast cancer involving four or more axillary nodes, *Semin Oncol* 22(6 suppl 15):18-23, 1995.

AVM–DOXORUBICIN-VINBLASTINE-MITOMYCIN

Doxorubicin. 30 mg/m^2 intravenously on days 1 and 29.

Vinblastine. 6 mg/m^2 intravenously on days 1 and 29.

Mitomycin. 10 mg/m^2 intravenously on day 1.

NOTE: Repeat the cycle every 8 weeks; a salvage regimen.

Selected Reading

Luikart SD, Witman GB, Portlock CS: Adriamycin (doxorubicin), vinblastine, and mitomycin C combination chemotherapy in refractory breast carcinoma, *Cancer* 54:1252-1255, 1984.

CAF–CYCLOPHOSPHAMIDE-DOXORUBICIN-FLUOROURACIL

Cyclophosphamide. 500 mg/m^2 intravenously on day 1.

Doxorubicin. 50 mg/m^2 intravenously on day 1.

5-Fluorouracil. 500 mg/m^2 intravenously on day 1.

NOTE: The regimen differs from FAC only in that 5-fluorouracil is given on days 1 and 8 in FAC but is given only once per course in this regimen. Drugs are given every 21 days.

Selected Readings

Smalley RV: A comparison of cyclophosphamide, Adriamycin, and 5-fluorouracil (CAF) and cyclophosphamide, methotrexate, 5-fluorouracil, vincristine, and pred-nisone (CMFVP) in patients with advanced breast cancer, *Breast Cancer Res Treat* 3:209-220, 1983.

Smalley RV et al: A comparison of cyclophosphamide, Adriamycin, 5-fluorouracil, vincristine, prednisone (CMFVP) in patients with metastatic breast cancer, *Cancer* 40:625-632, 1977.

CAF: HIGH DOSE

Cyclophosphamide. 600 mg/m^2 intravenously on day 1.

Doxorubicin. 60 mg/m^2 intravenously on day 1.

5-Fluorouracil. 600 mg/m^2 intravenously on days 1 and 8.

NOTE: CAF, high dose produces neutropenia in the majority of cases and this may require G-CSF. Repeat the courses every 28 days for four courses.

Selected Readings

Budman DR et al: Initial findings of CALGB 8541: a dose and dose intensity trial of cyclophosphamide, doxorubicin, and 5-fluorouracil as adjuvant treatment of stage II, node +, female breast cancer, *Proc Am Soc Clin Oncol* 11:51, 1992.

Wood WC et al: Dose and dose intensity of adjuvant chemotherapy for stage II, node-positive breast carcinoma, *N Engl J Med* 330:1253-1259, 1994.

CFP—CYCLOPHOSPHAMIDE-FLUOROURACIL-PREDNISONE

Cyclophosphamide. 150 mg/m^2 intravenously on days 1 to 5.

5-Fluorouracil. 300 mg/m^2 intravenously on days 1 to 5.

Prednisone. 40 mg/day orally tapered by 10 mg weekly to 10 mg/day.

NOTE: Repeat the cycle every 5 weeks.

Selected Reading

Rosner D, Nemoto T, Lane WW: A randomized study of intensive versus moderate chemotherapy programs in metastatic breast cancer, *Cancer* 59:874-883, 1987.

CMF (ADJUVANT)—CYCLOPHOSPHAMIDE-METHOTREXATE-FLUOROURACIL

Below the Age of 60 Years

Cyclophosphamide. 100 mg/m^2 orally on days 1 to 14.

Methotrexate. 40 mg/m^2 intravenously on days 1 and 8.

5-Fluorouracil. 600 mg/m^2 intravenously on days 1 and 8.

Above the Age of 60 Years

Cyclophosphamide. 100 mg/m^2 orally on days 1 to 14.

Methotrexate. 30 mg/m^2 intravenously on days 1 and 8.

5-Fluorouracil. 400 mg/m^2 intravenously on days 1 and 8.

NOTE: Repeat the cycle every 28 days. Many clinicians make no change in dosage for patients over 60 years of age and use the higher dose at all ages.

Selected Readings

Bonadonna G et al: Combination chemotherapy as an adjuvant treatment in operable breast cancer, *N Engl J Med* 294:405-410, 1976.

Bonadonna G et al: Adjuvant cyclophosphamide, methotrexate and fluorouracil in node-positive breast cancer: the results of 20 years of follow-up, *N Engl J Med* 332:901-906, 1995.

CMF (INTRAVENOUS)—21 DAY

Cyclophosphamide. 600 mg/m^2 intravenously every 21 days.

Methotrexate. 40 mg/m² intravenously every 21 days.

5-Fluorouracil. 600 mg/m² intravenously every 21 days.

Selected Reading

Weiss RB et al: Adjuvant chemotherapy after conservative surgery plus irradiation versus modified radical mastectomy, *Am J Med* 83:455-463, 1987.

CMF (INTRAVENOUS)—28 DAYS

Cyclophosphamide. 600 mg/m² intravenously on days 1 and 8.

Methotrexate. 40 mg/m² intravenously on days 1 and 8.

5-Fluorouracil. 600 mg/m² intravenously on days 1 and 8.

NOTE: The Milan group and Dr. Bonadonna now regard this as their new "standard CMF." Repeat every 28 days. For adjuvant therapy in patients at high risk with more than four involved nodes, doxorubicin → CMF is preferred (see Buzzoni et al, 1991, in "Doxorubicin → CMF," the third combination forward).

Selected Readings

Bonadonna G et al: Milan adjuvant and neoadjuvant studies in stage I and II resectable breast cancer. In Salmon SE, ed: *Adjuvant therapy of cancer VI*, Philadelphia, 1990, WB Saunders, pp 169-173.

CMFP—CYCLOPHOSPHAMIDE-METHOTREXATE-FLUOROURACIL-PREDNISONE

Cyclophosphamide. 100 mg/m² by mouth on days 1 to 14.

Methotrexate. 30 to 40 mg/m² intravenously on days 1 and 8.

5-Fluorouracil. 400 to 600 mg/m² intravenously on days 1 and 8.

Prednisone. 40 mg/m² by mouth on days 1 to 14.

NOTE: The lower dose is for patients over 65 years of age. Repeat the therapy every 28 days.

Selected Readings

Marschke RF et al: Randomized clinical trial of CFP versus CMFP in women with metastatic breast cancer, *Cancer* 63:1931-1937, 1989.

COOPER REGIMEN

5-Fluorouracil. 12 mg/kg intravenously every week for 8 weeks and then every other week for 7 additional months.

Methotrexate. 0.7 mg/kg intravenously every week for 8 weeks and then every other week for 7 months.

Vincristine. 0.035 mg/kg intravenously every week for 5 weeks and then once monthly.

Cyclophosphamide. 2 mg/kg/day by mouth for 9 months.

Prednisone. 0.75 mg/kg/day by mouth for 10 days, then 0.375 mg/kg/day for 10 days, then 0.1875 mg/kg/day for 10 days, then 5 mg/day for 20 days, and then discontinue.

NOTE: The severe neurotoxicity of vincristine and the frequent side effects of prednisone compared to their minimal contribution to the efficacy of the regimen have caused many clinicians to use CMF alone or other regimens.

Selected Reading
Cooper RG, Holland JF, Glidewell O: Adjuvant chemotherapy of breast cancer, *Cancer* 44:793-798, 1979.

DOXORUBICIN → CMF

Doxorubicin. 75 mg/m^2 by IV bolus every 21 days for four courses.

Cyclophosphamide. Beginning with course five, 600 mg/m^2 intravenously on days 1, 22, . . . to eight courses.

Methotrexate. 40 mg/m^2 intravenously on days 1, 22, . . . to eight courses.

Fluorouracil. 600 mg/m^2 intravenously on days 1, 22, . . . to eight courses.

NOTE: This protocol is published as adjuvant therapy for patients with four or more involved nodes. Therapy is given every 21 days at full dose unless the patient is too neutropenic or thrombocytopenic. In such a situation, therapy is postponed a week or, rarely, 2 weeks. The total therapy is 12 courses, four of doxorubicin and eight of CMF.

Selected Readings
Bonadonna G, Zambetti M, Valagussa P: Sequential or alternating doxorubicin and CMF regimens in breast cancer with more than three positive nodes, *JAMA* 273:542-547, 1995.
Buzzoni R et al: Adjuvant chemotherapy with doxorubicin plus cyclophosphamide, methotrexate, and fluorouracil in the treatment of resectable breast cancer with more than three positive axillary nodes, *J Clin Oncol* 9:2134-2140, 1991.

DUKE HIGH-DOSE INTENSITY AFM

5-Fluorouracil. 750 mg/m^2 daily by continuous IV infusion on days 1 to 5.

Doxorubicin. 25 mg/m^2 on days 3 to 5 by IV bolus.

Methotrexate. 250 mg/m^2 intravenously on day 15.

Leucovorin. 12.5 mg by mouth 24 hours after methotrexate and every 6 hours for six doses (total).

NOTE: Repeat every 21 days. The treatment can be given with an outpatient pump. The maximum doxorubicin dose (cumulative) is 400 mg/m^2. This program has been used for induction before high-dose chemotherapy with autologous bone marrow or peripheral stem cell support.

Selected Reading
Jones RB et al: The Duke AFM program: intensive induction chemotherapy for metastatic breast cancer, *Cancer* 66:431-436, 1990.

FEC—FLUOROURACIL-EPIRUBICIN-CYCLOPHOSPHAMIDE

5-Fluorouracil. 500 mg/m^2 intravenously on day 1.

Epirubicin. 60 mg/m^2 intravenously on day 1.

Cyclophosphamide. 500 mg/m^2 intravenously on day 1.

NOTE: Repeat every 28 days to a cumulative maximum epirubicin dose of 1000 mg/m^2 or to evidence of progression. Reduce all three drugs 20% to 40% in subsequent courses for leukocyte nadirs less than 1500 and 1000 µL, respectively.

Selected Reading

Blomquist C et al: Influence of treatment schedule on toxicity and efficacy of cyclophosphamide, epirubicin, and fluorouracil in metastatic breast cancer: a randomized trial comparing weekly and every four week administration, *J Clin Oncol* 11:467-473, 1993.

FEP—FLUOROURACIL-EPIRUBICIN-CISPLATIN

5-Fluorouracil. 200 mg/m^2 daily by continuous IV infusion on days 1 to 7.

Epirubicin. 50 mg/m^2 intravenously on day 1.

Cisplatin. 60 mg/m^2 intravenously on day 1.

NOTE: The 5-fluorouracil is begun 4 hours before the cisplatin, which is given over 1 hour after 4 hours of prehydration and with 6 hours of posthydration. Cycles are repeated every 3 weeks to a maximum of eight cycles (epirubicin 400 mg/m^2). A potent antiemetic regimen is necessary.

Selected Reading

Jones AL et al: Phase II study of continuous infusion fluorouracil with epirubicin and cisplatin in patients with metastatic and locally advanced breast cancer: an active new regimen, *J Clin Oncol* 12:1259-1265, 1994.

HOPKINS 16-WEEK DOSE-INTENSE REGIMEN

Cyclophosphamide. 100 mg/m^2 by mouth for 7 days (single daily AM dose).

Doxorubicin. 40 mg/m^2 by IV bolus on day 1.

Vincristine. 1 mg by IV bolus on day 1.

Methotrexate. 100 mg/m^2 intravenously on day 1, hour 0.

5-Fluorouracil. 600 mg/m^2 intravenously 20 hours after methotrexate on day 2.

Leucovorin. 10 mg/m^2 by mouth every 6 hours for six doses starting 24 hours after methotrexate.

NOTE: On weeks 1, 3, 5, 7, 9, 11, 13, and 15, give the above regimen. On weeks 2, 4, 6, 8, 10, 12, 14, and 16, substitute a continuous infusion of 5-fluorouracil, 300 mg/m^2/day, for the 5-fluorouracil and leucovorin on days 1 and 2.

Selected Readings

Abeloff MD et al: Sixteen-week dose-intense chemotherapy in the adjuvant treatment of breast cancer, *J Natl Cancer Inst* 82:570-574, 1990.

Beveridge RA et al: Sixteen-week dose intense chemotherapy for breast cancer, *Proc Am Soc Clin Oncol* 7:13, 1988.

IFOSFAMIDE-MITOXANTRONE

Ifosfamide. 2000 mg/m^2 intravenously over 1 hour on days 1 to 3.

Mesna. 400 mg/m^2 IV bolus immediately before and 4 hours after ifosfamide administration and then 2000 mg orally 8 hours after ifosfamide on days 1 to 3.

Mitoxantrone. 12 mg/m^2 IV bolus on day 3.

NOTE: Repeat course every 21 days.

Selected Reading

Perez JE et al: Ifosfamide and mitoxantrone as first line chemotherapy for metastatic breast cancer, *J Clin Oncol* 11:461-466, 1993.

MINI-ICE—IFOSFAMIDE-CARBOPLATIN-ETOPOSIDE

Ifosfamide. 3000 mg/m^2 intravenously on days 1 to 3.

Carboplatin. 200 mg/m^2 intravenously on days 1 and 2.

Etoposide. 150 mg/m^2 intravenously twice a day for 2 days.

Mesna. 1000 mg/m^2 30 minutes before and 4 and 8 hours after ifosfamide on days 1 to 3.

NOTE: Ifosfamide is begun at time zero for 1 hour and is followed by etoposide over 11 hours. Then carboplatin is given over 1 hour followed by etoposide over 11 hours. Day 2 is a repetition of day 1. Day 3 involves only the ifosfamide and mesna. Regimen is repeated every 28 days.

Selected Reading

Perkins JB, Fields KF, Elfenbein GJ: Ifosfamide/carboplatin/etoposide chemotherapy for metastatic breast cancer with or without autologous hematopoietic stem cell transplantation: evaluation of dose response relationship, *Semin Oncol* 22(3 suppl 7):5-8, 1995.

MITOXANTRONE-CYCLOPHOSPHAMIDE-FLUOROURACIL

Mitoxantrone. 10 mg/m^2 intravenously on day 1.

Cyclophosphamide. 500 mg/m^2 intravenously on day 1.

5-Fluorouracil. 1000 mg/m^2 intravenously on day 1.

NOTE: Repeat the cycle every 21 days.

Selected Reading

Holmes FA et al: Mitoxantrone, cyclophosphamide, and fluorouracil in metastatic breast cancer unresponsive to hormonal therapy, *Cancer* 59:1992-1999, 1987.

MITOXANTRONE–FLUOROURACIL–HIGH-DOSE LEUCOVORIN

Mitoxantrone. 12 mg/m^2 intravenously on day 1.

Leucovorin (high dose). 300 mg intravenously on days 1 to 3 over 1 hour before 5-Fluorouracil.

5-Fluorouracil. 350 mg/m^2 by IV push on days 1 to 3.

NOTE: Treatment courses are repeated every 21 days. Patients older than 65 years receive mitoxantrone, 9 mg/m^2, on day 1 unless the leukocyte count is greater than 2000/µL; if so, they get the full 12 mg/m^2.

Selected Reading

Hainsworth JD et al: Mitoxantrone, fluorouracil, and high-dose leucovorin: an effective, well-tolerated regimen for metastatic breast cancer, *J Clin Oncol* 9:1731-1736, 1991.

3M–MITOMYCIN-MITOXANTRONE-METHOTREXATE

Mitomycin. 7 mg/m^2 on day 1.

Mitoxantrone. 7 mg/m^2 on days 1 and 22.

Methotrexate. 35 mg/m^2 on days 1 and 22.

NOTE: Repeat course every 6 weeks. Those patients who have surgery first should receive four courses. Those who have neoadjuvant therapy should have two courses before surgery and radiation (if necessary), and two courses afterward. Tamoxifen 20 mg/day is given concomitantly with 3M and is then continued for 5 years. For those who sustain an adverse reaction between mitomycin and tamoxifen, the tamoxifen can be started after the completion of chemotherapy, or the mitomycin may be omitted and the mitoxantrone dose raised to 11 mg/m^2 (an equivalent dose intensity) and the tamoxifen given concomitantly (2M + T).

Selected Reading

Powles TJ et al: Randomized trial of chemoendocrine therapy started before or after surgery for treatment of primary breast cancer, *J Clin Oncol* 13:547-552, 1995.

MV–MITOMYCIN-VINBLASTINE

Mitomycin. 10 mg/m^2 intravenously on days 1 and 28.

Vinblastine. 5 mg/m^2 intravenously on days 1, 14, 28, and 42.

Subsequent cycles:

Mitomycin. 10 mg/m^2 intravenously on day 1.

Vinblastine. 5 mg/m^2 intravenously on days 1 and 21.

NOTE: Repeat subsequent cycles every 6 to 8 weeks. Do not exceed total cumulative dose of 50 mg/m^2 of mitomycin.

Selected Reading

Garewal HS et al: Treatment of advanced breast cancer with mitomycin C combined with vinblastine or vindisine, *J Clin Oncol* 1:772-775, 1983.

PACLITAXEL-CISPLATIN

Paclitaxel. 90 mg/m^2 intravenously over 3 hours on day 1.

Cisplatin. 60 mg/m^2 intravenously over 3 hours on day 1.

NOTE: Give the cisplatin after the paclitaxel infusion is completed. To avoid hypersensitivity reactions, premedicate with the usual dexamethasone, diphenhydramine, and cimetadine or ranitidine. Antiemetics and hydration are also important.

Selected Reading

Tolcher AW, Gelmon KA: Interim results of a phase I/II study of biweekly paclitaxel and cisplatin in patients with metastatic breast cancer, *Semin Oncol* 22(4 suppl 8):28-32, 1995.

PACLITAXEL-DOXORUBICIN

Doxorubicin. 50 mg/m^2 intravenously followed 4 hours later by the following:

Paclitaxel. 150 mg/m^2 over 24 hours by continuous infusion.

NOTE: To avoid hypersensitivity reactions to paclitaxel, premedicate with dexamethasone, diphenhydramine, and cimetadine or ranitidine. Repeat courses every 3 weeks as tolerated.

Selected Reading

Sledge GW Jr: Doxorubicin/paclitaxel combination chemotherapy for metastatic breast cancer: the Eastern Cooperative Oncology Group experience, *Semin Oncol* 22 (5 suppl 12):123-125, 1995.

PACLITAXEL–HIGH-DOSE FLUOROURACIL/LEUCOVORIN

Leucovorin. 500 mg/m^2 IV infusion over 2 hours followed by:

5-Fluorouracil. 2000 mg/m^2 IV infusion over 24 hours with both drugs given on days 1, 8, 15, 22, 29, and 36.

Paclitaxel. 175 mg/m^2 IV infusion over 3 hours before starting leucovorin on days 1 and 22.

NOTE: Usual premedication for paclitaxel. After a 2-week rest period, the regimen is repeated as many times as it is effective and tolerable.

Selected Reading

Klassen U et al: Phase I/II study with paclitaxel in combination with weekly high-dose 5-fluorouracil/folinic acid in the treatment of metastatic breast cancer: an interim analysis, *Semin Oncol* 22(6 suppl 14):7-11, 1995.

VATH–VINBLASTINE-DOXORUBICIN-THIOTEPA-FLUOXYMESTERONE

Vinblastine. 4.5 mg/m^2 intravenously on day 1.

Doxorubicin. 45 mg/m^2 intravenously on day 1.

Thiotepa. 12 mg/m^2 intravenously on day 1.

Fluoxymesterone. 30 mg/day by mouth for 21 days.

NOTE: Repeat the cycle every 21 days. Discontinue doxorubicin therapy at a cumulative dose of 550 mg/m^2.

Selected Reading

Hart RD, Perloff M, Holland JF: One-day VATH (vinblastine, Adriamycin, thiotepa and halotestin) therapy for advanced breast cancer refractory to prior chemotherapy, *Cancer* 48:1522-1527, 1981.

VINORELBINE-DOXORUBICIN

Doxorubicin. 50 mg/m^2 intravenously on day 1.

Vinorelbine. 25 mg/m^2 intravenously on days 1 and 28.

NOTE: Repeat cycles every 3 weeks up to toxicity or a maximum of 11 cycles (550 mg/m^2 of doxorubicin) or until recurrence.

Selected Readings

Hochster HS: A combined doxorubicin/vinorelbine (Navelbine) therapy in the treatment of advanced breast cancer, *Semin Oncol* 22(2 suppl 5):55-60, 1995.

Spielmann M et al: Phase II trial of vinorelbine/doxorubicin as first-line therapy of advanced breast cancer, *J Clin Oncol* 12:1764-1770, 1994.

CARCINOID (MALIGNANT) AND ISLET CELL CARCINOMA

These are not common tumors. The carcinoid syndrome occurs in about 10% of patients with malignant carcinoid. When it occurs, consider the use of the somatostatin analogue octreotide before chemotherapy for carcinoid. Symptom relief may sometimes be obtained at lesser cost with cyproheptadine and loperamide (Imodium) or diphenoxylate (Lomotil). For metastatic disease, the active palliative agents include doxorubicin, cisplatin, streptozocin, 5-fluorouracil, cyclophosphamide, and interferon alpha. There are no convincing randomized studies demonstrating the superiority of combination regimens over single-agent therapy, but combinations seem to be preferred by most experts.

NOTE: Consider the use of the somatostatin analogue octreotide before chemotherapy for symptomatic carcinoid.

CISPLATIN-ETOPOSIDE

Cisplatin. 100 mg/m^2 intravenously on day 1.

Etoposide. 120 mg/m^2 intravenously on day 1.

NOTE: Repeat the cycle every 28 days. A vigorous hydration regimen is needed for cisplatin.

Selected Reading

Davis S et al: Treatment of metastatic carcinoid and Merkel cell tumors with cisplatin and etoposide, *Proc Am Soc Clin Oncol* 6:73, 1987.

DOXORUBICIN-CISPLATIN

Doxorubicin. 50 mg/m^2 intravenously on day 1.

Cisplatin. 50 mg/m^2 intravenously on day 1 with hydration.

NOTE: Repeat the cycle every 3 or 4 weeks.

Selected Reading

Sridhar KS et al: Doxorubicin plus cisplatin in the treatment of apudomas, *Cancer* 55:2634-2637, 1985.

FAC-S—FLUOROURACIL-DOXORUBICIN-CYCLOPHOSPHAMIDE-STREPTOZOCIN

5-Fluorouracil. 400 mg/m^2 (300 mg/m^2) intravenously on days 1 and 8.

Doxorubicin. 30 mg/m^2 (15 mg/m^2) intravenously on day 1.

Cyclophosphamide. 75 mg/m^2 (50 mg/m^2) orally on days 1 to 14.

Streptozocin. 400 mg/m^2 (200 mg/m^2) intravenously on days 1 and 8.

NOTE: Poor-risk patients were given the doses in parentheses. Poor risk was defined by any one of the following: age older than 70 years, total bilirubin level greater than 1.5 mg/dL, SGOT level greater than three times normal, 5-hydroxyindoleacetic acid (5-HIAA) level greater than 150 mg/24 hr, carcinoid syndrome, or bone marrow involvement by tumor. Courses were given every 4 weeks. Patients with heart disease did not receive doxorubicin but were given the following:

5-Fluorouracil. 600 mg/m^2 (400 mg/m^2) intravenously on days 1 and 8.

Cyclophosphamide. 100 mg/m^2 (75 mg/m^2) orally on days 1 to 14.

Streptozocin. 600 mg/m^2 (400 mg/m^2) intravenously on days 1 and 8.

Selected Reading

Bukowski RM et al: A phase 2 trial of combination chemotherapy in patients with metastatic carcinoid tumors: a Southwest Oncology Group study, *Cancer* 60:2891-2895, 1987.

SC—STREPTOZOCIN-CYCLOPHOSPHAMIDE

Streptozocin. 500 mg/m^2 intravenously for 5 consecutive days.

Cyclophosphamide. 1000 mg/m^2 intravenously on day 1.

NOTE: Repeat streptozocin every 6 weeks and cyclophosphamide every 3 weeks. If the 5-HIAA level exceeds 150 mg/24 hr or there are florid manifestations of the carcinoid syndrome, begin with half doses and gradually work up to the recommended doses.

Selected Reading

Moertel CG, Hanley JA: Combination chemotherapy trials in metastatic carcinoid syndrome, *Cancer Clin Trials* 2:327-334, 1979.

SD—STREPTOZOCIN-DOXORUBICIN (ISLET CELL CARCINOMA OR CARCINOID)

Streptozocin. 500 mg/m^2 intravenously on days 1 to 5.

Doxorubicin. 50 mg/m^2 intravenously on days 1 and 22.

NOTE: Repeat every 42 days. The cumulative dose of doxorubicin should not exceed 500 mg/m^2. This drug combination has also been used for carcinoid.

Selected Reading

Moertel CG et al: Streptozocin-doxorubicin, streptozocin-fluorouracil, or chlorozotocin in the treatment of advanced islet-cell carcinoma, *N Engl J Med* 326:519-523, 1992.

SF–STREPTOZOCIN-FLUOROURACIL

Streptozocin. 500 mg/m^2/day intravenously on days 1 to 5.

5-Fluorouracil. 500 mg/m^2/day intravenously on days 1 to 5.

NOTE: Repeat the cycle every 28 days.

Selected Readings

Chernicoff D et al: Combination chemotherapy for islet cell carcinoma and metastatic carcinoid tumors with 5-fluorouracil and streptozotocin, *Cancer Treat Rep* 63:795-796, 1979.

CARCINOMA OF UNKNOWN PRIMARY

Carcinoma of unknown primary (CUP) accounts for about 5% to 10% of all cancer patients. These patients present with biopsy-proven metastatic disease, with no known primary organ involved. They should be designated as having neoplasia of unknown primary site. Some are poorly differentiated and with special histochemical studies (e.g., immunoperoxidase staining) will be found to be melanomas, sarcomas, neuroendocrine tumors, mesotheliomas, lymphomas, or germ cell tumors and should be treated as such. Some remain undiagnosed even at autopsy. Other more differentiated tumors that present in the axilla in women are usually breast cancers, whereas those that present in the lymph nodes of the neck are usually of respiratory origin (i.e., lung, pharynx, or larynx) or occasionally of thyroid or breast origin and are treated accordingly. Still others are fairly well differentiated adenocarcinomas below the diaphragm and are usually of pancreatic, prostatic, or ovarian origin.

Recently a group has been identified who have poorly differentiated carcinomas in the midline, usually mediastinum, retroperitoneum, or lymph nodes. Men predominate 3:1 and are usually age 30 to 55, with rapid progression of symptoms and objective evidence of rapid tumor growth. Only 20% have elevations of beta-HCG or alpha-fetoprotein. This group represents 30% of the total group of CUP. Active drugs for CUP include cisplatin, carboplatin, paclitaxel, etoposide, vinblastine, bleomycin, 5-fluorouracil–leucovorin, doxorubicin, and mitomycin. These drugs are used in combinations that usually (but not always) include a platinum compound. Some of the regimens used in testicular and extragonadal germ cell cancer are also effective for CUP.

In the poorly differentiated carcinoma and adenocarcinoma group, the patient's tumors are rapidly responsive to platinum-based chemotherapy, with one fourth achieving a complete response, two thirds an objective response, and one sixth going on to long-term survival (more than 5 years). High-dose chemotherapy with bone marrow or stem cell support is being evaluated for patients with refractory or recurrent disease.

PACLITAXEL-CARBOPLATIN-ETOPOSIDE

Paclitaxel. 200 mg/m^2 intravenously over 1 hour on day 1.

Carboplatin. Target dose to AUC 6 intravenously on day 1 (see Appendix A, Table A-6).

Etoposide. 50 mg/100 mg total dose, orally, alternating on days 1 to 10.

NOTE: Give four courses at 21-day intervals. Give usual premedication for paclitaxel.

Selected Reading

Hainsworth JD et al: Carcinoma of unknown primary site (CUP): a phase II trial of paclitaxel, carboplatin and etoposide, *Proc Am Soc Clin Oncol* 15:453, 1996.

PVB—CISPLATIN-VINBLASTINE-BLEOMYCIN AND PEB—CISPLATIN-ETOPOSIDE-BLEOMYCIN

Cisplatin. 20 mg/m^2 intravenously on days 1 to 5.

Vinblastine. 0.15 mg/kg intravenously on days 1 and 2.

Bleomycin. 30 units total, on days 2, 9, and 16 of each course.

NOTE: Courses are given every 3 weeks for three or four courses. The vinblastine may be replaced by etoposide 100 mg/m^2 intravenously on days 1 to 5 of each course. Many find PEB more efficacious and less toxic.

Selected Readings

Greco FA, Vaughn WK, Hainsworth JD: Advanced poorly differentiated carcinoma of unknown primary site: recognition of a treatable syndrome, *Ann Intern Med* 104:547-553, 1986.

Hainsworth JD, Johnson DH, Greco FA: The role of cisplatin/bleomycin-based chemotherapy in the treatment of poorly differentiated carcinoma of unknown primary site, *Semin Oncol* 19(2 suppl 5):54-57, 1992.

CERVICAL CARCINOMA

Cervical carcinoma is the most common malignancy of women worldwide and the third most common in the United States. Early diagnosis has dramatically reduced the death rate because early stage disease is frequently curable by surgery and/or radiation therapy. Current studies suggest that the efficacy of radiation is enhanced by the concomitant use of hydroxyurea or cisplatin. Neoadjuvant therapy is being evaluated. Recurrent or metastatic disease is treated with chemotherapy for palliation. Active drugs include, cisplatin, carboplatin, doxorubicin, epirubicin, ifosfamide, dibromodulcitol, bleomycin, vincristine, methotrexate, irinotecan, paclitaxel, and altretamine. There are no controlled studies demonstrating a superior response to combination chemotherapy compared with single-drug therapy, but several studies are in progress to evaluate some new combinations. Further considerations include histology, renal function, and the effect of prior radiation therapy, which may change the sensitivity of the tumor to therapeutic agents and can compromise the pelvic bone marrow.

ADENOCARCINOMA REGIMEN

5-Fluorouracil. 500 to 800 mg/m^2 by IV infusion over a 76-hour period.

Doxorubicin. 40 to 50 mg/m^2 by IV infusion over a 76-hour period.

Cisplatin. 50 to 60 mg/m^2 by IV infusion over a 76-hour period.

NOTE: Repeat cycle every 28 days as tolerated.

Selected Reading

Kavanagh JJ et al: Combination chemotherapy for metastatic or recurrent adenocarcinoma of the cervix, *J Clin Oncol* 10:1621-1623, 1987.

BIC–BLEOMYCIN-IFOSFAMIDE-CARBOPLATIN

Bleomycin. 30 units intravenously on day 1.

Ifosfamide. 2000 mg/m^2 intravenously over 2 hours on days 1 to 3.

Carboplatin. 200 mg/m^2 intravenously on day 1.

Mesna. 400 mg/m^2 intravenously at 15 minutes, at 4 hours, and at 8 hours (800 mg/m^2 if given orally) after the start of each dose of ifosfamide.

NOTE: Treatment is usually given on an outpatient basis every 28 days.

Selected Readings

Murad AM, Santiago FF, Triginelli SA: A phase II trial of BIC (bleomycin, ifosfamide, and carboplatin) in advanced cervical carcinoma, *Proc Am Soc Clin Oncol* 11:229, 1992.

Murad AM, Triginelli SA, Ribalta JCL: Phase II trial of bleomycin, ifosfamide, and carboplatin in metastatic cervical cancer, *J Clin Oncol* 12:55-59, 1994.

BIP–BLEOMYCIN-IFOSFAMIDE-CISPLATIN

Bleomycin. 30 units in 3 L of 5% dextrose or normal saline over a 24-hour period on day 1.

Cisplatin. 50 mg/m^2 by slow IV bolus on day 2.

Ifosfamide. 5000 mg/m^2 in 3 L of 5% dextrose or normal saline over a 24-hour period on day 2.

Mesna. 6000 mg/m^2 administered by continuous infusion concurrent with the ifosfamide and for 12 hours thereafter.

NOTE: During treatment, maintain the urine output at 100 mL/hr. Repeat the treatment every 21 days.

Selected Reading

Buxton EJ et al: Combination bleomycin, ifosfamide, and cisplatin chemotherapy in cervical cancer, *J Natl Cancer Inst* 81:359-361, 1989.

IFOSFAMIDE-CARBOPLATIN

Ifosfamide. 5000 mg/m^2 by continuous IV infusion on day 1.

Carboplatin. 300 mg/m^2 intravenously over 30 minutes on day 1.

Mesna. 9200 mg total dose by continuous 36-hour infusion starting on day 1.

NOTE: Repeat every 4 weeks if WBC count >3000/µL, platelet count >100,000/µL, and creatinine clearance >60 mL/min. If these levels are not reached, delay up to 2 weeks as necessary.

Selected Reading

Kuhnle H et al: Phase II study of carboplatin/ifosfamide in untreated advanced cervical cancer, *Cancer Chemother Pharmacol* 26:S33-S35, 1990.

MVAC–METHOTREXATE-VINBLASTINE-DOXORUBICIN-CISPLATIN

Methotrexate. 30 mg/m^2 intravenously on days 1, 15, and 22.

Vinblastine. 3 mg/m^2 intravenously on days 2, 15, and 22.

Doxorubicin. 30 mg/m^2 intravenously on day 2.

Cisplatin. 70 mg/m^2 intravenously on day 2.

NOTE: See discussion note of M-VAC in the section on bladder cancer.

Selected Reading

Long HJ, Cross WG, Wisead HS: MVAC: a highly active combination chemotherapy regimen in advanced/recurrent cancer of the uterine cervix and vagina, *Proc Am Soc Clin Oncol* 9:158, 1990.

COLON CARCINOMA

Colon carcinoma is the fourth most common type of cancer and the second most frequent cause of cancer death. This is a surgically treatable and often curable tumor when confined to the bowel. There is convincing evidence in stage III (Duke's C) that adjuvant chemotherapy with 5-fluorouracil and levamisole or 5-fluorouracil and leucovorin can significantly delay recurrence and may prolong life. It is not yet clear whether this is true of stage II (Duke's B). Metastatic disease (stage IV) may be palliated with chemotherapy with 5-fluorouracil plus leucovorin or interferon-alpha, as well as with other modulators (PALA) in a variety of combinations. Irinotecan is a new FDA-approved drug that has significant activity in patients who fail 5-fluorouracil therapy. Tomudex is a new experimental drug that shows promise for colon carcinoma. Gemcitabine, approved for pancreatic cancer, is being evaluated for colon cancer. The oral formulation UFT (tegafur and uracil) is completing its experimental trials in colon cancer and an FDA filing is planned for later this year.

ADJUVANT FLUOROURACIL-LEUCOVORIN

NOTE: Four large studies used somewhat different doses and schedules of the two drugs after surgery. The 3-year disease-free survivals and overall survivals were quite similar (Shulman and Schilsky, 1995). Doses are listed with references.

Selected Reading

Shulman K, Schilsky RL: Adjuvant therapy of colon cancer, *Semin Oncol* 22:600-610, 1995.

NSABP-CO3 Trial

5-Fluorouracil. 500 mg/m^2 by IV bolus.

Leucovorin. 500 mg/m^2 intravenously over 2 hours.

NOTE: Give leucovorin over 2 hours, then 1 hour later give 5-fluorouracil bolus. Both drugs are given 1 day a week for a 6-week course. After a 2-week rest, a new course is begun and pattern is repeated for six courses.

Selected Reading

Wolmark AN et al: The benefit of leucovorin-modulated fluorouracil as postoperative adjuvant therapy for primary colon cancer: results from National Surgical Adjuvant Breast and Bowel Project Protocol C-03, *J Clin Oncol* 11:1879-1887, 1993.

Impact Study

5-Fluorouracil. 370 to 400 mg/m^2/day intravenously on days 1 to 5.

Leucovorin. 200 mg/m^2/day intravenously on days 1 to 5.

NOTE: Drugs given every 28 days for six cycles.

Selected Reading

International Multicentre Pooled Analysis of Colon Cancer Trials (IMPACT) Investigators: efficacy of adjuvant fluorouracil and folinic acid in colon cancer, *Lancet* 345:939-944, 1995.

NCCTG Study

5-Fluorouracil. 425 mg/m^2 IV bolus on days 1 to 5.

Leucovorin. 20 mg/m^2 IV bolus on days 1 to 5.

NOTE: Drugs are repeated every 4 weeks for 6 months.

Selected Reading

O'Connell M et al: An intergroup trial of intensive course 5-FU and low dose leucovorin as surgical adjuvant therapy for high-risk colon cancer, *Proc Am Soc Clin Oncol* 12:190, 1993.

Italian Study

5-Fluorouracil. 400 mg/m^2 IV bolus on days 1 to 5.

Leucovorin. 200 mg/m^2 IV bolus on days 1 to 5.

NOTE: Drugs are repeated every 4 weeks for 12 cycles.

Selected Reading

Francini G et al: Folinic acid and 5-fluorouracil as adjuvant chemotherapy in colon cancer, *Gastroenterology* 106:899-906, 1994.

ADJUVANT FLUOROURACIL-LEVAMISOLE

5-Fluorouracil. 450 mg/m^2/day by IV bolus on days 1 to 5 and, beginning on day 28, 450 mg/m^2 intravenously weekly.

Levamisole. 150 mg/day (50 mg every 8 hours) orally on days 1 to 3, repeated every other week.

NOTE: Treatment is continued for 52 weeks. Recent studies suggest that 26 weeks of therapy yield approximately equivalent results.

Selected Readings

Laurie JA et al: Surgical adjuvant therapy of large-bowel carcinoma: an evaluation of levamisole and the combination of levamisole and fluorouracil, *J Clin Oncol* 7:1447-1456, 1989.

Moertel CG et al: Levamisole and fluorouracil for adjuvant therapy of resected colon carcinoma, *N Engl J Med* 322:352-358, 1990.

Moertel CG et al: Fluorouracil plus levamisole as effective adjuvant therapy after resection of stage III colon carcinoma: a final report, *Ann Intern Med* 122:321-326, 1995.

FLUOROURACIL–INTERFERON ALFA-2A

5-Fluorouracil. 750 mg/m^2/day by continuous IV infusion on days 1 to 5 and then 750 mg/m^2/wk by IV bolus beginning on day 15.

Interferon alfa-2a. 9 million units subcutaneously 3 times weekly beginning on day 1.

Selected Readings

Wadler S et al: Fluorouracil and recombinant alfa-2a-interferon: an active regimen against advanced colorectal carcinoma, *J Clin Oncol* 7:1769-1775, 1989.

Wadler S et al: Phase II trial of fluorouracil and recombinant interferon alfa-2a in patients with advanced colorectal carcinoma: an Eastern Cooperative Oncology Group study, *J Clin Oncol* 9:1806-1810, 1991.

FLUOROURACIL-LEUCOVORIN: HIGH DOSE

Leucovorin. 500 mg/m^2 in a 2-hour IV infusion in normal saline; repeat every week for 6 weeks.

5-Fluorouracil. 600 mg/m^2 by IV bolus 1 hour after the start of leucovorin; repeat every week for 6 weeks.

Selected Reading

Petrelli N et al: A prospective randomized trial of 5-fluorouracil versus 5-fluorouracil and high-dose leucovorin versus 5-fluorouracil and methotrexate in previously untreated patients with advanced colorectal carcinoma, *J Clin Oncol* 5:1559-1565, 1987.

FLUOROURACIL-LEUCOVORIN: LOW DOSE

5-Fluorouracil. 425 mg/m^2/day by IV bolus on days 1 to 5.

Leucovorin. 20 mg/m^2/day by IV bolus on days 1 to 5.

NOTE: Repeat the treatment at 4 weeks, 8 weeks, and then every 5 weeks.

Selected Readings

Poon MA et al: Biochemical modulation of fluorouracil: evidence of significant improvement of survival and quality of life in patients with advanced colorectal carcinoma, *J Clin Oncol* 7:1407-1418, 1989.

Poon MA et al: Biochemical modulation of fluorouracil with leucovorin: confirmatory evidence of improved therapeutic efficacy in advanced colorectal cancer, *J Clin Oncol* 9:1967-1972, 1991.

MOF-STREP—SEMUSTINE-VINCRISTINE-FLUOROURACIL-STREPTOZOCIN

Semustine. 30 mg/m^2 orally on days 1 to 5 every 10 weeks.

Vincristine. 1 mg intravenously on day 1 every 5 weeks.

5-Fluorouracil. 300 mg/m^2 intravenously on days 1 to 5 every 5 weeks.

Streptozocin. 500 mg/m^2 intravenously on day 1 and weekly.

NOTE: This regimen is now of historic interest only, but it is frequently referred to as a point of comparison for one of the "active" regimens for colon cancer. Semustine is no longer used in the United States for new patients.

Selected Reading

Kemeny N et al: Therapy for metastatic colorectal carcinoma with a combination of methyl-CCNU, 5-fluorouracil, vincristine, and streptozotocin (MOF-Strep), *Cancer* 45:876-881, 1980.

FLUOROURACIL-LEUCOVORIN CONTINUOUS INFUSION

Leucovorin. 500 mg/m^2/day by continuous IV infusion for 5.5 days.

5-Fluorouracil. 370 mg/m^2/day by IV bolus for 5 days (first dose given 24 hours after initiation of the leucovorin infusion).

NOTE: Repeat every 28 days.

Selected Reading

Doroshow JH et al: Prospective randomized comparison of fluorouracil versus fluorouracil and high-dose continuous infusion leucovorin calcium for the treatment of advanced measurable colorectal cancer in patients previously unexposed to chemotherapy, *J Clin Oncol* 8:491-501, 1990.

SEQUENTIAL METHOTREXATE-FLUOROURACIL-LEUCOVORIN

Methotrexate. 200 mg/m^2 intravenously over a 30-minute period on day 1.

5-Fluorouracil. 600 mg/m^2 by IV bolus 24 hours after methotrexate.

Leucovorin. 10 mg/m^2 orally every 6 hours for six doses beginning 24 hours after methotrexate.

NOTE: Courses are repeated every 2 weeks.

Selected Reading

Marsh JC et al: The influence of drug interval on the effect of methotrexate and fluorouracil in the treatment of advanced colorectal cancer, *J Clin Oncol* 9:371-380, 1991.

ENDOMETRIAL CANCER

Endometrial cancer is the most common malignancy of the female genital tract in the United States. Early disease is usually curable with surgery and/or radiation therapy. For recurrent or metastatic disease, a great many single agents have demonstrated some palliative efficacy. These include the hormonal agents, progestins and tamoxifen, and the cytotoxic chemotherapeutic drugs doxorubicin, epirubicin, cisplatin, carboplatin, fluorouracil, vincristine, and paclitaxel. Combination chemotherapy can also be palliative, including those regimens listed below and some others at various stages of investigation.

CAP–CYCLOPHOSPHAMIDE-DOXORUBICIN-CISPLATIN

Cyclophosphamide. 600 mg/m^2 intravenously on day 1.

Doxorubicin. 45 mg/m^2 intravenously on day 1.

Cisplatin. 50 mg/m^2 intravenously on day 1.

NOTE: Repeat the cycle every 4 weeks.

Selected Reading

DeOliveira CF et al: Phase 2 study of cyclophosphamide (C), Adriamycin (A), cisplatin (P) in recurrent or advanced endometrial cancer (EC), *Proc Am Soc Clin Oncol* 5:123, 1986.

CISPLATIN-DOXORUBICIN

Doxorubicin. 60 mg/m^2 intravenously on day 1.

Cisplatin. 50 mg/m^2 intravenously on day 1.

NOTE: Repeat every 3 weeks for eight cycles. Vigorous hydration and potent antiemetics are essential. More toxic than doxorubicin alone for a small, but statistically significant, therapeutic advantage.

Selected Reading

Thigpen T et al: Phase III trial of doxorubicin +/− cisplatin in advanced or recurrent endometrial carcinoma: a Gynecological Oncology Group study, *Proc Am Soc Clin Oncol* 12:261, 1993.

ESOPHAGEAL CARCINOMA

Esophageal carcinoma is the twentieth most frequent cancer but the thirteenth most common cause of cancer mortality. Upper esophageal (cervical) is primarily squamous cell carcinoma and associated with smoking and alcohol consumption. Lower (thoracic and gastroesophageal) cancer is less clearly so associated and may have other etiologies. At presentation, 50% of cases appear to be locoregional and 50% disseminated. After careful staging, about 80% are found to be disseminated. Active single agents include cisplatin, 5-fluorouracil, methotrexate, mitomycin, paclitaxel, and vindesine (desacetyl vinblastine). Bleomycin and mitoguazone are active but rarely used. Docetaxel and irinotecan look promising. Combination chemotherapy is most frequently used as neoadjuvant, concomitant with radiation, or after recurrence or metastasis.

CARBOPLATIN-CISPLATIN-FLUOROURACIL

Carboplatin. 300 mg/m^2 intravenously on day 1.

Cisplatin. 25 mg/m^2/day intravenously on days 2 to 5.

5-Fluorouracil. 750 mg/m^2/day by continuous IV infusion on days 1 to 4.

NOTE: Therapy is administered every 4 weeks for three courses, and patient is then reevaluated for surgery or other therapy.

Selected Reading

Cure H et al: Carboplatin plus cisplatin plus 5-fluorouracil: feasibility study in advanced esophageal cancer, *Proc Am Soc Clin Oncol* 11:178, 1992.

CISPLATIN-FLUOROURACIL-RADIATION THERAPY

5-Fluorouracil. 1000 mg/m^2/day by continuous IV infusion on days 1 to 4 of weeks 1, 5, 8, and 11.

Cisplatin. 75 mg/m^2 at 1 mg/min intravenously on day 1 of each course on weeks 1, 5, 8, and 11.

NOTE: Radiation therapy is given concurrently as 200 cGy 5 days a week with a total of 3000 cGy of regional treatment and 2000 cGy to a boost field (total 5000 cGy) in 5 weeks.

Selected Reading

Herskovic A et al: Combined chemotherapy and radiotherapy compared with radiotherapy alone in patients with cancer of the esophagus, *N Engl J Med* 326:1593-1598, 1992.

CISPLATIN-VINBLASTINE-FLUOROURACIL

Cisplatin. 20 mg/m^2/day by continuous IV infusion on days 1 to 5 and 17 to 21.

Vinblastine. 1 mg/m^2/day by IV bolus on days 1 to 4 and 17 to 20.

5-Fluorouracil. 300 mg/m^2/day by continuous IV infusion for the 21-day course.

NOTE: Radiation therapy is given in daily fractions of 250 cGy 5 days per week to a total of 3750 cGy over a period of 21 days. When possible, radiation therapy may be delivered at 150 cGy twice a day for 5 days a week to a total dose of 4500 cGy over the 21-day period. After a 3-week rest, surgery (transhiatal esophagectomy) is performed on day 42 if feasible.

Selected Readings

Forastiere AA et al: Concurrent chemotherapy and radiation therapy followed by transhiatal esophagectomy for local-regional cancer of the esophagus, *J Clin Oncol* 8:119-127, 1990.

Forastiere AA et al: Preoperative chemoradiation followed by transhiatal esophagectomy for carcinoma of the esophagus: final report, *J Clin Oncol* 11:1118-1123, 1993.

FAP–FLUOROURACIL-DOXORUBICIN-CISPLATIN

5-Fluorouracil. 600 mg/m² intravenously on days 1 and 8.

Doxorubicin. 30 mg/m² intravenously on day 1.

Cisplatin. 75 mg/m² intravenously on day 1 with hydration and mannitol diuresis.

NOTE: Repeat the course every 4 weeks as tolerated.

Selected Reading

Gisselbrecht C et al: Fluorouracil (F), Adriamycin (A), and cisplatin (P) (FAP): combination chemotherapy of advanced esophageal carcinoma, *Cancer* 52:974-977, 1983.

INTERFERON ALPHA–FLUOROURACIL

5-Fluorouracil. 750 mg/m²/day by continuous infusion on days 1 to 5 followed by a weekly outpatient bolus of 750 mg/m².

Interferon alfa-2a. 9 million units 3 times a week from day 1.

Selected Reading

Kelsen D et al: Interferon alfa-2a and fluorouracil in the treatment of patients with advanced esophageal cancer, *J Clin Oncol* 10:269-274, 1992.

M-F–MITOMYCIN-FLUOROURACIL

Mitomycin. 10 mg/m² intravenously on day 1.

5-Fluorouracil. 1000 mg/m² by continuous IV infusion on days 1 to 4 and 29 to 32.

NOTE: The cycle is usually followed by surgery or radiation therapy.

Selected Reading

Franklin R et al: Combined modality therapy for esophageal squamous cell carcinoma, *Cancer* 51:1062-1071, 1983.

NEOADJUVANT FLUOROURACIL-CISPLATIN

Cisplatin. 20 mg/m² intravenously over 1 hour on days 1 to 5.

5-Fluorouracil. 1000 mg/m^2/day by continuous IV infusion for 20 hours on days 1 to 5.

NOTE: The first course is given in the hospital. The 5-fluorouracil is given over 20 hours to allow the cisplatin to be administered. Doses are increased or decreased in subsequent courses (some of which may be given as outpatient therapy) depending on predetermined criteria of toxicity, which are outlined in the report. Two preoperative and three or four postoperative courses are given. Chemotherapy is repeated every 21 days for up to six courses maximum. For those not surgically resectable, a radiation therapy course is outlined with concomitant 5-fluorouracil.

Selected Reading

Ajami JA et al: Prolonged chemotherapy for localized squamous carcinoma of the esophagus, *Eur J Cancer* 28A:880-884, 1992.

PACLITAXEL-CISPLATIN-FLUOROURACIL

Paclitaxel. 250 mg/m^2 intravenously over 3 hours on day 1.

Cisplatin. 20 mg/m^2 intravenously on days 1 to 5.

5-Fluorouracil. 1000 mg/m^2/day by continuous IV infusion on days 1 to 5.

Filgrastim (G-CSF). 5 µg/kg/day subcutaneously on day 6 to adequate ANC recovery.

NOTE: This is a preliminary neoadjuvant regimen before surgery or radiation. If the first course is successful, a second course may be given after ANC recovery and before surgery. Give usual premedication for paclitaxel.

Selected Reading

Javed T et al: A regimen of paclitaxel, cisplatin and 5-fluorouracil followed by G-CSF is highly active against epidermoid and adenocarcinoma of esophagus, *Proc Am Soc Clin Oncol* 14:195, 1995.

GASTRIC ADENOCARCINOMA

Gastric adenocarcinoma is the thirteenth most common cancer and the ninth most frequent cause of cancer death in the United States but the second most frequent cause of cancer mortality worldwide. Treatment of choice is surgical attempt at cure when localized and resectable. Adjuvant therapy may be radiation or chemotherapy or a combination thereof. Active chemotherapy drugs include 5-fluorouracil with or without leucovorin, doxorubicin, epirubicin, methotrexate, mitomycin, cisplatin, and etoposide. Single-agent therapy with 5-fluorouracil alone has been used for 2 decades, but now combination chemotherapy is more frequently used at a small increase in efficacy and a large increase in toxicity. Radiation therapy is sometimes used as adjuvant alone, with concomitant 5-fluorouracil or cisplatin or the combination of both drugs.

FAM—FLUOROURACIL-DOXORUBICIN-MITOMYCIN

5-Fluorouracil. 600 mg/m^2 intravenously on days 1, 8, 29, and 36.

Doxorubicin. 30 mg/m^2 intravenously on days 1 and 29.

Mitomycin. 10 mg/m^2 intravenously on day 1.

NOTE: Repeat the cycle every 56 days. The efficacy and therapeutic index of this regimen has been questioned by a prospectively randomized trial showing no improvement in survival versus 5-fluorouracil alone (Cullinan et al, 1985).

Selected Readings

Cullinan SA et al: A comparison of three chemotherapeutic regimens in the treatment of advanced pancreatic and gastric carcinoma: fluorouracil versus fluorouracil and doxorubicin versus fluorouracil, doxorubicin, and mitomycin, *JAMA* 253:2061-2067, 1985.

Macdonald JS et al: 5-Fluorouracil, doxorubicin, and mitomycin (FAM) combination chemotherapy for advanced gastric cancer, *Ann Intern Med* 93:533-536, 1980.

EAP–ETOPOSIDE-DOXORUBICIN-CISPLATIN

Etoposide. 120 mg/m^2 intravenously on days 4 to 6.

Doxorubicin. 20 mg/m^2 intravenously on days 1 and 7.

Cisplatin. 40 mg/m^2 intravenously on days 2 and 8.

NOTE: Etoposide is reduced to 100 mg/m^2 for patients older than 60 years. Repeat the treatment every 4 weeks. Lerner et al (1992) found that EAP was highly toxic and afforded no better survival than less toxic regimens.

Selected Readings

Kelsen D et al: FAMTX versus etoposide, doxorubicin, and cisplatin: a random assignment trial in gastric cancer, *J Clin Oncol* 10:541-548, 1992.

Lerner A et al: Etoposide, doxorubicin and cisplatin chemotherapy for advanced gastric adenocarcinoma: results of a phase 2 trial, *J Clin Oncol* 10:536-540, 1992.

Preusser P et al: Phase II study with the combination etoposide, doxorubicin, and cisplatin in advanced metastatic gastric cancer, *J Clin Oncol* 7:1310-1317, 1989.

EAP-II–ETOPOSIDE-DOXORUBICIN-CISPLATIN

Etoposide. 100 mg/m^2 intravenously on days 1 to 3.

Doxorubicin. 40 mg/m^2 intravenously on day 1.

Cisplatin. 80 mg total given in divided doses over 1 to 3 days.

NOTE: Dose is reduced in patients over 65 years. Courses are repeated every 21 days as tolerated. Claimed to be less toxic than original EAP.

Selected Reading

Haim N, Tsalik M, Robinson E: Treatment of gastric adenocarcinoma with the combination of etoposide, adriamycin and cisplatin (EAP): comparison between two schedules, *Oncology* 51:102-107, 1994.

ELF–ETOPOSIDE-LEUCOVORIN-FLUOROURACIL

Etoposide. 120 mg/m^2 intravenously on days 1 to 3 over a 1-hour period.

Leucovorin. 300 mg/m^2 intravenously on days 1 to 3 over a 2-hour period.

5-Fluorouracil. 500 mg/m^2 by IV bolus midway through the leucovorin infusion.

NOTE: Give leucovorin immediately after etoposide. Repeat the course every 4 or 5 weeks.

Selected Readings

Geffen JR et al: Phase II trial of VP-16, leucovorin and fluorouracil (ELF) in advanced gastric carcinoma, *Proc Am Soc Clin Oncol* 11:195, 1992.

Wilke H et al: New developments in the treatment of gastric carcinoma, *Semin Oncol* 17(suppl 2):61-70, 1990.

FAMTX–FLUOROURACIL-DOXORUBICIN-METHOTREXATE

5-Fluorouracil. 1500 mg/m^2 intravenously on day 1 (given 1 hour after the end of the methotrexate infusion).

Methotrexate. 1500 mg/m^2 intravenously on day 1.

Leucovorin. 15 mg/m^2 orally every 6 hours for 48 hours starting 24 hours after methotrexate.

Doxorubicin. 30 mg/m^2 intravenously on day 15.

NOTE: Repeat the treatment every 4 weeks.

Selected Readings

Kelsen D et al: FAMTX versus etoposide, doxorubicin, and cisplatin: a random assignment trial in gastric cancer, *J Clin Oncol* 10:541-548, 1992.

Wils J et al: An EORTC Gastrointestinal Group evaluation of the combination of sequential methotrexate and 5-fluorouracil, combined with Adriamycin in advanced measurable gastric cancer, *J Clin Oncol* 4:1799-1803, 1986.

FAP–FLUOROURACIL-DOXORUBICIN-CISPLATIN

5-Fluorouracil. 300 mg/m^2 intravenously on days 1 to 5.

Doxorubicin. 40 mg/m^2 intravenously on day 1.

Cisplatin. 60 mg/m^2 intravenously on day 1 with hydration.

NOTE: Repeat the cycle every 5 weeks.

Selected Reading

Moertel CG et al: Phase II study of combined 5-fluorouracil, doxorubicin, and cisplatin in the treatment of advanced upper gastrointestinal adenocarcinoma, *J Clin Oncol* 4:1053-1057, 1986.

FLUOROURACIL-LEUCOVORIN

5-Fluorouracil. 340 to 400 mg/m^2 intravenously on days 1 to 5.

Leucovorin. 200 mg/m^2 intravenously on days 1 to 5.

NOTE: Repeat the cycle every 21 days.

Selected Reading

Machover D et al: Treatment of advanced colorectal and gastric adenocarcinomas with 5-fluorouracil and high-dose folinic acid, *J Clin Oncol* 4:685-696, 1986.

GESTATIONAL TROPHOBLASTIC DISEASE

Gestational trophoblastic disease (GTD) is a group of diseases that extends over the range of the relatively benign hydatidiform mole, invasive mole, or placental site trophoblastic tumor to the choriocarcinoma with its high potential for widespread metastasis and high mortality without therapy. Fortunately, the tumor is rare and when it occurs is sensitive to many chemotherapeutic agents including methotrexate, dactinomycin, cisplatin, etoposide, vincristine, cyclophosphamide, and chlorambucil. In good-prognosis cases, single-agent methotrexate or dactinomycin are usually sufficient. In more aggressive disease, combination chemotherapy is usually effective. Response to therapy can be followed by the fall in the human chorionic gonadotropin level or its beta-subunit, which serves as a marker for residual tumor. In experienced hands and with early therapy, the overall cure rate is 96%. Hence all patients with GTD should be referred promptly to a center with oncologists experienced in the management of this tumor.

APE–DACTINOMYCIN-CISPLATIN-ETOPOSIDE

Dactinomycin.   0.3 mg/m^2 intravenously on days 1 to 3 and 14 to 16.

Cisplatin.   100 mg/m^2 intravenously on day 1.

Etoposide.   100 mg/m^2 intravenously (or 200 mg/m^2 orally) on days 1 to 3 and 14 to 16.

NOTE: Repeat the cycles every 4 weeks.

Selected Reading

Theodore C et al: Treatment of high-risk gestational trophoblastic disease with chemotherapy combination containing cisplatin and etoposide, *Cancer* 64:1824-1828, 1989.

EMA-CO–ETOPOSIDE-METHOTREXATE-DACTINOMYCIN-CYCLOPHOSPHAMIDE-VINCRISTINE

Etoposide.   100 mg/m^2 intravenously on days 1 and 2.

Methotrexate.   300 mg/m^2 on day 1 as a 12-hour infusion.

Dactinomycin.   0.5 mg intravenously on days 1 and 2.

Leucovorin.   15 mg by mouth twice daily on days 2 and 3.

Cyclophosphamide.   600 mg/m^2 intravenously on day 8.

Vincristine.   1.0 mg/m^2 intravenously on day 8.

NOTE: For high-risk patients, this regimen is repeated every 2 weeks until remission or failure. After 12 courses, a rest period is frequently necessary.

Selected Reading

Newlands ES: VP-16 in combinations for first-line treatment of malignant germ-cell tumors and gestational choriocarcinoma, *Semin Oncol* 12(suppl 2):37-41, 1985.

EMA-CO: MODIFIED

Etoposide. 100 mg/m^2 intravenously over 30 minutes on days 1 and 2.

Methotrexate. 100 mg/m^2 IV bolus on day 1, then 200 mg/m^2 IV infusion over 12 hours.

Dactinomycin. 0.35 mg/m^2 IV bolus on days 1 and 2.

Leucovorin. 15 mg by mouth or intramuscularly every 12 hours for four doses starting 24 hours after the methotrexate bolus.

Cyclophosphamide. 600 mg/m^2 intravenously on day 8.

Vincristine. 1.0 mg/m^2 intravenously on day 8.

NOTE: Repeat cycle every 14 days.

Selected Reading

Soper JT et al: Alternating weekly chemotherapy with etoposide-methotrexate-dactinomycin/cyclophosphamide-vincristine for high risk gestational trophoblastic disease, *Obstet Gynecol* 83:113-117, 1994.

METHOTREXATE-LEUCOVORIN

Methotrexate. 1 mg/kg intramuscularly every other day for four doses.

Leucovorin. 10% of the methotrexate dose intramuscularly 24 hours after each methotrexate dose.

NOTE: A second course is given if the HCG titer does not fall by 1 log within 18 days, if the HCG level plateaus for more than 2 weeks or becomes reelevated, or if new sites of disease develop.

Selected Readings

Berkowitz RS, Goldstein DP, Bernstein MR: Methotrexate with citrovorum factor rescue as primary therapy for gestational trophoblastic disease, *Cancer* 50:2024-2027, 1982.

Berkowitz RS, Goldstein DP, Bernstein MR: Ten years experience with methotrexate and folinic acid as primary therapy for gestational trophoblastic disease. *Gynecol Oncol* 23:111-118, 1986.

PVB–CISPLATIN-VINBLASTINE-BLEOMYCIN

Vinblastine. 0.3 mg/kg intravenously on day 1.

Bleomycin. 15 units/day by continuous IV infusion on days 1 to 3.

Cisplatin. 100 mg/m^2 intravenously on day 2.

NOTE: Repeat at 21-day intervals.

Selected Reading

Azab M et al: Cisplatin, vinblastine, and bleomycin combination in the treatment of resistant high-risk gestational trophoblastic tumors, *Cancer* 64:1829-1832, 1989.

HEAD AND NECK SQUAMOUS CELL CARCINOMA

Head and neck squamous cell carcinoma accounts for 5% of all malignancies and ranks as the sixth most common cancer in men. The larynx is the most common site, followed by the oral cavity, pharynx, and salivary gland. Frequency is closely correlated with smoking and heavy alcohol intake (particularly the combination). Smokeless tobacco is an important factor in the cause of oral cancer, whereas pipe smoking and chronic sun exposure are linked to an increased incidence of lip cancer. Epstein-Barr virus is associated with nasopharyngeal carcinoma (NPC), which tends to be a lymphoepithelioma and does not usually behave the way squamous cell carcinomas do. NPC is usually treated with local and regional radiation therapy.

Surgery is the treatment of first choice when it can be curative, except in the case of laryngeal cancer where chemotherapy combined with radiation therapy gives equivalent results with preservation of the organ and hence of normal speech. Active drugs include cisplatin, methotrexate, bleomycin, carboplatin, 5-fluorouracil, vincristine, paclitaxel, ifosfamide, docetaxel, cyclophosphamide, and hydroxyurea. Chemotherapy may be used as neoadjuvant (therapy given before surgery or radiation), synchronous (usually single agent) with radiation, or postdefinitive (as adjuvant after surgery or radiation). Combination chemotherapy is usually neoadjuvant or postdefinitive. A recent metanalysis (Munro, 1995) shows that both synchronous and neoadjuvant chemotherapy prolong survival, the former more than the latter. It is more difficult to evaluate postdefinitive therapy because distant metastases are an uncommon cause of treatment failure. Most patients with head and neck cancer who die, do so because of locoregional failure. However, several studies indicate that combination chemotherapy results in better response rates and longer survival than single agents, but these studies have not demonstrated a superior survival rate.

Selected Reading
Munro AJ: An overview of randomized controlled trials of adjuvant chemotherapy in head and neck cancer, *Br J Cancer* 71:83-91, 1995.

BMC–BLEOMYCIN-METHOTREXATE-CISPLATIN

Bleomycin. 10 units intramuscularly on days 1, 8, and 15.

Methotrexate. 40 mg/m^2 intramuscularly on days 1 and 15.

Cisplatin. 50 mg/m^2 intravenously on day 4.

NOTE: Repeat the cycle every 21 days.

Selected Reading
Kuten A et al: Multidrug chemotherapy using bleomycin, methotrexate and cisplatin alone or combined with radiotherapy in advanced head and neck cancer, *Cancer Treat Rep* 67:573-574, 1983.

CABO–CISPLATIN-METHOTREXATE-BLEOMYCIN-VINCRISTINE

Cisplatin. 50 mg/m^2 intravenously on day 4.

Methotrexate. 40 mg/m^2 intravenously on days 1 and 15.

Bleomycin. 10 units intravenously on days 1, 8, and 15.

Vincristine. 2 mg intravenously on days 1, 8, and 15.

NOTE: Courses are given every 3 weeks. After three courses, weekly maintenance methotrexate is given. Vincristine therapy may be discontinued after 6 doses.

Selected Readings

Clavel M et al: Combination chemotherapy with methotrexate, bleomycin, and vincristine with or without cisplatin in advanced squamous cell carcinoma of the head and neck, *Cancer* 60:1173-1177, 1987.

Clavel M et al: Randomized comparison of cisplatin, methotrexate, bleomycin and vincristine (CABO) versus cisplatin and 5-FU (CF) versus cisplatin in recurrent or metastatic squamous cell carcinoma of the head and neck: a phase III study of the EORTC Head and Neck Cancer Cooperative Group, *Ann Oncol* 5:521-526, 1994.

CARBOPLATIN-FLUOROURACIL

Carboplatin. 300 mg/m^2 intravenously on day 1.

5-Fluorouracil. 1000 mg/m^2/day for 96 hours by continuous IV infusion.

NOTE: Repeat course every 28 days. Response rates are superior to methotrexate 40 mg/m^2 intravenously weekly, but toxicity is greater and there is no improvement in overall survival.

Selected Reading

Forastiere AA et al: Randomized comparison of cisplatin plus fluorouracil and carboplatin plus fluorouracil versus methotrexate in advanced squamous cell carcinoma of the head and neck: a Southwest Oncology Group study, *J Clin Oncol* 10:1245-1251, 1992.

CISPLATIN-FLUOROURACIL

Cisplatin. 100 mg/m^2 intravenously on day 1.

5-Fluorouracil. 1000 mg/m^2 by continuous IV infusion for 96 hours.

NOTE: Repeat every 3 weeks.

Selected Reading

Jacobs C et al: A phase III randomized study comparing cisplatin and fluorouracil as single agents and in combination for advanced squamous cell carcinoma of the head and neck, *J Clin Oncol* 10:257-263, 1992.

CFBM—CISPLATIN-FLUOROURACIL-BLEOMYCIN-METHOTREXATE

Cisplatin. 80 mg/m^2 by continuous IV infusion on day 1.

5-Fluorouracil. 800 mg/m^2/day by continuous IV infusion on days 2 to 6.

Bleomycin. 15 units intravenously on day 1.

Methotrexate. 100 mg/m^2 intravenously on day 16.

Leucovorin. 15 mg by mouth every 6 hours for six doses beginning 24 hours after the methotrexate.

NOTE: Cycles are 3 to 4 weeks apart, and at least two to four cycles must be completed to evaluate the response.

Selected Readings

Amrein PC: Cisplatin and 5-fluorouracil vs the same plus bleomycin and methotrexate in recurrent squamous cell carcinoma of the head and neck, *Proc Am Soc Clin Oncol* 9:175, 1990.

Amrein PC, Fabian RL: Treatment of recurrent head and neck cancer with cisplatin and 5-fluorouracil versus the same plus bleomycin and methotrexate, *Laryngoscope* 102:901-906, 1992.

PACLITAXEL-CISPLATIN

Paclitaxel. 200 mg/m^2 intravenously over 3 hours on day 1.

Cisplatin. 75 or 100 mg/m^2 intravenously over 1 hour on day 1.

NOTE: Paclitaxel should always be given before cisplatin to avoid excess toxicity. This is a phase I/II study and doses are preliminary. Repeat course every 3 weeks. Hanauske et al recommend cisplatin 100 mg/m2 whereas Hitt et al recommend 75 mg/m^2 and tend to give filgrastim (G-CSF) 5 µg/kg subcutaneously on days 4 through 12. Monitor for neutropenia and neurotoxicity. Give usual premedication for paclitaxel.

Selected Readings

Hanauske AR et al: Clinical phase I study of paclitaxel followed by cisplatin in advanced head and neck squamous cell carcinoma, *Semin Oncol* 22(6 suppl 14):35-39, 1995.

Hitt R et al: A phase I/II study of paclitaxel plus cisplatin as first line therapy for head and neck cancers: preliminary results, *Semin Oncol* 22(6 suppl 15):50-54, 1995.

PBF—CISPLATIN-BLEOMYCIN-FLUOROURACIL

Cisplatin. 100 mg/m^2 intravenously on day 1.

Bleomycin. 15 units IV bolus on day 1 and 16 units/m^2/day by continuous infusion on days 1 to 5.

5-Fluorouracil. 650 mg/m^2/day by continuous infusion on days 1 to 5.

NOTE: Three cycles are given at monthly intervals.

Selected Reading

Boussen H et al: Chemotherapy of metastatic and/or recurrent undifferentiated nasopharyngeal carcinoma with cisplatin, bleomycin and fluorouracil, *J Clin Oncol* 9:1675-1681, 1991.

PFL—CISPLATIN-FLUOROURACIL-LEUCOVORIN

Cisplatin. 25 mg/m^2/day intravenously on days 1 to 5.

5-Fluorouracil. 800 mg/m^2/day intravenously on days 2 to 6.

Leucovorin. 500 mg/m^2/day intravenously on days 1 to 6.

NOTE: All drugs are administered by continuous infusion and repeated once every 28 days.

Selected Reading

Dreyfuss AI et al: Continuous infusion high-dose leucovorin with 5-fluorouracil and cisplatin for untreated stage IV carcinoma of the head and neck, *Ann Intern Med* 112:167-172, 1990.

SIMULTANEOUS FLUOROURACIL-CISPLATIN-RADIATION

5-Fluorouracil. 1000 mg/m^2/day as a 96-hour infusion.

Cisplatin. 75 mg/m^2 intravenously on day 1.

NOTE: Simultaneous radiation of 3000 cGy in 15 fractions between days 1 and 19 is an integral part of the regimen. Repeat the chemotherapy course in 4 to 6 weeks. Operable patients go on to surgery.

Selected Readings

Adelstein DJ et al: Simultaneous versus sequential combined technique therapy for squamous cell head and neck cancer, *Cancer* 65:1685-1691, 1990.

Adelstein DJ et al: Simultaneous radiotherapy and chemotherapy with 5-fluorouracil and cisplatin for locally confined squamous cell head and neck cancer, *NCI Monogr* 6:347-351, 1988.

VINORELBINE-CISPLATIN

Cisplatin. 80 mg/m^2 intravenously on day 1.

Vinorelbine. 25 mg/m^2 intravenously on days 1 and 8.

NOTE: Repeat every 3 weeks. The cisplatin is given over 90 minutes with prehydration, posthydration, and antiemetics. If neutropenia is prolonged, delay an additional week before the next course and follow it with filgrastim (G-CSF).

Selected Reading

Gebbia V et al: Vinorelbine plus cisplatin in recurrent or previously unresectable squamous cell carcinoma of the head and neck, *Am J Clin Oncol* 18:293-296, 1995.

KAPOSI'S SARCOMA

Kaposi's sarcoma (KS) may present in any of five different modes:

1. Classic KS in elderly males of Italian or East European Jewish extraction; follows a relatively indolent course.
2. African KS in young or middle-aged males; may be indolent or aggressive.
3. Immunosuppressive treatment–related KS in patients with renal or other organ transplant on immunosuppressive drugs.
4. Epidemic KS in young male homosexuals with HIV and usually aggressive and disseminated disease.
5. Nonepidemic homosexual-related KS, which is usually indolent.

Local skin lesions may be treated with intralesional injections of drugs such as vinblastine or interferon alpha or with electron beam radiation therapy. Systemic disease is treated with active single agents such as vinblastine, etoposide, vincristine, bleomycin, liposomal daunorubicin, liposomal doxorubicin, or interferon alpha or with combination chemotherapy. Aggressiveness of the therapy is dependent on the extent of the underlying disease and residual immunocompetency.

ABV–DOXORUBICIN-BLEOMYCIN-VINBLASTINE

Doxorubicin. 40 mg/m^2 intravenously on day 1.

Bleomycin. 10 units total intravenously on days 1 and 15.

Vinblastine. 6 mg/m^2 intravenously on day 1.

NOTE: Repeat courses every 28 days to maximum safe dose of doxorubicin, about 11 courses. Do not exceed a bleomycin dose of 300 units/m^2. Although the lesions of Kaposi's sarcoma usually regress with therapy, the underlying AIDS usually progresses unless treated with effective anti-HIV combination chemotherapy. Opportunistic infections are the most frequent cause of mortality. Patients with early stage disease or those unable or unwilling to take intravenous therapy can be treated with etoposide orally, 150 mg/m^2 /day for 3 consecutive days repeated every 28 days, as tolerated.

Selected Reading

Laubenstein LJ et al: Treatment of epidemic Kaposi's sarcoma with etoposide or a combination of doxorubicin, bleomycin, and vinblastine, *J Clin Oncol* 2:1115-1120, 1984.

BLEOMYCIN-VINCRISTINE

Bleomycin. 10 units/m^2 intravenously every 2 weeks.

Vincristine. 1.4 mg/m^2 (maximum 2 mg) intravenously every 2 weeks.

NOTE: Vincristine doses are modified for peripheral neuropathy but not for neutropenia. Cycles can be repeated up to a maximum dose of bleomycin of 300 units, and vincristine is limited by peripheral neuropathy. Survival is limited by the underlying HIV and the development of opportunistic infections. The latter can be treated prophylactically and therapeutically.

Selected Reading

Gill P et al: Treatment of advanced Kaposi's sarcoma using a combination of bleomycin and vincristine, *Am J Clin Oncol* 13:315-319, 1990.

DOXORUBICIN-BLEOMYCIN-VINCRISTINE

Doxorubicin. 20 mg/m^2 intravenously on day 1.

Bleomycin. 10 units/m^2 on day 1.

Vincristine. 1.4 mg/m^2 (maximum 2 mg) day 1.

NOTE: Repeat every 2 weeks to complete remission or two cycles beyond maximum response. Do not exceed cumulative doxorubicin dose of 450 mg/m^2 or bleomycin dose of 300 units.

Selected Reading

Gill PS et al: Systemic treatment of AIDS-related Kaposi's sarcoma: results of a randomized trial, *Am J Med* 90:427-433, 1991.

VINCRISTINE-VINBLASTINE

Vincristine. 2 mg total intravenously during odd-numbered weeks.

Vinblastine. 0.1 mg/kg intravenously during even-numbered weeks.

NOTE: Alternate therapy as long as effective. Reduce dose of vinblastine for WBC counts <3000 or platelet counts <50,000. Discontinue for detectable to moderate muscle weakness or severe paresthesias.

Selected Reading

Kaplan L, Abrams D, Volberding P: Treatment of Kaposi's sarcoma in acquired immunodeficiency syndrome with an alternating vincristine-vinblastine regimen, *Cancer Treat Rep* 70:1121-1122, 1986.

LEUKEMIA: ACUTE LYMPHOBLASTIC

Acute lymphoblastic leukemia (ALL) accounts for about one third of childhood malignancies and afflicts approximately 2500 children per year. Fortunately, over the past 30 years it has changed from 100% fatal within 3 or 4 months of diagnosis to approximately 60% to 65% curable today. The major instruments of that progress have been new and better drugs used more effectively in systematic studies by cooperative groups. To get closer to our goal of a 100% cure rate with less toxicity, it is important to continue the systematic study of new and better therapies through the cooperative group mechanism. Hence no protocols are listed here for childhood ALL. All patients should be placed on a protocol of one of the national cooperative study groups (see Chapter 12). This will give the individual child the best possible chance to get the latest and best therapy, and will serve all children by advancing us to the goal of more cures with less acute and long-term toxicity.

ALL in adults does not respond as well to therapy. Although 60% to 80% of patients can be expected to attain a complete remission after induction therapy, only 35% to 40% can be expected to survive 2 years unless they also undergo an aggressive consolidation and maintenance program as well as central nervous system prophylaxis. Response is related to age, and older patients do not respond as well as younger patients. Adverse prognostic features for remission induction include age over 60; WBC count greater than 30,000; non-B, non-T phenotype; and poor performance status. Adverse prognostic features for remission duration include all of the foregoing plus age over 35, presence of the Philadelphia chromosome [t(9;22)]; other less common translocations [t(4;11), t(8;14)] and variants, and Burkitt's (L3) phenotype (SIg+).

The drugs that are active in ALL include vincristine, prednisone, L-asparaginase, daunorubicin, doxorubicin, idarubicin, mitoxantrone, cytarabine, methotrexate, 6-mercaptopurine, teniposide, 6-thioguanine, cyclophosphamide, and amsacrine. These drugs have been most effective in combinations of at least three drugs, usually given intensively over a short term with transfusional support and antiinfective therapy, and most recently with cytokines to stimulate neutrophil regeneration. After remission induction, further short-term intensive consolidation chemotherapy is given for one or more courses and then longer-term maintenance therapy at lower dose. For those in the high-risk group but younger than 55 years of age, high-dose marrow ablative chemotherapy (with or without radiation) followed by allogeneic transplantation is a consideration in first or second remission if there is a compatible donor. Autologous transplantation for those without a suitable donor is being evaluated because there is no convincing proof that its results so far are superior to a good, intensive chemotherapy program. For the group with standard risk ALL, there is no demonstrable survival advantage to the transplantation program, allogeneic or autologous. Because the optimal postremission therapy for patients with ALL is still unclear, participation in clinical trials should be considered.

AMSACRINE-CYTARABINE

Amsacrine. 200 mg/m^2/day intravenously on days 1 to 3.

Cytarabine. 3000 mg/m^2/day intravenously as a 3-hour infusion on days 1 to 5.

Selected Reading

Arlin ZA et al: Amsacrine with high-dose cytarabine is highly effective therapy for refractory and relapsed acute lymphoblastic leukemia in adults, *Blood* 72:433-435, 1988.

BAY AREA LEUKEMIA STUDY GROUP
Induction

Daunorubicin. 50 mg/m^2 intravenously on days 1 to 3.

Vincristine. 2 mg intravenously on days 1, 8, 15, and 22.

Prednisone. 60 mg/m^2 orally on days 1 to 28.

L-Asparaginase. 6000 units/m^2 intramuscularly on days 17 to 28.

Consolidation: Treatment A (Cycles 1, 3, 5, 7)

Daunorubicin. 50 mg/m^2 intravenously on days 1 and 2.

Vincristine. 2 mg intravenously on days 1 and 8.

Prednisone. 60 mg orally on days 1 to 14.

L-Asparaginase. 12,000 units/m^2 intramuscularly on days 2, 4, 7, 9, 11, and 14.

Consolidation: Treatment B (Cycles 2, 4, 6, 8)

Teniposide. 165 mg/m^2 intravenously on days 1, 4, 8, and 11.

Cytarabine. 300 mg/m^2 intravenously on days 1, 4, 8, and 11.

Consolidation: Treatment C (Cycle 9)

Methotrexate. 690 mg/m^2 intravenously over a 42-hour period.

Leucovorin. 15 mg/m^2 intravenously every 6 hours for 12 doses beginning at 42 hours (i.e., at the completion of methotrexate infusion).

NOTE: There are contingency treatments if the bone marrow shows residual leukemia on day 14 or 28. CNS prophylaxis is administered within 1 week of achieving complete remission and consists of 1800 cGy in 10 fractions over a period of 12 to 14 days and six weekly doses of methotrexate, 12 mg intrathecally.

Selected Reading
Linker CA et al: Treatment of adult acute lymphoblastic leukemia with intensive cyclical chemotherapy: a follow-up report, *Blood* 78:2814-2822, 1991.

CYTARABINE–HIGH-DOSE MITOXANTRONE
Induction
Mitoxantrone. 40 to 80 mg/m^2 intravenously on day 2.

Cytarabine. 3000 mg/m^2/day intravenously over a 3-hour period on days 1 to 5.

Vincristine. 1.4 mg/m^2 intravenously on day 15.

Prednisone. 60 mg/m^2/day orally for 35 days and then taper.

Consolidation
Vincristine. 1.4 mg/m^2 intravenously weekly for 6 weeks.

Prednisone. 60 mg/m^2 orally for 6 weeks.

L-Asparaginase. 20,000 units intravenously three times a week for six doses.

Methotrexate. 10 mg intravenously twice a week during the first, third, and fifth weeks.

Maintenance
Similar to the L-2 or L-10 Memorial Sloan-Kettering Protocol (*Cancer* 37:1256-1264, 1976) but being reevaluated to shorten the duration.

Selected Reading
Arlin ZA et al: Short course high dose mitoxantrone with high dose cytarabine is effective therapy for adult lymphoblastic leukemia, *Leukemia* 5:712-714, 1991.

ETOPOSIDE–HIGH-DOSE CYTARABINE
Etoposide. 100 mg/m^2/day intravenously on days 1 to 5.

Cytarabine. 2000 mg/m^2 intravenously over a 3-hour period twice a day on days 1 to 5.

Dexamethasone. 16 mg/day intravenously or by mouth on days 1 to 5.

NOTE: Steroid eye drops should be given every 2 to 4 hours for 7 days from the start of therapy. Only patients younger than 65 years old were treated. Patients with acute myelogenous leukemia were also treated, with more limited responses. Some patients received etoposide, 100 mg/m^2 twice a day, and had more toxicity without an apparent increase in response.

Selected Reading

Gore R et al: Treatment of relapsed and refractory acute leukemia with high-dose cytosine arabinoside and etoposide, *Cancer Chemother Pharmacol* 23:373-376, 1989.

FIVE-DRUG CANCER AND LEUKEMIA GROUP B INDUCTION REGIMEN

Cyclophosphamide. 1200 mg/m^2 intravenously on day 1.

Daunorubicin. 45 mg/m^2 intravenously on days 1 to 3.

Vincristine. 2 mg total intravenously on days 1, 8, 15, and 22.

Prednisone. 60 mg/m^2 orally on days 1 to 21.

L-Asparaginase. 6000 units/m^2 intravenously on days 5, 8, 11, 15, 18, and 22.

NOTE: Doses of cyclophosphamide, daunorubicin, and prednisone are reduced for patients over 60 years of age. Treatment lasts 24 months. Consolidation over 8 weeks is with cyclophosphamide, 6-mercaptopurine, cytarabine, vincristine, and L-asparaginase. CNS prophylaxis is given with 2400 cGy brain radiation and intrathecal methotrexate. Late intensification is with doxorubicin, vincristine, dexamethasone, cyclophosphamide, cytarabine, and 6-thioguanine. Maintenance is with vincristine, prednisone, 6-mercaptopurine, and methotrexate.

Selected Reading

Larson RA et al: A five-drug remission induction regimen with intensive consolidation for adults with acute lymphoblastic leukemia: Cancer and Leukemia Group B study 8811, *Blood* 85:2025-2037, 1995.

FRENCH MULTICENTER STUDY (PAME)
Induction

Cytarabine. 1000 mg/m^2 intravenously over a 2-hour period twice a day on days 1 to 5.

Mitoxantrone. 12 mg/m^2 intravenously over a 1-hour period on days 1 to 5.

Etoposide. 200 mg/m^2 intravenously over a 1-hour period on days 6 to 8.

Prednisone. 0.5 mg/kg orally on days 1 to 5.

Maintenance: Course A

Prednisone. 40 mg/m^2/day orally on days 1 to 7.

Vincristine. 1.5 mg/m^2/day intravenously on days 1 and 7.

Methotrexate. 3000 mg/m^2 intravenously over a 2-hour period on day 1.

Leucovorin. 15 mg/m^2 every 6 hours for six doses beginning 24 hours after the start of the methotrexate infusion.

L-Asparaginase. 10,000 units/m^2/day intramuscularly on days 15 to 21.

Maintenance: Course B

Amsacrine. 200 mg/m^2 intravenously on day 1.

Teniposide. 120 mg/m^2 intravenously on day 1.

Cytarabine. 25 mg/m^2 subcutaneously twice a day on days 15 to 21.

Prednisone. 40 mg/m^2/day by mouth on days 15 to 21.

Maintenance: Course C
Etoposide. 200 mg/m^2 intravenously on day 1.

Cyclophosphamide. 600 mg/m^2 intravenously on day 1.

Prednisone. 40 mg/m^2/day orally on days 15 to 21.

6-Mercaptopurine. 50 mg/m^2/day orally on days 15 to 21.

Selected Reading
Milpied N et al: Successful treatment of adult acute lymphoblastic leukemia after relapse with prednisone, intermediate-dose cytarabine, mitoxantrone, and etoposide (PAME) chemotherapy, *Cancer* 66:627-631, 1990.

GERMAN MULTISTUDY GROUP
Induction: Phase I
Prednisone. 60 mg/m^2 orally on days 1 to 28.

Vincristine. 1.5 mg/m^2 (maximum, 2.0 mg) intravenously on days 1, 8, 15, and 22.

Daunorubicin. 25 mg/m^2 intravenously on days 1, 8, 15, and 22.

L-Asparaginase. 5000 units/m^2 intravenously on days 1 to 14.

Induction: Phase II
Cyclophosphamide. 650 mg/m^2 intravenously on days 29, 43, and 57.

Cytarabine. 75 mg/m^2 intravenously on days 31 to 34, 38 to 41, 45 to 48, and 52 to 55.

6-Mercaptopurine. 60 mg/m^2 orally on days 29 to 57.

Methotrexate. 10 mg/m^2 (maximum, 15 mg) intrathecally on days 31, 38, 45, and 52.

Reinduction: Phase I
Dexamethasone. 10 mg/m^2 orally on days 1 to 28.

Vincristine. 1.5 mg/m^2 (maximum, 2.0 mg) intravenously on days 1, 8, 15, and 22.

Doxorubicin. 25 mg/m^2 intravenously on days 1, 8, 15, and 22.

Reinduction: Phase II
Cyclophosphamide. 650 mg/m^2 (maximum, 1000) intravenously on day 29.

Cytarabine. 75 mg/m^2 intravenously on days 31 to 34 and 38 to 41.

Thioguanine. 60 mg/m^2 orally on days 29 to 34.

Maintenance

6-Mercaptopurine. 60 mg/m^2 orally daily during weeks 10 to 18 and 29 to 130.

Methotrexate. 20 mg/m^2 orally or intravenously weekly during weeks 10 to 18 and 29 to 130.

NOTE: Cranial irradiation at 2400 cGy is instituted after remission is achieved.

Selected Readings

Freund M et al: Treatment of relapsed or refractory adult acute lymphocytic leukemia, *Cancer* 69:709-716, 1992. (This protocol is from the same group but somewhat more intense as befits relapsed or refractory disease.)

Hoelzer D et al: Prognostic factors in a multicenter study for treatment of acute lymphoblastic leukemia in adults, *Blood* 71:123-131, 1988.

MITOXANTRONE–HIGH-DOSE CYTARABINE

Mitoxantrone. 5 mg/m^2 intravenously over a 1-hour period on days 1 to 5.

Cytarabine. 3000 mg/m^2 intravenously over a 2-hour period every 12 hours for six doses.

GM-CSF. 125 µg/m^2 intravenously over a 4-hour period daily beginning 24 hours after chemotherapy until granulocytes number more than 2000/µL.

NOTE: A second course was administered at the same dose schedule in patients who did not obtain a complete remission after the first course and who did not have prohibitive toxicities.

Selected Reading

Kantarjian HM et al: Intensive chemotherapy with mitoxantrone and high-dose cytosine arabinoside followed by granulocyte-macrophage colony-stimulating factor in the treatment of patients with acute lymphocytic leukemia, *Blood* 79:876-881, 1992.

SALVAGE MITOXANTRONE-IFOSFAMIDE-ETOPOSIDE

Etoposide. 100 mg/m^2 intravenously on days 1 to 5.

Ifosfamide. 1500 mg/m^2 intravenously on days 1 to 5.

Mesna. 1500 mg/m^2 intravenously on days 1 to 5.

Mitoxantrone. 8 mg/m^2 intravenously on days 1 to 3.

Selected Reading

Schiller G et al: Phase II study of etoposide, ifosfamide and mitoxantrone for the treatment of resistant adult acute lymphoblastic leukemia, *Am J Hematol* 43:195-199, 1993.

LEUKEMIA: ACUTE NONLYMPHOCYTIC

Acute nonlymphocytic leukemia (ANLL) includes the eight subtypes as defined by the French-American-British (FAB) classification based on morphological, histochemical, and immunological criteria. Untreated, the disease is fatal in months. With aggressive therapy, 60% to 70% of patients will achieve remission, but only 15% to 20% will survive 3 or more years and may be cured. Adverse prognostic factors include older age, central nervous system involvement, systemic infection at diagnosis, WBC count greater than 100,000, certain cytogenetic abnormalities and the evolution of the ANLL from chronic myelocytic leukemia, the myelodysplastic syndrome, polycythemia vera, alkylating agent or radiation therapy, and the development of multiple drug resistance.

Active drugs include cytarabine, daunorubicin, doxorubicin, idarubicin, mitoxantrone, etoposide, methotrexate, 6-thioguanine, 6-mercaptopurine, amsacrine, and 5-azacytidine. New drugs being evaluated in ANLL include fludarabine, cladribine, paclitaxel, and topotecan. Effective induction therapy involves at least two or more active drugs. Acute promyelocytic leukemia (APL) therapy runs a high probability of severe hemorrhagic complications with disseminated intravascular coagulation, often in spite of low-dose heparinization. The recent use of all transretinoic acid in induction therapy of APL has increased the response rate and reduced the incidence of hemorrhagic complications. This method requires follow-up combination chemotherapy to induce and maintain a remission.

Allogeneic bone marrow transplantation can be considered in patients younger than 55 in first remission if a histocompatible sibling is available as a potential donor. It is the only potentially curative therapy after relapse. In such cases, the patient and the potential donor should be HLA typed early, and the potential marrow donor should not donate blood products to the patient. Such a procedure has the advantage that a graft-versus-leukemia effect can contribute to a possible cure. The disadvantage of an allograft is the potential for graft-versus-host disease, severe infection caused by immunosuppression, and the risk of posttransplant lymphoma. Studies exploring the utility of autologous transplants are in progress. They have the advantage of being possible to an older age (65), no HLA match is needed, and there is no graft-versus-host disease. The negative aspect is the absence of a graft-versus-leukemia effect, the likely marrow contamination by occult tumor cells, and the slow marrow reconstitution with the danger of infection and hemorrhage.

Since responses to combination chemotherapy in the elderly (those over age 60 or 65, depending on individual physiology) are so poor and toxicity and treatment-related mortality are so high, there is a tendency to not treat the elderly. Although some elderly patients have a relatively indolent disease that progresses slowly, several studies suggest that nontreatment leads to early mortality in most cases. However, combination chemotherapy with less intensive regimens often leads to equal response rates, fewer induction deaths, and a greater median survival rate.

ALL TRANSRETINOIC ACID (ATRA) IN PROMYELOCYTIC LEUKEMIA

ATRA.   45 mg/m^2/day orally until complete remission (CR) or 90 days.

Daunorubicin.   60 mg/m^2 intravenously on days 1 to 3 after CR.

Cytarabine. 200 mg/m^2 intravenously on days 1 to 7 after CR.

NOTE: Those patients who do not achieve CR with the first course get a second course of the same therapy. When CR is achieved, a consolidation or third course is given with daunorubicin 45 mg/m^2 on days 1 to 3 and cytarabine 1000 mg/m^2 every 12 hours on days 1 to 4.

Selected Reading

Fenaux P et al: Effect of all transretinoic acid in newly diagnosed acute promyelocytic leukemia: results of a multicenter randomized trial, *Blood* 82:3241-3249, 1993.

AMSA-AZA—AMSACRINE-AZACYTIDINE

Amsacrine. 150 mg/m^2 intravenously on days 1 to 5.

5-Azacytidine. 150 mg/m^2 intravenously on days 1 to 5.

NOTE: If a complete or partial remission is achieved, repeat both drugs at the same dosage level on 3 consecutive days monthly until relapse. These group C drugs may be obtained from the NCI for use on an approved protocol.

Selected Reading

Kahn SB et al: 4'-(9-Acridinylamino) methanesul-fon-*m*-anisidide (m-AMSA) and 5-azacytidine (AZA) in the treatment of relapsed adult acute leukemia, *Am J Clin Oncol* 6:493-502, 1983.

CD—CYTARABINE-DAUNORUBICIN

Cytarabine. 100 mg/m^2 by intravenously infusion over a 24-hour period for 7 days.

Daunorubicin. 45 mg/m^2 intravenously on days 1 to 3.

NOTE: Repeat the courses for further induction or consolidation, with cytarabine for 5 days and daunorubicin for 2 days.

Selected Readings

Yates J et al: Cytosine arabinoside with daunorubicin or Adriamycin for therapy of acute myelocytic leukemia: a CALGB study, *Blood* 60:454-462, 1982.

Yates JW et al: Cytosine arabinoside and daunorubicin therapy in acute nonlymphocytic leukemia, *Cancer Chemother Rep* 57:485-488, 1973.

DAT—DAUNORUBICIN-CYTARABINE-THIOGUANINE
Induction

Daunorubicin. 60 mg/m^2 intravenously on days 5 to 7.

Cytarabine. 100 mg/m^2 intravenously over a 30-minute period twice daily for 7 days.

6-Thioguanine. 100 mg/m^2 orally every 12 hours for 7 days.

Consolidation Therapy

Two cycles of cytarabine and thioguanine every 12 hours for 5 days, followed by a single injection of daunorubicin. Consolidation cycles were given at 21-day intervals.

Central Nervous System Therapy

Prophylactic 2400-cGy cranial irradiation. Cytarabine, 100 mg/m^2 intrathecally divided into five doses. The authors did *not* find that this increased survival. Cranial radiation frequently leads to cognitive loss; the extent depends on dose and age and associated therapy and comorbidity.

Maintenance Therapy

Monthly 5-day cycles of cytarabine and thioguanine alternating with a single dose of daunorubicin.

Selected Readings

Gale RP, Cline MJ: High remission-induction rate in acute myeloid leukemia, *Lancet* 1:497-499, 1977.

Gale RP et al: Intensive chemotherapy for acute myelogenous leukemia, *Ann Intern Med* 94:753-757, 1981.

DAUNORUBICIN–CYTARABINE–HIGH-DOSE CYTARABINE

Induction

Daunorubicin. 45 mg/m^2/day intravenously for 3 days.

Cytarabine. 200 mg/m^2/day by continuous infusion for 7 days.

Consolidation

Cytarabine. 3000 mg/m^2 every 12 hours intravenously over a 3-hour period for six doses on days 1, 3, and 5 for four courses.

Maintenance

Cytarabine. 100 mg/m^2 subcutaneously every 12 hours for 10 doses.

Daunorubicin. 45 mg/m^2 intravenously for 1 dose.

NOTE: If day 14 bone marrow after induction shows persistent disease, a second induction course is given with daunorubicin for 2 days and cytarabine for 5 days in same doses as in the original induction.

Selected Readings

Dillman RO et al: A comparative study of 2 different doses of cytarabine for acute myeloid leukemia: a phase III trial of CALGB, *Blood* 78:2520-2526, 1991.

Mayer RI et al: Intensive postremission chemotherapy in adults with acute myeloid leukemia, *N Engl J Med* 331:896-903, 1994.

IDARUBICIN-CYTARABINE, NO. 1

Induction

Idarubicin. 12 mg/m^2/day intravenously on days 1 to 3.

Cytarabine. 25 mg/m^2 by IV bolus followed immediately by 200 mg/m^2/day by continuous infusion on days 1 to 5.

Consolidation

Idarubicin. 12 mg/m^2/day intravenously on days 1 and 2.

Cytarabine. 25 mg/m² by IV bolus followed immediately by 200 mg/m²/ day by continuous infusion on days 1 to 4.

NOTE: Patients under 50 years of age with an HLA-identical sibling who achieve complete remission are considered for allogeneic bone marrow transplantation.

Selected Reading

Berman E et al: Results of a randomized trial comparing idarubicin and cytosine arabinoside with daunorubicin and cytosine arabinoside in adult patients with newly diagnosed acute myelogenous leukemia, *Blood* 77:1666-1674, 1991.

IDARUBICIN-CYTARABINE, NO. 2

Induction

Idarubicin. 13 mg/m² intravenously on days 1 to 3.

Cytarabine. 100 mg/m² by continuous IV infusion on days 1 to 7.

Postremission Therapy

Idarubicin. 13 mg/m² intravenously for 2 days.

Cytarabine. 100 mg/m² by continuous IV infusion for 5 days.

NOTE: If remission is not achieved with the first course, a second induction course is given. Two postremission courses are given as consolidation.

Selected Reading

Wiernik PH et al: Cytarabine plus idarubicin or daunorubicin as induction and consolidation therapy for previously untreated adult patients with acute myeloid leukemia, *Blood* 79:313-319, 1992.

INTENSIVE FIVE-DRUG THERAPY

Remission Induction

Daunorubicin. 70 mg/m² intravenously on days 1 to 3.

Cytarabine. 100 mg/m² intravenously every 12 hours on days 1 to 7.

6-Thioguanine. 100 mg/m² orally every 12 hours on days 1 to 7.

Prednisone. 40 mg/m² orally on days 1 to 7.

Vincristine. 1 mg/m² intravenously on days 1 and 7.

Consolidation

Daunorubicin. 70 mg/m² intravenously on days 1 and 2.

Cytarabine. 100 mg/m² intravenously every 12 hours on days 1 to 5.

6-Thioguanine. 100 mg/m² orally every 12 hours on days 1 to 5.

Prednisone. 40 mg/m² orally on days 1 to 5.

Vincristine. 1 mg/m² intravenously on day 1.

Monthly Maintenance

Cytarabine. 20 to 25 mg/m² subcutaneously every 6 hours on days 1 to 5.

6-Thioguanine. 100 mg/m² orally every 12 hours on days 1 to 5.

Prednisone. 40 mg/m^2 orally on days 1 to 5.

Vincristine. 1 mg/m^2 intravenously on day 1.

Intensification (Courses 6 and 12)
Same as remission induction.

Selected Reading
Glucksberg H: Intensification therapy for acute nonlymphoblastic leukemia in adults, *Cancer* 52:198-205, 1983.

MITOXANTRONE-CYTARABINE

Mitoxantrone. 12 mg/m^2 intravenously on days 1 to 3.

Cytarabine. 100 mg/m^2/day continuous IV infusion for 7 days.

NOTE: If not in bone marrow CR by day 10, a repeat course was given with the same drugs for 2 and 5 days, respectively. Consolidation begins when peripheral blood is normal, usually 6 weeks after induction. Consolidation consists of two courses of the same drugs for 2 and 5 days, respectively, and a second course of consolidation about 4 weeks later.

Selected Reading
Arlin Z et al: Randomized multicenter trial of cytosine arabinoside with mitoxantrone or daunorubicin in previously untreated adult patients with acute nonlymphocytic leukemia, *Leukemia* 4:177-183, 1990.

MEC–MITOXANTRONE-ETOPOSIDE-CYTARABINE

Mitoxantrone. 12 mg/m^2 intravenously on days 1 to 3.

Etoposide. 200 mg/m^2/day by continuous IV infusion on days 8 to 10.

Cytarabine. 500 mg/m^2/day by continuous IV infusion on days 1 to 3 and 8 to 10.

NOTE: Patients who have a partial or complete remission can receive a second course for reinduction or consolidation, respectively, or may be considered for bone marrow transplantation. Only patients younger than 60 years of age are treated with this regimen.

Selected Reading
Archimbaud E et al: Intensive sequential chemotherapy with mitoxantrone and continuous infusion etoposide and cytarabine for previously treated myelogenous leukemia, *Blood* 77:1894-1900, 1991.

MITOXANTRONE-ETOPOSIDE
Induction
Mitoxantrone. 10 mg/m^2 intravenously on days 1 to 5.

Etoposide. 100 mg/m^2 intravenously on days 1 to 3.

Consolidation
Mitoxantrone. 8 mg/m^2 intravenously on days 1 to 5.

Etoposide. 75 mg/m^2 intravenously on days 1 to 5.

Cytarabine. 75 mg/m^2 intravenously every 12 hours on days 1 to 5.

NOTE: Mitoxantrone is given over a 15-minute period and etoposide over approximately 45 minutes, with induction courses sometimes extended to a fourth or fifth day. Cytarabine is usually infused over a 1-hour period.

Selected Reading

Ho AD et al: Combination therapy with mitoxantrone and etoposide in refractory acute myelogenous leukemia, *Cancer Treat Rep* 70:1025-1027, 1986.

MITOXANTRONE-ETOPOSIDE-INTERDOSE CYTARABINE

Mitoxantrone. 6 mg/m^2/day by IV bolus on days 1 to 6.

Etoposide. 80 mg/m^2/day intravenously over a 1-hour period on days 1 to 6.

Cytarabine. 1000 mg/m^2/day intravenously over a 6-hour period on days 1 to 6.

NOTE: Etoposide was given first each day over a 1-hour period and followed immediately by the 6-hour cytarabine infusion, which was followed 3 hours later by a bolus of mitoxantrone. Complete responders were given a 4-day repeat course as consolidation and then individualized for long-term therapy.

Selected Reading

Amadori S et al: Mitoxantrone, etoposide, and intermediate-dose cytarabine: an effective and tolerable regimen for the treatment of refractory acute myeloid leukemia, *J Clin Oncol* 9:1210-1214, 1991.

MITOXANTRONE–HIGH-DOSE ETOPOSIDE

Mitoxantrone. 7.5 mg/m^2 intravenously on days 1 to 5.

Etoposide. 500 mg/m^2 intravenously on days 1 to 4.

NOTE: Mucositis is severe with this regimen. Repeat in 4 weeks or when pancytopenia or thrombocytopenia recovers.

Selected Reading

O'Brien S et al: Mitoxantrone and high-dose etoposide for patients with relapsed or refractory acute leukemia, *Cancer* 68:691-694, 1991.

SALVAGE REGIMEN

Cytarabine. 3000 mg/m^2 by 1-hour infusion in D$_5$W every 12 hours on days 1 to 6.

Amsacrine. 100 mg/m^2 intravenously on days 7 to 9.

Pyridoxine. 150 mg intravenously every 12 hours on days 1 to 6.

Selected Reading

Hines JD et al: High dose cytosine arabinoside and m-AMSA is effective therapy in relapsed acute nonlymphocytic leukemia, *J Clin Oncol* 2:545-549, 1984.

VAPA–VINCRISTINE-DOXORUBICIN-PREDNISOLONE-CYTARABINE

Induction

Vincristine. 1.5 mg/m² intravenously on days 1 and 5.

Doxorubicin. 30 mg/m² intravenously on days 1 to 3.

Prednisolone. 40 mg/m² intravenously on days 1 to 5 every 12 hours.

Cytarabine. 100 mg/m² by continuous IV infusion on days 1 to 7.

NOTE: If the bone marrow on day 14 is hypoplastic with fewer than 5% blasts, the second induction course is delayed until remission or until blasts repopulate the marrow. If day 14 marrow blasts exceed 5% with cellularity greater than 25%, the second induction is given immediately. It consists of the same dose of the above drugs, but vincristine only on day 1, doxorubicin only on days 1 and 2, and cytarabine only on days 1 to 5. Patients who go into remission are then treated with intensive sequential maintenance therapy.

Sequence I

Doxorubicin. 45 mg/m² intravenously on day 1.

Cytarabine. 200 mg/m² by continuous IV infusion on days 1 to 5.

NOTE: Sequence I is given 4 times at 3- to 4-week intervals.

Sequence II

Doxorubicin. 30 mg/m² intravenously on day 1.

Azacytidine. 150 mg/m² by continuous IV infusion on days 1 to 5.

NOTE: Sequence II is given 4 times at 4-week intervals.

Sequence III

Vincristine. 1.5 mg/m² intravenously on day 1.

Methylprednisolone. 800 mg/m² intravenously on days 1 to 5.

6-Mercaptopurine. 500 mg/m² intravenously on days 1 to 5.

Methotrexate. 7.5 mg/m² intravenously on days 1 to 5.

NOTE: Sequence III is given 4 times at 3-week intervals.

Sequence IV

Cytarabine. 200 mg/m² by continuous IV infusion on days 1 to 5.

NOTE: Sequence IV is given 4 times at 3- to 4-week intervals.

Selected Readings

Weinstein HJ et al: Treatment of acute myelogenous leukemia in children and adults, *N Engl J Med* 303:473-478, 1980.

Weinstein HJ et al: Chemotherapy for acute myelogenous leukemia in children and adults: VAPA update, *Blood* 62:315-319, 1983.

LEUKEMIA: CHRONIC GRANULOCYTIC (MYELOCYTIC)

Chronic granulocytic leukemia (myelocytic) (CML) is the most common of the myeloproliferative disorders. It is not currently curable with conventional chemotherapy. Average survival is 3 or 4 years in the chronic phase; after development of an accelerated phase, survival is usually less than a year, and after blastic transformation, it is only a few months. CML is characterized by the presence of the Philadelphia (Ph) chromosome, which results from the reciprocal translocation between the long arms of chromosomes 9 and 22. It is seen in all hematopoietic precursors. This translocation results in the transfer of the abelson (abl) oncogene to an area of chromosome 22 termed the *breakpoint cluster region (bcr)*. This in turn results in a fused bcr-abl gene. Molecular techniques can now be used to supplement cytogenetic studies to detect the presence of the 9;22 translocation in patients without a visible Ph chromosome (Ph). Patients with Ph− CML (5% of all CML patients) have a poorer response to therapy and a shorter survival than Ph+ patients. Some believe that Ph+ defines CML and those who are Ph− have another disease.

Treatment of CML for cure is initiated early in the chronic phase for patients who have an appropriate bone marrow donor. BMT is less successful in the accelerated phase and almost never in the blastic phase. In the blastic phase, those patients whose cells are lymphoblastic and positive for the enzyme terminal deoxynucleotidyl transferase (TdT) can be treated with combination chemotherapy and often go into remission for 4 to 8 months, which may provide time to do a bone marrow transplantation. For those who have no donor, high-dose chemotherapy with autologous bone marrow transplantation may give some additional time by returning the patient to an earlier stage of disease. For standard-dose chemotherapy, active drugs include interferon-alpha, hydroxyurea, busulfan, cytarabine, mitoxantrone, daunorubicin, 5-azacytidine, and plicamycin. They are frequently used as single agents and sometimes in combination. Interferon alpha will often induce a disappearance of the Ph chromosome and a clinical remission for a time. Hydroxyurea may prolong survival but never achieves a cure. Busulfan was once standard therapy but is difficult to use safely and has more toxicity than the other two agents. Combination chemotherapy seems to give some increased palliation in small series but needs more study.

CVAD—CONTINUOUS VINCRISTINE-DOXORUBICIN-DEXAMETHASONE

Vincristine. 0.4 mg/day continuous IV infusion on days 1 to 4.

Doxorubicin. 12 mg/m²/day continuous IV infusion on days 1 to 4.

Dexamethasone. 40 mg/day total orally on days 1 to 4, 9 to 12, and 17 to 20.

NOTE: Course two is started on day 24 with the addition of cyclophosphamide 1000 mg/m² intravenously that day, and the above regimen is repeated.

Selected Reading

Derderian PM et al: Chronic myelogenous leukemia in the lymphoid blastic phase: characteristics, treatment, response and prognosis, *Am J Med* 94:69-74, 1993.

DAUNORUBICIN-CYTARABINE

Daunorubicin. 120 mg/m^2 intravenously over 2 hours on day 1.

Cytarabine. 500 mg/m^2 intravenously over 2 hours followed by 1500 mg/m^2 by continuous IV infusion over 24 hours on days 1 to 4.

Methylprednisolone. 100 mg/day intravenously on days 1 to 5.

Sargramostim (GM-CSF). 125 µg/m^2/day intravenously beginning 24 hours after completion of chemotherapy until ANC above 200/µL.

NOTE: Results are not spectacular, and toxicity is severe. However, 25% to 33% of those in accelerated or severe blast phase CML can be expected to achieve a transient complete hematological remission, with a lesser percent experiencing a transient cytogenetic response. Patients may then be treated as chronic phase and perhaps qualify for allogeneic bone marrow transplantation.

Selected Reading

Kantarjian HM et al: Treatment of chronic myelogenous leukemia in accelerated and blastic phases with daunorubicin, high-dose cytarabine and granulocyte-macrophage colony-stimulating factor, *J Clin Oncol* 10:398-405, 1992.

MITOXANTRONE-AZACYTIDINE

Mitoxantrone. 12 mg/m^2 intravenously on days 1 to 3.

5-Azacytidine. 150 mg/m^2/day intravenously in three divided doses.

Selected Reading

Dutcher JP et al: Phase II study of mitoxantrone and 5-azacytidine for accelerated and blast crisis of chronic myelogenous leukemia: a study of the Eastern Cooperative Oncology Group, *Leukemia* 6:770-775, 1992.

PLICAMYCIN-HYDROXYUREA

Plicamycin. 25 µg/kg intravenously over a 2- to 4-hour period every other day for 3 weeks.

Hydroxyurea. 4000 mg/day for WBC counts more than 100,000; 3000 mg/day for WBC counts more than 75,000; 2000 mg/day for WBC counts more than 50,000; 1500 mg/day for WBC counts more than 30,000; 1000 mg/day for WBC counts more than 15,000; 500 mg/day for WBC counts more than 7500; hold for WBC counts less than 7500.

NOTE: After 3 weeks, maintenance consisted of plicamycin infusions 1 to 3 times weekly, as well as hydroxyurea according to the above schedule. Plicamycin was withheld for moderate or severe nausea or vomiting, decreased platelet counts, prolongation of prothrombin times, increasing levels of serum glutamic-oxaloacetic transaminase (SGOT) or serum glutamate pyruvic transaminase (SGPT), and symptomatic hypocalcemia refractory to supplementation with oral calcium.

Selected Reading

Koller CA, Miller DM: Preliminary observations on the therapy of the myeloid blast phase of chronic granulocytic leukemia with plicamycin and hydroxyurea, *N Engl J Med* 315:1433-1438, 1986.

VP–VINCRISTINE-PREDNISONE IN LYMPHOID BLAST CRISIS

Vincristine. 2 mg/m² intravenously weekly.

Prednisone. 60 mg/m²/day orally for 14 days and then tapered.

Selected Reading

Canellos GP et al: Hematologic and cytogenetic remission of blastic transformation in chronic granulocytic leukemia, *Blood* 38:671-679, 1971.

LEUKEMIA: CHRONIC LYMPHOCYTIC

Chronic lymphocytic leukemia (CLL) is the most common of the lymphoid leukemias with about 10,000 new cases a year in the United States. It is a disorder of morphologically mature but immunologically less mature lymphocytes and is manifested by progressive accumulation of these cells in the blood, bone marrow, and lymphatic tissues. In most series, 95% of patients have a clonal proliferation of B-lymphocytes, with the remainder having T-cell CLL as determined by cell surface antigen studies. There is no curative therapy. Overall 5-year survival is approximately 60% depending on stage of disease. In early-stage disease, antileukemic therapy is frequently unnecessary. Confusion with prolymphocytic leukemia, hairy cell leukemia, splenic lymphoma, chronic T-cell lymphocytosis, non-Hodgkin's lymphoma, Sezary syndrome, and adult T-cell leukemia/lymphoma may be avoided by determination of cell surface markers and by the clinical presentation. Although CLL is a disease of the elderly, about 15% of patients are younger than 50.

In more advanced stages, especially with immune destruction of red cells and platelets or bulky nodes and/or spleen, therapy is indicated. Active drugs include chlorambucil, cyclophosphamide, prednisone, fludarabine, cladribine, vincristine, and pentostatin. Currently being evaluated are irinotecan, 9-aminocamptothecin, topotecan, paclitaxel, and biological response modifiers. Occasionally, local radiation therapy to bulky nodes or an enlarged spleen is indicated. On occasion, bone marrow transplantation is a consideration, allogeneic or autologous. Whether combination chemotherapy is more efficacious than single-agent therapy is as yet unresolved.

CP VERSUS CVP–CHLORAMBUCIL-PREDNISONE VERSUS CYCLOPHOSPHAMIDE-VINCRISTINE-PREDNISONE

Chlorambucil. 30 mg/m² orally on day 1.

Prednisone. 80 mg total daily dose orally on days 1 to 5.

versus

Cyclophosphamide. 300 mg/m² orally on days 1 to 5.

Vincristine. 1.4 mg/m² intravenously on day 1.

Prednisone. 100 mg/m² orally on days 1 to 5.

NOTE: Repeat every 3 weeks up to 18 months or maximal response. There are no significant differences between these two regimens in complete remission or duration of remission.

Selected Reading

Raphael B et al: Comparison of chlorambucil and prednisone versus cyclophosphamide, vincristine and prednisone as initial treatment for chronic lymphocytic leukemia: long-term follow-up of an Eastern Cooperative Oncology Group randomized clinical trial, *J Clin Oncol* 9:770-776, 1991.

LUNG CANCER: NON–SMALL-CELL CARCINOMA

Non–small-cell lung carcinoma (NSCLC) is the designation that is used to include squamous cell carcinoma, adenocarcinoma, and large-cell undifferentiated carcinoma of the lung when considering therapy because these diseases tend to respond similarly to treatment. They account for about 80% of lung cancers, whereas small-cell cancers comprise almost all of the rest. Unlike many cancers, the cause of lung cancer is clear—85% to 87% of cases are the result of the direct effects of smoking tobacco, 3% to 5% are caused by passive smoking, 3% to 4% are caused by radon, and 4% to 9% are the result of other causes. Thus 90% of lung cancer cases are preventable by avoiding tobacco.

NSCLC is staged by the TNM staging system; stages I and II are surgically resectable and frequently curable but account for only 25% of cases at diagnosis. There is no evidence that chemotherapy is indicated after surgery for stage I. However, several studies demonstrate that platinum-based adjuvant chemotherapy increases the time to tumor recurrence and prolongs survival in stage II disease. About 35% of cases are stage III. Platinum-based neoadjuvant chemotherapy plus radiation therapy in ambulatory patients with good performance in this stage sometimes makes previously inoperable lesions surgically resectable, with prolongation of survival. Stage IV patients are incurable but may derive some palliative benefit from systemic chemotherapy or local radiation therapy to painful metastatic sites or brain metastases.

Single agents that have demonstrated efficacy include cisplatin, ifosfamide, mitomycin, vinblastine, vindisine, and carboplatin. Lesser responses are seen with cyclophosphamide, doxorubicin, epirubicin, etoposide, 5-fluorouracil, and methotrexate. New drugs that show promise and are being evaluated include vinorelbine, irinotecan, edatrexate, fotemustine, gemcitabine, paclitaxel, docetaxel, and topotecan. However, single agents are rarely used except in combination with radiation therapy. Various combination chemotherapy regimens include two, three, four, five, or six drugs or more used concurrently or in sequence. Some regimens are used as first line, others in attempts at salvage to prolong survival. Choice is based on efficacy, toxicity, underlying pathology (that contraindicates some drugs), and physiological age. Some drugs that are favorites in other countries are not yet approved or commercially available in the United States as this was being written. Others are available but insufficiently studied in lung cancers.

CAP–CYCLOPHOSPHAMIDE-DOXORUBICIN-CISPLATIN

Cyclophosphamide. 400 mg/m^2 intravenously on day 1.

Doxorubicin. 40 mg/m^2 intravenously on day 1.

Cisplatin. 60 mg/m^2 intravenously on day 1.

Mannitol. 25 g intravenously with cisplatin.

NOTE: Repeat the cycle every 4 weeks.

Selected Readings

Eagan RT et al: Phase II trial of cyclophosphamide, Adriamycin, and *cis*-dichloro-diammine-platinum II by infusion in patients with adenocarcinoma and large cell carcinoma of the lung, *Cancer Treat Rep* 64:1589-1591, 1979.

Feld R, Rubenstein L, Thomas PA: Adjuvant chemotherapy with cyclophosphamide, doxorubicin and cisplatin in patients with completely resected stage I non–small cell lung cancer, *Chest* 106(6 suppl):307S-309S, 1994.

CARBOPLATIN-IFOSFAMIDE-ETOPOSIDE

Carboplatin. 300 to 350 mg/m^2 intravenously on day 1.

Ifosfamide. 1500 mg/m^2 intravenously on days 1, 3, and 5.

Mesna. 2000 mg (400-mg IV bolus and 1600-mg continuous IV infusion over a 24-hour period) on days 1, 3, and 5.

Etoposide. 60 to 100 mg/m^2 intravenously on days 1, 3, and 5.

NOTE: Repeat every 28 days until progression or a maximum of six courses. Chang et al (1995) gave ifosfamide 1250 mg/m^2 and mesna on days 1 to 3 and etoposide 80 mg/m^2 on days 1 to 3.

Selected Readings

Chang AY et al: Ifosfamide/carboplatin/etoposide chemotherapy in patients with metastatic non–small cell lung cancer, *Semin Oncol* 22(3 suppl 7):9-12, 1995.

van Zandwijk N et al: Dose-finding studies with carboplatin, ifosfamide, etoposide, and mesna in non–small cell lung cancer, *Semin Oncol* 17(suppl 2):16-19, 1990.

CISPLATIN-CYCLOPHOSPHAMIDE-MITOMYCIN

Cisplatin. 75 mg/m^2 intravenously on day 1.

Mitomycin. 10 mg/m^2 intravenously on day 1.

Cyclophosphamide. 400 mg/m^2 intravenously on day 1.

NOTE: Treatment is repeated at 3-week intervals with attention to adequate hydration and antiemetics. A maximum of six cycles is given if there is no progression or unacceptable toxicity. No dose reductions are made, but supportive care is active. This careful, prospective, randomized study showed a highly statistically significant prolongation of survival in the chemotherapy group compared with the supportive care group. The chemotherapy patients, most of whom were treated as outpatients, had only mild toxicity.

Selected Reading

Cartei G et al: Cisplatin-cyclophosphamide-mitomycin combination chemotherapy with supportive care versus supportive care alone for treatment of metastatic non–small cell lung cancer, *J Natl Cancer Inst* 85:794-800, 1993.

CISPLATIN-VINBLASTINE

Cisplatin.   100 mg/m^2 intravenously on days 1 and 29.

Vinblastine.   5 mg/m^2 intravenously on days 1, 8, 15, 22, and 29.

NOTE: Begin radiation therapy on day 50, and give 6000 cGy over a 6-week period. The chemotherapy plus radiation arm showed a survival advantage over the radiation therapy alone arm.

Selected Reading

Dillman RO et al: A randomized trial of induction chemotherapy plus high-dose radiation versus radiation alone in stage III non–small cell lung cancer, *N Engl J Med* 323:940-945, 1990.

ETOPOSIDE WITH CISPLATIN OR CARBOPLATIN

Cisplatin.   120 mg/m^2 intravenously on day 1.

Etoposide.   100 mg/m^2 intravenously on days 1 to 3 *or*

Carboplatin.   325 mg/m^2 intravenously on day 1.

Etoposide.   100 mg/m^2 intravenously on days 1 to 3.

NOTE: Courses may be repeated every 3 or 4 weeks.

Selected Reading

Klastersky J et al: A randomized study comparing cisplatin or carboplatin with etoposide in patients with advanced non–small-cell lung cancer: European Organization for Research and Treatment of Cancer protocol 07861, *J Clin Oncol* 8:1556-1562, 1990.

ORAL ETOPOSIDE-CYCLOPHOSPHAMIDE

Etoposide.   50 mg/m^2/day orally on days 1 to 14.

Cyclophosphamide.   50 mg/m^2/day orally on days 1 to 14.

NOTE: Repeat course every 28 days and adjust for myelosuppression. This outpatient treatment is well tolerated in stage IV patients with survivals comparable to those with more intensive regimens.

Selected Reading

Grunberg SM et al: Extended administration of oral etoposide and oral cyclophosphamide for the treatment of advanced non–small-cell lung cancer: a Southwest Oncology Group study, *J Clin Oncol* 11:1598-1601, 1993.

MIP–MITOMYCIN-IFOSFAMIDE-CISPLATIN

Mitomycin. 6 mg/m^2 intravenously on day 1.

Ifosfamide. 3000 mg/m^2 mixed with mesna 1000 mg/m^2 intravenously on day 1.

Cisplatin. 50 mg/m^2 intravenously on day 1.

NOTE: Additional mesna should be given (e.g., 400 mg/m^2 before, 4 and 8 hours after starting ifosfamide). Three MIP courses are given at 3-week intervals before surgery. The preoperative chemotherapy group had a better survival than the surgery only group.

Selected Reading

Rosell R et al: A randomized trial comparing preoperative chemotherapy plus surgery with surgery alone in patients with non–small-cell lung cancer, *N Engl J Med* 330:153-158, 1994.

MVP–MITOMYCIN-VINBLASTINE-CISPLATIN

Mitomycin. 8 mg/m^2 intravenously on day 1.

Vinblastine. 6 mg/m^2 (maximum 10 mg) intravenously on day 1.

Cisplatin. 50 mg/m^2 intravenously on day 1.

NOTE: Courses repeated every 21 days, but mitomycin given only every other course.

Selected Reading

Ellis PA et al: Symptom relief with MVP (mitomycin C, vinblastine and cisplatin) chemotherapy in advanced non–small-cell lung cancer, *Br J Cancer* 71:366-370, 1995.

PACLITAXEL-CARBOPLATIN

Paclitaxel. 135 mg/m^2 24-hour continuous IV infusion on day 1.

Carboplatin. Dose targeted to AUC 7.5 intravenously on day 1.

Filgrastim (G-CSF). 5 µg/kg subcutaneously on days 3 to 17 in cycles two to six.

NOTE: Paclitaxel can be gradually escalated in increments of 40 mg/m^2 to a maximum of 215 mg/m^2 if well tolerated. Courses are given every 3 weeks to a total of six courses unless the patient relapses sooner. Thirty minutes before starting the paclitaxel infusion, give hypersensitivity prophylaxis with dexamethasone 20 mg intravenously, diphenhydramine 50 mg orally, and cimetidine 300 mg orally. Give carboplatin after the paclitaxel.

Selected Reading

Langer CJ et al: Paclitaxel and carboplatin in combination in the treatment of advanced non–small-cell lung cancer: a phase II toxicity response and survival analysis, *J Clin Oncol* 13:1860-1870, 1995.

VINBLASTINE-CISPLATIN

Vinblastine. 4 mg/m² by IV bolus on days 1 and 2.

Cisplatin. 20 mg/m² intravenously on days 1 to 3.

NOTE: Cisplatin is given over a 2-hour period in 1000 mg of 5% dextrose in ¹/₂ normal saline with appropriate antiemetics. Cycles are repeated every 3 weeks to relapse or limiting toxicity.

Selected Reading

Blum RH et al: Cisplatin and vinblastine chemotherapy for metastatic non–small-cell carcinoma followed by irradiation in patients with regional disease, *Cancer Treat Rep* 70:333-337, 1986.

VINDESINE-CISPLATIN

Vindesine. 3 mg/m² intravenously weekly for 4 weeks and then every 2 weeks.

Cisplatin. 120 mg/m² intravenously on days 1 and 29 and then every 6 weeks.

NOTE: Neurotoxicity may be limiting.

Selected Reading

Rapp E et al: Chemotherapy can prolong survival in patients with advanced non–small-cell lung cancer: report of a Canadian multicenter randomized trial, *J Clin Oncol* 6:633-641, 1988.

VINORELBINE-CISPLATIN

Vinorelbine. 30 mg/m² intravenously over 20 minutes weekly.

Cisplatin. 120 mg/m² intravenously over 1 hour on days 1 and 29, then every 6 weeks.

Selected Reading

LeChevalier T et al: Randomized study of vinorelbine and cisplatin versus vindesine and cisplatin versus vinorelbine alone in advanced non–small-cell lung cancer: results of a European multicenter trial including 612 patients, *J Clin Oncol* 12:360-367, 1994.

VIP–VINORELBINE-IFOSFAMIDE-CISPLATIN

Vinorelbine. 25 mg/m² intravenously on days 1 and 28.

Ifosfamide. 3000 mg/m² intravenously on day 1.

Cisplatin. 80 mg/m² intravenously on day 1.

Mesna. 600 mg/m² intravenously just before and 4 and 8 hours after ifosfamide.

NOTE: Repeat course every 21 days.

Selected Reading

Baldini E et al: Combination chemotherapy with vinorelbine, ifosfamide, and cisplatin: a phase II study in stage III B-IV non–small-cell lung cancer, *Semin Oncol* 21(3 suppl 4):12-15, 1994.

LUNG CANCER: SMALL-CELL CARCINOMA

Small-cell lung cancer (SCLC) comprises 20% of new lung cancer cases and is primarily the result of smoking tobacco. Because it spreads so rapidly, the majority of cases are metastatic at the time of diagnosis. Hence the TNM system has not generally been used, and patients are classified as having limited disease (confined to one lung and the ipsilateral lymph nodes that can be included in a reasonable radiation field) or extensive disease (anything beyond the definition of limited). The natural history of untreated SCLC is 4-month survival in limited-stage disease and 2-month survival in extensive-stage disease. The tumor is very sensitive to multiple chemotherapy drugs and to radiation, with a complete response (CR) rate of 40% to 70% and an overall response (OR) rate of 80% to 95% in limited-stage disease, and a 15% to 30% CR and a 65% to 85% OR rate in extensive-stage disease. In spite of these encouraging response rates, the median survival is 12 to 20 months in limited-stage disease with a 2-year survival of 10% to 40% and a 5-year survival of 6% to 12%. In extensive-stage disease, median survival is 5 to 7 months and a 2-year survival of up to 5% and only anecdotal 5-year survivals.

Active drugs include cisplatin, carboplatin, etoposide, lomustine, carmustine, cyclophosphamide, epirubicin, altretamine, ifosfamide, methotrexate, mechlorethamine, teniposide, and vincristine. Drugs being evaluated include cytarabine, idarubicin, mitomycin, mitoxantrone, vinblastine, gemcitabine, paclitaxel, lonidamine, vinorelbine, docetaxel, irinotecan, and topotecan. However, chemotherapy is used as a single agent only as a radiation sensitizer and is otherwise used therapeutically in combinations of two to six drugs concomitantly or sequentially. Usually, six courses are given. In limited-stage disease, concurrent or sequential radiation therapy is frequently given to the involved thoracic area. Prophylactic cranial radiation used to be given routinely, but since the recognition of postradiation cognitive impairment, radiation is given less frequently to the brain and usually only if the patient has a CR and understands the potential for cognitive impairment. In extensive-stage disease, radiation is used for palliation of bone pain, for bronchial obstruction, for superior vena cava syndrome not responsive to chemotherapy, and for brain metastases. Surgery plays a minor role. Paraneoplastic syndromes include Cushing's, Eaton-Lambert (myasthenic), and secretion of inappropriate antidiuretic hormone (SIADH).

NOTE: Cisplatin-etoposide regimens used in non–small-cell lung cancer are frequently used for small-cell lung cancer.

CAE–CYCLOPHOSPHAMIDE-DOXORUBICIN-ETOPOSIDE

Cyclophosphamide. 1000 mg/m^2 intravenously on day 1.

Doxorubicin. 45 mg/m² intravenously on day 1.

Etoposide. 50 mg/m² intravenously on days 1 to 5.

NOTE: Repeat the cycles every 3 weeks. Patients achieving a complete response receive 3000 cGy of whole-brain irradiation. Patients with limited-stage disease who are not in complete remission after four courses receive 3000 cGy to residual intrathoracic tumor.

Selected Readings

Bunn PA Jr, Greco FA, Einhorn L: Cyclophosphamide, doxorubicin, and etoposide as first line therapy in the treatment of small-cell lung cancer, *Semin Oncol* 13(3 suppl 3):45-53, 1986.

Rudolph A et al: Cytoxan, Adriamycin and etoposide (CAE) versus Cytoxan, Adriamycin and vincristine (CAV) in the treatment of small-cell carcinoma of the lung (SCCL), *Proc Am Soc Clin Oncol* 2:192, 1983.

CARBOPLATIN-ETOPOSIDE

Carboplatin. 300 mg/m² intravenously on day 1.

Etoposide. 100 mg/m² intravenously on days 1 to 3.

NOTE: Repeat every 28 days for four courses. Bishop et al give carboplatin 100 mg/m² intravenously days 1 to 3 and etoposide 120 mg/m² intravenously on days 1 to 3 and give up to six courses if progression free.

Selected Readings

Bishop JF et al: Carboplatin (CBDCA, JM-8) and VP 16-213 in previously untreated patients with small-cell lung cancer, *J Clin Oncol* 5:1574-1578, 1987.

Smith IE et al: Carboplatin (Paraplatin; JM-8) and etoposide (VP-16) as first-line combination therapy for small-cell lung cancer, *J Clin Oncol* 5:185-189, 1987.

CARBOPLATIN-ETOPOSIDE-VINCRISTINE

Carboplatin. 300 mg/m² intravenously on day 1.

Etoposide. 140 mg/m² intravenously on days 1 to 3.

Vincristine. 1.4 mg/m² intravenously (maximum, 2.0) on days 1, 8, and 15.

NOTE: Repeat every 4 weeks for six cycles.

Selected Reading

Gatzemeier U et al: Combination chemotherapy with carboplatin, etoposide, and vincristine as first-line treatment in small-cell lung cancer, *J Clin Oncol* 10:818-823, 1992.

CARBOPLATIN-IFOSFAMIDE

Carboplatin. 300 mg/m² intravenously over a 30-minute period on day 1.

Ifosfamide. 4000 mg/m² by continuous IV infusion over a 24-hour period with hyperhydration on day 1.

Mesna. 450 mg/m² intravenously every 4 hours for nine injections.

Selected Reading

LeChevalier T et al: A phase II study of the combination of carboplatin and ifosfamide in previously untreated metastatic small-cell lung carcinoma, *Cancer*
67:2980-2983, 1991.

CAV—CYCLOPHOSPHAMIDE-DOXORUBICIN-VINCRISTINE

Cyclophosphamide. 1000 mg/m^2 intravenously on day 1.

Doxorubicin. 40 mg/m^2 intravenously on day 1.

Vincristine. 1.0 mg/m^2 (maximum, 2.0 mg) intravenously on day 1.

NOTE: Repeat every 3 weeks for six cycles.

Selected Reading

Roth BJ et al: Randomized study of cyclophosphamide, doxorubicin, and vincristine versus etoposide and cisplatin versus alternation of these two regimens in
extensive small-cell lung cancer: a phase III trial of the Southeastern Cancer Study
Group, *J Clin Oncol* 10:282-291, 1992.

CISPLATIN-ORAL ETOPOSIDE

Cisplatin. 100 mg/m^2 intravenously on day 1.

Etoposide. 50 mg/m^2 by mouth daily for 21 days.

*NOTE: Repeat the treatment every 28 days. Since etoposide is only available as a 50-
mg capsule, dose "rounding" may be necessary.*

Selected Reading

Murphy PB et al: A phase II trial of cisplatin and prolonged administration of oral
etoposide in extensive-stage small cell lung cancer, *Cancer* 69:370-375, 1992.

CISPLATIN-ETOPOSIDE

Etoposide. 80 mg/m^2 intravenously on days 1 to 3.

Cisplatin. 80 mg/m^2 intravenously on day 1.

*NOTE: Repeat every 3 weeks. The high-dose schedule with etoposide given for 5 days
increases toxicity but not the response or survival rates.*

Selected Reading

Ihde DC et al: Prospective randomized comparison of high-dose and standard-dose
etoposide and cisplatin chemotherapy in patients with extensive-stage small-cell
lung cancer, *J Clin Oncol* 12:2022-2034, 1994.

CODE—CISPLATIN-VINCRISTINE-DOXORUBICIN-ETOPOSIDE

Cisplatin. 25 mg/m^2 intravenously on day 1 every week for 9 weeks.

Vincristine. 1 mg/m^2 intravenously on day 1 of weeks 1, 2, 4, 6, and 8.

Doxorubicin. 40 mg/m^2 intravenously on day 1 of weeks 1, 3, 5, 7, and 9.

Etoposide. 80 mg/m^2 intravenously on day 1 of weeks 1, 3, 5, 7, and 9.

Etoposide. 80 mg/m^2 orally on days 2 and 3 of weeks 1, 3, 5, 7, and 9.

Prednisone. 50 mg by mouth daily for 5 weeks, then alternate days to 9 weeks, and then taper over a 2-week period.

Cimetidine. 600 mg orally twice daily for 9 weeks.

Cotrimoxazole. One double-strength tablet twice daily on weeks 2 to 11.

Ketoconazole. 200 mg by mouth daily on weeks 2 to 11.

NOTE: When using ketoconazole, do not allow terfenadine (Seldane) or astemizole (Hismanal) to be administered.

Selected Reading

Murray N et al: Intensive weekly chemotherapy for the treatment of extensive-stage small-cell lung cancer, *J Clin Oncol* 9:1623-1628, 1991.

CPE—CARBOPLATIN-PACLITAXEL-ETOPOSIDE

Paclitaxel. 135 mg/m^2 intravenously by 1-hour infusion on day 1.

Carboplatin. To AUC 5 intravenously on day 1.

Etoposide. 50 mg alternating with 100 mg orally on days 1 to 10.

NOTE: Always give paclitaxel before carboplatin. Premedicate with usual paclitaxel hypersensitivity regimen. Cycles are given every 21 days. Patients with limited-stage disease receive concurrent radiation therapy (4500 cGy/25 fractions) beginning with the third chemotherapy cycle (week 6).

Selected Reading

Hainsworth JD et al: Treatment of small cell lung cancer (SCLC) with paclitaxel (one-hour infusion), carboplatin, and low dose daily etoposide, *Proc Am Soc Clin Oncol* 14:384, 1996.

ECCO—ETOPOSIDE-CARBOPLATIN-CYCLOPHOSPHAMIDE-VINCRISTINE

Etoposide. 120 mg/m^2 intravenously on days 1 to 3.

Carboplatin. 100 mg/m^2 intravenously on days 1 to 3.

Cyclophosphamide. 750 mg/m^2 intravenously on day 1.

Vincristine. 1.4 mg/m^2 intravenously on day 1.

NOTE: Courses given every 28 days for six courses.

Selected Reading

Bishop JF et al: Etoposide, carboplatin, cyclophosphamide and vincristine in previously untreated patients with small-cell lung cancer, *Cancer Chemother Pharmacol* 25:367-370, 1990.

ETOPOSIDE-IFOSFAMIDE-CISPLATIN

Etoposide. 75 mg/m^2/day intravenously on days 1 to 4.

Ifosfamide. 1200 mg/m^2/day intravenously on days 1 to 4.

Cisplatin. 20 mg/m²/day intravenously on days 1 to 4.

Mesna. 300 mg/m² by IV bolus just before ifosfamide and then 1200 mg/m²/day by continuous IV infusion on days 1 to 4.

NOTE: Repeat every 21 days for four cycles.

Selected Reading

Loehrer PJ et al: Etoposide, ifosfamide, and cisplatin in extensive small cell lung cancer, *Cancer* 69:669-673, 1992.

PACLITAXEL-CISPLATIN-ETOPOSIDE

Paclitaxel. 170 mg/m² intravenously over 3 hours on day 1.

Cisplatin. 60 mg/m² intravenously on days 1 to 3.

Etoposide. 80 mg/m² intravenously on days 1 to 3.

Filgrastim (G-CSF). 5 µg/kg subcutaneously on days 5 to 14.

NOTE: Courses given every 21 days. Premedicate with paclitaxel hypersensitivity regimen and give paclitaxel before cisplatin.

Selected Reading

Levitan N et al: Results of phase I dose escalation trial of paclitaxel, etoposide, and cisplatin followed by filgrastim in the treatment of patients with extensive-stage small-cell lung cancer, *Proc Am Soc Clin Oncol* 14:379, 1995.

VICCE—VINCRISTINE-IFOSFAMIDE-CISPLATIN-CARBOPLATIN-ETOPOSIDE

Carboplatin. 300 mg/m² intravenously on day 1 of cycles 1, 3, and 5.

Etoposide. 120 mg/m² intravenously on days 1 and 2, 240 mg/m² orally on day 3.

Ifosfamide. 5000 mg/m² as 24-hour IV infusion mixed with mesna 5000 mg/m² and given on day l.

Mesna. 3000 mg/m² intravenously in 1 L saline over 12 hours at completion of ifosfamide-mesna infusion.

Vincristine. 1 mg/m² intravenously on day 14.

Cisplatin. 100 mg/m² intravenously on day 1 of cycles 2, 4, and 6.

NOTE: Repeat cycles every 3 weeks after cisplatin courses and every 4 weeks after carboplatin cycles. Prophylactic cotrimoxazole 960 mg is given orally twice daily. Check adequate hydration for cisplatin course. Prophylactic cranial irradiation may be given on day 5 of first cycle and thoracic radiation may be given on day 5 of third cycle.

Selected Reading

Prendiville J et al: Intensive therapy for small-cell lung cancer using carboplatin alternating with cisplatin, ifosfamide, etoposide, midcycle vincristine and radiotherapy, *J Clin Oncol* 9:1446-1452, 1991.

VIP—ETOPOSIDE-IFOSFAMIDE-CISPLATIN

Cisplatin. 20 mg/m^2 intravenously on days 1 to 4.

Etoposide. 75 mg/m^2 intravenously on days 1 to 4.

Ifosfamide. 1200 mg/m^2 intravenously on days 1 to 4.

Mesna. 300 mg/m^2 intravenously before first dose ifosfamide and 1200 mg/m^2 by continuous IV infusion on days 1 to 4.

NOTE: Repeat courses every 3 weeks for four cycles. Hydration and antiemetics per routine for cisplatin.

Selected Reading

Loehrer PJ et al: Cisplatin plus etoposide with and without ifosfamide in extensive small-cell lung cancer: a Hoosier Oncology Group study, *J Clin Oncol* 13:2594-2599, 1995.

LYMPHOMA: HODGKIN'S DISEASE

The treatment regimen for Hodgkin's disease (HD) is one of the great success stories of combination chemotherapy. The development of the four-drug regimen with the acronym MOPP produced long-lasting, disease-free intervals that appeared to be cures. This set the stage for the evaluation of combination chemotherapy because single agents almost never produced cures. There are about 8000 new cases of HD each year in the United States. Most are in adults, with a bimodal pattern with peak incidence in people ages 20 to 24 and 80 to 84. HD seems to have an increased incidence in patients with HIV, but it is not an AIDS-defining condition.

Staging is very important in directing therapy, and the Ann Arbor modification of the Rye staging system is generally used. In addition to the four stages, disease is also described as A or B, the latter characterized by fever, night sweats, and a 10% loss of body weight without obvious other cause. The stages are sometimes modified with the designation E to indicate that an organ has been directly invaded by disease from a lymph node. Since the tumor is contiguous and can be included in a reasonable radiation field, it does not downstage the condition. However, one must be sure that the disease in the organ is an extension from the node; otherwise involvement of a nonlymphoid organ indicates stage IV disease and a worse prognosis. Even in stage III-IV disease, combination chemotherapy can lead to cure in 75% of cases.

The usual treatment for stage I and stage IIA is radiation therapy to the area of involvement and one lymph node group beyond, as it is thought that HD spreads in an orderly fashion. Treatment of stage IIB is controversial because the condition is rare and there are no large randomized trials of treatment of this stage. It is important to emphasize, however, that initial therapy should aim for cure and that it should not be compromised to minimize toxicity with the idea that relapse can be salvaged later with aggressive chemotherapy. It is true that combination chemotherapy cures about two thirds of those who relapse after radiation therapy and a lesser percentage of those who relapse after induction chemotherapy, but it ultimately results in more toxicity and a lower cure rate than initial curative therapy.

Active single agents include mechlorethamine, chlorambucil, vincristine, vinblastine, etoposide, procarbazine, prednisone, doxorubicin, idarubicin, epirubicin, daunorubicin, mitoxantrone, cyclophosphamide, ifosfamide, cisplatin, carboplatin, cytarabine, 5-fluorouracil, and methotrexate. Single-agent therapy in HD is never used, and since the development of MOPP, combinations of three, four, or more drugs are the routine initial therapies. Even though overall cure rates are high, one has to consider the cost in toxicity and have contingent plans for the possibility that cure will not occur and a salvage regimen will be necessary. Accordingly, there is now a tendency to use less mechlorethamine and chlorambucil up front. This may reduce the incidence of sterility, of later development of leukemia, and the development of long-term marrow impairment. This would also reduce the chance of having problems with autologous stem cell collection if needed in the future.

One must be aware of the potential lung damage from bleomycin, carmustine, and radiation and of the potential cardiac damage of anthracyclines and high-dose cyclophosphamide. Many salvage regimens are listed because each has its own problems. In some cases a salvage regimen will be used to try to induce another complete response, and in other cases it will be used to demonstrate sensitivity to chemotherapy, for cytoreduction, and for priming for a peripheral blood stem cell (PBSC) collection for high-dose chemotherapy with stem cell and cytokine support. Some regimens for high-dose therapy with autologous bone marrow transplantation (ABMT) or PBSC support are listed in Chapter 9, High-Dose Chemotherapy With Stem Cell Support.

ABDIC—DOXORUBICIN-BLEOMYCIN-DACARBAZINE-LOMUSTINE-PREDNISONE

Doxorubicin. 45 mg/m^2 intravenously on day 1.

Bleomycin. 5 units/m^2 intravenously on days 1 and 5.

Dacarbazine. 200 mg/m^2 intravenously on days 1 to 5.

Lomustine. 50 mg/m^2 orally on day 1.

Prednisone. 40 mg/m^2 orally on days 1 to 5.

NOTE: Repeat every 28 days.

Selected Readings

Rogers RW et al: Adriamycin, bleomycin, DIC, CCNU, and prednisone (ABDIC) chemotherapy in MOPP-resistant Hodgkin's disease, *Cancer* 46:2349-2355, 1980.

Tannir N et al: Long-term follow-up with ABDIC salvage chemotherapy of MOPP-resistant Hodgkin's disease, *J Clin Oncol* 1:432-439, 1983.

ABVD—DOXORUBICIN-BLEOMYCIN-VINBLASTINE-DACARBAZINE

Doxorubicin. 25 mg/m^2 intravenously on days 1 and 15.

Bleomycin. 10 units/m^2 intravenously on days 1 and 15.

Vinblastine. 6 mg/m^2 intravenously on days 1 and 15.

Dacarbazine. 375 mg/m^2 intravenously on days 1 and 15.

NOTE: In the original 1975 report, dacarbazine was given at 150 mg/m^2 intravenously on days 1 to 5. Cycles are repeated every 4 weeks. For patients with poor prognoses, alternating ABVD and MOPP at 4-week intervals has been effective.

Selected Readings

Bonadonna G et al: Combination chemotherapy of Hodgkin's disease with Adriamycin, bleomycin, vinblastine and imidazole carboxamide (ABVD) vs. MOPP, *Cancer* 36:252-259, 1975.

Santoro A, Bonfante V, Bonadonna G: Salvage chemotherapy with ABVD in MOPP-resistant Hodgkin's disease, *Ann Intern Med* 96:139-143, 1982.

B-CAVe—BLEOMYCIN-LOMUSTINE-DOXORUBICIN-VINBLASTINE

Bleomycin. 2.5 units/m^2 intravenously on days 1, 28, and 35.

Lomustine. 100 mg/m^2 orally on day 1.

Doxorubicin. 60 mg/m^2 intravenously on day 1.

Vinblastine. 5 mg/m^2 intravenously on day 1.

NOTE: Cycles are repeated every 6 weeks (if blood cell counts permit) to a total of nine cycles.

Selected Readings

Harker GW, Kuslan P, Rosenberg SA: Combination chemotherapy for advanced Hodgkin's disease after failure of MOPP: ABVD and B-CAVe, *Ann Intern Med* 101:440-446, 1984.

Porzig KJ et al: Treatment of advanced Hodgkin's disease with B-CAVe following MOPP failure, *Cancer* 41:1670-1675, 1978.

BVCPP—CARMUSTINE-VINBLASTINE-CYCLOPHOSPHAMIDE-PROCARBAZINE-PREDNISONE

Carmustine. 100 mg/m^2 intravenously on day 1.

Vinblastine. 5 mg/m^2 intravenously on day 1.

Cyclophosphamide. 600 mg/m^2 intravenously on day 1.

Procarbazine. 100 mg/m^2 orally on days 1 to 10.

Prednisone. 60 mg/m^2 orally on days 1 to 10.

NOTE: Repeat the cycle every 28 days.

Selected Reading

Durant JR et al: BCNU, velban, cyclophosphamide, procarbazine and prednisone (BVCPP) in advanced Hodgkin's disease, *Cancer* 42:2101-2110, 1978.

CEP—LOMUSTINE-ETOPOSIDE-PREDNIMUSTINE

Lomustine. 80 mg/m^2 orally on day 1.

Etoposide. 100 mg/m^2/day orally on days 1 to 5.

Prednimustine. 60 mg/m^2/day orally on days 1 to 5.

NOTE: Repeat every 28 days. As this chapter was written, prednimustine was still experimental in the United States.

Selected Reading

Santoro A et al: CCNU, etoposide and prednimustine (CEP) in refractory Hodgkin's disease, *Semin Oncol* 13(suppl 1):23-26, 1986.

CHLVPP—CHLORAMBUCIL-VINBLASTINE-PROCARBAZINE-PREDNISONE

Chlorambucil. 6 mg/m^2/day orally on days 1 to 14.

Vinblastine. 6 mg/m^2 intravenously on days 1 and 8.

Procarbazine. 100 mg/m^2 orally on days 1 to 14.

Prednisone. 40 mg/day (total) orally on days 1 to 14.

NOTE: Repeat every 28 days for six courses.

Selected Readings

Druker BJ, Rosenthal DS, Canellos GP: Chlorambucil, vinblastine, procarbazine and prednisone: an effective but less toxic regimen than MOPP for advanced-stage Hodgkin's disease, *Cancer* 63:1060-1064, 1989.

Selby P et al: ChlVPP combination chemotherapy for Hodgkin's disease: long term results, *Br J Cancer* 62:279-285, 1990,

CVPP—LOMUSTINE-VINBLASTINE-PROCARBAZINE-PREDNISONE

Lomustine. 75 mg/m^2 orally on day 1.

Vinblastine. 4 mg/m^2 intravenously on days 1 and 8.

Procarbazine. 100 mg/m^2 orally on days 1 to 14.

Prednisone. 40 mg/m^2 orally on days 1 to 14.

NOTE: Repeat the cycle every 28 days. Prednisone is given in cycles 1 and 4 only.

Selected Reading

Cooper MR et al: A new effective four-drug combination of CCNU (1-[2-chloroethyl]-3-cyclohexyl-1-nitrosourea) (NSC-79038), vinblastine, prednisone and procarbazine for the treatment of advanced Hodgkin's disease, *Cancer* 46:654-662, 1980.

CVPP—CYCLOPHOSPHAMIDE-VINBLASTINE-PROCARBAZINE-PREDNISONE

Cyclophosphamide. 300 mg/m^2 intravenously on days 1 and 8.

Vinblastine. 10 mg intravenously on days 1, 8, and 15.

Procarbazine. 100 mg/m² orally on days 1 to 15.

Prednisone. 40 mg/m² orally on days 1 to 15.

NOTE: Repeat the cycle every 28 days. Prednisone is given in cycles 1 and 4 only.

Selected Reading

Gibbs GE et al: Long-term survival of patients with Hodgkin's disease: treatment with cyclophosphamide, vinblastine, procarbazine, and prednisone, *Arch Intern Med* 141:897-900, 1981.

LOPP/EVAP
LOPP—Chlorambucil-Vincristine-Procarbazine-Prednisone
Chlorambucil. 10 mg (total) orally on days 1 to 10.

Vincristine. 1.4 mg/m² (maximum, 2.0 mg) intravenously on days 1 and 8.

Procarbazine. 100 mg/m²/day (maximum, 200 mg) orally on days 1 to 10.

Prednisone. 25 mg/m²/day (maximum, 60 mg) orally on days 1 to 14.

EVAP—Etoposide-Vinblastine-Doxorubicin-Prednisone
Etoposide. 150 mg/m²/day (maximum, 200 mg) orally on days 1 to 3.

Vinblastine. 6 mg/m² (maximum, 10 mg) intravenously on days 1 and 8.

Doxorubicin. 25 mg/m² intravenously on days 1 and 8.

Prednisone. 25 mg/m²/day (maximum, 60 mg) orally on days 1 to 14.

NOTE: Give four courses of LOPP alternating with four courses of EVAP (LOPP, EVAP, LOPP, EVAP . . .) until complete remission (CR) and then a total of four additional alternating courses to a maximum response (e.g., if CR occurred after the sixth course, give a total of 10 courses; if CR occurred after the eighth course, give a total of 12 courses).

Selected Reading

Hancock BW et al: LOPP alternating with EVAP is superior to LOPP alone in the initial treatment of advanced Hodgkin's disease: results of a British National Lymphoma Investigational Trial, *J Clin Oncol* 10:1252-1258, 1992.

MOPP—MECHLORETHAMINE-VINCRISTINE-PROCARBAZINE-PREDNISONE
Mechlorethamine. 6 mg/m² intravenously on days 1 and 8.

Vincristine. 1.4 mg/m² intravenously on days 1 and 8.

Procarbazine. 100 mg/m² orally on days 1 to 14.

Prednisone. 40 mg/m² orally on days 1 to 14.

NOTE: Usually six courses are given or two courses beyond complete remission. C-MOPP simply replaces the mechlorethamine with cyclophosphamide, 650 mg/m², on days 1 and 8. Repeat every 28 days.

Selected Reading

DeVita VT Jr, Serpick AA, Carbone PO: Combination chemotherapy in the treatment of advanced Hodgkin's disease, *Ann Intern Med* 73:881-895, 1970.

MOPP/ABV HYBRID

Mechlorethamine. 6 mg/m^2 intravenously on day 1.

Vincristine. 1.4 mg/m^2 (maximum dose, 2.0 mg) intravenously on day 1.

Procarbazine. 100 mg/m^2 orally on days 1 to 7.

Prednisone. 40 mg/m^2 orally on days 1 to 14.

Doxorubicin. 35 mg/m^2 intravenously on day 8.

Bleomycin. 10 units/m^2 intravenously on day 8.

Vinblastine. 6 mg/m^2 intravenously on day 8.

NOTE: Repeat the cycle every 28 days. Each dose of bleomycin is preceded by 100 mg of hydrocortisone intravenously. If chemical phlebitis occurs from mechlorethamine, 600 mg/m^2 of cyclophosphamide may be substituted.

Selected Reading

Klimo P, Connors JM: MOPP/ABV hybrid program: combination chemotherapy based on early introduction of seven effective drugs for advanced Hodgkin's disease, *J Clin Oncol* 3:1174-1182, 1985.

MOP-BAP–MECHLORETHAMINE-VINCRISTINE-PROCARBAZINE-BLEOMYCIN-DOXORUBICIN-PREDNISONE

Mechlorethamine. 6 mg/m^2 intravenously on day 1.

Vincristine. 1.4 mg/m^2 intravenously on days 1 and 8 (maximum, 2.0 mg).

Procarbazine. 100 mg/m^2 orally on days 2 to 7 and days 9 to 12 (total, 10 days).

Bleomycin. 2 units/m^2 intravenously on days 1 and 8.

Doxorubicin. 30 mg/m^2 intravenously on day 8.

Prednisone. 40 mg/m^2 on days 2 to 7 and 9 to 12 (total, 10 days).

NOTE: Repeat the cycles every 4 weeks for 10 courses. Prednisone is given during the first, fourth, seventh, and tenth courses of therapy.

Selected Reading

Jones SE et al: Comparison of Adriamycin-containing chemotherapy (MOP-BAP) with MOPP-bleomycin in the management of advanced Hodgkin's disease, *Cancer* 51:1339-1347, 1983.

MVPP–MECHLORETHAMINE-VINBLASTINE-PROCARBAZINE-PREDNISONE

Mechlorethamine. 6 mg/m^2 intravenously on days 1 and 8.

Vinblastine. 6 mg/m^2 intravenously on days 1 and 8.

Procarbazine. 100 mg/m^2 orally on days 1 to 14.

Prednisone. 40 mg/m^2 orally on days 1 to 14.

NOTE: Repeat every 28 days.

Selected Reading

Nicholson WM et al: Combination chemotherapy in generalized Hodgkin's disease, *Br Med J* 3:7-10, 1970.

PAVe—PROCARBAZINE-MELPHALAN-VINBLASTINE

Procarbazine. 100 mg/m^2/day orally on days 1 to 14.

Melphalan. 7.5 mg/m^2 orally on days 1, 2, 8, and 9.

Vinblastine. 6.0 mg/m^2 intravenously on days 1 and 8.

NOTE: Patients receive radiation therapy plus six cycles of PAVe at monthly intervals.

Selected Readings

Horning SJ et al: The Stanford experience with procarbazine, alkeran and vinblastine (PAVe) and radiotherapy for locally extensive and advanced stage Hodgkin's disease, *Ann Oncol* 3:747-754, 1992.

Thompson JM et al: Current Stanford results utilizing MOP(P) vs. PAVe as adjuvant chemotherapy for Hodgkin's disease, *Proc Am Soc Clin Oncol* 2:212, 1983.

SCAB—STREPTOZOCIN-LOMUSTINE-DOXORUBICIN-BLEOMYCIN

Streptozocin. 500 mg/m^2 intravenously on days 1 to 5.

Lomustine. 100 mg/m^2 orally on day 1.

Doxorubicin. 45 mg/m^2 intravenously on day 1.

Bleomycin. 15 units/m^2 IM on days 1 and 8.

NOTE: Repeat the cycle every 28 days.

Selected Reading

Diggs CH, Wiernik PH, Sutherland JC: Treatment of advanced untreated Hodgkin's disease with SCAB: an alternative to MOPP, *Cancer* 47:224-228, 1981.

STANFORD V REGIMEN

Doxorubicin. 25 mg/m^2 intravenously on days 1 and 15.

Vinblastine. 6 mg/m^2 intravenously on days 1 and 15.

Mechlorethamine. 6 mg/m^2 intravenously on day 1.

Vincristine. 1.4 mg/m^2 (maximum 2 mg) on days 8 and 22.

Bleomycin. 5 units/m^2 intravenously on days 8 and 22.

Etoposide. 60 mg/m² intravenously on days 15 and 16.

Prednisone. 40 mg/m² orally every other day.

NOTE: Treatment cycle is repeated every 28 days for three cycles. In the third cycle, vinblastine dose is decreased to 4 mg/m² and vincristine to 1 mg/m² for patients 50 years and older. Prednisone is tapered for all patients by 10 mg every other day starting at week 10. All patients receive cotrimoxazole, acyclovir, and ketoconizole as prophylaxis against infection. An H-2 blocker is used to prevent corticosteroid gastritis, and stool softeners prevent constipation from vinca alkaloids. Two weeks after the completion of chemotherapy, radiation (3600 cGy) is given to areas of initially bulky disease.

Selected Reading

Bartlett NL et al: Brief chemotherapy, Stanford V, and adjuvant radiotherapy for bulky or advanced stage Hodgkin's disease: a preliminary report, *J Clin Oncol* 13:1080-1088, 1996.

VBM–VINBLASTINE-BLEOMYCIN-METHOTREXATE

Vinblastine. 6 mg/m² intravenously on days 1 and 8.

Bleomycin. 10 units/m² intravenously on days 1 and 8.

Methotrexate. 30 mg/m² intravenously on days 1 and 8.

NOTE: Treatment is given every 28 days for six courses.

Selected Reading

Horning SJ et al: Vinblastine, bleomycin, and methotrexate: an effective adjuvant in favorable Hodgkin's disease, *J Clin Oncol* 6:1822-1831, 1988.

VEEP–VINCRISTINE-EPIRUBICIN-ETOPOSIDE-PREDNISOLONE

Vincristine. 1.4 mg/m² (maximum 2 mg) intravenously on days 1 and 8.

Epirubicin. 50 mg/m² intravenously on day 1.

Etoposide. 100 mg/m² intravenously days 1 to 4, or 200 mg orally on days 1 to 4.

Prednisolone. 100 mg total orally on days 1 to 8.

NOTE: Prednisone may be substituted for prednisolone. Epirubicin was selected for its reputed lesser toxicity compared with doxorubicin. If the WBC count is greater than 1500/μL and the platelet count greater than 100,000/μL on days 8 and 15, then etoposide is given for 5 days in the next course. If the WBC count is less than 1000/μL or platelets less than 50,000/μL, then etoposide is given for only 3 days in the next course. Therapy is given for two courses beyond a complete remission.

Selected Reading

Hill M et al: Evaluation of the efficacy of the VEEP regimen in adult Hodgkin's disease with assessment of gonadal and cardiac toxicity, *J Clin Oncol* 13:387-395, 1995.

LYMPHOMA: NON-HODGKIN'S DISEASE

Non-Hodgkin's lymphoma (NHL) is the sixth most common cause of cancer and the sixth most common cause of cancer deaths in the United

States in 1996. There are over 52,000 new cases a year and 23,300 deaths a year. Survival is improving, but there is room for more information, better therapy, and better survival.

Treatment is based on accurate staging and pathology. As mentioned in the introduction to the Hodgkin's disease section, the E designation is for disease spread from lymph nodes to other organs by direct extension. As the understanding of lymphoma pathology improved with the characterization of B and T cells and the antibodies that are raised to them, new classification schemes have evolved. Although most in the United States preferred the Rappaport morphological classification initially, it was soon challenged by the Lukes-Butler immunological approach in the United States and by the Kiel classification in Europe. Finally, to be able to translate the understanding of the pathology from one laboratory to another and from one country to another, an international working formulation was cooperatively developed and published in 1982 under the auspices of the NCI. This was intended to serve only as a way to translate with understanding from one system to another, but it soon became a classification itself and, in fact, the dominant one. Recently, a new international classification has been developed, the Revised European-American Lymphoma (REAL) Classification (Harris NL et al: A revised European-American classification of lymphoid neoplasms: a proposal from the International Lymphoma Study Group, *Blood* 84:1361-1392, 1994).

Active drugs for treatment of NHL include chlorambucil, cyclophosphamide, doxorubicin, idarubicin, epirubicin, mitoxantrone, vincristine, vinblastine, procarbazine, methotrexate, cytarabine, bleomycin, etoposide, teniposide, fludarabine, cladribine, pentostatin, cisplatin, carboplatin, prednisone, and dexamethasone. New agents are currently being evaluated in clinical trials. After the dramatic success of combination chemotherapy in producing long-term, disease-free complete remissions in a high percentage of cases of advanced Hodgkin's disease, the same principles and some of the same chemotherapy regimens were applied to the treatment of stages II, III, and IV non-Hodgkin's lymphomas. Results were very encouraging in intermediate- and high-grade lymphomas with a series of first-generation regimens: MOPP, C-MOPP, BACOP, CVP, CHOP, and COMLA. In an attempt to improve both the response rates and survival, a series of second-generation protocols evolved: COPBLAM, M-BACOD, m-BACOD, and ProMACE-MOPP. Although better results were claimed for these regimens in small, uncontrolled studies, the results were not convincing, and a third generation of new protocols was introduced with claims of great superiority in uncontrolled studies for these new regimens: COPBLAM-III, MACOP-B, ProMACE-CytaBOM, and CODBLAM IV. After several small two-arm randomized prospective cooperative studies failed to demonstrate a statistically significant superiority of some second-generation regimens over first generation, and third generation over second, a four-arm large intergroup cooperative study was launched. The report of that study showed no significant difference in response rate, time to treatment failure, or overall survival between CHOP, m-BACOD, Pro-MACE-CytaBOM, and MACOP-B (Fisher RI et al: Comparison of a standard regimen (CHOP) with three intensive chemotherapy regimens for advanced non-Hodgkin's lymphoma, *N Engl J Med* 328:1002-1006,1993).

Therapy has been based largely on stage and pathology. To develop a more accurate prognostic index, an international group pooled its case material and evaluated outcomes after doxorubicin-based combination chemotherapy. They found that prognosis was most predictable if based on pathological stage, level of lactic dehydrogenase (LDH), performance status, and age (under or over 60 years). This helps in selecting initial therapy and salvage therapy when necessary. Various attempts to salvage patients who failed initial therapy led to large numbers of salvage regimens. A few of the more widely used are listed in addition to the first-, second-, and third-generation regimens because they offer opportunities to treat patients who may have cardiac, renal, or pulmonary contraindications to the use of some of the drugs. In addition, some of the salvage regimens are used to debulk relapsed disease and demonstrate continued drug sensitivity before an attempt at high-dose chemotherapy with autologous bone marrow transplantation or stem cell support to reinduce a sustained remission. The high-dose transplantation-associated regimens with or without radiation therapy vary from one transplantation center to another and on average yield a 20% to 40% cure rate. They are listed in Chapter 9, High-Dose Chemotherapy With Stem Cell Support. The dizzying plethora of regimens indicates a lack of clear superiority of any one at this time. However, anyone treating bulky lymphomas must be prepared to deal with the tumor lysis syndrome (Cohen LF et al: Acute tumor lysis syndrome, *Am J Med* 68:486-491, 1980).

Although cures can be achieved in about 50% of patients with intermediate and high-grade lymphoma, cures are rare in low-grade lymphoma. They may be indolent and progress slowly over 5 to 8 years, but eventually kill the patient. It is not yet clear what therapeutic approach is best. A few patients are best observed until they show signs of progression. Others are well served with single-agent chemotherapy. Most are treated with mild combination chemotherapy, and several regimens are listed for that purpose. High-dose chemotherapy with stem cell support is strictly experimental in this setting.

High-grade B-cell non-Hodgkin's lymphoma in HIV-infected patients is an AIDS-defining morbidity, just as an opportunistic infection is. Because these patients are generally immunodepressed from their HIV infection and 30% to 50% of their tumors are associated with Epstein-Barr virus (EBV), the therapy of their aggressive lymphoma is particularly difficult. The chemotherapy itself further compromises the immune system, increasing the likelihood of opportunistic infection. Hence lower dose intensity treatment is used most often, and some of these regimens are listed. About half of these patients have some regression of their lymphoma, but it is usually brief, and about 50% die of their lymphoma and the remainder succumb to an opportunistic infection.

AIDS-related primary central nervous system lymphoma is 100% EBV associated and is usually an aggressive B-cell neoplasm in patients with far-advanced AIDS. Radiation therapy alone is the usual palliative therapy. Attempts to breach the blood-brain barrier and deliver effective chemotherapy are being tried in a few centers under carefully defined experimental protocols for patients with primary non-Hodgkin's lymphoma of the brain that is *not* HIV-associated. It may also be treated with combination chemotherapy followed by radiation therapy.

The problems of lymphoblastic lymphoma and Burkitt's lymphoma are not addressed with detailed regimens here. They are seen more frequently in children, and although very aggressive, they are fortunately uncommon and potentially curable. Useful regimens are long and complex and are available in several references, including the following.

Selected Readings

Lymphoblastic lymphoma

Anderson JR et al: Childhood non-Hodgkin's lymphoma: the results of a randomized therapeutic trial comparing a 4-drug regimen (COMP) with a 10-drug regimen (LSA$_2$-L$_2$), *N Engl J Med* 308:559-565,1983.

Coleman CN et al: Treatment of lymphoblastic lymphoma in adults, *J Clin Oncol* 4:1628-1637, 1986.

Hvizdala EV et al: Lymphoblastic lymphoma in children: a randomized trial comparing LSA$_2$-L$_2$ with the A-COP + therapeutic regimen: a Pediatric Oncology Group study, *J Clin Oncol* 6:26-33, 1988.

Levine AM et al: Successful therapy of convoluted T-lymphoblastic lymphoma in the adult, *Blood* 61:92-99, 1983.

Magrath IT et al: An effective therapy for both undifferentiated (including Burkitt's) lymphomas and lymphoblastic lymphomas in children and young adults, *Blood* 63:1102-1111, 1984.

Salloum E et al: Lymphoblastic lymphoma in adults: a clinicopathological study of 34 cases treated at the Institut Gustave-Roussy, *Eur J Cancer Clin Oncol* 24:1609-1616, 1988.

Slater DE et al: Lymphoblastic lymphoma in adults, *J Clin Oncol* 4:57-67, 1986.

Voak JB, Jones SE, McKelvey EM: The chemotherapy of lymphoma, *Blood* 57: 186-188, 1981.

Weinstein HJ, Cassady JR, Levey R: Long-term results of the APO protocol (vincristine, doxorubicin [Adriamycin], and prednisone) for the treatment of mediastinal lymphoblastic lymphoma, *J Clin Oncol* 1:537-541, 1983.

Noncleaved cell lymphomas

Bernstein JI et al: Combined modality therapy for adults with small noncleaved cell lymphoma (Burkitt's and non-Burkitt's type), *J Clin Oncol* 4:847-858, 1986.

Lopez TM et al: Small non-cleaved cell lymphoma in adults: superior results for stages I-III disease, *J Clin Oncol* 8:615-622, 1990.

McMaster ML et al: Effective treatment of small non-cleaved-cell lymphoma with high density, brief duration chemotherapy, *J Clin Oncol* 9:941-946, 1991.

For pediatric lymphomas, leukemias, and solid tumors, abundant material is available in the following books.

Fernbach DJ, Vietti TJ: *Clinical pediatric oncology*, ed 4, St. Louis, 1991, Mosby.

Miller DR, Baehner RL: *Blood diseases of infancy and childhood*, St. Louis, 1995, Mosby.

Nathan DG, Oski F: *Hematology of infancy and childhood*, ed 4, Philadelphia, 1992, WB Saunders.

Pizzo PA, Poplack DG: *Principles and practice of pediatric oncology*, ed 3, Philadelphia, 1997, Lippincott-Raven.

ACOB–DOXORUBICIN-CYCLOPHOSPHAMIDE-VINCRISTINE-BLEOMYCIN-PREDNISONE

Doxorubicin.   50 mg/m^2 intravenously on day 1 of weeks 1, 3, and 5.

Cyclophosphamide. 350 mg/m² intravenously on day 1 of weeks 1, 3, and 5.

Vincristine. 1.4 mg/m² (2 mg maximum) intravenously on day 1 of weeks 2, 4, and 6.

Bleomycin. 10 units/m² intravenously on day 1 of weeks 2, 4, and 6.

Prednisone. 50 mg by mouth daily for 28 days and then taper.

Cotrimoxazole. 1 double-strength tablet orally twice daily for 6 weeks.

Ketoconazole. 200 mg by mouth daily for 6 weeks.

NOTE: Patients taking ketoconazole should avoid use of terfenadine (Seldane) and astemizole (Hismanal).

Selected Readings

Connors JM et al: Brief chemotherapy and involved field radiation therapy for limited stage, histologically aggressive lymphoma, *Ann Intern Med* 107:25-30, 1987.

Connors JM et al: ACOB: 6 week chemotherapy and involved field radiotherapy (IFRT) for limited stage large cell lymphoma: initial results, *Proc Am Soc Clin Oncol* 7:224, 1988.

ACOMLA–DOXORUBICIN-CYCLOPHOSPHAMIDE-VINCRISTINE-METHOTREXATE-LEUCOVORIN-CYTARABINE

Doxorubicin. 40 mg/m² intravenously on day 1.

Cyclophosphamide. 1000 mg/m² intravenously on day 1.

Vincristine. 2.0 mg intravenously on days 1, 8, and 15.

Methotrexate. 120 mg/m² intravenously on days 22, 29, 36, 43, 50, 57, 64, and 71.

Cytarabine. 300 mg/m² intravenously 1 hour after the methotrexate on days 22, 29, 36, 43, 50, 57, 64, and 71.

Leucovorin. 25 mg orally 24 hours after each methotrexate dose and repeated every 6 hours for six doses.

NOTE: Administer three cycles, each lasting 3 months.

Selected Reading

Newcomer LN et al: Randomized study comparing doxorubicin, cyclophosphamide, vincristine, methotrexate with leucovorin rescue, and cytarabine (ACOMLA) with cyclophosphamide, doxorubicin, vincristine, prednisone, and bleomycin (CHOP-B) in the treatment of diffuse histiocytic lymphoma, *Cancer Treat Rep* 66:1279-1284, 1982.

AIDS-RELATED ORAL REGIMEN

Lomustine (CCNU). 100 mg/m² orally on day 1 of cycles 1, 3, and 5.

Etoposide. 200 mg/m² orally on days 1 to 3.

Cyclophosphamide. 100 mg/m² orally on days 22 to 31.

Procarbazine. 100 mg/m^2 orally on days 22 to 31.

NOTE: Each cycle is 42 days.

Selected Readings

Remick S et al: Novel oral combination chemotherapy (CT) in the management of AIDS-related non-Hodgkin lymphoma (NHL): longer follow-up, *Proc Am Soc Clin Oncol* 11:48, 1992.

Remick SC et al: Novel oral combination chemotherapy in the treatment of inter-mediate-grade and high-grade AIDS-related non-Hodgkin's lymphoma, *J Clin Oncol* 11:1691-1702, 1993.

AIDS-RELATED INTRAVENOUS REGIMEN

Cyclophosphamide. 300 mg/m^2 intravenously on day 1.

Doxorubicin. 25 mg/m^2 intravenously on day 1.

Vincristine. 1.4 mg/m^2 intravenously (maximum, 2.0 mg) on day 1.

Bleomycin. 4 units/m^2 intravenously on day 1.

Dexamethasone. 3 mg/m^2/day orally on days 1 to 5.

Methotrexate. 500 mg/m^2 intravenously on day 15.

Leucovorin. 25 mg orally every 6 hours for four doses beginning 6 hours after the completion of methotrexate.

Cytarabine. 50 mg intrathecally on days 1, 8, 21, and 28.

NOTE: For patients with known CNS involvement, give helmet-field radiotherapy to 4000 cGy; with known marrow involvement alone, give 2400 cGy to same field. Chemotherapy cycles are given at 28-day intervals for four to six cycles. Zidovudine may be resumed after chemotherapy. Proteases need not be interrupted.

Selected Reading

Levine AM et al: Low-dose chemotherapy with central nervous system prophylaxis and zidovudine maintenance in AIDS-related lymphoma, *JAMA* 266:84-88, 1991.

AIDS-RELATED INFUSIONAL REGIMEN

Cyclophosphamide. 187.5 mg/m^2/day IV infusion on days 1 to 4.

Doxorubicin. 12.5 mg/m^2/day IV infusion on days 1 to 4.

Etoposide. 60 mg/m^2/day IV infusion on days 1 to 4.

NOTE: All drugs administered as a continuous infusion over 4 days. Therapy is repeated every 28 or more days for up to six cycles.

Selected Reading

Sparano JA et al: Infusional cyclophosphamide, doxorubicin, and etoposide in human immunodeficiency virus and human T-cell leukemia virus type I–related non-Hodgkin's lymphoma: a highly active regimen, *Blood* 81:2810-2815, 1993.

BACOP—BLEOMYCIN-DOXORUBICIN-CYCLOPHOSPHAMIDE-VINCRISTINE-PREDNISONE

Bleomycin. 4 units/m^2 intravenously on days 1, 5, 8, 12, 15, and 19.

Doxorubicin. 45 mg/m^2 intravenously on day 1.

Cyclophosphamide. 600 mg/m^2 intravenously on day 1.

Vincristine. 1.2 mg/m^2 intravenously on days 1, 8, and 15.

Prednisone. 40 mg/m^2 orally on days 1 to 21 and then taper.

NOTE: Repeat the cycle every 21 days.

Selected Reading

Skarin AT et al: Combination chemotherapy of advanced non-Hodgkin's lymphoma with bleomycin, Adriamycin, cyclophosphamide, vincristine, and prednisone (BACOP), *Blood* 49:759-770, 1977.

CAP-BOP—CYCLOPHOSPHAMIDE-DOXORUBICIN-PROCARBAZINE-BLEOMYCIN-VINCRISTINE-PREDNISONE

Cyclophosphamide. 650 mg/m^2 intravenously on day 1.

Doxorubicin. 50 mg/m^2 intravenously on day 1.

Procarbazine. 100 mg/m^2 orally on days 1 to 7.

Bleomycin. 10 units/m^2 subcutaneously on day 15.

Vincristine. 1.4 mg/m^2 intravenously on day 15.

Prednisone. 100 mg orally on days 15 to 21.

NOTE: Repeat at 21- to 28-day intervals to documented complete remission, and then give two more courses. In patients older than 70 years of age, give two-thirds doses of all drugs except prednisone.

Selected Reading

Armitage JO et al: Chemotherapy for diffuse large-cell lymphoma: rapidly responding patients have more durable remissions, *J Clin Oncol* 4:160-164, 1986.

CHOEP—CYCLOPHOSPHAMIDE-DOXORUBICIN-VINCRISTINE-ETOPOSIDE-PREDNISOLONE

Cyclophosphamide. 750 mg/m^2 intravenously on day 1.

Doxorubicin. 50 mg/m^2 intravenously on day 1.

Vincristine. 2 mg total intravenously on day 1.

Etoposide. 100 mg/m^2 intravenously on days 1 to 3.

Prednisolone. 100 mg total orally on days 1 to 5.

NOTE: Repeat every 21 days for four courses. Prednisone can replace prednisolone. Some patients may need granulocyte colony-stimulating factor for the second and subsequent courses.

Selected Reading

Koppler H et al: Sequential versus alternating chemotherapy for high-grade non-Hodgkin's lymphomas: a randomized multicentre trial, *Hematol Oncol* 1:217-223, 1991.

CHOP—CYCLOPHOSPHAMIDE-DOXORUBICIN-VINCRISTINE-PREDNISONE

Cyclophosphamide. 750 mg/m^2 intravenously on day 1.

Doxorubicin. 50 mg/m^2 intravenously on day 1.

Vincristine. 1.4 mg/m^2 intravenously on day 1.

Prednisone. 100 mg/m^2 orally on days 1 to 5.

NOTE: Repeat the cycle every 3 weeks.

Selected Reading

McKelvey EM et al: Hydroxydaunomycin (Adriamycin) combination chemotherapy in malignant lymphoma, *Cancer* 38:1484-1493, 1976.

CHOP-BLEO—CYCLOPHOSPHAMIDE-DOXORUBICIN-VINCRISTINE-PREDNISONE-BLEOMYCIN

Cyclophosphamide. 750 mg/m^2 intravenously on day 1.

Doxorubicin. 50 mg/m^2 intravenously on day 1.

Vincristine. 2 mg intravenously on days 1 and 5.

Prednisone. 100 mg orally on days 1 to 5.

Bleomycin. 15 units intravenously on days 1 and 5.

NOTE: Repeat the cycle every 21 or 28 days.

Selected Reading

Rodriguez V et al: Combination chemotherapy (CHOP-Bleo) in advanced (non-Hodgkin's) malignant lymphoma, *Blood* 49:325-333, 1977.

C-MOPP—CYCLOPHOSPHAMIDE-VINCRISTINE-PROCARBAZINE-PREDNISONE

Cyclophosphamide. 650 mg/m^2 intravenously on days 1 and 8.

Vincristine. 1.4 mg/m^2 intravenously on days 1 and 8.

Procarbazine. 100 mg/m^2 orally on days 1 to 14.

Prednisone. 40 mg/m^2 orally on days 1 to 14.

NOTE: Cycles are 14 days with 14-day rest period.

Selected Readings

DeVita VT Jr et al: Advanced diffuse histiocytic lymphoma, a potentially curable disease, *Lancet* 1:248-250, 1975.

CNOP–CYCLOPHOSPHAMIDE-MITOXANTRONE-VINCRISTINE-PREDNISONE

Cyclophosphamide. 750 mg/m² intravenously on day 1.

Mitoxantrone. 10 mg/m² intravenously on day 1.

Vincristine. 1.4 mg/m² intravenously on day 1.

Prednisone. 50 mg/m² orally on days 1 to 5.

NOTE: Repeat at 4-week intervals for six courses or two courses beyond a complete remission.

Selected Readings

Pavlovsky S et al: Results of a randomized study of previously-untreated intermediate and high grade lymphoma using CHOP versus CNOP, *Ann Oncol* 3:205-209, 1992.

Sonneveld P, Michiels JJ: Full dose chemotherapy in elderly patients with non-Hodgkin's lymphoma: a feasibility study using a mitoxantrone containing regimen, *Br J Cancer* 62:105-108, 1990.

COP-BLAM–CYCLOPHOSPHAMIDE-VINCRISTINE-PREDNISONE-BLEOMYCIN-DOXORUBICIN-PROCARBAZINE

Cyclophosphamide. 400 mg/m² intravenously on day 1.

Vincristine. 1.0 mg/m² intravenously on day 1.

Prednisone. 40 mg/m² orally on days 1 to 10.

Bleomycin. 15 units intravenously on day 14.

Doxorubicin. 40 mg/m² intravenously on day 1.

Procarbazine. 100 mg/m² orally on days 1 to 10.

NOTE: Repeat the cycle every 21 days. Graded intensification of the induction phase is described in the report below. Cumulative maximum doses are 550 mg/m² of doxorubicin and 250 units/m² of bleomycin.

Selected Reading

Laurence J et al: Combination chemotherapy of advanced diffuse histiocytic lymphoma with the six-drug COP-BLAM regimen, *Ann Intern Med* 97:190-195, 1982.

COP-BLAM III

COP-BLAM III is a more intensive modification of COP-BLAM, incorporates continuous daily IV infusions of vincristine and bleomycin for up to 5 days, and thus requires considerable periods of hospitalization.

Selected Reading

Coleman M et al: The COP-BLAM programs: evolving chemotherapy concepts in large cell lymphoma, *Semin Hematol* 23(2 suppl 2):23-33, 1988.

COPP–CYCLOPHOSPHAMIDE-VINCRISTINE-PROCARBAZINE-PREDNISONE

Cyclophosphamide. 600 mg/m^2 intravenously on days 1 and 8.

Vincristine. 1.4 mg/m^2 intravenously on days 1 and 8.

Procarbazine. 100 mg/m^2 intravenously on days 1 to 10.

Prednisone. 40 mg/m^2 intravenously on days 1 to 14.

NOTE: Cycles are 14 days with a 14-day rest period.

Selected Reading

Stein RS et al: Combination chemotherapy of lymphomas other than Hodgkin's disease, *Ann Intern Med* 81:601-609, 1974.

CVP–CYCLOPHOSPHAMIDE-VINCRISTINE-PREDNISONE

Cyclophosphamide. 400 mg/m^2 orally on days 1 to 5.

Vincristine. 1.4 mg/m^2 intravenously on day 1.

Prednisone. 100 mg/m^2 orally on days 1 to 5.

NOTE: Repeat the cycle every 21 days.

Selected Reading

Bagley CM Jr et al: Advanced lymphosarcoma: intensive cyclical combination chemotherapy with cyclophosphamide, vincristine, and prednisone, *Ann Intern Med* 76:227-234, 1972.

DHAP–CISPLATIN-CYTARABINE-DEXAMETHASONE

Cisplatin. 100 mg/m^2 intravenously as a continuous infusion for 24 hours on day 1.

Cytarabine. 2000 mg/m^2 on day 2 every 12 hours (two doses for a total of 4000 mg/m^2).

Dexamethasone. 40 mg total intravenously or orally on days 1 to 4.

NOTE: DHAP requires vigorous hydration and adequate antiemetics. Repeat every 3 or 4 weeks. For patients over 70 years of age, use only 1000 mg/m^2 cytarabine.

Selected Reading

Cabanillas F, Velasquez WS, McLaughlin P: Results of recent salvage chemotherapy regimens for lymphoma and Hodgkin's disease, *Semin Hematol* 25(suppl 2):47-50, 1988.

Velasquez WS et al: Effective salvage therapy for lymphoma with cisplatin in combination with high-dose ara-C and dexamethasone (DHAP), *Blood* 71:117-122, 1988.

DICE–DEXAMETHASONE-IFOSFAMIDE-CISPLATIN-ETOPOSIDE

Dexamethasone. 10 mg by IV bolus every 6 hours on days 1 to 4.

Ifosfamide. 1000 mg/m^2 (maximum, 1750 mg) intravenously in 100 mL of normal saline over a 20-minute period on days 1 to 4.

Cisplatin. 25 mg/m^2 intravenously in 250 mL of normal saline over a 60-minute period on days 1 to 4.

Etoposide. 100 mg/m^2 intravenously in 250 mL of normal saline over a 60-minute period on days 1 to 4.

Mesna. 200 mg/m^2 in 50 mL of normal saline over a 10-minute period 1 hour before each ifosfamide infusion on days 1 to 4. Immediately after first ifosfamide infusion, give mesna, 900 mg/m^2/24 hr (i.e., mesna, 300 mg/m^2 per liter of normal saline), and continue mesna for 12 hours after the last dose of ifosfamide.

NOTE: Courses are repeated every 3 or 4 weeks, CBC, platelet count, and creatinine clearance values permitting.

Selected Readings

Goss PE: New perspectives in the treatment of non-Hodgkin's lymphoma, *Semin Oncol* 19(suppl 12):23-30, 1992.

Goss PE et al: Dexamethasone/ifosfamide/cisplatin/etoposide (DICE) as therapy for patients with advanced refractory non-Hodgkin's lymphoma: preliminary report of a phase II study, *Ann Oncol* 2(suppl 1):43-46, 1991.

DICEP—DOSE-INTENSIVE CYCLOPHOSPHAMIDE–ETOPOSIDE–CISPLATIN

Cyclophosphamide. 2500 mg/m^2 intravenously on days 1 and 2.

Etoposide. 500 mg/m^2 intravenously on days 1 to 3.

Cisplatin. 50 mg/m^2 intravenously on days 1 to 3.

NOTE: Courses repeated every 5 weeks for four courses. Antibacterial, antifungal, anti-diarrheal, and antiemetic therapy are essential as is hydration. GM-CSF or G-CSF may be used to control neutropenia.

Selected Readings

Neidhardt JA et al: Granulocyte colony stimulating factor (rhG-CSF) stimulates recovery of granulocytes in patients receiving dose-intensive chemotherapy without bone marrow transplantation, *J Clin Oncol* 7:1685-1692, 1989.

Neidhart JA et al: Multiple courses of dose-intensive cyclophosphamide, etoposide and cisplatinum (DICEP) produce durable responses in refractory non-Hodgkin's lymphoma, *Cancer Invest* 12:1-11, 1994.

DVIP—DEXAMETHASONE-ETOPOSIDE-IFOSFAMIDE-CISPLATIN

Dexamethasone. 20 mg intravenously for two doses on days 1 to 4.

Etoposide. 75 mg/m^2/day intravenously on days 1 to 4.

Ifosfamide. 1200 mg/m^2/day intravenously on days 1 to 4.

Mesna. 720 mg/m^2/day intravenously in three divided daily doses on days 1 to 4.

Cisplatin. 20 mg/m²/day intravenously on days 1 to 4.

NOTE: During the first cycle, full doses were given only to patients under 60 years of age whose Eastern Cooperative Oncology Group (ECOG) performance status was 0 to 2 and who had received no prior extensive radiation therapy and no prior chemotherapy. Courses were repeated every 3 weeks when the WBC count was over 4000 and the platelet count was over 100,000.

Selected Reading

Haim N et al: Salvage therapy for non-Hodgkin's lymphoma with a combination of dexamethasone, etoposide, ifosfamide and cisplatin, *Cancer Chemother Pharmacol* 30:243-244, 1992.

EPIC—ETOPOSIDE-PREDNISOLONE-IFOSFAMIDE-CARBOPLATIN

Etoposide. 100 mg/m² intravenously over 1 hour on days 1 to 4.

Ifosfamide. 1000 mg/m² intravenously over 15 minutes on days 1 to 5.

Mesna. 1000 mg/m² intravenously in 3 L saline on days 1 to 5.

Prednisolone. 100 mg total orally on days 1 to 5.

Carboplatin. 240 mg/m² intravenously over 30 minutes on day 12.

NOTE: This program is for patients who fail induction chemotherapy or relapse and need to have their tumor mass reduced to benefit from subsequent high-dose ablative chemotherapy with ABMT or PBSC support. Supportive services include allopurinol, hydration, antiemetics, antifungal agents, and H-2 blockers. Carboplatin is not given on day 12 if the WBC count is less than 1000/µL or the platelet count less than 100,000/µL. A similar EPIC program using cisplatin instead of carboplatin has been reported by Hickish et al (1993).

Selected Readings

Hickish T et al: EPIC: an effective low toxicity regimen for relapsing lymphoma, *Br J Cancer* 68:599-604, 1993.

Richardson DS et al: Salvage chemotherapy for relapsed and resistant lymphoma with a carboplatin containing schedule—EPIC, *Hematol Oncol* 12:125-128, 1994.

EPOCH—ETOPOSIDE-PREDNISONE-VINCRISTINE-CYCLOPHOSPHAMIDE-DOXORUBICIN

Etoposide. 50 mg/m²/day intravenously on days 1 to 4.

Vincristine. 0.4 mg/m²/day intravenously on days 1 to 5.

Doxorubicin. 10 mg/m²/day intravenously on days 1 to 5.

Cyclophosphamide. 750 mg/m² intravenously on day 6.

Prednisone. 60 mg/m²/day orally on days 1 to 14.

NOTE: Administer etoposide, vincristine, and doxorubicin by continuous infusion, and repeat the treatment every 21 days.

Selected Readings

Wilson WH et al: Infusional etoposide, vincristine and Adriamycin with cyclophosphamide, prednisone (EPOCH) and *R*-verapamil in relapsed lymphoma, *Proc Am Soc Clin Oncol* 10:275, 1991.

Wilson WH et al: EPOCH chemotherapy: toxicity and efficacy in relapsed and refractory non-Hodgkin's lymphoma, *J Clin Oncol* 11:1573-1582, 1993.

F-MACHOP—FLUOROURACIL-METHOTREXATE-CYTARABINE-CYCLOPHOSPHAMIDE-DOXORUBICIN-VINCRISTINE-PREDNISONE

Vincristine. 0.5 mg/m^2 intravenously at time 0 and at 12 hours on day 1.

Cyclophosphamide. 800 mg/m^2 intravenously at 36 hours (i.e., middle of day 2).

5-Fluorouracil. 15 mg/kg by continuous IV infusion for 6 hours starting at 36 hours.

Cytarabine. 1000 mg/m^2 by continuous IV infusion for 6 hours immediately after 5-fluorouracil infusion.

Doxorubicin. 60 mg/m^2 intravenously at 48 hours (end of day 2).

Methotrexate. 500 mg/m^2 by continuous IV infusion for 6 hours beginning at hour 60 (middle of day 3).

Prednisone. 60 mg/m^2/day orally for 14 days.

Leucovorin. 20 mg/m^2 intravenously 18 hours after the methotrexate infusion and repeated every 12 hours for four doses.

NOTE: Prophylactic intrathecal methotrexate, 12 mg total dose, plus cytarabine, 30 mg/m^2, is given to patients considered at high risk of CNS infiltration (advanced stage, marrow involvement, younger than 30 years of age) on day 10 of each course. A course is administered every 3 or 4 weeks for a total of six cycles. During the last three cycles, the dose of doxorubicin is reduced to 40 mg/m^2 and that of methotrexate to 300 mg/m^2.

Selected Readings

Amadori S et al: Treatment of diffuse aggressive non-Hodgkin's lymphomas with an intensive multidrug regimen including high dose cytosine arabinoside (F-MACHOP), *Semin Oncol* 12(suppl 3):218-222, 1985.

Guglielmi C et al: Combination chemotherapy for the treatment of diffuse aggressive lymphomas: F-MACHOP update, *Semin Oncol* 14(suppl 1):104-109, 1987.

FMP—FLUDARABINE-MITOXANTRONE-PREDNISONE

Fludarabine. 25 mg/m^2 intravenously on days 1 to 3.

Mitoxantrone. 10 mg/m^2 intravenously on day 1.

Prednisone. 40 mg total orally on days 1 to 5.

NOTE: The regimen of McLaughlin et al (1996) (FND) differs from FMP only in the substitution of dexamethasone 20 mg orally or intravenously on days 1 to 5 for the prednisone. Courses are repeated every 4 weeks. Give cotrimoxazole double strength twice a day as prophylaxis.

Selected Readings

McLaughlin P et al: Fludarabine, mitoxantrone, and dexamethasone: an effective new regimen for indolent lymphoma, *J Clin Oncol* 14:1262-1268, 1996.

Zinzani PL, Bendandi M, Tura S: FMP regimen (fludarabine, mitoxantrone, prednisone) as therapy in recurrent low-grade non-Hodgkin's lymphoma, *Eur J Haematol* 55:262-266, 1995.

IMVP-16—IFOSFAMIDE-METHOTREXATE-ETOPOSIDE

Ifosfamide. 1000 mg/m^2 intravenously on days 1 to 5.

Methotrexate. 30 mg/m^2 intramuscularly on days 3 and 10.

Etoposide. 100 mg/m^2 intravenously on days 1 to 3.

NOTE: Repeat the cycle every 21 days. Give ifosfamide in 1000 mL of D$_5$W over a 1-hour period, and give etoposide in 1000 mL of normal saline over a 2-hour period. The authors did not use mesna, which was not available at the time. A standard recommended dose of mesna should be added to prevent hemorrhagic cystitis. Mesna should be given intravenously, 200 mg/m^2 every 4 hours for three doses beginning before each daily dose of ifosfamide.

Selected Reading

Cabanillas F et al: An effective regimen for patients with lymphoma who have relapsed after initial combination chemotherapy, *Blood* 60:693-697, 1982.

LNH-80 AND LNH-84
Induction

Cyclophosphamide. 1200 mg/m^2 intravenously on day 1.

Doxorubicin. 75 mg/m^2 intravenously on day 1.

Vindesine. 2 mg/m^2 intravenously on days 1 and 5.

Bleomycin. 5 units/m^2 intravenously on days 1 and 5.

Methylprednisolone. 60 mg/m^2/day intravenously on days 1 to 5.

Methotrexate. 15 mg total intrathecally once per course.

NOTE: Courses are given every 15 days or when polymorphonuclear neutrophils exceed 1500/µL. A consolidation course is given 1 month after the final induction course and includes cytarabine, high-dose methotrexate with leucovorin rescue, and L-asparaginase. A final intensification course is started 2 months after the last injection of L-asparaginase. It includes cyclophosphamide, teniposide, cytarabine, bleomycin, and methylprednisolone. Total therapy requires 8 months. Consult the original article for details. LNH-84 has a slightly different consolidation schedule with ifosfamide and etoposide added.

Selected Readings

Coiffier B et al: Intensive and sequential combination chemotherapy for aggressive malignant lymphomas (protocol LNH-80), *J Clin Oncol* 4:147-153, 1986.

Coiffier B et al: LNH-84 regimen: a multicenter study of 737 patients with aggressive malignant lymphoma, *J Clin Oncol* 7:1018-1026, 1989.

MACOP-B—METHOTREXATE-DOXORUBICIN-CYCLOPHOSPHAMIDE-VINCRISTINE-PREDNISONE-BLEOMYCIN

Methotrexate. 400 mg/m^2 intravenously during weeks 2, 6, and 10.

Leucovorin. 15 mg orally every 6 hours for six doses given 24 hours after each dose of methotrexate.

Doxorubicin. 50 mg/m^2 intravenously during weeks 1, 3, 5, 7, 9, and 11.

Cyclophosphamide. 350 mg/m^2 intravenously during weeks 1, 3, 5, 7, 9, and 11.

Vincristine. 1.4 mg/m^2 to a maximum of 2 mg intravenously during weeks 2, 4, 6, 8, 10, and 12.

Bleomycin. 10 units/m^2 intravenously during weeks 4, 8, and 12.

Prednisone. 75 mg orally daily; dose tapered over last 15 days.

Cotrimoxazole. Two double-strength tablets orally twice daily throughout.

Ketoconazole. 200 mg orally daily throughout.

Hydrocortisone. 100 mg intravenously given just before each dose of bleomycin.

NOTE: The methotrexate is given as a 100-mg/m^2 IV bolus with the remaining 300 mg/m^2 infused over a 4-hour period. The authors recently switched the methotrexate to weeks 4, 8, and 12 and are testing a new program, VACOP-B, in which etoposide replaces methotrexate and leucovorin (see VACOP-B description). If the creatinine clearance is less than 60 mL/min, bleomycin replaces methotrexate for that course. Do not allow the use of astemizole (Hismanal) or terfenadine (Seldane) when using ketoconazole.

Selected Readings

Klimo P, Connors JM: MACOP-B chemotherapy for the treatment of advanced diffuse large cell lymphoma, *Ann Intern Med* 102:596-602, 1985.

Klimo P, Connors JM: Updated clinical experience with MACOP-B, *Semin Hematol* 24(suppl 1):26-34, 1987.

m-BACOD—METHOTREXATE-BLEOMYCIN-DOXORUBICIN-CYCLOPHOSPHAMIDE-VINCRISTINE-DEXAMETHASONE

Methotrexate. 200 mg/m^2 intravenously on days 8 and 15.

Leucovorin. 10 mg/m^2 orally every 6 hours for eight doses beginning on days 9 and 16.

Bleomycin. 4 mg/m^2 intravenously on day 1.

Doxorubicin. 45 mg/m^2 intravenously on day 1.

Cyclophosphamide. 600 mg/m^2 intravenously on day 1.

Vincristine. 1.0 mg/m^2 intravenously on day 1.

Dexamethasone. 6.0 mg/m^2 orally on days 1 to 5.

NOTE: Repeat the cycle on day 22 for 10 cycles.

Selected Readings

Shipp MA et al: Identification of major prognostic subgroups of patients with large-cell lymphoma treated with m-BACOD or M-BACOD, *Ann Intern Med* 104:757-765, 1986.

Skarin AT et al: Moderate dose methotrexate (m) combined with bleomycin (B), Adriamycin (A), cyclophosphamide (C), Oncovin (O) and dexamethasone (D), m-BACOD, in advanced, diffuse histiocytic leukemia, *Proc Am Soc Clin Oncol* 2:220, 1983.

MINE-ESHAP

MINE—Mesna-Ifosfamide-Mitoxantrone-Etoposide

Mesna. 1330 mg/m^2/day intravenously over a 1-hour period on days 1 to 3 and 500 mg orally 4 hours after the ifosfamide dose.

Ifosfamide. 1330 mg/m^2/day intravenously over a 1-hour period on days 1 to 3.

Mitoxantrone. 8 mg/m^2 intravenously on day 1.

Etoposide. 65 mg/m^2/day intravenously on days 1 to 3.

NOTE: Repeat every 21 days for six courses, and then start ESHAP.

ESHAP—Etoposide—Methylprednisolone—High-Dose Cytarabine—Cisplatin

Etoposide. 60 mg/m^2 intravenously on days 1 to 4.

Methylprednisolone. 500 mg intravenously on days 1 to 4.

High-dose cytarabine. 2000 mg/m^2 intravenously over a 2-hour period on day 5 after cisplatin.

Cisplatin. 25 mg/m^2/day intravenously on days 1 to 4 by continuous infusion.

NOTE: If complete remission is achieved with MINE, consolidate with three courses of ESHAP. If there is only a partial MINE response, then give six courses of ESHAP.

Selected Readings

Cabanillas F: Experience with salvage regimens at M.D. Anderson Hospital, *Ann Oncol* 2(suppl 1):31-32, 1991.

Cabanillas F et al: Salvage therapy with non–cross resistant regimens (MINE-ESHAP) for transformed and low grade lymphomas, *Proc Am Soc Clin Oncol* 10:273, 1991.

Rodriguez MA et al: Results of a salvage treatment program for relapsing lymphoma: MINE consolidated with ESHAP, *J Clin Oncol* 13:1734-1741, 1995.

---

m-BNCOD—METHOTREXATE-BLEOMYCIN-MITOXANTRONE-VINCRISTINE-DEXAMETHASONE

Cyclophosphamide. 600 mg/m^2 intravenously on day 1.

Bleomycin.   4 units/m^2 intravenously on day 1.

Vincristine.   1 mg/m^2 intravenously on day 1.

Mitoxantrone.   10 mg/m^2 intravenously on day 1.

Dexamethasone.   6 mg/m^2 orally on days 1 to 5.

Methotrexate.   200 mg/m^2 intravenously on days 8 and 15.

Leucovorin.   15 mg/m^2 orally every 6 hours on days 9, 10, 16, and 17.

NOTE: Repeat the cycle every 21 days.

Selected Reading

Guglielmi C et al: A phase III comparative trial of m-BACOD vs. m-BNCOD in the treatment of stage II-IV diffuse non-Hodgkin's lymphomas, *Haematologica* 74:563-569, 1989.

NOAC–MITOXANTRONE-CYTARABINE

Mitoxantrone.   10 mg/m^2/day intravenously on days 2 and 3.

Cytarabine.   3000 mg/m^2 intravenously over a 3-hour period every 12 hours on day 1 (total, two doses).

NOTE: Repeat the cycle every 4 weeks. Give glucocorticoid eye drops to prevent ocular toxicity with high-dose cytarabine.

Selected Readings

Ho AD et al: Mitoxantrone and high-dose cytarabine as salvage therapy for refractory non-Hodgkin's lymphoma, *Cancer* 64:1388-1392, 1989.

PRO-MACE-CYTABOM–METHOTREXATE-DOXORUBICIN-CYCLOPHOSPHAMIDE-ETOPOSIDE-CYTARABINE-VINCRISTINE

Cyclophosphamide.   650 mg/m^2 intravenously on day 1.

Doxorubicin.   25 mg/m^2 intravenously on day 1.

Etoposide.   120 mg/m^2 intravenously over a 60-minute period on day 1.

Prednisone.   60 mg/m^2 orally on days 1 to 14.

Cytarabine.   300 mg/m^2 intravenously on day 8.

Bleomycin.   5 units/m^2 intravenously on day 8.

Vincristine.   1.4 mg/m^2 intravenously on day 8.

Methotrexate.   120 mg/m^2 intravenously on day 8.

Leucovorin.   25 mg/m^2 orally every 6 hours for four doses beginning on day 9.

NOTE: The next cycle begins on day 22. At least six cycles are given, two cycles beyond a complete remission. This regimen was associated with an increased incidence of diffuse interstitial pneumonia with four deaths. Hence all patients now receive prophylactic trimethoprim-sulfamethoxazole (cotrimoxazole), one double-strength tablet twice daily.

Selected Readings

Fisher RI et al: Randomized treatment of Pro-MACE-MOPP vs Pro-MACE-CytaBOM in previously untreated advanced stage diffuse aggressive lymphomas, *Proc Am Soc Clin Oncol* 3:242, 1984.

Longo DL et al: Superiority of Pro-MACE-CytaBOM over ProMACE-MOPP in the treatment of advanced diffuse aggressive lymphoma: results of a prospective randomized trial, *J Clin Oncol* 9:25-38, 1991.

VACOP-B—ETOPOSIDE-DOXORUBICIN-CYCLOPHOSPHAMIDE-VINCRISTINE-PREDNISONE-BLEOMYCIN

Etoposide.   50 mg/m^2 intravenously on day 1 of weeks 3, 7, and 11.

Etoposide.   100 mg/m^2 orally on days 2 and 3 of weeks 3, 7, and 11.

Doxorubicin.   50 mg/m^2 intravenously on day 1 of weeks 1, 3, 5, 7, 9, and 11.

Cyclophosphamide.   350 mg/m^2 intravenously on day 1 of weeks 1, 5, and 9.

Vincristine.   1.2 mg/m^2 intravenously on day 1 of weeks 2, 4, 6, 8, 10, and 12.

Bleomycin.   10 units/m^2 intravenously on day 1 of weeks 2, 4, 6, 8, 10, and 12. Give hydrocortisone, 100 mg intravenously, with each dose of bleomycin.

Prednisone.   45 mg/m^2 orally daily for 1 week and then every other day.

Cotrimoxazole.   1 double-strength tablet orally twice a day for 14 weeks.

Ketoconazole.   200 mg orally daily for 1 week and then every other day. Do not allow the use of astemizole (Hismanal) or terfenadine (Seldane).

Cimetidine.   600 mg orally twice a day for 1 week and then every other day.

NOTE: This regimen was relatively safe in the hands of its originators, but highly toxic when used by Sobrevilla-Calvo et al (1992).

Selected Readings

Connors JM et al: VACOP-B: 12-week chemotherapy for advanced stage diffuse large cell lymphoma: efficacy is sustained and toxicity reduced compared to MACOP-B, *Proc Am Soc Clin Oncol* 9:254, 1990.

Sobrevilla-Calvo P et al: Unexpected high rate of fatal toxicity of the VACOP-B regimen for malignant lymphoma, *Proc Am Soc Clin Oncol* 11:335, 1992.

VIM—ETOPOSIDE-IFOSFAMIDE-MITOXANTRONE

Etoposide.   65 mg/m^2 intravenously on days 1 to 3.

Ifosfamide.   650 mg/m^2 intravenously with equal dose mesna on days 1 to 3.

Mitoxantrone.   3 mg/m^2 intravenously on days 1 to 3.

NOTE: Repeat cycle every 3 weeks.

Selected Reading

Hopfinger G et al: Ifosfamide, mitoxantrone and etoposide (VIM) as salvage therapy of low toxicity in non-Hodgkin's lymphoma, *Eur J Haematol* 55:223-227, 1995.

PRIMARY NON-HODGKIN'S LYMPHOMA OF THE CENTRAL NERVOUS SYSTEM—CHEMORADIOTHERAPY WITH CHOD/BVAM

CHOD—CYCLOPHOSPHAMIDE-DOXORUBICIN-VINCRISTINE-DEXAMETHASONE

Cyclophosphamide. 750 mg/m^2 intravenously on day 1.

Doxorubicin. 50 mg/m^2 intravenously on day 1.

Vincristine. 1.4 mg/m^2 intravenously on day 1.

Dexamethasone. 4 mg orally 4 times daily on days 1 to 7.

NOTE: After a single cycle of CHOD, start BVAM.

BVAM—CARMUSTINE-VINCRISTINE-CYTARABINE-METHOTREXATE

Carmustine. 100 mg/m^2 intravenously on days 8 and 50.

Vincristine. 1.4 mg/m^2 intravenously on days 15, 29, 43, 57, 71, and 85.

Methotrexate. 1500 mg/m^2 intravenously on days 15, 29, 43, 57, 71, and 85.

Leucovorin. 15 mg 4 times daily for 3 days, 24 hours after each dose of methotrexate.

Cytarabine. 3000 mg/m^2 intravenously on days 16, 30, 44, 58, 72, and 86.

NOTE: Radiotherapy begins 10 to 14 days after day-86 cytarabine with whole-brain radiation 4500 cGy in 25 fractions in 5 weeks. An interesting and promising alternative approach involves osmotic disruption of the blood-brain barrier to allow enhanced delivery of chemotherapy without cognitive loss and without radiotherapy. Neuwelt et al (1991) and Dahlborg et al (1996) describe their experiences, and it is clear that this is a technique that requires a trained and experienced team to accomplish therapy successfully and safely.

Selected Readings

Bessell EM et al: Primary non-Hodgkin's lymphoma of the CNS treated with BVAM or CHOD/BVAM chemotherapy before radiotherapy, *J Clin Oncol* 14:945-954, 1996.

Dahlborg SA et al: Non-AIDS primary CNS lymphoma: first example of a durable response in a primary brain tumor using enhanced chemotherapy delivery without cognitive loss and without radiotherapy, *The Cancer J from Sci Am* 2:166-174, 1996.

Neuwelt EA et al: Primary CNS lymphoma treated with osmotic blood brain barrier disruption: prolonged survival and preservation of cognitive function, *J Clin Oncol* 9:1580-1590, 1991.

REGIMENS FOR THE ELDERLY (AGE 70 AND OLDER)

CAP/BOP—CYCLOPHOSPHAMIDE-DOXORUBICIN-PROCARBAZINE-BLEOMYCIN-VINCRISTINE-PREDNISONE

Cyclophosphamide. 650 mg/m^2 intravenously on day 1.

Doxorubicin. 50 mg/m^2 intravenously on day 1.

Procarbazine. 100 mg/m^2 orally on days 1 to 7.

Bleomycin. 10 units/m^2 subcutaneously on day 15.

Vincristine. 1.4 mg/m^2 (maximum 2 mg) intravenously on day 15.

Prednisone. 100 mg total orally on days 15 to 21.

NOTE: Regimen is repeated every 21 to 28 days as tolerated to two cycles beyond a complete response or a maximum of nine cycles.

Selected Reading

Vose JM et al: The importance of age in survival of patients treated with chemotherapy for aggressive non-Hodgkin's lymphoma, *J Clin Oncol* 6:1838-1844, 1988.

LD-ACOP-B—LOW DOSE DOXORUBICIN-CYCLOPHOSPHAMIDE-VINCRISTINE-BLEOMYCIN-PREDNISONE

Doxorubicin. 25 mg/m^2 intravenously on days 1, 15, 28, 42, 56, and 70.

Cyclophosphamide. 250 mg/m^2 intravenously on days 1, 15, 28, 42, 56, and 70.

Vincristine. 1.2 mg/m^2 (maximum 2 mg) on days 8, 22, 35, 49, 63, and 77.

Bleomycin. 10 units/m^2 intravenously on days 8, 22, 35, 49, 63, and 77.

Prednisone. 50 mg total/day orally for 6 weeks then q.o.d. 6 weeks.

Cotrimoxazole DS. One tablet twice a day orally for 12 weeks.

Cimetadine. 600 mg twice a day orally for 12 weeks.

Ketoconazole. 200 mg total/day orally for 12 weeks. Do not allow use of terfenadine (Seldane) or astemizole (Hismanal).

NOTE: Give hydrocortisone 100 mg total intravenously with each dose bleomycin.

Selected Reading

O'Reilly SE, Klimo P, Connors JM: Low-dose ACOP-B and VABE: weekly chemotherapy for elderly patients with advanced-stage diffuse large-cell lymphoma, *J Clin Oncol* 9:741-747, 1991.

P/DOCE—PREDNISONE-DOXORUBICIN-VINCRISTINE-CYCLOPHOSPHAMIDE-ETOPOSIDE

Doxorubicin. 40 mg/m^2 intravenously days 1, 8, 28, 29, and 56 *or*

Epirubicin. 50 mg/m^2, but not both.

Vincristine. 1.2 mg/m^2 intravenously on days 1, 28, and 49.

Etoposide. 50 mg/m^2 intravenously day 28.

Etoposide. 100 mg/m^2 orally on days 2, 3, 4, and 5.

Prednisone. 50 mg total orally on days 1 to 10, 28 to 37, and 49 to 58.

Cotrimoxazole DS. One tablet orally twice a day.

Ketoconazole. 200 mg total orally on days 1 to 10, 28 to 37, and 49 to 58. Do not allow use of terfenadine (Seldane) or astemizole (Hismanal).

Cimetadine. 600 mg twice a day on days 1 to 10, 28 to 37, and 49 to 58.

Selected Reading

O'Reilly SE et al: In search for an optimal regimen for elderly patients with advanced-stage diffuse large-cell lymphoma: results of a phase II study of P/DOCE chemotherapy, *J Clin Oncol* 11:2250-2257, 1993.

P-VABEC—PREDNISONE-VINCRISTINE-DOXORUBICIN-BLEOMYCIN-ETOPOSIDE-CYCLOPHOSPHAMIDE

Doxorubicin. 30 mg/m^2 intravenously on day 1 of weeks 1, 3, 5, 7, 9, and 11.

Etoposide. 100 mg/m^2 intravenously on day 1 of weeks 1, 3, 5, 7, 9, and 11.

Cyclophosphamide. 350 mg/m^2 on day 1 of weeks 1, 3, 5, 7, 9, and 11.

Vincristine. 1.2 mg/m^2 (maximum 2 mg) intravenously on day 1 of weeks 2, 4, 6, 8, 10, and 12.

Bleomycin. 5 units/m^2 intravenously on day 1 of weeks 2, 4, 6, 8, 10, and 12.

Prednisone. 50 mg/day during treatment period and tapered thereafter.

Selected Reading

Martelli M et al: P-VABEC: a prospective study of a new weekly chemotherapy regimen for elderly aggressive non-Hodgkin's lymphoma, *J Clin Oncol* 11:2362-2369, 1993.

MELANOMA

Melanoma accounts for about 3% of all new cancer cases in the United States, and the rate is increasing along with increased sun exposure. Prognosis is affected by clinical and histological factors and by anatomical location of the lesion. Thickness and/or level of invasion of the melanoma, mitotic index, tumor-infiltrating lymphocytes, ulceration or bleeding at the primary site, and involvement of regional lymph nodes all affect the prognosis. Wide local excision and in some cases regional nodal dissection (early prophylactic or late palliative) can prolong survival, as can adjuvant immunotherapy with interferon alpha-2. Once distant metastases occur, cure is unlikely, but palliation with immunotherapy and/or chemotherapy may be worthwhile. Active agents include dacarbazine, lomustine, cisplatin, carboplatin, carmustine, dactinomycin, paclitaxel, procarbazine, vincristine, vinblastine, bleomycin, interleukin-2, and interferon alpha-2. Hormonal agents such as megestrol and tamoxifen have been used with some chemotherapy regimens with uncertainty about their contribution to efficacy. At present, response rates and survival are only marginally improved by combination chemotherapy with or without immunotherapy. However, new vaccines, monoclonal antibodies, and new chemoimmunotherapy approaches are in clinical trials. In the absence of any high response rates in current therapy, patients should be encouraged to participate in clinical trials to evaluate new therapeutic approaches.

CHEMOIMMUNOTHERAPY

Dacarbazine. 750 mg/m^2 intravenously on day 1 of weeks 1 and 4.

Carboplatin. 400 mg/m^2 intravenously on day 1 of weeks 1 and 4.

Interleukin-2. 4.8 million IU/m^2 subcutaneously 3 times/day, on day 1 of weeks 7 and 10; 2.4 million IU/m^2 subcutaneously 2 times/day, on days 3 to 5 of weeks 7 and 10; 2.4 million IU/m^2 subcutaneously 2 times/day, on days 1 to 5 of weeks 8, 9, 11, and 12.

Interferon alpha. 3 million U/m^2 subcutaneously on days 3 and 5 of weeks 7 and 10; 6 million U/m^2 subcutaneously on days 1, 3, and 5 of weeks 8, 9, 11, and 12.

NOTE: Therapy can all be given as outpatient treatment. Toxicity is tolerable with adequate antiemetics.

Selected Reading

Atzpodien J et al: Chemoimmunotherapy of advanced malignant melanoma: sequential administration of subcutaneous interleukin-2 and interferon-alpha after intravenous dacarbazine and carboplatin or intravenous dacarbazine, cisplatin, carmustine and tamoxifen, *Eur J Cancer* 31A:876-881, 1995.

DACARBAZINE-DACTINOMYCIN

Dacarbazine. 800 mg/m^2 intravenously every 3 weeks.

Dactinomycin. 1.2 mg/m^2 intravenously every 3 weeks.

Selected Reading

Hochster H et al: Single-dose dacarbazine and dactinomycin in advanced malignant melanoma, *Cancer Treat Rep* 69:39-42, 1985.

DACARBAZINE-CARMUSTINE-CISPLATIN-TAMOXIFEN

Dacarbazine. 220 mg/m^2 intravenously on days 1 to 3.

Carmustine. 150 mg/m^2 intravenously on day 1.

Cisplatin. 25 mg/m^2 intravenously on days 1 to 3.

Tamoxifen. 10 mg orally twice daily.

NOTE: Repeat the treatment with DTIC and cisplatin every 3 weeks. Repeat the treatment with carmustine every 6 weeks. Rusthoven et al (1996) have called into question the value of adding tamoxifen to this regimen. Nathanson, Meelu, and Losada use megestrol acetate 160 mg/day orally instead of tamoxifen.

Selected Readings

DelPrete SA et al: Combination chemotherapy with cisplatin, carmustine, dacarbazine, and tamoxifen in metastatic melanoma, *Cancer Treat Rep* 68:1403-1405, 1984.

McClay EF et al: The importance of tamoxifen to a cisplatin-containing regimen in the treatment of metastatic melanoma, *Cancer* 63:1292-1295, 1991.

Nathanson L, Meelu MA, Losada R: Chemohormone therapy of metastatic melanoma with megestrol acetate plus dacarbazine, carmustine and cisplatin, *Cancer* 78:93-102, 1994.

Richards JM et al: Effective chemotherapy for melanoma after treatment with interleukin-2, *Cancer* 69:427-429, 1992.

Rusthoven JJ et al: Randomized, double-blind, placebo-controlled trial comparing the response rates of carmustine, dacarbazine and cisplatin with and without tamoxifen in patients with metastatic melanoma, *J Clin Oncol* 14:2083-2090, 1996.

POC–PROCARBAZINE-VINCRISTINE-LOMUSTINE

Procarbazine. 100 mg/m^2/day (max. 150 mg/day) orally on days 1 to 10.

Vincristine. 1.4 mg/m^2 (max. 2 mg) intravenously on days 1 and 8.

Lomustine. 150 mg/m^2 (max. 200 mg) orally on day 1.

NOTE: Repeat the cycle every 4 to 6 weeks.

Selected Readings

Carmo-Pereira J, Costa FO, Henriques E: Combination cytotoxic chemotherapy with procarbazine, vincristine, and lomustine (POC) in disseminated malignant melanoma: 8 years follow-up, *Cancer Treat Rep* 68:1211-1214, 1984.

Samuel LM et al: Phase II trial of procarbazine, vincristine and lomostine (POC) chemotherapy in metastatic cutaneous melanoma, *Eur J Cancer* 30A:2054-2056, 1994.

VDP–VINBLASTINE-DACARBAZINE-CISPLATIN

Vinblastine. 5 mg/m^2 intravenously on days 1 and 2.

Dacarbazine. 150 mg/m^2 intravenously on days 1 to 5.

Cisplatin. 75 mg/m^2 intravenously on day 5.

NOTE: Repeat every 21 to 28 days.

Selected Reading

Luikart SD, Kennedy TMS, Kirkwood JM: Randomized phase III trial of vinblastine, bleomycin, and *cis*-dichlorodiammine platinum versus dacarbazine in malignant melanoma, *J Clin Oncol* 2:164-168, 1984.

MALIGNANT MESOTHELIOMA

Malignant mesothelioma afflicts about 2200 and kills 2000 patients yearly in the United States. A history of asbestos exposure is reported in about 70% to 80% of all cases. Pleural mesothelioma may progress more slowly than peritoneal mesothelioma, but this difference may reflect earlier diagnosis by chest x-ray studies. In many cases the tumor grows through the diaphragm, making the site of origin difficult to assess. Major prognostic factors are age, stage, performance status, histology, and nodal status. Aggressive surgical approaches may provide long-term survival (without cure) when performed in centers with experienced teams. Intracavitary chemotherapy or palliative radiotherapy may follow resection. Active first-line chemotherapy drugs include doxorubicin, epirubicin, ifosfamide, cyclophosphamide, cisplatin, carboplatin, mitomycin, methotrexate, and edatrexate. In general, combination chemotherapy gives response rates only marginally better than single agents (Ong ST, Vogelzang NJ: Chemotherapy in malignant pleural mesothelioma: a review, *J Clin Oncol* 14:1007-1017, 1996).

CISPLATIN-MITOMYCIN

Cisplatin. 75 mg/m^2 intravenously once every 4 weeks.

Mitomycin. 10 mg/m^2 intravenously once every 4 weeks.

NOTE: Hydration and antiemetics are important. Maximum cumulative dose of mitomycin is 50 mg/m^2.

Selected Reading

Chahinian AP et al: Randomized phase II trial of cisplatin with mitomycin or doxorubicin for malignant mesothelioma by the Cancer and Leukemia Group B, *J Clin Oncol* 11:1559-1565, 1993.

CD–CYCLOPHOSPHAMIDE-DOXORUBICIN

Cyclophosphamide. 400 mg/m^2 intravenously on days 1 and 8.

Doxorubicin. 40 mg/m^2 intravenously on days 1 and 8.

NOTE: Repeat the cycle every 28 days. Discontinue doxorubicin therapy after 450 mg/m^2.

Alternative Program Given Every 21 Days

Cyclophosphamide. 1000 mg/m^2 intravenously on day 1.

Doxorubicin. 45 mg/m^2 intravenously on day 1.

Selected Reading

Antman KH et al: Peritoneal mesothelioma: natural history and response to chemotherapy, *J Clin Oncol* 1:386-391, 1983.

CYCLOPHOSPHAMIDE-DOXORUBICIN-CISPLATIN

Cyclophosphamide. 500 mg/m^2 intravenously on day 1.

Doxorubicin. 50 mg/m^2 intravenously on day 1.

Cisplatin. 80 mg/m^2 intravenously on day 1.

NOTE: Courses were given every 3 weeks for three cycles, and then the cisplatin dose was reduced to 50 mg/m^2 and additional courses given as tolerated. Vigorous hydration and antiemetics are needed.

Selected Reading

Shin DM et al: Prospective study of combination chemotherapy with cyclophosphamide, doxorubicin and cisplatin for unresectable or metastatic malignant pleural mesothelioma, *Cancer* 76:2230-2236, 1995.

DOXORUBICIN-CISPLATIN

Doxorubicin. 60 mg/m² intravenously on day 1.

Cisplatin. 60 mg/m² intravenously on day 1.

NOTE: Repeat every 3 or 4 weeks.

Selected Reading

Ardizzoni A et al: Activity of doxorubicin and cisplatin combination chemotherapy in patients with diffuse malignant pleural mesothelioma, *Cancer* 67:2984-2987, 1991.

MULTIPLE MYELOMA

Multiple myeloma is also called *plasma cell neoplasm* because it is essentially a collection of plasma cells derived from a single transformed B-cell lymphocyte. A solitary plasmacytoma is sometimes curable by resection or radiation therapy, but multiple myeloma, although highly treatable, is rarely curable. Diagnosis is based on detection of an M-protein in the serum or urine, demonstration of more than 10% plasma cells on a bone marrow examination, detection of lytic bone lesions, or generalized osteoporosis with anemia and an elevated beta-microglobulin. Variants falling within the spectrum of plasma cell neoplasm include Waldenstrom's macroglobulinemia, heavy-chain disease (Franklin's disease), and monoclonal gammopathy of undetermined significance.

Active drugs include melphalan, prednisone, carmustine, doxorubicin, vincristine, dexamethasone, cyclophosphamide, chlorambucil, cisplatin, and interferon alpha-2. Bone destruction can often be decreased or slowed with the use of gallium nitrate or biphosphonates such as pamidronate. Vigorous therapy of infection is essential because the major causes of death in myeloma are infection and renal failure. Although melphalan and prednisone were the standard treatment for several decades, other combination chemotherapy is beginning to be used more often to avoid early melphalan use. This avoids excessive destruction of early stem cells so that they will be available if high-dose chemotherapy (with melphalan or other drugs) is selected for rescue. Although it appears that high-dose chemotherapy with stem cell and cytokine support can frequently prolong life, there is no convincing evidence that it is curative in a high proportion of cases. For further information, see Chapter 9, which discusses high-dose chemotherapy with stem cell support.

ABC-P–DOXORUBICIN-CARMUSTINE-CYCLOPHOSPHAMIDE-PREDNISONE

Carmustine. 50 mg/m² intravenously on day 1.

Cyclophosphamide. 200 mg/m² intravenously on day 1.

Doxorubicin. 20 mg/m² intravenously on day 2.

Prednisone. 60 mg/m² orally on days 1 to 5.

NOTE: Repeat the cycle every 4 weeks.

Selected Reading

Presant CA, Klahr C: Adriamycin, 1,3-bis(2-chloroethyl)-1-nitrosourea (BCNU, NSC-409962), cyclophosphamide plus prednisone (ABC-P) in melphalan resistant multiple myeloma, *Cancer* 42:1222-1227, 1978.

BAP—CARMUSTINE-DOXORUBICIN-PREDNISONE

Carmustine. 75 mg/m² intravenously on day 1.

Doxorubicin. 30 mg/m² intravenously on days 1 and 22.

Prednisone. 0.6 mg/kg orally in three equally divided doses daily for 7 days every 3 weeks.

NOTE: Repeat the cycle every 6 weeks.

Selected Reading

Kyle RA et al: Multiple myeloma resistant to melphalan: treatment with doxorubicin, cyclophosphamide, carmustine (BCNU) and prednisone, *Cancer Treat Rep* 66:451-456, 1982.

CBCP—CISPLATIN-CARMUSTINE-CYCLOPHOSPHAMIDE-PREDNISONE

Cisplatin. 50 mg/m² intravenously on day 1.

Carmustine. 50 mg/m² intravenously on day 1.

Cyclophosphamide. 300 mg/m² intravenously on day 1.

Prednisone. 75 mg/day orally on days 1 to 7.

NOTE: Repeat the cycle every 4 weeks.

Selected Reading

Broun GO Jr et al: Cisplatin, BCNU, cyclophosphamide and prednisone in multiple myeloma, *Cancer Treat Rep* 66:237-242, 1982.

CYCLOPHOSPHAMIDE-PREDNISONE

Cyclophosphamide. 150 to 250 mg/m² (500 mg maximum) intravenously or orally weekly.

Prednisone. 100 mg orally every other day.

Selected Reading

Wilson K et al: Weekly cyclophosphamide and alternate-day prednisone: an effective secondary therapy in multiple myeloma, *Cancer Treat Rep* 71:981-982, 1987.

M-2–VINCRISTINE-CARMUSTINE-CYCLOPHOSPHAMIDE-MELPHALAN-PREDNISONE

Vincristine. 0.03 mg/kg intravenously on day 1.

Carmustine. 0.5 mg/kg intravenously on day 1.

Cyclophosphamide. 10 mg/kg intravenously on day 1.

Melphalan. 0.25 mg/kg orally for 4 days.

Prednisone. 1.0 mg/kg/day orally for 7 days, and then 0.5 mg/kg/day orally for 7 days.

NOTE: Repeat the cycle every 35 days.

Selected Reading

Case BC Jr, Lee BJ, Clarkson BD: Improved survival times in multiple myeloma treated with melphalan, prednisone, cyclophosphamide, vincristine, and BCNU: M-2 protocol, *Am J Med* 63:897-903, 1977.

MP–MELPHALAN-PREDNISONE

Melphalan. 10 mg/m^2 orally on days 1 to 4.

Prednisone. 60 mg/m^2 orally on days 1 to 4.

NOTE: Repeat the cycle every 6 weeks.

Selected Reading

Southwest Oncology Group Study: Remission maintenance therapy for multiple myeloma, *Arch Intern Med* 135:147-152, 1975.

VAD–VINCRISTINE-DOXORUBICIN-DEXAMETHASONE

Vincristine. 0.4 mg/day continuous IV infusion on days 1 to 4.

Doxorubicin. 9 mg/m^2/day continuous IV infusion on days 1 to 4.

Dexamethasone. 40 mg orally on days 1 to 4, 9 to 12, and 17 to 20.

NOTE: All patients received prophylactic antacid treatment with cimetidine and antibiotic prophylaxis with cotrimoxazole. Cycles were repeated every 25 days until a maximum reduction in myeloma protein levels had occurred. Four additional courses were given after the myeloma protein levels disappeared or stabilized.

Selected Reading

Barlogie B, Smith L, Alexanian R: Effective treatment of advanced multiple myeloma refractory to alkylating agents, *N Engl J Med* 310:1353-1356, 1984.

VAP–VINCRISTINE-DOXORUBICIN-PREDNISONE

Vincristine. 1.5 mg intravenously on day 1.

Doxorubicin. 35 mg/m^2 intravenously on day 1.

Prednisone. 45 mg/m^2/day orally on days 1 to 5, 9 to 13, and 17 to 21.

NOTE: Cycles were repeated every 25 days. Patients who responded were maintained on monthly courses of VCAP.

Selected Reading

Alexanian R, Yap BS, Bodey GP: Prednisone pulse therapy for refractory myeloma, *Blood* 62:572-577, 1983.

VBAP–VINCRISTINE-CARMUSTINE-DOXORUBICIN-PREDNISONE

Vincristine. 1 mg intravenously on day 1.

Carmustine. 30 mg/m^2 intravenously on day 1.

Doxorubicin. 30 mg/m^2 intravenously on day 1.

Prednisone. 100 mg orally on days 1 to 4.

NOTE: Repeat the cycle every 21 days.

Selected Reading

Bonnet J et al: Vincristine, BCNU, doxorubicin, and prednisone (VBAP) combination in the treatment of relapsing or resistant multiple myeloma: a Southwest Oncology Group study, *Cancer Treat Rep* 66:1267-1271, 1982.

VMCP ALTERNATING WITH VCAP
VMCP–Vincristine-Melphalan-Cyclophosphamide-Prednisone

Vincristine. 1.0 mg/m^2 (maximum, 1.5 mg) intravenously on day 1.

Melphalan. 6 mg/m^2 orally on days 1 to 4.

Cyclophosphamide. 125 mg/m^2 orally on days 1 to 4.

Prednisone. 60 mg/m^2 orally on days 1 to 4.

NOTE: Alternate every 3 weeks with the VCAP regimen.

VCAP–Vincristine-Cyclophosphamide-Doxorubicin-Prednisone

Vincristine. 1.0 mg/m^2 (maximum, 1.5 mg) intravenously on day 1.

Cyclophosphamide. 125 mg/m^2 orally on days 1 to 4.

Doxorubicin. 30 mg/m^2 intravenously on day 1.

Prednisone. 60 mg/m^2 orally on days 1 to 4.

Selected Reading

Salmon SE et al: Alternating combination chemotherapy and levamisole improves survival in multiple myeloma: a Southwest Oncology Group study, *J Clin Oncol* 1:453-461, 1983.

OSTEOSARCOMA

Osteosarcoma is a malignant spindle cell tumor that produces osteoid and is the most common primary malignant adult bone tumor (with the exception of multiple myeloma, which is usually grouped with the hematopoietic malignancies). Site of the primary is a significant prognostic factor. Distal tumors have a more favorable prognosis, whereas axial skeleton primaries have a poor prognosis. Other prognostic factors include age, histology, duration of symptoms, size of tumor, LDH level, alkaline phosphatase level, and tumor ploidy.

Patients whose tumors can be resected and whose metastases (primarily to lung) can be removed may have a long survival, especially with adjuvant chemotherapy. Active agents include doxorubicin, high-dose methotrexate, vincristine, cyclophosphamide, cisplatin, bleomycin, dactinomycin, etoposide, and ifosfamide. Activity is significantly enhanced by their use in various combination chemotherapy regimens, which may permit limb-sparing surgery.

CISPLATIN-DOXORUBICIN

Cisplatin. 90 mg/m^2 intravenously over a 6-hour period with hydration.

Doxorubicin. 75 mg/m^2 intravenously 48 hours after cisplatin.

NOTE: Pretreatment and posttreatment hydration is an essential element of the protocol. Bramwell et al (1992) used a similar program with the doxorubicin given as a 25 mg/m^2 bolus on 3 consecutive days and the cisplatin as 100 mg/m^2 by 24-hour infusion. Treatments were repeated at 3-week intervals for six cycles.

Selected Readings

Bramwell VHC et al: A comparison of two short intensive adjuvant chemotherapy regimens in operable osteosarcoma of limbs in children and young adults: the first study of the European Osteosarcoma Intergroup, *J Clin Oncol* 10:1579-1591, 1992.

Pratt CB et al: Treatment of unresectable or metastatic osteosarcoma with cisplatin or cisplatin-doxorubicin, *Cancer* 56:1930-1933, 1985.

DFCI-TCH STUDY III

Vincristine. 2.0 mg/m^2 (maximum, 2.0 mg) intravenously; 30 minutes later, give the drugs below.

Methotrexate. 7500 mg/m^2 intravenously over a 6-hour period.

Leucovorin. 15 mg intravenously (beginning 2 hours after the methotrexate dose is completed) every 3 hours for eight doses and then 15 mg of oral leucovorin every 6 hours for eight doses.

Doxorubicin. 75 mg/m^2 intravenously every 3 weeks for six courses beginning with the fifth course of vincristine-methotrexate.

NOTE: The vincristine-methotrexate-leucovorin (VML) protocol is administered every week for 4 weeks, then every 3 weeks with the addition of doxorubicin for six courses, then VML every week for 4 weeks, then every 3 weeks for six courses, and then every week for a final four courses.

Selected Reading

Goorin AM et al: Weekly high dose methotrexate and doxorubicin for osteosarcoma: the Dana-Farber Cancer Institute/The Children's Hospital–Study III, *J Clin Oncol* 5:1178-1184, 1987.

T-10

Methotrexate. 8000 to 12,000 mg/m^2 on days 1, 8, 15, 22, 64, 71, 99, and 106.

Leucovorin. 10 to 15 mg orally every 6 hours for 10 doses starting 20 hours after each methotrexate dose.

Bleomycin. 15 units/m^2 on days 43 and 44.

Cyclophosphamide. 600 mg/m^2 on days 43 and 44.

Dactinomycin. 0.6 mg/m^2 on days 43 and 44.

Doxorubicin. 30 mg/m^2 on days 78, 79, and 80.

NOTE: On day 29, resection or amputation is performed if indicated; otherwise an endoprosthesis is placed on day 113. If tissue then shows grade I or II tumor (see the references for a definition), the patient's chemotherapy consists of three cycles of cisplatin plus doxorubicin, bleomycin, cyclophosphamide, and dactinomycin (T-10A). If the tumor is grade III or IV after chemotherapy, three cycles of bleomycin, cyclophosphamide, dactinomycin, methotrexate, and doxorubicin (T-10B) are given. This program requires extensive facilities and experience to perform it safely and successfully. In some later trials, cisplatin was sometimes added and the regimen individualized.

Selected Readings

Meyers PA et al: Chemotherapy for nonmetastatic osteogenic sarcoma: the Memorial Sloan-Kettering experience, *J Clin Oncol* 10:5-15, 1992.

Rosen G et al: Preoperative chemotherapy for osteogenic sarcoma: selection of postoperative adjuvant chemotherapy based on the response of the primary tumor to preoperative chemotherapy, *Cancer* 49:1221-1230, 1982.

ETOPOSIDE-CYCLOPHOSPHAMIDE-CISPLATIN-DOXORUBICIN

Etoposide. 200 mg/m^2/day by 72-hour continuous IV infusion during weeks 0, 3, 13, 19, 25, and 31.

Cyclophosphamide. 300 mg/m^2 intravenously every 12 hours for six doses during weeks 0, 3, 13, 19, 25, and 31.

Cisplatin. 100 mg/m^2 intravenously during weeks 6, 8, 16, 22, 28, and 34.

Doxorubicin. 40 mg/m^2 intravenously during weeks 6, 8, 16, 22, 28, and 34.

NOTE: Surgery is performed during week 10.

Selected Reading

Cassano WF, Graham-Pole J, Dickson N: Etoposide, cyclophosphamide, cisplatin, and doxorubicin as neoadjuvant chemotherapy for osteosarcoma, *Cancer* 68:1899-1902, 1991.

OVARIAN CARCINOMA

Ovarian carcinoma is the fourth most common cause of cancer death in women and the leading cause of all female genital cancer deaths in the United States. One in 70 women will develop ovarian cancer in her lifetime. The incidence has increased sixfold over the last 70 years. The cause is not clear but may be related to nulliparity, infertility, or a family hereditary pattern. Three general types have been identified: ovarian cancer alone, ovarian and breast cancers, or ovarian and colon cancers. The highest risk factor is a family history of a first-degree relative (mother, daughter, or sister) with the disease.

Favorable prognosis in ovarian cancer is associated with younger age; good performance status; cell type other than mucinous and clear-cell; lower-stage, well-differentiated tumor; smaller disease volume before surgical debulking; absence of ascites; and platinium-based therapy. Because the disease is often asymptomatic in its early stages, most patients have widespread disease at the time of diagnosis. Hence the yearly mortality rate is approximately 65% of the incidence rate. Nevertheless, early stages of the disease are curable in a high percentage of patients.

Therapy involves surgical exploration by an experienced gynecological oncologist with debulking of all grossly visible tumor, including the area just under the diaphragm and leaving behind of minimal tumor—lesions less than 1 cm. This is followed by chemotherapy as soon as adequate surgical healing has taken place. Active agents include paclitaxel, cisplatin, carboplatin, cyclophosphamide, ifosfamide, doxorubicin, altretamine, etoposide, and tamoxifen. Investigational agents that appear to have some activity include docetaxel, topotecan, irinotecan, and gemcitabine. Therapy is most successful as combination chemotherapy. Recently, it has been demonstrated that paclitaxel plus cisplatin gives a higher complete and overall response rate than cyclophosphamide plus cisplatin. It was also shown that the combination of cyclophosphamide, doxorubicin, and cisplatin has a minimally better response rate than the combination without doxorubicin, but the investigators concluded that the added toxicity of the doxorubicin outweighed the advantage and recommended the two drugs rather than the three-drug regimen. The Gynecological Oncology Group (GOG) is currently comparing carboplatin plus paclitaxel to earlier combinations to determine whether its lesser toxicity will still yield equivalent responses. For patients who fail first-line regimens, there are a variety of salvage regimens, some of which are listed. High-dose chemotherapy with bone marrow or peripheral stem cell support is the subject of several experimental trials. The role of radiation therapy is controversial, but is generally reserved for palliation or special situations. For patients who have low-volume disease or minimum residual disease after debulking and systemic chemotherapy, intraperitoneal chemotherapy with cisplatin, paclitaxel, cytarabine, or a combination thereof is frequently successful in prolonging disease-free survival.

Ovarian germ cell tumor is a clinically and histologically different disease although it afflicts the same organ. It has a different clinical course, prognosis, and therapy and is discussed in a separate section.

CARBOPLATIN-CISPLATIN

Carboplatin. 480 mg/m^2 intravenously on day 1.

Cisplatin. 50 mg/m^2 intravenously on day 3.

NOTE: Segelov et al (1994) used carboplatin 300 mg/m^2 in a similar regimen.

Selected Readings

Gill I et al: Phase I study of carboplatin (CB) day 1 and cisplatin (CP) day 3, *Proc Am Soc Clin Oncol* 9:74, 1990.

Segelov E et al: A phase II study of carboplatin and cisplatin in advanced ovarian cancer, *Eur J Gynaecol Oncol* 15:277-282, 1994.

CHAD—CYCLOPHOSPHAMIDE-DOXORUBICIN-ALTRETAMINE-CISPLATIN

Cyclophosphamide. 600 mg/m^2 intravenously on day 1.

Altretamine. 150 mg/m^2 orally on days 8 to 22.

Doxorubicin. 25 mg/m^2 intravenously on day 1.

Cisplatin. 50 mg/m^2 intravenously on day 1.

NOTE: Repeat the cycle every 28 days.

Selected Reading

Vogl SE et al: Cisplatin based combination chemotherapy for advanced ovarian cancer: high overall response rate with curative potential only in women with small tumor burdens, *Cancer* 51:2024-2030, 1983.

CHAP-5—CYCLOPHOSPHAMIDE-ALTRETAMINE-DOXORUBICIN-CISPLATIN

Cyclophosphamide. 100 mg/m^2 orally on days 15 to 28.

Altretamine. 150 mg/m^2 orally on days 15 to 28.

Doxorubicin. 35 mg/m^2 intravenously on day 1.

Cisplatin. 20 mg/m^2 intravenously on days 1 to 5.

NOTE: Starting on day 36, repeat the cycle.

Selected Readings

Neijt JP et al: Combination chemotherapy with Hexa-CAF and CHAP-5 in advanced ovarian carcinoma: a randomized study of the Netherlands Joint Study Group for ovarian cancer, *Proc Am Soc Clin Oncol* 2:148, 1983.

Neijt JP et al: Randomized trial comparing two combination chemotherapy regimens (CHAP-5 v CP) in advanced ovarian carcinoma, *J Clin Oncol* 5:1157-1168, 1987.

CIC—CARBOPLATIN-IFOSFAMIDE-CISPLATIN

Carboplatin. 200 mg/m^2 intravenously on day 1.

Ifosfamide. 1500 mg/m^2/day intravenously on days 1 to 3.

Cisplatin. 50 mg/m^2 intravenously on days 2 and 3.

Mesna. 900 mg/m^2/day intravenously in three divided doses on days 1 to 3.

NOTE: Repeat every 4 weeks for six courses.

Selected Reading

Lund B et al: Combined high-dose carboplatin and cisplatin, and ifosfamide in previously untreated ovarian cancer patients with residual disease, *J Clin Oncol* 8:1226-1230, 1990.

CYCLOPHOSPHAMIDE WITH CISPLATIN OR CARBOPLATIN

Cisplatin-Cyclophosphamide

Cisplatin. 75 mg or 100 mg/m^2 intravenously on day 1.

Cyclophosphamide. 600 mg/m^2 intravenously on day 1.

Carboplatin-Cyclophosphamide

Carboplatin. 300 mg/m^2 intravenously on day 1.

Cyclophosphamide. 600 mg/m^2 intravenously on day 1.

NOTE: Repeat every 28 days for six courses. There is evidence to suggest that the equivalence ratio of carboplatin to cisplatin is 4 to 1. The Southwest group used 100 mg/m^2 cisplatin, and the Canadian group used 75 mg/m^2.

Selected Readings

Albert D et al: Improved therapeutic index of carboplatin plus cyclophosphamide versus cisplatin plus cyclophosphamide: final report by the Southwest Oncology Group of phase III, randomized trial in stages III and IV ovarian cancer, *J Clin Oncol* 10:706-717, 1992.

Swenerton K et al: Cisplatin-cyclophosphamide versus carboplatin-cyclophosphamide in advanced ovarian cancer: a randomized phase III study of the National Cancer Institute of Canada Clinical Trials Group, *J Clin Oncol* 10:718-726, 1992.

CISPLATIN-CARBOPLATIN-CYCLOPHOSPHAMIDE

Cyclophosphamide. 600 mg/m^2 intravenously on day 1.

Carboplatin. 280 mg/m^2 intravenously on day 1.

Cisplatin. 50 mg/m^2 intravenously on day 1.

NOTE: This protocol requires appropriate hydration and antiemetics. Use carboplatin before giving cisplatin (i.e., use in the order listed). Repeat every 4 weeks.

Selected Reading

Grem J et al: Cisplatin, carboplatin, and cyclophosphamide combination chemotherapy in advanced-stage ovarian carcinoma: an Eastern Cooperative Oncology Group pilot study, *J Clin Oncol* 9:1793-1800, 1991.

H-CAP—ALTRETAMINE-CYCLOPHOSPHAMIDE-DOXORUBICIN-CISPLATIN

Altretamine. 150 mg/m^2/day orally on days 1 to 14.

Cyclophosphamide. 350 mg/m^2 intravenously on days 1 and 8.

Doxorubicin. 20 mg/m^2 intravenously on days 1 and 8.

Cisplatin. 60 mg/m² intravenously on day 1.

NOTE: Repeat every 4 weeks.

Selected Readings

Greco FA, Johnson DH, Hainsworth JD: A comparison of hexamethylmelamine (altretamine), cyclophosphamide, doxorubicin, and cisplatin (H-CAP) vs cyclophosphamide, doxorubicin, and cisplatin (CAP) in advanced ovarian cancer, *Cancer Treat Rev* 18(suppl A):47-55, 1991.

Hainsworth JD et al: Advanced ovarian cancer: long-term results of treatment with intensive cisplatin-based chemotherapy of brief duration, *Ann Intern Med* 108:165-170, 1988.

HEXA-CAF—ALTRETAMINE-CYCLOPHOSPHAMIDE-METHOTREXATE-FLUOROURACIL

Altretamine. 150 mg/day orally for 14 days.

Cyclophosphamide. 150 mg/day orally for 14 days.

Methotrexate. 40 mg/m² intravenously on days 1 and 8.

5-Fluorouracil. 600 mg/m² intravenously on days 1 and 8.

NOTE: Repeat the cycle every 28 days.

Selected Reading

Young RC et al: Advanced ovarian adenocarcinoma: a prospective clinical trial of melphalan (L-PAM) versus combination chemotherapy, *N Engl J Med* 299:1261-1266, 1978.

INTRAPERITONEAL CISPLATIN-CYTARABINE

Cisplatin. 200 mg/m² intraperitoneally over a 30-minute period.

Cytarabine. 2000 mg/2 L of normal saline intraperitoneally over a 30-minute period.

Sodium thiosulfate. 4000 mg/m² in 250 mL of sterile water by IV bolus and then 12,000 mg/m² in sterile water over a 6-hour period by IV infusion.

NOTE: Repeat the cycle every 28 days. The cisplatin is mixed with the cytarabine in 2 L of normal saline over a 30- to 50-minute period and drained over a 4-hour span.

Selected Reading

Markman M et al: Intraperitoneal chemotherapy with high-dose cisplatin and cytosine arabinoside for refractory ovarian carcinoma and other malignancies principally involving the peritoneal cavity, *J Clin Oncol* 3:925-931, 1985.

PAC VERSUS PC
PAC—Cisplatin-Doxorubicin-Cyclophosphamide

Cisplatin. 50 mg/m² intravenously on day 1.

Doxorubicin. 45 mg/m² intravenously on day 1.

Cyclophosphamide. 600 mg/m^2 intravenously on day 1.

NOTE: Repeat every 28 days for six courses.

PC–Cisplatin-Cyclophosphamide
Cisplatin. 50 mg/m^2 intravenously on day 1.

Cyclophosphamide. 600 mg/m^2 intravenously on day 1.

NOTE: Repeat every 28 days for six courses.

Selected Readings
Bruzzone M et al: A randomized trial comparing PC vs PAC chemotherapy in epithelial ovarian cancer: 7 years follow-up, *Proc Am Soc Clin Oncol* 9:157, 1990.

Conte PF et al: A randomized trial comparing cisplatin plus cyclophosphamide versus cisplatin, doxorubicin and cyclophosphamide in advanced ovarian cancer, *J Clin Oncol* 4:965-971, 1986.

PACLITAXEL-CISPLATIN

Paclitaxel. 135 mg/m^2 over 3 hours on day 1.

Cisplatin. 75 mg/m^2 intravenously over 1 hour on day 1.

NOTE: This protocol is repeated every 3 weeks. Paclitaxel is always given before cisplatin. Premedication for paclitaxel is essential; use the standard three-drug regimen. Usual hydration and antiemetic procedures are also necessary before and after cisplatin. This program was superior to cisplatin-cyclophosphamide in a Gynecologic Oncology Group study.

Selected Readings
McGuire WP et al: Cyclophosphamide and cisplatin compared with paclitaxel and cisplatin in patients with stage III and stage IV ovarian cancer, *N Engl J Med* 334:1-6, 1996.

Rowinsky EK et al: Sequences of taxol and cisplatin: a phase I and pharmacologic study, *J Clin Oncol* 9:1692-1703, 1991.

PACLITAXEL-CARBOPLATIN

Paclitaxel. 185 mg/m^2 intravenously over 3 hours on day 1.

Carboplatin. Target dose to AUC 6 intravenously over 1 hour on day 1.

NOTE: Repeat every 21 days up to six courses. Premedicate with usual paclitaxel antihypersensitivity regimen. The Gynecologic Oncology Group is piloting a regimen with paclitaxel 175 mg/m^2 over 3 hours with carboplatin at AUC 7.5 with both drugs given every 21 days for six cycles.

Selected Readings
Meerpohl HG et al: Paclitaxel combined with carboplatin in the first line treatment of advanced ovarian cancer, *Semin Oncol* 22 (6 suppl 15):7-12, 1995.

Ozols RF: Combination regimens of paclitaxel and platinum drugs as first-line regimens for ovarian cancer, *Semin Oncol* 22 (6 suppl 15):1-6, 1995.

PACLITAXEL-CISPLATIN-CYCLOPHOSPHAMIDE

Paclitaxel. 250 mg/m² intravenously over 3 hours on day 1.

Cisplatin. 75 mg/m² intravenously on day 1.

Cyclophosphamide. 750 mg/m² intravenously on day 1.

NOTE: Repeat every 21 days. Use filgrastim (G-CSF) as indicated. Pay special attention to hydration, antiemetics, and premedication to avoid allergic reactions. Give paclitaxel first.

Selected Reading

Kohn EC et al: A pilot study of cyclophosphamide, paclitaxel and cisplatin with G-CSF for newly diagnosed ovarian cancer patients, *Proc Am Soc Clin Oncol* 15:281, 1996.

OVARIAN GERM CELL CANCER

Ovarian germ cell cancer accounts for about 5% of all ovarian malignancies in the United States. The incidence is much higher in the Orient, where up to 15% of ovarian cancers are of the germ cell type. They are generally classified as dysgerminomas and nondysgerminomas. The latter include embryonal carcinoma, endodermal sinus tumor, choriocarcinoma, mature teratoma, immature teratoma, and mixed germ cell tumor. After surgical removal in stages I, II, and III, even when it is complete, chemotherapy is indicated as adjuvant, except in stage IA grade I immature teratoma and stage IA pure dysgerminoma. Progress of the disease may often be followed with titers of beta-human chorionic gonadotropin (beta-HCG) or alpha-fetoprotein (AFP). Incomplete removal of stage III disease and all stage IV disease requires active chemotherapy. Active drugs include cisplatin, carboplatin, bleomycin, etoposide, vinblastine, dactinomycin, vincristine, cyclophosphamide, and ifosfamide. The three most commonly used combinations in order of their efficacy and inverse order of their development are BEP (bleomycin, etoposide, cisplatin), PVB (cisplatin, vinblastine, bleomycin) and VAC (vincristine, dactinomycin, cyclophosphamide). Long-term survival rates with this type of therapy range from 85% for dysgerminoma down to 50% to 70% for the nondysgerminomas.

ADJUVANT VAC–VINCRISTINE-DACTINOMYCIN-CYCLOPHOSPHAMIDE

Vincristine. 1.5 mg/m² intravenously on days 1 and 15.

Dactinomycin. 0.35 mg/m² intravenously on days 1 to 5.

Cyclophosphamide. 150 mg/m² intravenously on days 1 to 5.

NOTE: Courses given every 4 weeks. Gershenson et al (1985) give vincristine on day 1 of each cycle and dactinomycin 0.5 mg/m².

Selected Readings

Gershenson DM et al: Treatment of malignant non-dysgerminomatous germ cell tumors of the ovary with vincristine, dactinomycin and cyclophosphamide, *Cancer* 56:2756-2761, 1985.

Williams SD et al: Chemotherapy of advanced dysgerminoma: trials of the Gynecologic Oncology Group (GOG), *J Clin Oncol* 9:1950-1955, 1991.

ADJUVANT BEP—BLEOMYCIN-ETOPOSIDE-CISPLATIN

Bleomycin. 20 unit/m^2/wk intravenously.

Etoposide. 100 mg/m^2/day intravenously on days 1 to 5.

Cisplatin. 20 mg/m^2/day intravenously on days 1 to 5.

NOTE: Three courses are given over a 9-week period (i.e., every 21 days).

Selected Readings

Williams S et al: Ovarian germ cell tumors: adjuvant trials of the Gynecologic Oncology Group (GOG), *Proc Am Soc Clin Oncol* 8:150, 1989.

Williams S et al: Adjuvant therapy of ovarian germ cell tumors with cisplatin, etoposide and bleomycin: a trial of the Gynecologic Oncology Group, *J Clin Oncol* 12:701-706, 1994.

ADVANCED AND RECURRENT: PVB—CISPLATIN-VINBLASTINE-BLEOMYCIN

Cisplatin. 20 mg/m^2/day intravenously on days 1 to 5.

Vinblastine. 12 mg/m^2 intravenously on day 1.

Bleomycin. 20 units/m^2 intravenously weekly.

NOTE: Three or four courses are given at 3-week intervals.

Selected Reading

Williams SD et al: Cisplatin, vinblastine, and bleomycin in advanced and recurrent ovarian germ-cell tumors, *Ann Intern Med* 111:22-27, 1989.

PANCREATIC CARCINOMA

Pancreatic carcinoma is the twelfth most common cancer in the United States, but it is the fifth most common cause of cancer death. It is an insidious malignancy that causes late symptoms and hence late diagnosis, so that cure is uncommon. In the rare instances when early diagnosis is made, surgical pancreaticodudodenectomy with curative intent may be attempted by those skilled and experienced in performance of this challenging procedure. Although operative mortality rates are much improved, survival is only slightly improved. Adjuvant chemoradiation therapy has prolonged survival in some trials and not in others. Toxicity of the combined modality therapy is severe. Active drugs (response rate 10% or better) include 5-fluorouracil, mitomycin, streptozocin, ifosfamide, and doxorubicin. Gemcitabine appears to have some activity and has been FDA approved. Although several combinations have been reported to have activity greater than single agents (and are listed below with dosages), this has not been demonstrated in prospective clinical trials. In fact, FAM (fluorouracil, doxorubicin, mitomycin [doses listed in gastric cancer section]) was no more effective than 5-fluorouracil alone or mitomycin alone. Many clinicians use single agents or supportive palliative therapy, or enter willing patients into clinical trials.

FAM-S—FLUOROURACIL-DOXORUBICIN-MITOMYCIN-STREPTOZOCIN

5-Fluorouracil. 600 mg/m^2 intravenously on days 1, 8, 29, and 36.

Doxorubicin. 30 mg/m^2 intravenously on days 1 and 29.

Mitomycin. 10 mg/m^2 intravenously on day 1.

Streptozocin. 400 mg/m^2 intravenously on days 1, 8, 29, and 36.

NOTE: Repeat the cycle every 8 weeks. Reduce doses for poor-risk patients. This is a toxic regimen and may not be better than 5-fluorouracil alone.

Selected Reading
Bukowski RM et al: Phase II trial of 5-fluorouracil, Adriamycin, mitomycin C and streptozotocin (FAM-S) in pancreatic carcinoma, *Cancer* 50:197-200, 1982.

FAC—FLUOROURACIL-DOXORUBICIN-CISPLATIN

5-Fluorouracil. 300 mg/m^2 intravenously on days 1 to 5.

Doxorubicin. 40 mg/m^2 intravenously on day 1.

Cisplatin. 60 mg/m^2 intravenously on day 1.

NOTE: Repeat the cycle every 35 days.

Selected Reading
Moertel CG et al: A phase II study of combined 5-fluorouracil, doxorubicin and cisplatin in the treatment of advanced upper gastrointestinal adenocarcinomas, *J Clin Oncol* 4:1053-1057, 1986.

FAP—FLUOROURACIL-DOXORUBICIN-CISPLATIN

5-Fluorouracil. 300 mg/m^2 intravenously on days 1 to 5.

Doxorubicin. 50 mg/m^2 intravenously on day 1.

Cisplatin. 20 mg/m^2 intravenously on days 1 to 5.

NOTE: Repeat the cycle every 21 days. After six cycles, split-course radiation is administered at 200 cGy/day, 5 days/wk for 2 weeks separated by a 2-week rest period and then 2 more weeks of the same radiation (total dose, 4000 cGy). Each 2-week course includes 500 mg/m^2 of 5-fluorouracil intravenously on days 1 to 3 of therapy.

Selected Reading
Wagener D et al: A phase 2 study of 5-FU, Adriamycin and cisplatin (FAP) followed by a split course irradiation in combination with 5-FU for locally advanced pancreatic cancer (LAP), *Proc Am Soc Clin Oncol* 6:77, 1987.

SMF–STREPTOZOCIN-MITOMYCIN-FLUOROURACIL

Streptozocin. 1000 mg/m² intravenously on days 1, 8, 29, and 35.

Mitomycin. 10 mg/m² intravenously on day 1.

5-Fluorouracil. 600 mg/m² intravenously on days 1, 8, 29, and 35.

NOTE: Repeat the cycle every 56 days. This is a highly toxic regimen.

Selected Readings

Oster MW et al: Chemotherapy for advanced pancreatic cancer: a comparison of 5-fluorouracil, Adriamycin and mitomycin (FAM) with 5-fluorouracil, streptozocin, and mitomycin (FSM), *Cancer* 57:29-33, 1986.

Wiggans RG et al: Phase II trial of streptozotocin, mitomycin-C, and 5-fluorouracil (SMF) in the treatment of advanced pancreatic cancer, *Cancer* 41:387-391, 1978.

PROSTATIC CARCINOMA

Prostatic carcinoma is now the most common cause of cancer in the United States and the fourth most frequent cause of cancer death. Although it is true that prostate cancer is found microscopically in most men by age 90 (of those who come to autopsy), it was the cause of death in more than 41,000 men in the United States in 1996. With the wide availability of the prostate specific antigen test (PSA), earlier diagnosis is possible, and potentially increased survival will occur with earlier therapy.

The disease is most frequent in older men with the median at age 72, but it is known to afflict men in their late 40s and early 50s. Screening is with digital rectal examination and PSA, but there is controversy about the age at which it is appropriate to begin screening with each modality. The American Cancer Society recommends that they both begin at age 50. Therapy is usually surgical under age 70 in those with localized tumor and no comorbidity. Other alternatives are external beam radiation therapy or brachytherapy with radioactive seed implantation, which is still being clinically evaluated. For advanced or metastatic disease, hormonal therapy is preferred. Chemotherapy is used only after hormonal resistance or relapse occurs and even then is only marginally successful. The FDA recently approved mitoxantrone (with steroids) as chemotherapy for treatment of pain related to advanced prostate cancer that has progressed despite hormone therapy.

CEE–CISPLATIN-EPIRUBICIN-ESTRAMUSTINE

Cisplatin. 60 mg/m² intravenously on day 1.

Epirubicin. 60 mg/m² intravenously on day 1.

Estramustine. 10 mg/kg/day orally.

NOTE: Treated patients were younger than 70 years of age with metastatic hormone-resistant cancer and had not previously received chemotherapy. The cisplatin and epirubicin were repeated every 3 weeks for six cycles or until progression. Estramustine was given until progression.

Selected Reading

Lo Re G et al: Combination chemotherapy in "non-elderly" patients with hormone refractory prostatic carcinoma, *Proc Am Soc Clin Oncol* 11:211, 1992.

CFM–CYCLOPHOSPHAMIDE-FLUOROURACIL-MEGESTROL

Cyclophosphamide. 350 mg/m^2 intravenously every 2 weeks for six doses.

5-Fluorouracil. 350 mg/m^2 intravenously every 2 weeks for six doses.

Megestrol. 40 mg orally 3 times a day.

NOTE: After six doses, administer every 3 weeks.

Selected Reading

Gala KV et al: Cyclophosphamide, 5-fluorouracil and megestrol acetate in treatment of stage D prostate cancer, *Proc Am Soc Clin Oncol* 4:101, 1985.

DS–DOXORUBICIN-STILPHOSTROL

Doxorubicin. 60 mg/m^2 intravenously on day 1.

Stilphostrol. 1000 mg intravenously daily the first week and then twice weekly.

NOTE: Repeat the cycle every 3 weeks.

Selected Reading

Citrin DL, Hogan TF, Davis TE: Chemohormonal therapy of metastatic prostate cancer, *Cancer* 52:410-414, 1983.

ESTRAMUSTINE-ETOPOSIDE

Estramustine. 15 mg/kg/day orally in four divided doses.

Etoposide. 50 mg/m^2/day orally in two divided doses.

NOTE: Both drugs given daily for 21 days of every 28-day cycle. Therapy is continued until evidence of disease progression. Watch out for thromboembolic problems and neutropenia.

Selected Readings

Pienta KJ et al: A combination of oral estramustine and oral etoposide for the treatment of hormone refractory prostate cancer, *J Clin Oncol* 12:2005-2012, 1994.

Pienta KJ et al: Inhibition of prostate cancer growth by estramustine and etoposide, *Cancer* 75:1920-1926, 1995.

ESTRAMUSTINE-PACLITAXEL

Estramustine. 600 mg/m^2/day orally.

Paclitaxel. 120 mg/m^2 IV infusion for 96 hours starting on day 2.

NOTE: Repeat courses every 3 weeks. Use paclitaxel allergy prophylaxis regimen.

Selected Reading

Hudes GR et al: Paclitaxel plus estramustine in metastatic hormone-refractory prostate cancer, *Semin Oncol* 22(5 suppl 12):41-55, 1995.

ESTRAMUSTINE-VINBLASTINE

Estramustine. 600 mg/m² orally on days 1 to 42.

Vinblastine. 4 mg/m² intravenously weekly for 6 weeks.

NOTE: Repeat course every 8 weeks or until evidence of progression. Seidman et al (1992) use 10 mg/kg estramustine.

Selected Readings

Hudes GR: Phase II study of estramustine and vinblastine, two microtubule inhibitors, in hormone-refractory prostate cancer, *J Clin Oncol* 10:1754-1761, 1992.

Seidman AD et al: Estramustine and vinblastine: use of prostate specific antigen as a clinical trial end point for hormone refractory prostate cancer, *J Urol* 147:931-934, 1992.

GOSERELIN-FLUTAMIDE

Goserelin. 3.6 mg subcutaneously every 28 days.

Flutamide. 250 mg orally three times a day.

Most physicians use the new goserelin 10.8 mg implant every 90 days in patients who have done well for several months with the 3.6 mg preparation.

Selected Readings

Denis LJ et al: Goserelin acetate and flutamide versus bilateral orchiectomy: a phase III EORTC study (30853), *Urology* 42:119-130, 1993.

Jurincic CD, Horlbeck R, Klippel KF: Combined treatment (goserelin plus flutamide) versus monotherapy (goserelin alone) in advanced prostate cancer: a randomized study, *Semin Oncol* 18(suppl 6):21-25, 1991.

KETOCONAZOLE-HYDROCORTISONE

Ketoconazole. 400 mg orally 3 times a day.

Hydrocortisone. 30 mg each morning and 20 mg each evening orally.

NOTE: It is important to dose between meals and to avoid H-2 blockers, sucralfate, and antacids because ketoconazole requires an acid environment for absorption. Do not allow use of astemizole (Hismanal) or terfenadine (Seldane) when using ketoconazole.

Selected Reading

Muscato JJ et al: Optimal dosing of ketoconazole and hydrocortisone leads to long responses in hormone refractory prostate cancer, *Proc Am Soc Clin Oncol* 13:229, 1994.

LEUPROLIDE-FLUTAMIDE

Leuprolide. 1.0 mg/day subcutaneously daily.

Flutamide. 250 mg orally three times a day.

NOTE: Most physicians use leuprolide depot, 7.5 mg every 28 days, instead of the daily injections. A new 22.5-mg preparation has recently become available for injection every 90 days.

Selected Readings

Benson RC Jr et al: National Cancer Institute study of luteinizing hormone–releasing hormone plus flutamide versus luteinizing hormone–releasing hormone plus placebo, *Semin Oncol* 18(suppl 6):26-28, 1991.

Crawford ED et al: A controlled trial of leuprolide with and without flutamide in prostatic carcinoma, *N Engl J Med* 321:419-424, 1989.

Eisenberger MA et al: Prognostic factors in stage D2 prostate cancer: important implications for future trials, results of a cooperative intergroup study (INT 0036), *Semin Oncol* 21:613-619, 1994.

LHRH-ANALOGUE-BICALUTAMIDE

Goserelin acetate. 3.6 mg total subcutaneously every 28 days.

Bicalutamide. 50 mg orally every day, *or*

Leuprolide acetate. 7.5 mg total intramuscularly every 28 days.

Bicalutamide. 50 mg orally every day.

Selected Reading

Schellhammer P et al: A controlled trial of bicalutamide versus flutamide, each in combination with luteinizing hormone–releasing hormone analogue therapy in patients with advanced prostate cancer, *Urology* 45:745-752, 1995.

MITOXANTRONE-PREDNISONE

Mitoxantrone. 12 mg/m^2 intravenously on day 1.

Prednisone. 5 mg orally twice a day.

NOTE: Mitoxantrone is given every 21 days and prednisone daily. Watch for neutropenia and cardiac toxicity. Do not exceed total cumulative lifetime mitoxantrone dose of 140 mg/m^2.

Selected Reading

Tannock I et al: Chemotherapy with mitoxantrone and prednisone palliates patients with hormone-resistant prostate cancer: results of a randomized Canadian trial, *Proc Am Soc Clin Oncol* 14:245, 1995.

RENAL CELL CARCINOMA

Renal cell carcinoma is an adenocarcinoma that arises from the parenchyma of the kidney and accounts for 2.3% of all cancers and 85% of kidney cancers. The American Cancer Society estimates that kidney and other urinary cancers (excluding bladder) afflicted 30,600 and killed 12,000 in 1996, marking the diagnosis as the tenth most common malignancy and the eleventh most frequent cause of cancer death in the United States. The male:female ratio is about 3:2. Average age at presentation has been 55 to 60 years, but the diagnosis is being made earlier because of the serendipitous discovery of tumor masses on ultrasonography, CT scans, or MRIs of the abdomen being done for another indication. This also makes it possible to operate on stage I lesions, which have a high cure rate. Genetic abnormalities are a major risk factor, and many cases are the result of familial or Lindau–von Hippel disease (associated loss of a tumor-suppresser gene involving the short arm of chromosome 3). The histology in more than 75% of cases is a clear cell carcinoma. Dissemination is usually hematogenous with frequent metastases to lung, bone, brain, liver, thyroid, and other sites. Regional lymph node involvement is found in 15% to 30% of cases. If the tumor has not penetrated the renal capsule, local recurrence is rare.

In previous editions, we did not mention renal cell carcinoma because there was no therapy for metastatic or recurrent disease worth mentioning. A comprehensive review of the chemotherapy of renal cell carcinoma (Yagoda A, Abi-Rached B, Petrylak D: Chemotherapy for advanced renal-cell carcinoma: 1983-1993, *Semin Oncol* 22:42-60, 1995) found response rates under 8% for all drugs except floxuridine (14.6%) and 5-fluorouracil (10%). Responses with biological response modifiers have been much more encouraging. Early remissions with monoclonal antibodies and interferon-alpha seemed encouraging but have been eclipsed by better responses with interleukin-2 (IL-2). In 1992, the Food and Drug Administration approved the marketing of IL-2 for the treatment of renal cell carcinoma based on the studies of Rosenberg and colleagues at the NCI Surgery Branch (*N Engl J Med* 313:1485-1492, 1985, and 316:889-897, 1987) and subsequently updated (*JAMA* 271:907-913, 1944) using high-dose IL-2, which is very toxic but is the regimen listed in the product brochure. Since then, low-dose IL-2 has been shown to be equally efficacious and less toxic by NCI Surgery Branch investigators (Yang JC et al: Randomized comparison of high-dose and low-dose intravenous interleukin-2 for the therapy of metastatic renal cell carcinoma: an interim report, *J Clin Oncol* 12:1572-1576, 1994). Early reports of the use of subcutaneous IL-2 alone or of subcutaneous IL-2 with subcutaneous interferon alpha seem promising and less toxic than high-dose IL-2.

Autolymphocyte therapy (ALT) is an outpatient, low-toxicity approach to the adoptive immunotherapy of renal cell carcinoma in which patients are treated with autologous memory T-cells activated ex vivo by a mitogenic monoclonal antibody directed against the CD3 portion of the T-cell receptor, in combination with a mixture of previously generated autologous cytokines (Graham S et al: The use of ex vivo–activated memory T cells (autolymphocyte therapy) in the treatment of metastatic renal cell carcinoma: final results from a randomized, controlled, multisite study, *Semin Urol* 11:27-34, 1993). Results have been interesting because the tumor response rate in the treatment group compared with the control group was only (P = .04), but the survival comparison was highly statistically significant (P = .007), a survival advantage of approximately 2.4-fold. Further studies are in progress, including a comparison of ALT versus interferon alpha. At this point in time, it is advisable to have patients with renal cell carcinoma enter into an experimental protocol so that better treatments can be developed and the existing promising agents can be compared with each other in controlled trials. Worthwhile therapy for this disease is now available, and we must sort out the better approaches while we try to develop newer and better therapies.

SARCOMA

Sarcoma is a relatively uncommon tumor with a heterogeneous and complex histology and a classification that is not entirely accepted by many of the experts in the field. Sarcoma pathology is a field of its own. Generally, small, low-grade tumors can be surgically resected with a high cure rate. Large tumors (greater than 5 cm) are usually high grade, spread to lymph nodes and distant sites (most often lung), and have a poor prognosis. Nonetheless, some of these tumors are amenable to limb-sparing combined-modality therapy with neoadjuvant radiation with or without chemotherapy followed by surgery with long-term survival. If the metastases (usually lung) are isolated and can be resected, cure may be possible.

Active chemotherapeutic agents include doxorubicin, dacarbazine, cyclophosphamide, methotrexate, ifosfamide, etoposide, and vincristine. Both single-agent and combination chemotherapy are unproved by randomized prospective trials, so most patients should be entered into investigational protocols when possible.

AD–DOXORUBICIN-DACARBAZINE
Adequate Marrow

Doxorubicin. 60 mg/m^2 intravenously on day 1.

Dacarbazine. 250 mg/m^2 intravenously on days 1 to 5.

Inadequate Marrow

Doxorubicin. 45 mg/m^2 intravenously on day 1.

Dacarbazine. 200 mg/m^2 intravenously on days 1 to 5.

NOTE: Repeat the cycle every 22 days.

Selected Reading
Gottlieb JA et al: Adriamycin used alone and in combination for soft tissue and bony sarcomas, *Cancer Chemother Rep* 6:271-282, 1975.

CAD–CYCLOPHOSPHAMIDE-DOXORUBICIN-DACARBAZINE

Cyclophosphamide. 500 mg/m^2 intravenously on day 1.

Doxorubicin. 60 mg/m^2 intravenously on day 2.

Dacarbazine. 400 mg/m^2 intravenously on days 1 and 2.

NOTE: Cycles are repeated at 21 days. Doxorubicin is deleted after a total dose of 450 mg/m^2. Radiation therapy is administered between the third and fourth courses of chemotherapy.

Selected Reading
Antman KH et al: Survival of patients with localized high-grade soft tissue sarcoma with multimodality therapy, *Cancer* 51:396-401, 1983.

CY-VA-DIC—CYCLOPHOSPHAMIDE-VINCRISTINE-DOXORUBICIN-DACARBAZINE
Adequate Marrow
Cyclophosphamide. 500 mg/m^2 intravenously on day 1.

Vincristine. 1 mg/m^2 intravenously on days 1 and 5 (maximum, 1.5 mg/dose).

Doxorubicin. 50 mg/m^2 intravenously on day 1 only.

Dacarbazine. 250 mg/m^2 intravenously on days 1 to 5.

NOTE: Repeat cycle every 21 days. Bramwell et al used vincristine 1.4mg/m^2 intravenously on day 1 and dacarbazine 400 mg/m^2/day on days 1 to 3.

Selected Readings
Bramwell V et al: Adjuvant CYVADIC chemotherapy for adult soft-tissue sarcoma—reduced local recurrence but no improvement in survival: a study of the European Organization for Research and Treatment of Cancer Soft Tissue and Bone Sarcoma Group, *J Clin Oncol* 12:1137-1149, 1994.

Yap BS et al: Cyclophosphamide, vincristine, Adriamycin, and DTIC (CYVADIC) combination chemotherapy for the treatment of advanced sarcomas, *Cancer Treat Rep* 64:93-98, 1980.

DOXORUBICIN-IFOSFAMIDE
Doxorubicin. 75 mg/m^2 intravenously on day 1.

Ifosfamide. 5000 mg/m^2 continuous 24-hour infusion on day 1.

Mesna. 2500 mg/m^2 mixed with the ifosfamide and 1250 mg/m^2 over 12 hours following it.

rh GM-CSF. 250 μg/m^2/day subcutaneously beginning 24 hours after ifosfamide up to 14 days.

NOTE: The rh GM-CSF is discontinued once the WBC count equals or exceeds 10,000/μL. Therapy is continued for seven cycles or two cycles beyond a complete response, whichever comes first.

Selected Reading
Steward WP et al: Granulocyte-macrophage colony stimulating factor allows safe escalation of the dose-intensity of chemotherapy in metastatic adult soft tissue sarcomas: a study of the European Organization for Research and Treatment of Cancer Soft Tissue and Bone Sarcoma Group, *J Clin Oncol* 11:15-21, 1993.

DOXORUBICIN-DACARBAZINE-IFOSFAMIDE
Doxorubicin. 60 mg/m^2 by continuous IV infusion over 4 days (15 mg/m^2 per day).

Dacarbazine. 1000 mg/m^2 by continuous IV infusion over 4 days (250 mg/m^2 per day).

Ifosfamide. 6000 mg/m^2 intravenously over 3 days (2000 mg/m^2 per day).

Mesna. 10,000 mg/m^2 over 4 days (2500 mg/m^2 per day).

NOTE: Courses are repeated every 21 days if WBC count exceeds 3000/μL and platelet count reaches 100,000/μL.

Selected Reading

Antman K et al: An intergroup phase III randomized study of doxorubicin and dacarbazine with or without ifosfamide and mesna in advanced soft tissue and bone sarcomas, *J Clin Oncol* 11:1276-1285, 1993.

IFOSFAMIDE-(MESNA)-ETOPOSIDE

Etoposide. 100 mg/m^2 intravenously on days 1 to 5.

Ifosfamide. 1800 mg/m^2 intravenously on days 1 to 5.

NOTE: Etoposide is administered over a 1-hour period, followed immediately by ifosfamide and the loading dose of mesna (360 mg/m^2) mixed together and given over a 1-hour span. Subsequently, mesna is given by continuous infusion for 3 hours and then by bolus infusions over a period of 15 minutes every 3 hours for six doses at hours 5, 8, 11, 14, 17, and 20. Mesna doses after hour 5 were given orally; all earlier doses were intravenous. After four cycles, sites of residual metastatic disease in responding patients were treated with either surgery or radiation therapy to consolidate the response and achieve a complete remission. A total of 12 chemotherapy cycles at 3-week intervals was the planned goal.

Selected Reading

Miser JS et al: Ifosfamide with mesna uroprotection and etoposide: an effective regimen in the treatment of recurrent sarcomas and other tumors of children and young adults, *J Clin Oncol* 5:1191-1198, 1987.

MAI—MESNA-DOXORUBICIN-IFOSFAMIDE

Mesna. 300 mg/m^2 intravenously every 4 hours for three doses. Repeat daily for 5 days.

Doxorubicin. 16.6 mg/m^2/day intravenously on days 1 to 3.

Ifosfamide. 1500 mg/m^2/day intravenously on days 1 to 5.

NOTE: Repeat the treatment every 21 days.

Selected Reading

Hartlapp JH, Illiger HJ, Wolder H: Alternatives to CYVADIC combination therapy for soft tissue sarcoma. In Brade WP, Nagel GA, Seeber S, eds: Ifosfamide in tumor therapy. In *Contributions to oncology*, vol 26. Basel, Switzerland, 1987, Karger, pp 159-167.

MAID—MESNA-DOXORUBICIN-IFOSFAMIDE-DACARBAZINE

Mesna. 2500 mg/m^2/day intravenously on days 1 to 4.

Doxorubicin. 20 mg/m^2/day intravenously on days 1 to 3.

Ifosfamide. 2500 mg/m^2/day intravenously on days 1 to 3.

Dacarbazine. 300 mg/m^2/day intravenously on days 1 to 3.

NOTE: All drugs are administered by continuous infusion; doxorubicin is mixed with dacarbazine, and ifosfamide is mixed with mesna. Repeat the treatment every 21 days. Antman et al use very slightly different doses of ifosfamide and dacarbazine.

Selected Reading

Antman K et al: An intergroup phase III randomized study of doxorubicin and dacarbazine with or without ifosfamide and mesna in advanced soft tissue and bone sarcomas, *J Clin Oncol* 11:1276-1285, 1993.

Elias A et al: Response to mesna, doxorubicin, ifosfamide, and dacarbazine in 108 patients with metastatic or unresectable sarcoma and no prior chemotherapy, *J Clin Oncol* 7:1208-1216, 1989.

TESTICULAR AND EXTRAGONADAL GERM CELL CANCER

Testicular and extragonadal germ cell cancer is the most common cancer in males between 15 and 35. It accounts for 1% of cancers in males and is highly treatable and usually curable. Tumors are generally designated as seminoma or nonseminomatous. Pure seminomas (normal alfa-fetoprotein [AFP]) are very radiation sensitive, and stages I and II are treated with radiation, whereas stage III tumors are curable with combination chemotherapy. Nonseminomatous stage I is treated with resection and careful observation and small-volume stage II tumors are treated with resection, retroperitoneal lymph node dissection (RPLND), and careful observation. The observation should include monthly examinations, chest x-ray studies, AFPs and human beta-chorionic gonadotropin (beta-HCG) for the first year, and examinations every other month and tests the second year. Many clinicians also obtain an abdominal CT every other month the first year and every fourth month the second year. Bulky stage II and all stage III tumors are treated with combination chemotherapy.

Active chemotherapy drugs include cisplatin, bleomycin, etoposide, vinblastine, carboplatin, doxorubicin, dactinomycin, cyclophosphamide, and ifosfamide. They are always used in combinations of two or more drugs. The most frequently used combination in good-prognosis disease is bleomycin, etoposide, and cisplatin (BEP) given every 3 weeks for three courses. The results are worse if bleomycin is omitted, but the results are about the same if bleomycin is omitted and a fourth etoposide-cisplatin course is given. In poor-prognosis disease, four courses of BEP are essential, and high-dose cisplatin does not improve the results. For refractory or recurrent disease, high-dose therapy with ABMT or PBSC support is being evaluated.

BEP–BLEOMYCIN-ETOPOSIDE-CISPLATIN

Cisplatin. 20 mg/m^2 intravenously over a period of 15 to 30 minutes on days 1 to 5.

Bleomycin. 30 units by IV bolus on days 2, 9, and 16.

Etoposide.   100 mg/m^2 intravenously over a 30-minute period on days 1 to 5.

NOTE: Normal saline (100 mg/hr) is given on the days of cisplatin therapy. Watch for hypotension if etoposide is given too rapidly. Patients receive three or four courses at 3-week intervals on schedule, regardless of the granulocyte count. The dose of etoposide is reduced 20% for patients who received previous radiotherapy or had granulocytopenia and fever after an earlier course. A later paper showed equivalent efficacy with less toxicity using three courses instead of four.

Selected Readings

Einhorn LH et al: Evaluation of optimal duration of chemotherapy in favorable-prognosis disseminated germ cell tumors: a SECSG protocol, *J Clin Oncol* 7:387-391, 1989.

Williams SD et al: Treatment of disseminated germ-cell tumors with cisplatin, bleomycin, and either vinblastine or etoposide, *N Engl J Med* 316:1435-1440, 1987.

CEB—CARBOPLATIN-ETOPOSIDE-BLEOMYCIN

Carboplatin.   Target dose to AUC 5 intravenously on day 1.

Etoposide.   120 mg/m^2 intravenously on days 1 to 3.

Bleomycin.   30 units total intravenously on days 2, 9, and 16.

NOTE: Repeat cycles every 21 days for a total of four cycles. Diphenhydramine is given concomitantly with each dose of bleomycin to prevent febrile reactions. Carboplatin dose is adjusted to nadir WBC and platelet counts as described in report.

Selected Readings

Bajorin DF et al: Randomized trial of etoposide and cisplatin versus etoposide and carboplatin in patients with good-risk germ cell tumors: a multiinstitutional study, *J Clin Oncol* 11:598-606, 1993.

Horwich A et al: Effectiveness of carboplatin, etoposide and bleomycin combination chemotherapy in good-prognosis metastatic testicular nonseminomatous germ cell tumors, *J Clin Oncol* 9:62-69, 1991.

ETOPOSIDE-CISPLATIN

Cisplatin.   20 mg/m^2 intravenously on days 1 to 5 every 3 weeks.

Etoposide.   100 mg/m^2 intravenously on days 1 to 5 every 3 weeks.

NOTE: Usually use four courses every 3 weeks, depending on stage and retroperitoneal lymph node dissection results. Consider surgery after (if there is radiologic evidence of residual disease after four courses).

Selected Reading

Bosl GJ et al: A randomized trial of etoposide and cisplatin versus vinblastine, + bleomycin + cisplatin + cyclophosphamide + dactinomycin in patients with good prognosis germ cell tumors, *J Clin Oncol* 6:1231-1238, 1988.

HOP—IFOSFAMIDE-VINCRISTINE-CISPLATIN FOR RELAPSED SEMINOMA

Ifosfamide.   1200 mg/m^2 intravenously on days 1 to 5.

Vincristine.   2 mg total intravenously on day 1.

Cisplatin. 20 mg/m^2 intravenously on days 1 to 5.

NOTE: Cycles repeated every 21 days for a total of four cycles. This therapy is for bulky (>10 cm) pure seminoma (with normal AFP), extragonadal seminoma, or relapsed disease after previous radiotherapy. Mesna 300 mg/m^2 intravenously should be given 15 minutes before and 4 and 8 hours after starting ifosfamide.

Selected Reading

Fossa SD et al: Cisplatin, vincristine and ifosfamide combination chemotherapy of metastatic seminoma: results of EORTC trial 30874, *Br J Cancer* 71:619-624, 1995.

ICE–IFOSFAMIDE-CISPLATIN-ETOPOSIDE

Cisplatin. 20 mg/m^2 intravenously on days 1 to 5.

Etoposide. 100 mg/m^2 intravenously on days 1 to 5.

Ifosfamide. 1200 mg/m^2 intravenously on days 1 to 5.

Mesna. 200 mg/m^2 by IV bolus 30 minutes before and 4 and 8 hours after each dose of ifosfamide.

NOTE: Repeat every 3 weeks.

Selected Reading

Harstrick A et al: Cisplatin, etoposide, and ifosfamide salvage therapy for refractory or relapsing germ cell carcinoma, *J Clin Oncol* 9:1549-1555, 1991.

PVB–CISPLATIN-VINBLASTINE-BLEOMYCIN

Cisplatin. 20 mg/m^2 intravenously for 5 days.

Vinblastine. 0.15 mg/kg intravenously on days 1 and 2.

Bleomycin. 30 units intravenously on day 2 and then weekly for 12 consecutive weeks.

NOTE: Repeat every 3 weeks for a total of four courses.

Selected Reading

Stoter G et al: High-dose versus low-dose vinblastine in cisplatin-vinblastine-bleomycin combination chemotherapy of non-seminomatous testicular cancer: a randomized study of the EORTC Genitourinary Tract Cancer Cooperative Group, *J Clin Oncol* 4:1199-1206, 1986.

VAB VI–VINBLASTINE-DACTINOMYCIN-BLEOMYCIN-CYCLOPHOSPHAMIDE-CISPLATIN

Induction

Cyclophosphamide. 600 mg/m^2 intravenously on day 1.

Vinblastine. 4 mg/m^2 intravenously on day 1.

Dactinomycin. 1 mg/m^2 intravenously on day 1.

Bleomycin. 30 units intravenously on day 1 by IV push.

Bleomycin. 20 units/m^2/day by continuous IV infusion for 3 days.

Cisplatin. 120 mg/m^2 intravenously on day 4.

NOTE: The cycle is repeated every 3 or 4 weeks for two additional cycles, except that bleomycin is omitted from the third cycle.

Selected Reading

Vugrin D et al: VAB-6 combination chemotherapy in disseminated cancer of the testis, *Ann Intern Med* 95:59-61, 1981.

VeIP—VINBLASTINE-IFOSFAMIDE-CISPLATIN

Cisplatin. 20 mg/m^2/day intravenously for 5 days.

Ifosfamide. 1200 mg/m^2/day intravenously for 5 days.

Vinblastine. 0.11 mg/kg/day intravenously for 2 days.

Mesna. 120 mg/m^2 as an initial IV bolus and then 1200 mg/m^2/day by continuous IV infusion for 5 days.

NOTE: Repeat every 3 weeks for four courses.

Selected Reading

Munshi NC et al: Vinblastine, ifosfamide and cisplatin (VeIP) as second line chemotherapy in metastatic germ cell tumors (GCT), *Proc Am Soc Clin Oncol* 9:134, 1990.

VIP—ETOPOSIDE-IFOSFAMIDE-CISPLATIN

Etoposide. 75 mg/m^2/day intravenously on days 1 to 5.

Ifosfamide. 1200 mg/m^2/day intravenously on days 1 to 5.

Mesna. 400 mg intravenously before the day-1 ifosfamide dose and then 1200 mg/day by continuous IV infusion on days 1 to 5 (120 hours).

Cisplatin. 20 mg/m^2/day intravenously on days 1 to 5.

NOTE: Repeat the treatment every 21 days.

Selected Reading

Loehrer PJ et al: Salvage therapy in recurrent germ cell cancer: ifosfamide and cisplatin plus either vinblastine or etoposide, *Ann Intern Med* 109:540-546, 1988.

VPV—VINBLASTINE-CISPLATIN-ETOPOSIDE

Vinblastine. 8 mg/m^2 intravenously on day 1.

Cisplatin. 120 mg/m^2 intravenously on day 3.

Etoposide. 50 mg/m^2 intravenously on days 2 to 5.

NOTE: Repeat every 3 weeks for a total of four courses.

Selected Reading

Wozniak J et al: A randomized trial of cisplatin, vinblastine, and bleomycin versus vinblastine, cisplatin, and etoposide in the treatment of advanced germ cell tumors of the testis: a Southwest Oncology Group Study, *J Clin Oncol* 9:70-76, 1991.

THYMOMA (MALIGNANT)

Malignant thymoma is a rare tumor that is slow growing and frequently diagnosed as an incidental finding of chest radiography. The term is generally restricted to neoplasms of the thymic epithelial cells and excludes pure lymphomas of the organ. Verification of malignancy is often difficult and is based on the presence of invasion of the tumor capsule, surrounding tissue, or metastasis. Myasthenia gravis is associated in about 30% of thymoma patients, but its presence is not an adverse prognostic factor in terms of eradication of the tumor. Therapy is surgical if the tumor is localized, and recurrence is only 2% if it is encapsulated. If the tumor is invasive, the recurrence rate is 40%, and radiation therapy is given locally. For metastatic disease, chemotherapy is used, but only a few phase II studies have been reported. Active drugs include cisplatin, doxorubicin, cyclophosphamide, ifosfamide, etoposide, and prednisone. They are usually given in combinations.

ADOC—DOXORUBICIN-CISPLATIN-VINCRISTINE-CYCLOPHOSPHAMIDE

Doxorubicin. 40 mg/m^2 intravenously on day 1.

Vincristine. 0.6 mg/m^2 intravenously on day 3.

Cyclophosphamide. 700 mg/m^2 intravenously on day 4.

Cisplatin. 50 mg/m^2 intravenously on day 1.

NOTE: Repeat the cycle every 3 weeks if blood counts permit.

Selected Readings

Fornasiero A et al: Chemotherapy of invasive or metastatic carcinoma: report of 11 cases, *Cancer Treat Rev* 68:1205-1210, 1984.

Fornasiero A et al: Chemotherapy for invasive thymoma: a 13 year experience, *Cancer* 68:30-33, 1991.

BAPP—BLEOMYCIN-DOXORUBICIN-CISPLATIN-PREDNISONE

Bleomycin. 12 units/m^2 intravenously on day 1.

Doxorubicin. 50 mg/m^2 intravenously on day 1.

Cisplatin. 50 mg/m^2 intravenously on day 1.

Prednisone. 40 mg/m^2 orally on days 1 to 5.

NOTE: Repeat the cycle every 4 weeks to a total cumulative dose of 540 mg/m^2 of doxorubicin and 175 units of bleomycin.

Selected Reading

Chahinian AP et al: Treatment of invasive or metastatic thymoma: report of eleven cases, *Cancer* 47:1752-1761, 1981.

CEE

Cisplatin.   75 mg/m^2 intravenously on day 1.

Etoposide.   120 mg/m^2/day intravenously on days 1, 3, and 5.

Epirubicin.   100 mg/m^2 intravenously on day 1.

NOTE: Repeat every 3 weeks for three cycles, and then perform surgery followed by radiation therapy with 4600 to 6000 cGy.

Selected Reading

Macchiarini P et al: Neoadjuvant chemotherapy, surgery, and postoperative radiation therapy for invasive thymoma, *Cancer* 68:706-713, 1991.

CISPLATIN-ETOPOSIDE

Cisplatin.   60 mg/m^2 intravenously on day 1.

Etoposide.   120 mg/m^2 intravenously on days 1 to 3.

NOTE: Repeat courses every 3 weeks for six or more courses.

Selected Reading

Giaccone G et al: Cisplatin and etoposide combination chemotherapy for locally advanced or metastatic thymoma: a phase II study of the EORTC Lung Cancer Cooperative Group, *J Clin Oncol* 14:814-820, 1996.

COLP–CYCLOPHOSPHAMIDE-VINCRISTINE-LOMUSTINE-PREDNISONE

Cyclophosphamide.   1000 mg/m^2 intravenously on day 1.

Vincristine.   1.3 mg/m^2 intravenously (maximum, 2.0 mg) on day 1.

Lomustine.   70 mg/m^2 intravenously on day 1.

Prednisone.   40 mg/m^2 orally on days 1 to 7.

NOTE: Repeat the cycle every 4 weeks.

Selected Reading

Daugaard G, Hansen HH, Rorth M: Combination chemotherapy for malignant thymoma, *Ann Intern Med* 99:189-190, 1983.

PAC–CISPLATIN-DOXORUBICIN-CYCLOPHOSPHAMIDE

Cisplatin.   50 mg/m^2 intravenously on day 1.

Doxorubicin.   50 mg/m^2 on day 1.

Cyclophosphamide.   500 mg/m^2 intravenously on day 1.

NOTE: Cycles repeated every 21 days for up to eight cycles. Adequate hydration and antiemetics are essential.

Selected Reading

Loehrer PJ et al: Cisplatin plus doxorubicin plus cyclophosphamide in metastatic or recurrent thymoma: final results of an intergroup trial, *J Clin Oncol* 12:1164-1168, 1994.

THYROID CARCINOMA

Thyroid carcinoma is responsible for 1% of all cancers in the United States and is the most common endocrine malignancy. It is seen more often in women than men and in patients who had head and neck radiation in childhood. It is now being seen in a 100-fold or more increase in children in the area around Chernobyl after the nuclear reactor release of radiation. Generally, well-differentiated tumors (papillary or follicular) are highly treatable and usually curable. Poorly differentiated cancers (medullary or anaplastic) are less common but are aggressive, metastasize early, and have a poor prognosis.

The recommended therapy for localized disease, depending on histology, is total thyroidectomy (some advocate lobectomy in stage I papillary cancer) plus exogenous thyroid suppression, and in some cases 131-iodine ablation. Regional (stage III) involvement with nodal metastases requires total thyroidectomy, involved node removal or radical neck dissection, and 131-iodine ablation if the tumor demonstrates adequate uptake of the isotope. If not, then external beam radiation is used. Distant metastases are treated with 131-iodine ablation if uptake is adequate. If not, then external beam radiation is given to control local disease, and patients are considered for investigational chemotherapy protocol or chemotherapy regimens in the literature. Active agents include doxorubicin, cisplatin, bleomycin, and etoposide. Combinations are usually used, but their efficacy has not been demonstrated in prospective randomized trials.

BAP–BLEOMYCIN-DOXORUBICIN-CISPLATIN

Bleomycin. 30 units/day for 3 days by continuous IV infusion.

Doxorubicin. 60 mg/m^2 intravenously on day 5.

Cisplatin. 60 mg/m^2 intravenously on day 5.

NOTE: Repeat every 3 or 4 weeks. Usual antiemetic and hydration and maximum tolerated dose guidelines all apply.

Selected Reading

De Besi P et al: Combined chemotherapy with bleomycin, Adriamycin, and platinum in advanced thyroid cancer, *J Endocrinol Investig* 14:475-480, 1991.

DOXORUBICIN-CISPLATIN

Doxorubicin. 60 mg/m^2 intravenously on day 1.

Cisplatin. 40 mg/m^2 intravenously on day 1.

NOTE: The dose of doxorubicin was adjusted for hematological or hepatic dysfunction. Treatment was given every 3 weeks to a total dose of 550 mg/m² of doxorubicin or until evidence of failure of therapy.

Selected Reading

Shimaoka K et al: A randomized trial of doxorubicin versus doxorubicin plus cisplatin in patients with advanced thyroid carcinoma, *Cancer* 56:2155-2160, 1985.

DMBV–DOXORUBICIN-MELPHALAN-BLEOMYCIN-VINCRISTINE

Doxorubicin.   40 mg/m² intravenously on day 1.

Melphalan.   6 mg/m² orally on days 3 to 6.

Bleomycin.   15 units/m² intramuscularly on day 15.

Vincristine.   1.0 mg/m² intravenously on day 15.

NOTE: Repeat the cycle every 28 days.

Selected Reading

Durie BGM et al: High risk thyroid cancer: prolonged survival with early multimodality therapy, *Cancer Clin Trials* 4:67-73, 1981.

ADDITIONAL NOTE

In compiling this list of protocols, many fine programs were omitted. In some cases, those omitted may be superior to some included. Since the compilation was completed, many additional useful protocols have been published, and more will be forthcoming every week.

Conscientious physicians are urged to check the NCI's PDQ for the most up-to-date listings of the state of the art treatments. At the risk of being repetitious (albeit, repetition is a fine educational tool), we would urge clinicians to check the availability of ongoing protocols with the cooperative and/or institutional clinical research groups with whom they may be affiliated for eligibility of their patients to participate in suitable research projects. This would make available to them the latest (and optimally the best) possible therapy and newest drugs. When a good research protocol is matched to an appropriate patient, then the best interests of the patient and society are served simultaneously.

7

Ethical Considerations in Cancer

The role of the physician and associated health professionals is to cure illness and preserve life whenever possible. This is often not possible, especially in the field of oncology. Inherent in that role is also the relief of pain and suffering without doing any harm. The goals of prolongation of survival and pain relief are sometimes in conflict, and a sensitive balance must be achieved, considering the wishes of the patient and the constraints of the law. These decisions are frequently difficult and must be based on ethical considerations. Until recently, little was written about ethics in oncology (Fischer and Duffy, 1992).

MAJOR PRINCIPLES OF MEDICAL ETHICS

Although there are diverse value systems, several principles have been established to guide ethical decision making (Beauchamp and Childress, 1989):

1. *Autonomy* is allowing the patient to make a personal choice. The physician may collaborate with the patient on all substantive decisions, but the patient is the final authority (except when a decision is made contrary to the civil law). When the patient chooses a course of action that is contrary to the moral principles of the physician (e.g., cessation of therapy, suicide, abortion), the physician may withdraw from the physician-patient relationship after providing an acceptable substitute.
2. *Beneficence* means that one ought to prevent and remove harm and promote good (e.g., preserve life, relieve pain, restore health, and ameliorate suffering).
3. *Nonmaleficence* is best characterized by the injunction to "first do no harm."
4. *Justice* is the fair allocation of medical resources. Some people get more and some get less. Rationing is a fact of life. The problem is the basis for the decision that leads to "who gets what." As medications, technology, and hospitalization become more expensive, health care is rationed by inconveniencing the patient (Grumet, 1989), by hassling the physician (American Society of Internal

Medicine, 1990), and by denying insurance coverage for what should be funded (Eastman, 1991).

Adequate and often excessive care is given to the wealthy because they can afford it and to the elderly because they have Medicare. The very poor usually get adequate care because they have Medicaid (welfare), although there is an effort to reduce that entitlement. Inadequate care is sometimes given to the working poor who have no health insurance or to the middle-class people with less comprehensive, third-party coverage.

As the costs of health care escalate and the public demands universal health care at bargain prices, hard choices will have to be made between what is a reasonable expense and what may be desirable but is not cost effective (Ubel et al, 1996; Callahan, 1992). Oregon attempted to come to grips with this problem in a highly controversial change of its welfare laws that sets priorities (Garland, 1992). The change is an attempt to maximize the benefits of limited resources (Eddy, 1991). However, implementation has been delayed by challenges in the courts. This is unfortunate because this nation is better served by allowing individual states to run their own experiments to learn what is useful and what is problematic. If this approach is allowed to proceed, we may all learn some valuable lessons that may serve as models for the nation. In the meantime, the physician, among others, must protect the medical commons (i.e., the fair distribution of resources) (Hiatt, 1975). If a sensible health care system is to be crafted, physicians must have major input as ombudsmen for the patients and not as self-serving entrepreneurs (Thier, 1991). While we wait for this to happen, the nation's health care system is floundering. Congress is trying to improve the budget deficit by reducing benefits under Medicare and turning Medicaid over to the individual states. Meanwhile, a rapidly growing network of private insurance-industry managed care is beginning to dominate the health care system of the country.

MANAGED CARE

Managed care was advertised as a means to reduce the costs of health care for the nation, reduce waste, maintain the quality of care, and return the cost savings to society or to the individuals insured. In most areas, managed care has restricted access to care, especially to necessary hospitalization and to consultation by specialists. In fact, many managed care companies have forced physicians to be "double agents." The companies pay their physicians extra for not hospitalizing patients and for denying them referrals to specialists and to expensive modalities of diagnosis or therapy. Some companies go so far as to write into their contracts that physicians must agree not to tell patients when there is therapy available that the insurance provider will not fund, even when the physician thinks it is the best therapy for the patient—a technique known as the "gag rule." In other words, some physicians have to promise to withhold relevant information under threat of not being admitted to the managed care panel or if on the panel, being "decertified" or not reappointed for "disloyalty" to the company by putting the interests of the patient ahead of that of the insurer. The American Medical Association (AMA) protested the "gag rule" and urged legislation to require full disclosure to patients (Associated Press, 1996).

Medical care under the "gag rule" system leads to a negation of the physician-patient relationship and the obligation of the physician to make the welfare of the patient the prime consideration. Any other priority is unethical. The imperative of abiding by the physician-patient covenant was recently restated. It has been endorsed by the American College of Physicians, the American Board of Internal Medicine, and numerous other societies (Cassel, 1996; Crawshaw et al, 1995).

Physicians are advised to work through their medical organizations as patient advocates to remove all contract clauses that are contrary to the welfare of patients. It must be remembered that "the physician-patient relationship is the cornerstone for achieving, maintaining, and improving health" (Emanuel and Dubler, 1995). Indeed, the physician is a therapeutic agent when there is a good physician-patient bond, and the disruption of that relationship by closed panels is counter to good medical care. Patients are not well served when the insurer treats physicians as economic cost centers to be moved around, substituted, or excluded simply for a perceived cost-saving benefit to the insurer.

Hospitals are feeling the restrictions of managed care as acutely as physicians (Anders, 1994). It is clear to hospital administrators that managed care is a misnomer—it is not concerned with *care* but with *cost*. As a result, many hospitals have had to drastically reduce the number of professional nurses on their staffs and substitute unlicensed assistive personnel. Some clinics are being closed, equipment maintenance is being deferred, purchases of newer state-of-the-art equipment are on "hold," and the numbers of full-time medical staff personnel (pathologists, radiologists, anesthesiologists) are being reduced by attrition or by discharging personnel and replacing them with independent vendors at market-negotiated rates.

TO TELL THE TRUTH

The problem of whether and when to tell the patient the truth has gone through an interesting metamorphosis. Thirty years ago physicians rarely told patients that they had cancer, and if specifically questioned, they routinely lied "to protect the patient" (Oken, 1961). Today it is general practice to tell a competent adult the truth (Novack et al, 1979). Since patients know the truth more often than families suspect, a "conspiracy of misinformation" serves to isolate the patient from his or her family and physician when the patient needs them the most. It is essential for the patient to know and understand the nature of the clinical problem to give an informed consent for therapy, whether routine or experimental. To deny the patient the truth, regardless of the wishes of other family members who may profess the desire to protect the patient, may place the physician in legal jeopardy. The courts in the United States "generally require that the patient be told the diagnosis, the nature of the contemplated treatment, the risks inherent in such treatment, the prognosis if the proposed treatment is not undertaken, and the alternative methods of treatment, if any" (Miller, 1980).

Disclosure is best given in the presence of a family member or friend because the patient may not understand all that is being told. It is desirable to have another member of the health team present, not only as a witness, but as a knowledgeable confidante who can rediscuss the information and reinterpret it to the patient and family. The oncology nurse is in an excellent position to fulfill this role (Otte and Allen, 1987). When the patient is considering consent for an experimental program, it is essential that the consent be informed, or it is not valid or legal. Strict guidelines have been proposed for consent forms (Levine, 1974), and most refereed journals will not accept an article for publication unless the consent process is stated and fulfills the guidelines. However, patients under the stress of a cancer diagnosis are often unable to make valid, rational decisions quickly and are at the mercy of their health care professionals (Tabak, 1995). The patients need compassion, information, and the feeling that they can say "no." The 1978 World Medical Assembly proposal concerning informed consent has been summarized as follows (McGrath, 1995):

1. There should be an explanation of the proposed treatment, obviously in words readily understood by the patient.
2. The risks and benefits of the treatment should be clearly stated.
3. Any alternatives to treatment should be included in the discussion.
4. There should be adequate time for the patient's questions.
5. The patient should be aware of the option to withdraw at any time from treatment or to refuse treatment entirely. The patient should be assured that such a decision will be respected and that there will be continued support from the health professionals involved.

The physician must always remember the implied contract with the patient who places his or her life in the trust of the physician. The physician is expected to exercise good judgment to protect the quality of the patient's life for as long as he or she lives. If, in the honest opinion of the physician, this can best be done with an experimental program, then it should be recommended. If it can best be done with conventional therapy, then that should be recommended. The goal of the researcher is to find new knowledge. The goal of the physician must be the best interests of the patient.

"DO NOT RESUSCITATE" ORDERS

One of the major complaints of the public about physicians, and about oncologists and surgeons in particular, is their tendency to ignore the wishes of cancer patients. In spite of carefully executed advance directives and specific and clear indications by patients of their desire not to have resuscitation or prolongation of their terminal illness, patients frequently end up with unwanted IV lines, feeding tubes, and even respiratory assistance in an intensive care unit (Gilligan and Raffin, 1996).

Lay critics accuse physicians and hospitals of persisting with unauthorized therapy in an unethical manner as a device for extracting professional fees and keeping hospital beds filled. In actuality, this is too simplistic an explanation and unlikely to be true most of the time. The problem is that those who become physicians do so to save lives and make sick people well. Death symbolizes physicians' personal failures as professionals. Many physicians have difficulty dealing with death and need to learn to let go when there is nothing more to do for the patient and the patient is ready to die and wants nothing more to be done.

The majority of the public now generally recognizes that there comes a time in the treatment of a terminally ill patient when further therapy is not beneficial and may compromise the quality of the patient's remaining life. The oncologist must be ready to decrease and then discontinue active therapy as it becomes clear that it is not helpful and may even be harmful (Duffy, 1992). In such situations, it is more humane to withhold further therapy and not resuscitate when a cardiopulmonary arrest occurs (Blackhall, 1987). The Judicial Council of the American Medical Association (1981) says that "with informed consent a physician may do what is medically necessary to alleviate severe pain, or cease or omit treatment to let a terminally ill patient die, but he should not intentionally cause death." Many people agree with this. The recommendation of the President's Commission for the Study of Ethical Problems in Medicine and Biomedical and Behavioral Research (1983) also states that "a competent and informed patient or an incompetent patient's surrogate is entitled to decide with the attending physician that an order against resuscitation should be written in the chart."

DISCONTINUING CARE

Far more controversial is the question of discontinuing or not starting IV fluids under specific circumstances in dying patients who are comatose (Micetich, Steinecker, and Thomasma, 1983). It was and is hard to remove a functioning IV line, but it is easier not to restart one that has infiltrated or produced inflammation at the insertion site.

The next issue is the discontinuance or the failure to initiate nutritional feeding lines (enteral or parenteral) for the terminally ill comatose patient (Emanuel, 1992). Enteral and parenteral support can no longer be dismissed as simple, automatically applied components of medical care. As in other areas of intervention, health care professionals must confront the ethical and legal questions that may arise concerning nourishing seriously ill, unconscious patients (Dresser and Boisaubin, 1985). Decisions will have to be made on a case-by-case basis consistent with any prior "living will" or other expression of patient wishes or in cooperation with the legal next of kin. It should be unnecessary to take cases to court if the physicians and family can agree on what is best for the patient. The following guidelines given by Fry (1986) seem reasonable.

1. If the patient is mentally and legally competent, the wishes of the patient should be respected.
2. If the patient is incompetent but has made a living will or has made known his or her wishes to family or friends, the patient's decision made when competent should be respected.
3. If the patient is incompetent and has never made his or her wishes known, health care personnel should be guided by the best interests of the patient (consistent with the directives of the next of kin).

ADVANCED DIRECTIVES

The Patient Self-Determination Act became federal law on December 1, 1991 (White and Fletcher, 1991). It requires hospitals to ask patients if they have indicated their health care preferences in writing in case at some time the patient is unable to communicate competently. This process is known as *advanced directives*. The specific laws differ by state, and physicians need to check the law in effect in the local jurisdiction. Generally, there are three types of advanced directives.

1. The living will.
2. Appointment of a health care agent.
3. Durable power of attorney for health care decisions.

The living will is a document that is signed when the patient is competent and specifies preference about life-prolonging medical treatment should the patient become permanently unconscious and terminally ill (Annas, 1991). One can specify that no resuscitative measures be taken, and the patient may choose to be allowed to die without specified interventions. The document can be revised or revoked at any time that one is still competent.

Another alternative is to appoint a "health care agent." This individual is empowered to state the patient's wishes about prolonging medical care if the patient is unable to do so. He or she simply tells the physician the wishes of the patient.

A durable power of attorney for health care designates a person to make medical decisions for the patient who is incapacitated or incompetent. The various states allow different degrees of authority (LaPuma, Orentlicher, and Moss, 1991). Physicians and hospitals who ignore their patient's end-of-life instructions will do so at their legal and financial peril.

HOSPICE

When primary or secondary therapy for the cancer patient has failed, there is often no worthwhile further therapy, and physicians are required to explain this honestly and compassionately. Some patients may still wish to try an additional or experimental therapy, even if the chances of success are small or unknown. As long as patients are fully informed of the facts and the potential for response or failure of the additional therapy, alternatives should be offered. However, the patient and family need to be warned that their managed care company may decline to pay for what it considers futile therapy. The patient and family may still choose to proceed and pay for the therapy from their own assets. At this point, some families begin to look for miracles and start chasing alternative therapies that are often largely unproved and available only in remote and exotic locations. However, most patients faced with repeated therapeutic failures elect to forego further therapy with a low potential for benefit. These patients have traditionally received supportive care from home health agencies that are recognized by Medicare and other third-party payers. As described by Bulkin and Lukashok (1988):

> It is important to distinguish between hospice care and traditional home care. The latter is geared toward active therapy for acute problems; the individual patient is

the unit of care, and services and benefits are specified accordingly. In hospice, the unit of care is the entire family, and mandated benefits include the services of physicians, nurses, social workers, and other health professionals in the home; medication for pain relief and symptom control; medical appliances and equipment; nutrition counseling; extensive health and support services in the home; and bereavement counseling for the patient's family for up to one year.

Some patients in terminal phases may request physician-assisted suicide or voluntary euthanasia (Brock, 1992). These issues are now before the courts or the voters in referendums.

PHYSICIAN-ASSISTED SUICIDE

Second only to abortion, physician-assisted suicide is the most talked about high-profile controversy before the public and the medical profession. In a survey of Rhode Island physicians, 65% reported that they had been asked by patients to turn off a respirator, and 12% had been asked by a patient to administer a lethal dose of medication to end the suffering (Fried et al, 1993). In the state of Washington, 26% of physicians who responded to a questionnaire had received one or more requests for help to hasten death. Within a single calendar year, 12% had received at least one explicit request for physician-assisted suicide; some physicians reported between one and 20 such individual requests and up to 10 individual requests for euthanasia (Back et al, 1996). In England, a survey of National Health Service physicians revealed that 60% of those who responded had been asked by one or more patients to hasten their deaths and 45% had been asked to take active steps to hasten death. Although physician-assisted suicide is still illegal in England, 32% of those asked said they had complied with the request at least once (Ward and Tate, 1994).

In any large oncology practice, one may expect a suffering patient with terminal illness to say, "Doctor, I want to die. Will you help me?" (Quill, 1993). What should one do ethically? What can one do legally?

These questions have generated emotional discussion, articles, books, and some legislative and judicial attempts to respond to the issue. Judeo-Christian authorities more than a thousand years ago condemned suicide (although some other major religions have not). Synagogues and churches would not permit burial in the hallowed ground of their cemeteries of a person who had committed suicide. This practice is based on the idea that God gave life and only God can take life. It remains an article of faith of Catholicism and Orthodox Judaism. However, it is interesting that there is no specific prohibition of suicide per se in the Hebrew bible, and the six probable suicides (Samson, Saul and his armor bearer, and Achitophel) are never condemned in scripture for their suicides. Nor is the suicide of Judas in the New Testament criticized in that document. Nevertheless, the origin of suicide as an English common law offense was clearly ecclesiastical, based on the writings of St. Augustine and the disregard of earlier church approbation of Christian martyrdom. Initially, the suicide's goods were forfeited to his liege lord. Later suicide was made a crime against the state so that the king could receive the forfeited estate of the suicide as punishment for the offense (CeloCruz, 1992). More recently, English law and the laws of many of the individual states in the United States have decriminalized suicide and attempted suicide. However, they continue to regard assisting a suicide as a crime. Thus assisting in a non-criminal act is a crime in some states. It was under this concept of the common law that the state of Michigan attempted to convict Dr. Jack Kevorkian after two previous attempts had failed when he was charged under specific Michigan legislation aimed at criminalizing his activity in assisting suicides. In May 1996, Dr. Kevorkian was acquitted of the charges brought under the common law. He had explained his philosophy some years earlier (Kevorkian, 1991).

The difficult issue of physician-assisted suicide has been made more obscure by a confusion of terms. The following clear definitions have been published (Emanuel, 1994):

1. *Physician-assisted suicide* consists of a physician providing medications or other interventions to a patient with the understanding that the patient intends to use them to commit suicide.
2. *Terminating life-sustaining treatments (passive euthanasia)* is the withholding or withdrawing of life-sustaining medical treatments to allow a patient to die.
3. *Indirect euthanasia* is the administration of narcotics or other medications to relieve pain with the incidental consequence of causing sufficient respiratory depression to hasten the patient's death (the so-called *double effect*).
4. *Voluntary active euthanasia* is the intentional administration of medication or other interventions to cause the patient's death at the patient's explicit request and with full informed consent.
5. *Involuntary euthanasia* is euthanasia of a competent patient without that patient's explicit request or fully informed consent (e.g., the patient may not have been asked).
6. *Nonvoluntary euthanasia* is euthanasia of an incompetent patient who is incapable of explicitly requesting it (e.g., a mentally incompetent or comatose patient).

It is now generally agreed that it is both moral and legal, perhaps even mandatory, to withhold life-sustaining treatment under certain circumstance (President's Commission, 1983; Council on Ethical and Judicial Affairs, 1991; Hastings Center, 1987; Fischer, 1992; Pope Pius XII, 1973). Nurses have been more attuned to the need for compassion than physicians and have been less hesitant to participate in end-of-life decisions.

Many people feel that passive euthanasia is not much different than indirect euthanasia and that the two methods are very close to physician-assisted suicide. Indeed, 53% of respondents to a *New York Times*-CBS poll (1990) and 63% of respondents in a *Boston Globe*-Harvard School of Public Health survey (Blendon, Szalay and Knox, 1992; Knox, 1991) believed that doctors should be allowed to assist a terminally ill patient in taking his or her own life. Although the American Medical Association is opposed to physician-assisted suicide (Council on Scientific Affairs, 1996; *New York Times*-CBS, 1990), public support for this procedure is strong and growing. Interest was reflected in the rise to the top of the *New York*

Times best seller list of the book *Final Exit* (Humphry, 1991). In Oregon, the Death with Dignity Act passed in 1994 and became law. At this writing, its implementation has been blocked by a district court order after a legal challenge.

The state of Washington passed a law specifically criminalizing physician-assisted suicide. This was declared unconstitutional by the U.S. District Court in Washington and sustained by a vote of 8 to 3 in the Ninth Circuit U.S. Court of Appeals in San Francisco because the statute violates the "liberty interest" of the 14th amendment to the U.S. constitution. Less than a month later, the U.S. Second Circuit Court of Appeals in New York City ruled in *Quill v. Vacco* that two New York state statutes that ban physician-assisted suicide violate the "equal protection clause" of the 14th amendment because they unconstitutionally discriminate against persons who are terminally ill but are not on life-support systems that patients can have discontinued on request.

The U.S. Supreme Court has accepted the Washington case for review. If it sustains the Circuit Courts, then the laws of the states will have to come into conformity. Many of the strongest supporters of these decisions feel that it is important to have clear procedural safeguards similar in many respects to those in the Netherlands. Physician-assisted suicide and voluntary euthanasia are still illegal in Holland and punishable by a 12-year prison term if the physician is convicted (de Wachter, 1989). However, under an unofficial policy of the judiciary and the legislature, physicians (and only physicians) will *not* be prosecuted if they adhere to the guidelines of the Royal Dutch Medical Association (KNMG) and the State Commission on Euthanasia (Rigter, 1989; Gevers, 1987; Netherlands State Commission, 1987). Basically, these organizations require that:

1. There be an explicit and repeated request by the patient that leaves no reasonable doubt about the desire to die;
2. The mental or physical suffering of the patient must be very severe with no prospect of relief;
3. The patient's decision be well-informed, free, and enduring;
4. All options for other care to relieve the suffering adequately have been exhausted, or refused by the patient; and
5. The doctor consult another physician not involved in the case who must concur. In addition, nurses, pastors, and others may also be consulted.

The Dutch continue to examine and reexamine their policies in this matter, especially institutional guidelines and procedures (Haverkate and van der Wal, 1996).

Many suggestions have been made for safeguards and guidelines in the United States (Benrubi, 1992; Quill, Cassel, and Meier, 1992; Miller et al, 1994). They follow the Dutch guidelines in most respects but tend to add restrictions such as prospective committee review to ensure public accountability and the requirement for a palliative care consultation before a decision is made. There is some disagreement about whether to permit voluntary active euthanasia or only physician-assisted suicide. There is also diversity of opinion on the question of whether to restrict these choices only to terminally ill patients with fewer than 6 months to live or to include patients who are suffering with no foreseeable chance for improvement (e.g., those who are suffering from diseases such as amyotrophic lateral sclerosis). One would hope that patients could and would seek assistance when needed from their primary care physician or primary specialist who knows them well. It is important to be certain that no patient be induced to commit suicide whose needs may be met by appropriate palliative care. This is one reason that many hospice professionals have been in the forefront of opposition to legalization or acceptance of physician-assisted suicide. They frequently invoke the argument of "the slippery slope" and suggest that physicians may be induced to help patients kill themselves for family convenience, to save money for the insurance company or the heirs, or simply to get rid of an annoying patient for whom "nothing more can be done." There is always more that can be done to support the patient, the patient's family, and the patient's caregivers. The quality of mercy is something we all need, however we interpret our role in its delivery.

REFERENCES

American Society of Internal Medicine: The hassle factor: America's health care system strangling in red tape, *The Internist* 31(suppl): 3-31, 1990.

Anders G: Required surgery: health plans force even elite hospitals to cut costs sharply, *Wall Street J,* March 8, 1994.

Annas GJ: The health care proxy and the living will, *N Engl J Med* 324:1210-1213, 1991.

Associated Press: Doctors assail HMO gag rules, *New Haven Register,* June 28, 1996.

Back AL et al: Physician-assisted suicide and euthanasia in Washington State, *JAMA* 275:919-925, 1996.

Beauchamp TL, Childress JF: *Principles of biomedical ethics,* ed 3, New York, 1989, Oxford University Press.

Benrubi GI: Euthanasia—the need for procedural safeguards, *N Engl J Med* 326:197-199, 1992.

Blackhall LJ: Must we always use CPR? *N Engl J Med* 317:1281-1285, 1987.

Blendon RJ, Szalay US, Knox RA: Should physicians aid their patients in dying?: the public perspective, *JAMA* 267:2658-2662, 1992.

Brock DW: Euthanasia, *Yale J Biol Med* 65:121-129, 1992.

Bulkin W, Lukashok H: Rx for dying: the case for hospice, *N Engl J Med* 318:376-378, 1988.

Callahan D: Symbols, rationality, and justice: rationing health care, *Am J Law Med* 18:1-13, 1992.

Cassel CK: The patient-physician covenant: an affirmation of Asklepios, *Ann Intern Med* 124:604-606, 1996.

CeloCruz MT: Aid in dying: should we decriminalize physician-assisted suicide and physician-committed euthanasia? *Am J Law Med* 18:369-394, 1992.

Council on Ethical and Judicial Affairs, American Medical Association: Guidelines for the appropriate use of do-not-resuscitate orders, *JAMA* 265:1868-1871, 1991.

Council on Scientific Affairs, American Medical Association: Good care of the dying patient, *JAMA* 275:474-478, 1996.

Crawshaw R et al: Patient-physician covenant, *JAMA* 273:1553, 1995.

de Wachter MAM: Active euthanasia in the Netherlands, *JAMA* 262:3316-3319, 1989.

Dresser RS, Boisaubin EV Jr: Ethics, law and nutritional support, *Arch Intern Med* 145:122-124, 1985.

Duffy TP: When to let go, *N Engl J Med* 326:933-935, 1992.

Eastman P: Health insurance turndowns–a growing problem, *Oncology Times* May 1991.

Eddy DM: What's going on in Oregon? *JAMA* 266:417-420, 1991.

Emanuel EJ: Securing patients' right to refuse medical care: in praise of the Cruzan decision, *Am J Med* 92:307-312, 1992.

Emanuel EJ: Euthanasia: historical, ethical and empiric perspectives, *Arch Intern Med* 154:1890-1901, 1994.

Emanuel EJ, Dubler NN: Preserving the physician-patient relationship in the era of managed care , *JAMA* 273:323-328, 1995.

Fischer DS: Observations on ethical problems and terminal care, *Yale J Biol Med* 65:105-120, 1992.

Fischer DS, Duffy TP, eds: Ethics in hematology and oncology, *Yale J Biol Med* 65:63-142, 1992.

Fried TR et al: Limits of patient autonomy: physician attitudes and practices regarding life sustaining treatments and euthanasia, *Arch Intern Med* 153:722-728, 1993.

Fry ST: Ethical aspects of decision-making in the feeding of cancer patients, *Semin Oncol Nurs* 2:59-62, 1986.

Garland MJ: Justice, politics and community: expanding access and rationing health services in Oregon, *Law Med Health Care* 20:67-81, 1992.

Gevers JKM: Legal developments concerning active euthanasia on request in the Netherlands, *Bioethics* 1:156-162, 1987.

Gilligan T, Raffin TA: Whose death is it anyway? *Ann Intern Med* 125:137-141, 1996.

Grumet GW: Health care rationing through inconvenience, *N Engl J Med* 321:607-611, 1989.

Hastings Center: *Guidelines on the termination of life-sustaining treatment and the care of the dying,* Bloomington, Ind, 1987, Indiana University Press.

Haverkate I, van der Wal G: Policies on medical decisions concerning the end of life in Dutch health care institutions, *JAMA* 275:435-439, 1996.

Hiatt HH: Protecting the medical commons: who is responsible? *N Engl J Med* 293:235-241, 1975.

Humphry D: *Final exit,* New York, 1991, Dell.

Judicial Council of the American Medical Association: *Current opinions,* Chicago, 1981, American Medical Association.

Kevorkian J: *Prescription: medicide,* Buffalo, New York, 1991, Prometheus Books.

Knox RA: Poll: Americans favor mercy killing, *Boston Globe,* Nov 3, 1991.

LaPuma J, Orentlicher D, Moss RJ: Advance directives on admission: clinical implications and analysis of the patient self-determination act of 1990, *JAMA* 266:402-405, 1991.

Levine RJ: Guidelines for negotiating informed consent with prospective human subjects of experimentation, *Clin Res* 22:42-46, 1974.

McGrath P: It's OK to say no! *Cancer Nurs* 18:97-103, 1995.

Micetich KC, Steinecker PH, Thomasma DC: Are intravenous fluids morally required for a dying patient? *Arch Intern Med* 143:975-978, 1983.

Miller LJ: Informed consent, *JAMA* 244:2100-2103, 1980.

Miller FG et al: Regulating physician-assisted death, *N Engl J Med* 331:119-123, 1994.

Netherlands State Commission: Final report of the Netherlands State Commission on euthanasia: an English summary, *Bioethics* 1:163-174, 1987.

New York Times-CBS: Giving death a hand: rending issue, *New York Times* June 14, 1990.

Novack DH et al: Changes in physicians' attitudes toward telling the patient, *JAMA* 241:897-900, 1979.

Oken D: What to tell cancer patients: a study of medical attitudes, *JAMA* 175:1120-1128, 1961.

Otte DM, Allen KS: Ethical principles in the nursing care of the terminally ill patient, *Oncol Nurs Forum* 14:87-91, 1987.

Pope Pius XII: The prolongation446 of life. In Reiser SJ, Dyck AJ, Cirram MJ, eds: *Ethics in medicine: historical perspectives and contemporary concerns,* Cambridge, Mass, 1973, MIT Press.

President's Commission for the Study of Ethical Problems in Medicine and Biomedical and Behavioral Research: *Deciding to forego life sustaining treatment: ethical, medical and legal issues in treatment decisions,* Washington, DC, 1983, US Government Printing Office.

Quill TE: Doctor, I want to die. Will you help me? *JAMA* 270:870-873, 1993.

Quill TE, Cassel CK, Meier DE: Care of the hopelessly ill: proposed clinical criteria for physician-assisted suicide, *N Engl J Med* 327:1380-1384, 1992.

Rigter H: Euthanasia in the Netherlands: distinguishing facts from fiction, *Hastings Center Report* 19:(1, suppl) 31-32, 1989.

Tabak N: Decision making in consenting to experimental cancer therapy, *Cancer Nurs* 18:89-96, 1995.

Thier SO: Health care reform: who will lead? *Ann Intern Med* 115:54-58, 1991.

Ubel PA et al: Cost-effectiveness analysis in a setting of budget constraints: is it equitable? *N Engl J Med* 334:1174-1177, 1996.

Ward BJ, Tate PKA: Attitudes among NHS doctors to requests for euthanasia, *Br Med J* 308:1332-1334, 1994.

White ML, Fletcher JC: The patient self-determination act: on balance, more help than hindrance, *JAMA* 266:410-412, 1991.

8

Cancer Pain
Management

Many cancer patients, perhaps most, fear severe intractable pain even more than death. The physician and the health care team are able to cure cancer sometimes and prolong life frequently, but must relieve pain and suffering always. Although we are given the privilege of relieving pain and suffering, the public perception is that cancer patients are frequently in great pain, and some are reluctant to seek medical attention because of fear of pain. Too often, physicians and nurses do not fully understand the nature and proper treatment of pain in the cancer patient (Patt, 1993; Portenoy, 1993), which is quite different from the management of acute postoperative or posttraumatic pain (Sinatra et al, 1992).

UNDERESTIMATING NEED

Although 60% to 80% of cancer patients have moderate to severe pain at some time before death, a large proportion of them receive inadequate amounts of analgesics. The Eastern Cooperative Oncology Group (ECOG) study of pain management (Von Roenn et al, 1993) showed that only 50% of physicians believed that pain control was good or very good in their treatment center, and 86% believed that most cancer patients in the United States are undermedicated for their pain. The problems were identified as:

1. Poor pain assessment (69%)
2. Patient reluctance to report pain (49%)
3. Patient reluctance to take medication (49%)
4. Physician reluctance to give medication (46%)

To improve the systematic assessment of pain, a visual analogue scale with ratings from 0 to 5 or verbal ratings are frequently used to help the patient convey to the health care professional the degree of suffering that needs to be relieved. Three types of scales are popular—a visual analogue scale as a continuum (Table 8-1), a numeric rating scale (Table 8-2), and a categorical scale with verbal descriptors (Table 8-3).

TABLE 8-1
Visual Analogue Scale

No pain		Most pain

TABLE 8-2
Numeric Rating Scale

0	1	2	3	4	5	6	7	8	9	10

0 = No pain
10 = Worst pain imaginable

TABLE 8-3
Categorical Scale

0	1	2	3	4	5
No pain	Mild	Discomforting	Distressing	Intense	Excruciating
	Annoying, nagging	Troublesome, grueling, numbing, nauseating	Miserable, agonizing, gnawing	Horrible, dreadful, vicious, cramping	Unbearable, torturing, crushing, tearing

Pain is what the patient says it is. Neither pain nor the patient experiencing the pain can be fit into a clear-cut category with a predictable response. Indeed, the most helpful evaluations of severity of pain and pain relief come from patients themselves.

Concern about drug addiction by health care professionals and patients is understandable and appropriate. Although drug abuse is a national problem, it is important to discriminate between personalities who have psychological instability that influences them to abuse drugs and become addicted and patients who have physical symptoms that require interventions. Development of addiction is rare in medical patients who have pain and who have no history of addiction. Fear of such a rare phenomenon is not an adequate basis for withholding appropriate doses of narcotics for cancer patients (Porter and Jick, 1980).

Public and professional appreciation of the inadequate use of available drugs and techniques for pain relief led to a decade of attempts to educate physicians, nurses, and the laity in how to manage cancer pain. Since the World Health Organization (1986) published its guidelines and popularized its WHO analgesic ladder (Fig. 8-1), in the small number of situations it which its use has been evaluated (Jadad and Browman, 1995), analgesia was adequate in 69% to 100% of the patients analyzed. However, the authors pointed out that the evidence is insufficient to estimate confidently the WHO ladder's effectiveness. Other guidelines worth consulting are those of The American Pain Society (1992), the Ad Hoc Committee on

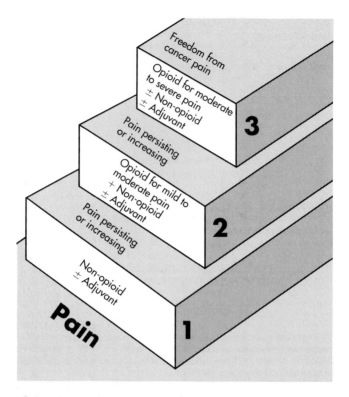

FIG. 8-1 The WHO three-step analgesic ladder. (World Health Organization, 1990.)

Cancer Pain of the American Society of Clinical Oncology (1992), and the Agency for Health Care Policy and Research (1994). The last is considered by many to be the current standard of care and can be obtained from the NCI Cancer Information Service by calling 1-800-4-CANCER. Also available from the same source are a Patient Guide, a Quick Reference Guide for Clinicians, and an Acute Pain Management Guide for Clinicians. Clinicians need to use these guides in their practice and should make the patient guides available to their patients who suffer from pain.

ASSESSMENT OF PAIN

The initial treatment of pain should be to both eliminate the cause and relieve the symptoms (Foley, 1989). The cause of the pain must be determined by carefully evaluating each complaint. In those cancer patients who do have chronic prolonged pain, it may be caused by one of the following mechanisms:

1. Partial or complete obstruction of a blood supply by tumor, leading to venous engorgement or arterial ischemia
2. Compression of the nerves, roots, or trunks by tumor or by metastatic fracture of bones adjacent to the nerves
3. Infiltration of the nerves, nerve roots, or nerve endings and blood vessels by tumor
4. Obstruction of a viscus by tumor
5. Infiltration and tumefaction in tissue enclosed by fascia or periosteum
6. Necrosis, infarction, or inflammation because of tumor

In addition to establishing the cause of the pain, assessment should include documentation of how pain is manifested behaviorally and symptomatically. Nevertheless, one cannot always verify a patient's statement of pain with a physiological sign (McCaffery, 1979). In chronic pain, a patient's pain expression may be minimized as a result of adaptive behavioral responses. A written pain history should include descriptions of:

1. Onset
2. Location
3. Duration
4. Intensity
5. Radiation
6. Relieving and aggravating factors
7. Cognitive response to pain

The many factors known to affect the pain response include anxiety, stress, family reactions, and the reaction of staff members. The impact of pain on the patient's sleep and eating habits also requires assessment. If the pain is not being controlled, it may dominate every aspect of the patient's life.

One should note the unique pains of tamoxifen therapy, sometimes associated with an exacerbation of bone pain after use. The alcohol-induced pain associated with the presence of Hodgkin's disease deserves note as well. Hypercalcemia may also precipitate or exacerbate pain.

Pain is a complex phenomenon that is very personal and at times an undefinable occurrence. Cancer pain instills feelings of helplessness, has a direct impact on emotions, and thus causes suffering. Therefore approaches to pain management and the relief of suffering need to be holistic and multidimensional (Cassel, 1982).

USING ANALGESICS FOR MILD PAIN

All pain is best relieved by removing the underlying cause (Fischer, 1984) with hormones or chemotherapy, surgery, or radiation. If that is not possible, however, and if the patient is ambulatory and the pain is mild, it may respond to simple analgesics such as aspirin, acetaminophen, diflunisal, choline magnesium trisalicylate, salsalate, propoxyphene, or a nonsteroidal antiinflammatory drug (NSAID) (Table 8-4). Although aspirin is the standard against which all other analgesics for mild pain have been

TABLE 8-4
Oral Analgesics for Mild or Moderate Pain: Approximate Equianalgesic Doses

Drug	Common brand name	Duration of analgesia (hr)	Oral dose (mg)	Plasma half life (hr)	Antiinflammatory	Platelet problems	Significant adverse effects
Aspirin	Many	3–5	650	3–5	Yes	Yes	GI, renal
Acetaminophen	Tylenol	3–4	650	1–4	No	No	Hepatic
Sodium salicylate	Generic	3–4	650	3–5	Yes	No	GI
Diflunisal	Dolobid	8–12	500	8–12	Yes	Mild	GI
Choline magnesium trisalicylate	Trilisate	8–12	1000	9–17	Yes	No	Tinnitis
Salsalate	Disalcid	16	750	1–2	Yes	Mild	Tinnitis
Ibuprofen	Motrin	3–5	400	2–3	Yes	Yes	GI
Fenoprofen	Nalfon	4–5	300	3–4	Yes	Yes	GI
Diclofenac	Voltaren	4–6	50	1–2	Yes	Yes	GI
Flurbiprofen	Ansaid	6–8	50	3–9	Yes	Yes	GI
Ketoprofen	Orudis	5–7	50	1–4	Yes	Yes	GI
Naproxen	Naprosyn	2–8	250	12–15	Yes	Yes	GI

Naproxen sodium	Anaprox	7–8	275	12–15	Yes	Yes	GI
Indomethacin	Indocin	3–4	25	3–11	Yes	Yes	GI, CNS
Tolmetin	Tolectin	3–4	200–400	1–2	Yes	Yes	GI
Sulindac	Clinoril	7	150	7–16	Yes	Yes	GI
Mefenamic acid	Ponstel	6	250	3–4	Yes	Yes	Marrow, GI
Meclofenamate	Meclomen	8	50	1–5	Yes	Yes	GI
Piroxicam	Feldene	24	20	30–86	Yes	Yes	GI
Etodolac	Lodine	4–12	200	7	Yes	Yes	GI
Propoxyphene	Darvon	4–6	65	6–12	No	No	CNS
Propoxyphene napsylate	Darvon-N	4–6	100	6–12	No	No	CNS
Pentazocine	Talwin Nx	3–4	50	2–3	No	No	CNS
Codeine	Many	3–5	32	2–3	No	No	Constipation, CNS
Hydrocodone	Many	3–4	5	3–4	No	No	Constipation, CNS
Oxycodone	Roxicodone	3–6	5	3–6	No	No	Constipation, CNS
Meperidine	Demerol	3–4	50	3–4	No	No	CNS

GI, Gastrointestinal; *CNS*, central nervous system.

compared, there is a tendency to avoid aspirin in many patients because of its propensity to cause gastrointestinal (GI) hemorrhage and because it irreversibly acetylates platelets so that they lose the ability to undergo viscous metamorphosis, an essential step in platelet aggregation and hemostasis. Aspirin may also interfere with the excretion of methotrexate by the kidney and may displace protein-bound methotrexate, increasing the possibility of drug toxicity.

Acetaminophen is usually the mild analgesic of first choice. Except for inflammatory conditions or bone pain, acetaminophen is as potent as aspirin but with fewer and more tolerable side effects. However, overdosage can be toxic or even fatal, particularly for small children. Acetaminophen does not inhibit platelet aggregation and has a duration of action of 3 to 4 hours. Three long-acting salicylates that have less GI toxicity than aspirin are available. Choline magnesium trisalicylate does not appear to interfere with platelet function at all, and diflunisal and salsalate exhibit only transient and reversible platelet inhibition. The drugs are generally given in the doses listed in Table 8-4 every 8 to 12 hours and, if taken at bedtime, will usually last through the night.

NSAIDs are helpful in controlling mild pain in general and moderate pain caused by inflammation or bone metastases. This reaction appears to involve, at least in part, an effect on prostaglandins. Ibuprofen and naproxen are available as generics. In some cases, a long-acting preparation such as piroxicam 20 mg is desirable because of its once-a-day dose, and 50 mg of flurbiprofen twice a day is popular as well. NSAIDS can produce severe GI hemorrhage and should be used cautiously, intermittently, and for brief periods.

USING ANALGESICS FOR MODERATE PAIN

When the cancer patient does not achieve adequate relief with nonnarcotics, a stronger analgesic is used, such as a narcotic in combination with aspirin or acetaminophen. This is a rational combination because narcotics act centrally and aspirin and acetaminophen act peripherally (Twycross and Lack, 1990). Oxycodone is available as a single agent, in combination, and as a new slow release, OxyContin, which appears to be a major addition to armamentarium used to treat intermediate and severe pain, providing excellent 12-hour pain relief. Dihydrocodeine and hydrocodone are available only in combinations. Narcotics predictably produce constipation, so patients need to be educated to use a stool softener and a laxative on a regular basis and to add bulk or fiber to their diet when possible.

Pentazocine is an agonist-antagonist drug with moderate analgesic effects that at one time was considered nonaddictive and potent. Greater experience has demonstrated substantial side effects, including sedation, drowsiness, nausea, vomiting, blurring of vision, respiratory depression (Catalano, 1985), and in older patients, a propensity to produce central nervous system (CNS) disturbances, including hallucinations, vertigo, and bad dreams. Like the other agonist-antagonist drugs (i.e., nalbuphine and butorphanol, and the partial agonist buprenorphine), it can also cause withdrawal symptoms if given to a patient receiving long-term narcotic analgesics. These drugs are not recommended for treatment of cancer pain because they block the analgesic effects of narcotics, they have an analgesic ceiling, and they may precipitate psychotomimetic effects.

Meperidine is one of the most popular analgesics and is widely used, but it should not be used for cancer pain. Its duration of action is short, and it is usually used in doses that are ineffective. Orally, 200 to 300 mg is required for severe pain and parenterally, at least 75 mg is required in average-sized adults. Parenterally, subcutaneous (SC) administration is suitable for occasional use, but it is painful and therefore it is usually given intramuscularly, which is also painful, or intravenously. Its toxic metabolite, normeperidine, can accumulate, especially when renal function is impaired, and can cause CNS stimulation that may lead to seizures. Because meperidine has atropine-like properties, it is a useful drug for renal colic and biliary colic. It has also been used intravenously to relieve shaking chills associated with transfusion reactions and IL-2 and amphotericin administration.

USING ANALGESICS FOR SEVERE PAIN

Strong narcotics are used in the management of severe pain. After more than 1000 years, there is no better group of drugs for this purpose than the opiates derived from the *Papaver somniferum* plant, more commonly known as the *poppy*. Morphine is the standard to which all other narcotic drugs are compared (Table 8-5), and so far there is none that is better overall. Morphine is effective, relatively inexpensive, and available as an oral, intramuscular, subcutaneous, rectal, intravenous, or intrathecal preparation. It is available in tablets, capsules, and oral liquid preparations; immediate- or controlled-release preparations; and in parenteral form in several strengths.

Whenever practical, narcotics should be given orally for chronic pain. It is important to give adequate doses on a regular schedule. Use of dosing as required leads to peaks and valleys of analgesia, whereas regular preventive therapy erases the memory and fear of pain and ultimately results in a lower total daily dose of narcotic. The as-needed schedule leads to anxiety about pain, results in overutilization and habituation, and is not recommended.

Although morphine is not absorbed as well by the oral route as some other narcotics (it is one third to one half absorbed), it can be given in an oral dose 2 to 3 times the parenteral dose. A starting dose of 10 mg for an average-size individual (5 mg in a debilitated elderly or low-body-mass individual) every 4 hours is recommended, with escalation of the dose if pain relief is inadequate or recurs before 4 hours is over. Pain for most patients is well controlled on an oral dose of 10 to 30 mg every 4 hours. Once the total daily dose has been determined using immediate-release morphine and verified over an additional 24 hours, sustained-release morphine (e.g., MS Contin, Oramorph-SR) may be substituted, assuming a ratio of 1:3 for parenteral to oral morphine. The 24-hour dose is divided into two doses given every 12 hours. An extra dose of immediate-release

TABLE 8-5
Strong Analgesics: Approximate Equianalgesic Doses

Drug	Brand name	Parenteral dose (mg)	Oral dose (mg)	Duration of analgesia (hr)	Plasma half-life (hr)
Morphine	Generic	10	30	4–5	2–4
Controlled-release morphine	MS Contin, Oramorph SR	—	30	8–12	—
Hydromorphone	Dilaudid	1.5	4	3–4	2–3
Oxymorphone	Numorphan	1.5	5 (rectal)	3–6	2–3
Methadone	Dolophine	10	20	5–6	30–60
Levorphanol	Levo-Dromoran	2	4	4–6	12–16
Meperidine	Demerol	100	300	2–4	3–4
Fentanyl	Duragesic	0.1	0.025/hr patch	1–2*	1.5–6
Oxycodone	Roxicodone	—	5	3–6	3–6
Controlled-release oxycodone	OxyContin	—	10	12	—
Ketorolac†	Toradol	30	10	5–6	5
Codeine	Generic	120	200	2–4	3–4
Tramadol	Ultram	—	50–100	4–6	7

*IV.
†Nonopiate, nonsteroidal antiinflammatory inhibitor.

morphine can be given for breakthrough pain. If this becomes frequent, the dose may be added to the calculation of the 12-hour sustained-release medication. Generally, a smaller total dose is used when the 12-hour schedule is satisfactory. Drowsiness and lethargy are usually transient, but in cases of sustained sedation, a mild stimulant such as 5 mg of methylphenidate (Ritalin) twice daily may be helpful. Nausea and vomiting usually respond to an antiemetic. The superiority of this approach and the improvement in the quality of life of cancer patients has been documented (Khojasteh et al, 1987; Warfield, 1993). OxyContin appears to have similar advantages as a long-acting analgesic.

A transdermal preparation of fentanyl (Duragesic) has become available in patches that release the analgesic over 72 hours. Patients usually reach a steady state in 12 hours and then maintain that level of analgesia for 72 hours. Thus a new patch has to be applied every 3 days. The patches come in four strengths: 25, 50, 75, and 100 µg/hr.

With careful attention to detail and a cooperative patient, smooth analgesic control can be achieved with transdermal fentanyl and periodic morphine for breakthrough pain. This avoids use of a continuous IV infusion and a pump. The patches are inconspicuous and can be titrated to the patient's needs, providing a continuous pain-free experience for those who cannot or prefer not to use slow-release oral morphine or develop nausea and/or experience vomiting from the oral preparation. Although fentanyl can cause nausea and vomiting, it is less emetogenic than an equianalgesic dose of morphine for most patients. This is a welcome and important addition to the analgesic armamentarium for the cohort of patients who will benefit from it. Unfortunately, it may not be effective in patients who perspire excessively or who are very hirsute.

When morphine is not desired for some reason, levorphanol or hydromorphone can be used in the equianalgesic doses as indicated in Table 8-5. It is important to be familiar with several pain drugs in each category (Omoigui, 1995). Methadone is favored by many because it is long acting. Although this is often desirable, there is danger of long-term accumulation. With a plasma half-life of 30 to 60 hours and with an analgesic effect of only 5 or 6 hours, drug accumulation can lead to progressively higher drug levels in plasma until a peak is reached in 4 days, at which time the patient may be lethargic or comatose. Since the antagonist naloxone is effective for 1 to 2 hours, several doses are needed before the excessive amount of methadone is eliminated from the body. The introduction of the oral narcotic antagonist naltrexone, which has an action duration of 10 hours, may be the treatment of choice after an initial one or two doses of naloxone. Clonidine (Catapres) has been used for opiate withdrawal with some success (Gold et al, 1980). Methadone may be useful for treating IV drug addicts who develop chronic pain for simultaneous analgesia and detoxification, but appropriate dosing is very difficult.

An attempt to improve the efficacy of morphine or heroin and reduce respiratory depression by adding cocaine, alcohol, and chloroform (the Brompton cocktail) gained great popularity when it was used in St. Christopher's Hospice in London. Studies since then by the major protagonist have demonstrated that the cocktail is no more effective than an equivalent dose of oral morphine solution (Twycross and Lack, 1984), and they now use the oral morphine solution and give a phenothiazine, if needed, for nausea or vomiting. The Brompton cocktail is not recommended for cancer pain because alcohol, cocaine, and chloroform may have deleterious effects.

Increased analgesic effect and decreased sedation have been reported with the use of 10 mg of methylphenidate with breakfast and 5 mg with lunch (Bruera et al, 1987). Decreased nausea and vomiting may be achieved with prophylactic use of prochlorperazine, haloperidol, thiethylperazine, lorazepam, or metoclopramide (Levy, 1985).

ADDITIONAL MEASURES FOR PAIN CONTROL

In some circumstances, the pharmacological approaches to pain control already described may not provide adequate relief. Additional therapeutic approaches are then used. Continuous IV or subcutaneous morphine is an effective and safe therapy, but may require rapid escalation of infusion rates and should be preceded by a period of repetitive IV boluses with the same drug. Patient-controlled analgesia with a variety of devices permits patients to treat their pain by directly activating doses of IV narcotics (Bruera and Schoeller, 1992; Citron et al, 1992). By simply pressing a button on a preprogrammed device, the patient may titer the analgesic dose to immediate needs. This decreases patient anxiety resulting from delays in receiving pain medication and the slow onset of relief when it is finally received. Generally, patients using this technique report a near-optimal state of analgesia with a minimum of sedation and fewer side effects. Potential overdosage can be minimized by preprogramming the device to deliver small bolus doses with a mandatory lockout interval between each dose. Although this therapy is popular for inpatients, it is being supplanted by fentanyl patches and sustained-release morphine for outpatient use because of the greater convenience of the patches and pills and the lesser cost compared with an ambulatory pump and its servicing.

Epidural and intrathecal administration of narcotics can produce localized selective analgesia without motor blockade. This avoids the side effects of systemic therapy. The infusions can be simplified with an implanted reservoir or with an exterior epidural catheter for self-administration. When tolerance develops or the procedure fails, electrical stimulation of the brain with implanted electrodes is sometimes successful.

Various noninvasive procedures may be employed to help control the pain itself or to relieve the emotional distress caused by the pain. These procedures are listed in Table 8-6. They also have the added benefit of helping the patient regain some sense of control in a situation plagued by feelings of helplessness.

Coping mechanisms used to reduce the intensity of pain include heat, cold, distraction, position change, massage, and exercise. Distraction techniques that included watching television, praying, and reading provided some relief for 89% of the patients who used the techniques and reported their results (McCaffery, 1979). Position change was thought to be beneficial by 86% of those who used the method. Less frequently used methods

TABLE 8-6
Noninvasive Pain-Relief Measures

Type	Technique	Examples
Distraction	Focus attention on stimuli other than pain sensation	Slow rhythmic breathing; visual concentration point; auditory stimulation (McCaffery, 1979)
Cutaneous stimulation	Skin stimulation activates large-diameter fibers, provoking an inhibition of pain messages carried by small fibers	Massage, heat/cold, menthol preparations, TENS units (McCaffery, 1979)
Relaxation	Mental and physical freedom from tension or stress	Heartbeat breathing, slow rhythmic breathing, relaxation with a trainer (McCaffery, 1979)
Imagery	Development of images involving all senses	Healing exercises, breathing out pain (Donovan, 1980)
Hypnosis	Directly blocks awareness of pain through suggestion of analgesia	Self-hypnosis, hypnosis with a therapist (Barber 1978)

TENS, Transcutaneous electrical nerve stimulation.

included exercise, application of cold, massage, nonnarcotic medications, and specific foods.

Invasive neurosurgical analgesic interventions may be employed for refractory pain, uncontrolled pain, or pain not controlled well enough with pharmacological interventions. These procedures include the following:

1. *Rhizotomy:* Spinal nerve roots severed; used in pain originating from the neck, shoulder, thorax, or abdominal wall.
2. *Cordotomy:* Divides spinal cord tracts; treats pain in the torso and extremities.
3. *Sympathectomy:* Segment of sympathetic nerve or ganglia excised; treats causalgia (constant burning sensation).
4. *Nerve blocks:* Can be neurolytic or nonneurolytic. Neurolytic blocks are done by injecting neurodestructive agents (phenol and absolute alcohol) on or near the target nerves. Nonneurolytic blocks are done with local anesthetic injection (lidocaine, procaine, and occasionally a corticosteroid) into nerve trunks. Neurolytic blocks have been particularly useful in cancer pain syndromes that are visceral or involve the torso (Marshall, 1996). Celiac plexus block is frequently used for pain associated with pancreatic cancer and other upper abdominal malignant diseases. Efficacy is 80% to 90% and lasts for 2 to more than 6 months. Hypogastric plexus block for pelvic malignant disease is less frequently used for pelvic malignant lesions.

A special pain situation that is particularly troublesome is postherpetic neuralgia. Herpes zoster is seen with increased frequency in patients with cancer and is unusually common in patients with lymphoma and other immunosuppression syndromes. There is some evidence that moderate-dose corticosteroids and the antiviral agent acyclovir (Zovirax) shorten the course of the disease and may reduce the incidence or intensity of post-herpetic neuralgia. For those who do develop pain, treatment with topical capsaicin (Zostrix) is sometimes effective. Most patients get relief from the usual analgesics, especially the long-acting ones, but reports of good adjunct responses with antidepressants such as amitriptyline, doxepin, or others (Walsh, 1983) and with carbamazepine (Tegretol) (Gerson, Jones, and Luscombe, 1977) are noted. The patient will be most grateful for any pain relief from this chronic, enervating pain that may afflict the "cured" patient as unmercifully as the terminal patient.

PEARLS TO REMEMBER

1. Believe the patient's complaint of pain.
2. Take a careful history of the pain complaint.
3. Perform a careful medical, psychological, and neurological examination.
4. Order and *personally* review the appropriate diagnostic studies.
5. Consider the full range of available therapeutic options and the opiate equivalency information provided.
6. Reassess the patient's response to therapy.
7. Discuss advance directives with the patient and family.
8. Do not be easily dissuaded from providing adequate doses of opiates for pain relief.

Since cancer patients rarely become addicted, one should not worry about addiction in the terminally ill patient.

REFERENCES

Ad Hoc Committee on Cancer Pain of the American Society of Clinical Oncology: Cancer pain assessment and treatment curriculum guidelines, *J Clin Oncol* 10:1976-1982, 1992.

Agency for Health Care Policy and Research: *Management of cancer pain: clinical practice guidelines,* Rockville, Md, 1994, US Dept of Health and Human Services.

American Pain Society: Principles of analgesic use in the treatment of acute pain and cancer pain, ed 3, Skokie, Ill, 1992, the society.

Barber J: Hypnosis as a psychological technique in the management of cancer pain, *Cancer Nurs* 1:361-363, 1978.

Bruera E, Schoeller T: Patient-controlled analgesia in cancer pain. In DeVita VT Jr, Hellman S, Rosenberg SA, eds: *Principles and practice of oncology. PPO updates* 6:1-7, 1992.

Bruera E et al: Methylphenidate associated with narcotics for the treatment of cancer pain, *Cancer Treat Rep* 71:67-70, 1987.

Cassel EJ: The nature of suffering and the goals of medicine, *N Engl J Med* 306:639-645, 1982.

Catalano RB: Pharmacology of analgesic agents used to treat cancer pain, *Semin Oncol Nurs* 1:126-140, 1985.

Citron ML et al: Patient-controlled analgesia for cancer pain: long term study of inpatient and outpatient use, *Cancer Invest* 10:335-341, 1992.

Donovan JI: Relaxation with guided imagery: a useful technique, *Cancer Nurs* 3:27-32, 1980.

Fischer DS: Hormonal and chemical therapy. In Twycross RG, ed: Pain relief in cancer, *Clin Oncol* 3:55-74, 1984.

Foley KM: Management of cancer pain, *Cancer* 63(suppl):2257-2386, 1989.

Gerson GR, Jones RB, Luscombe DK: Studies on the concomitant use of carbamazepine and clomipramine for the relief of postherpetic neuralgia, *Postgrad Med J* 53(suppl 4):104-109, 1977.

Gold MS et al: Opiate withdrawal using clonidine: a safe, effective and rapid nonopiate treatment, *JAMA* 243:343-346, 1980.

Jadad AR, Browman GP: The WHO analgesic ladder for cancer pain management, *JAMA* 274:1870-1873, 1995.

Khojasteh A et al: Controlled-release oral morphine sulfate in the treatment of cancer pain with pharmacokinetic correlation, *J Clin Oncol* 5:956-961, 1987.

Levy M: Pain management in advanced cancer, *Semin Oncol* 12:394-410, 1985.

Marshall KA: Managing cancer pain: basic principles and invasive treatments. *Mayo Clin Proc* 71:472-477, 1996.

McCaffery M: *Nursing management of the patient with pain*, Philadelphia, 1979, JB Lippincott.

Omoigui S: *The pain drugs handbook,* St. Louis, 1995, Mosby.

Patt RB: *Cancer pain,* Philadelphia, 1993, JB Lippincott.

Portenoy RK: Cancer pain management, *Semin Oncol* 20(2 suppl 1):19-36, 1993.

Porter J, Jick H: Addiction rare in patients treated with narcotics, *N Engl J Med* 302:123, 1980.

Sinatra RS et al: *Acute pain: mechanisms and management,* St. Louis, 1992, Mosby.

Twycross RG, Lack SA: *Symptom control in far advanced cancer: pain relief,* London, 1984, Pitman.

Twycross RG, Lack SA: *Therapeutics in terminal cancer,* Edinburgh, 1990, Churchill Livingstone.

Von Roenn JH et al: Physician attitudes and practice in cancer pain management: a survey from the Eastern Cooperative Oncology Group, *Ann Intern Med* 119:121-126, 1993.

Walsh TD: Antidepressants in chronic pain, *Clin Neuropharmacol* 6:271-295, 1983.

Warfield C: Guidelines for routine use of controlled-release oral morphine sulfate tablets, *Semin Oncol* 20(2 suppl 1):36-47, 1993.

World Health Organization: *Cancer pain relief,* Geneva, 1986, World Health Organization.

9

High-Dose Chemotherapy With Stem Cell Support

The concept of "dose intensity" is based on the theory that increasing the intensity of chemotherapy with active drugs by giving higher doses per unit of time or the same cumulative dose in a shorter period will lead to increased tumor-cell kill. This in turn should lead to improved responses and survival rates and increased survival durations (Hryniuk and Bush, 1984). There are data to suggest that this theory is probably valid with conventional dose chemotherapy (Hryniuk, 1988), although some reports raise doubts about that validity and question whether success rates are derived from total dose or dose intensity (Wood et al, 1994).

For those who believed that increased dose intensity was a panacea and that bone marrow toxicity was the dose-limiting factor, it was natural to look for ways to overcome the dose-limiting toxicity. Replacement of the damaged bone marrow was the obvious answer, either with human leukocyte antigen (HLA)–compatible donor marrow (allogeneic) or the patient's own (autologous) preserved pretreatment marrow. Autologous bone marrow transplant (ABMT) has been a widely practiced technique for a decade, but proof of its efficacy with randomized studies has just begun with only a few published randomized reports (Bezwoda, Seymour, and Dansey, 1995; Philip et al, 1995). Bone marrow damage leads to anemia, leukopenia with a high risk of infection, and thrombocytopenia with a risk of bleeding. However, before discussing rescue of the bone marrow, one must develop high-dose chemotherapy (HDCT) programs with or without radiation therapy (RT) that can eliminate virtually all neoplastic cells that can regrow or potentially metastasize. A reconstituted marrow is a Pyrrhic (i.e., useless) victory if the cancer recurs and kills the patient, and that still happens frequently after HDCT with or without RT, even with stem-cell rescue. We obviously need better regimens.

Destruction of a malignant tumor is best done with drugs that exhibit a dose-response effect, that are cell-cycle independent, and that have hematological toxicity as their major side effect. The alkylating agents meet these

TABLE 9-1
Cytotoxic Drugs Used in Hematopoietic Transplantation

Drug	Typical standard dose in combination	Typical transplant dose in combination
ALKYLATING AGENTS		
Cyclophosphamide	1000 mg/m^2	7500 mg/m^2
Ifosfamide	4000 mg/m^2	18,000 mg/m^2
Thiotepa	15 mg/m^2	800 mg/m^2
Mechlorethamine	6 mg/m^2	60 mg/m^2
Melphalan	16 mg/m^2	60 mg/m^2
Chlorambucil	0.4 mg/kg	6 mg/kg
Busulfan	4 mg/day	16 mg/kg
Carmustine	150 mg/m^2	450 mg/m^2
Cisplatin	60 mg/m^2	165 mg/m^2
Carboplatin	400 mg/m^2	1200 mg/m^2
PLANT ALKALOIDS		
Etoposide	300 mg/m^2	2400 mg/m^2
Teniposide	165 mg/m^2	600 mg/m^2
Paclitaxel	175 mg/m^2	775 mg/m^2
PLANT ANTIBIOTICS		
Mitoxantrone	12 mg/m^2	75 mg/m^2
Mitomycin	10 mg/m^2	90 mg/m^2

requirements best, and they are the drugs most often used for this purpose (Table 9-1). However, the plant alkaloids etoposide, teniposide, and paclitaxel are being tried in combination with alkylating agents and show promise in several regimens. The plant antibiotics mitoxantrone and mitomycin, and the antimetabolites cytarabine and thioguanine have also been combined in a few successful combinations of HDCT. Dose escalation continues until nonhematological toxicity becomes dose limiting.

With HDCT and bone marrow transplantation (BMT) or peripheral blood stem cell transplantation (PBSCT), the main dose-limiting nonhematological toxicities (Table 9-2) become the ultimate dose-limiting toxicity (DLT). In selecting preparative HDCT regimens, one must be mindful of the patient's associated disease, the patient's prior chemotherapy and radiation therapy (if any), and potential subsequent therapy that may be planned (e.g., avoid carmustine, busulphan, and cyclophosphamide if posttransplant radiation therapy to the lung area is likely). Single-agent HDCT (e.g., melphalan) has been used, but runs the risk of failing to eradicate all tumors cells and selecting a resistant population.

The list of HDCT preparative regimens in this chapter represents a small selection from a large group of published trials (Antman et al, 1992; Cohen and Krigel, 1995; and others in the general references listed at the end of this chapter). The list is not meant to suggest that these are necessarily the best, but they do seem to be those that are more frequently used

TABLE 9-2
Dose-Limiting Nonhematological Toxicity

Toxicity	Drugs
Pulmonary fibrosis and pneumonitis	Carmustine, busulfan, cyclophosphamide
Cystitis	Cyclophosphamide, ifosfamide
Myocarditis	Cyclophosphamide
Nephrotoxicity	Cisplatin, ifosfamide, carmustine, carboplatin, cyclophosphamide
Ototoxicity	Cisplatin, carboplatin
Hepatotoxicity and venoocclusive disease	Carboplatin, mitomycin, carmustine, busulfan
Mucositis	Thiotepa, melphalan, etoposide, mitoxantrone, busulfan
Neurological	Mechlorethamine, chlorambucil, busulfan, carmustine
Peripheral neuropathy	Carboplatin, paclitaxel, cisplatin

at this time. Each is used for a particular neoplasm but under some circumstances is equally suitable for other cancers. The field of HDCT regimen research is still young and growing, and indications by tumor type and stage and special characteristics are being evaluated by outcome, which will take several years to sort out. The best regimen has not yet been identified; perhaps it has not even been developed. New and better drugs may be in the pipeline.

It is regrettable that some leaders in the field have encouraged patients through media publicity and other avenues to demand HDCT with ABMT long before the indications for its use were clear. Others (Henderson, Hayes, and Gelman, 1988) suggested that the use of ABMT should be confined to well-designed, randomized, controlled trials until its place in the therapeutic armamentarium was more clearly defined. Alas, those calling for trials were ignored, and as a result only a few prospective randomized trials have been done. Perhaps too much money has been spent on litigation brought by patients who tried to force an insurer to pay for an off-trial BMT of unproved value, rather than using the resources in good scientific clinical research to clarify the role of ABMT in cancer management (Davidson, 1992). One would hope that this will be rectified in the future. Three high-priority phase III clinical trials testing HDCT with ABMT have had such low enrollment that the accrual deadline had to be extended from mid-1995 to mid-1997. Survival data will not be available from those trials until the year 2000 (Mathews, 1995). With HDCT with ABMT or PBSCT available off study, many oncologists and patients prefer to go that route on the assumption that the results with ABMT are always better. In addition, patients do not have to sign an informed consent because they and the insurance companies are told that this is now standard therapy. Whether it is, and for which neoplasms it is used and under what particular circumstances, was a point of some controversy at the most recent American

Society of Clinical Oncology (ASCO) meeting. The answers, however, will only be determined by future studies.

Not all randomized trials of HDCT with ABMT have shown a superiority over more conventional dose therapy without stem cell support. In patients in first complete remission with intermediate- and high-grade non-Hodgkin's lymphoma, results with HDCT and ABMT were not superior to sequential chemotherapy (Haioun et al, 1994). In childhood acute myelogenous leukemia (AML), encouraging results with ABMT in first remission were reported from nonrandomized trials, and HDCT with ABMT seemed to be the treatment of choice. However, a multicenter randomized trial of ABMT in children with AML in first remission failed to show a significant advantage over intensive consolidation chemotherapy (Ravindranath et al, 1996). High-dose allogeneic therapy does seem to give a higher response rate, probably because of a graft versus leukemia (GVL) immunological reaction. The early use of HDCT with or without RT with ABMT does not seem to improve the outcome in patients with aggressive non-Hodgkin's lymphoma who respond slowly to CHOP chemotherapy (Verdonck et al, 1995). The interpretation of each of these studies has been questioned. It is clear that many additional careful prospective randomized trials need to be done to clarify the role of and indications for HDCT with ABMT or PBSCT in a variety of cancers. We would encourage investigators and cooperative groups to set up such prospective randomized trials. Hopefully, the NCI, insurance companies, and HMOs will support the trials financially, physicians will refer patients to them, and patients will agree to participate in them. Only when the data that such trials generate are analyzed will we have a better appreciation of the role of HDCT in cancer care.

To support patients with aplastic anemia, congenital marrow aplasia, or bone marrow suppression, allogeneic BMT was developed using marrow donated from a sibling, parent, or an unrelated donor with a close match (i.e., at least 5 or 6 of the major histocompatibility complex [MHC] loci). Later, allogeneic BMT was extended to support patients with systemic cancer after the anticipated bone marrow aplasia following HDCT. However, the acute death rate caused by the HDCT with BMT was unacceptably high at around 20% to 50% with allogeneic transplants, and only 30% of patients who were advised to have a BMT could find a compatible donor. Greater experience and the development and availability of adequate quantities of recombinant DNA–generated cytokines (G-CSF and GM-CSF) have made autologous BMT feasible, and better infection control has reduced the allogeneic BMT death rate to 10% to 25% and the ABMT rate to less than 5% in major transplantation centers.

Technological progress in cell-separation equipment and the use of cytokines and postchemotherapy rebound enhancement of neutrophil production have made it possible to collect large numbers of peripheral blood stem cells. These cells are as effective as BMT in repopulating the marrow and relieve the neutropenia and thrombocytopenia in a shorter period of time. Accordingly, many centers are using PBSCT preferentially.

To avoid reinfusing viable neoplastic cells, a variety of "purging" techniques have been developed, such as treating the ABMT/PBSCT with monoclonal antibodies to the tumor cell antigens and using chemicals such as 4-hydroperoxy-cyclophosphamide.

New technology with adherence immunoaffinity columns is leading to still better therapy. CD34+ cells can be separated, concentrated, and then reinfused. The CD34+ cell concentrates are freer of contaminating tumor cells and provide a preparation "purged" of neoplastic cells. Many of the cells in this population have the properties of pluripotential (hematopoietic) stem cells (PPSC) and can provide engraftment after what would otherwise be lethal chemoradiotherapy. These concentrates can reduce the toxicity of PBSCT procedures by reducing the volume of cells infused.

In the treatment of acute leukemia with allogeneic BMTs or PBSCTs, the reduction of GVL may be a negative, with fewer patients becoming long-term survivors as happened with T-cell depletion and syngeneic (twin) transplants. With ABMT, there is no GVL or graft-versus-host disease (GVHD), but engraftment takes longer and the patient is at increased risk of infection or hemorrhage for a longer period. PBSCT reduces that period of vulnerability somewhat but when used for ABMT does not change the GVL or GVHD phenomena.

HDCT with ABMT or PBSCT has been used in the treatment of a variety of malignancies (Box 9-1). Critical to its success is the appropriate selection of an HDCT program. In the previous edition of this book, we considered HDCT to be experimental and did not list any HDCT regimens for fear that they would be used improperly by those without special training and in institutions lacking an adequate transplantation program with a dedicated unit and a trained cadre of nurses, physicians, and support personnel.

Today, one would hope that all HDCT with BMTs and PBSCTs is administered in conformity with the criteria of ASCO and the American Society of Hematology (ASH) (1990). Among other criteria, the two organizations suggest that "a sufficient number of patients must be treated each year to allow the development of a designated transplant unit with an experienced, full-time nursing team. This would require, in general, at least 10 to 20 transplants per year. Sufficient transplants must be performed to never have the unit empty. . . . If allogeneic bone marrow transplantation is performed, the transplant unit must demonstrate access to a certified histocompatibility laboratory for the necessary tissue typing." The nursing team "is the most important single aspect of a successful bone marrow transplantation unit. There need to be nurses committed full time to this program. There should be a high ratio of nurses to patients with the nurse-to-patient ratio not more than 1:2 on average. The number of patients transplanted must be sufficient to develop and maintain a full-time nursing team. . . . Bone marrow transplantation is a rapidly evolving therapeutic modality. Physicians performing this procedure should report their data to available registries (e.g., International Bone Marrow Transplant Registry) and, when appropriate, publish important observations in the medical literature." One might add that there is now an Autologous Blood and Marrow Transplantation Registry of North America to which data may be sent.

BOX 9-1
Neoplasms Treated With High-Dose Chemotherapy
Under Special and Appropriate Circumstances

LEUKEMIAS
Acute myeloblastic leukemia
Acute lymphoblastic leukemia
Chronic myelogenous leukemia
Myelodysplastic syndromes
Acute myelofibrosis

LYMPHOPROLIFERATIVE DISORDERS
Hodgkin's lymphoma
Non-Hodgkin's lymphoma
Chronic lymphocytic leukemia
Multiple myeloma

SOLID TUMORS
Neuroblastoma
Breast carcinoma
Germ cell tumors
Testicular carcinoma

BEING EVALUATED
Lung cancers
Melanoma
Astrocytomas
Osteosarcoma
Ewing's sarcoma
Ovarian carcinoma

Now that HDCT with ABMT or PBSCT is being used (and hopefully evaluated) in large numbers of cases, we have compiled a few of the more common HDCT preparative regimens and we list them separately from those regimens that require no stem cell support. Whole-body radiation therapy (WBRT) is being used less often as a preparative regimen, and accordingly, we have omitted regimens using both WBRT and HDCT. An increasing number of centers are using a double transplantation program such as HDCT with ABMT or PBSCT followed (after marrow cell recovery) by a second HDCT with the same or different HDCT regimen and rescue with PBSCT (Dunphy et al, 1990; Ayash et al, 1994). In selecting an HDCT regimen, it is generally important to demonstrate that the tumor is still inherently drug sensitive to standard (induction) drug therapy because those tumors that are not inherently drug sensitive have a low rate of response and/or short duration of response to HDCT with

ABMT or PBSCT. There should also be an expectation that the tumors selected for HDCT with ABMT or PBSCT are potentially curable (e.g., germ cell tumors, leukemias, lymphomas, and multiple myeloma) or at least highly responsive (e.g., breast and testicle carcinomas). Needless to say, these brief summaries of complex regimens should not be used without reviewing the original reports, and they should be administered only by individuals adequately trained and in institutions that meet the recommended criteria of ASCO and ASH.

REFERENCES

American Society of Clinical Oncology and American Society of Hematology: Recommended criteria for the performance of bone marrow transplantation, *J Clin Oncol* 8:563:564, 1990 and *Blood* 75:1209, 1990.

Antman K et al: Dose-intensive therapy in breast cancer, *Bone Marrow Transplant* 10(Suppl 1):67-73, 1992.

Ayash LJ et al: Double dose intensive chemotherapy with autologous marrow and peripheral-blood progenitor-cell support for metastatic breast cancer: a feasibility study, *J Clin Oncol* 12:37-44, 1994.

Bezwoda WR, Seymour L, Dansey RD: High-dose chemotherapy with hematopoietic rescue as primary treatment for metastatic breast cancer: a randomized trial, *J Clin Oncol* 13:2483-2489, 1995.

Cohen SC, Krigel RL: High-dose therapy with stem-cell infusion in lymphoma, *Semin Oncol* 22:218-229, 1995.

Davidson N: Out of the courtroom and into the clinic, *J Clin Oncol* 10:517-519, 1992 (editorial).

Dunphy FR et al: Treatment of estrogen receptor negative or hormonally refractory breast cancer with double high-dose chemotherapy intensification and bone marrow support, *J Clin Oncol* 8:1207-1216, 1990.

Haioun C et al: Comparison of autologous bone marrow transplantation with sequential chemotherapy for intermediate-grade and high-grade non-Hodgkin's lymphoma in first complete remission: a study of 464 patients, *J Clin Oncol* 12:2543-2551, 1994.

Henderson IC, Hayes DF, Gelman R: Dose-response in the treatment of breast cancer: a critical review, *J Clin Oncol* 6:1501-1515, 1988.

Hryniuk WM: More is better, *J Clin Oncol* 6:1365-1367,1988 (editorial).

Hryniuk W, Bush H: The importance of dose-intensity in chemotherapy of breast cancer, *J Clin Oncol* 2:1281-1288,1984.

Mathews J: NCI survey explores the M.D.'s perspective on ABMT trials, *J Natl Cancer Inst* 87:1510-1511, 1995.

Philip T et al: Autologous bone marrow transplantation as compared with salvage chemotherapy in relapses of chemotherapy-sensitive non-Hodgkin's lymphoma, *N Engl J Med* 333:1540-1545, 1995.

Ravindranath Y et al: Autologous bone marrow transplantation versus intensive consolidation chemotherapy for acute myeloid leukemia in childhood, *N Engl J Med* 334:1428-1434, 1996.

Verdonck LF et al: Comparison of CHOP chemotherapy with autologous bone marrow transplantation for slowly responding patients with aggressive non-Hodgkin's lymphoma, *N Engl J Med* 332:1045-1051, 1995.

Wood W et al: Dose and dose intensity of adjuvant chemotherapy for stage II, node-positive breast cancer, *N Eng J Med* 330:1253-1259, 1994.

High-Dose Chemotherapy Preparative Regimens for Use With Bone Marrow or Peripheral Blood Stem Cell Transplantation

LEUKEMIAS

BUCY–BUSULFAN-CYCLOPHOSPHAMIDE

Busulfan. 4 mg/kg/day in divided doses orally on days -7, -6, -5, and -4.

Cyclophosphamide. 60 mg/kg/ intravenously on days -3, and -2.

NOTE: All patients with leukemia are given methotrexate intrathecally (10 mg/m² but not more than 12 mg total). Allogeneic bone marrow is infused on day 0. Use of mesna should be considered.

Selected Readings

O'Donnell MR et al: Busulfan/cyclophosphamide as conditioning regimen for allogeneic bone marrow transplantation for myelodysplasia, *J Clin Oncol* 13:2973-2979, 1995.

Tutschka PJ, Copelan EA, Klein JP: Bone marrow transplantation for leukemia following a new busulfan and cyclophosphamide regimen, *Blood* 70:1382-1388, 1987.

BAVC–CARMUSTINE-AMSACRINE-ETOPOSIDE-CYTARABINE

Carmustine. 800 mg/m² intravenously on day -6.

Amsacrine. 150 mg/m² intravenously on days -5, -4, and -3.

Etoposide. 150 mg/m² intravenously on days -5, -4, and -3.

Cytarabine. 300 mg/m² continuous IV infusion on days -5, -4, and -3.

NOTE: Bone marrow infusion is given on day 0.

Selected Reading

Meloni G et al: BAVC regimen and autologous bone marrow transplantation in patients with acute myelogenous leukemia in second remission, *Blood* 75:2282-2285, 1990.

BUVP–BUSULFAN-ETOPOSIDE

Busulfan. 1 mg/kg every 6 hours orally on days -7, -6, -5, and -4.

Etoposide. 60 mg/kg intravenously over 6 to 10 hours on day -3.

NOTE: Autologous bone marrow was treated in vitro with 100 µg/mL 4-hydroperoxy-cyclophosphamide and infused on day 0.

Selected Readings

Chao NJ et al: Busulfan/etoposide: initial experience with a new preparatory regimen for autologous bone marrow transplantation in patients with acute nonlymphocytic leukemia, *Blood* 81:319-323, 1993.

Linker CA et al: Autologous bone marrow transplantation for acute myeloid leukemia using busulfan plus etoposide as a preparative regimen, *Blood* 81:311-318, 1993.

LYMPHOMAS

BEAM–CARMUSTINE-ETOPOSIDE-CYTARABINE-MELPHALAN

Carmustine. 300 mg/m^2 intravenously on day -6.

Etoposide. 200 mg/m^2 intravenously on days -5, -4, -3, and -2.

Cytarabine. 400 mg/m^2 intravenously on days -5, -4, -3, and -2.

Melphalan. 140 mg/m^2 intravenously on day -1.

NOTE: Bone marrow infusion is given on day 0. Carmustine has been given in a dose of 600 mg/m^2 but caused unacceptable toxicity. It has been used by some in a dose of 450 mg/m^2 as a compromise dose.

Selected Readings

Gribben JG et al: Successful treatment of refractory Hodgkin's disease by high-dose combination chemotherapy and autologous bone marrow transplantation, *Blood* 73:340-344, 1989.

Mills W et al: BEAM chemotherapy and autologous bone marrow transplantation for patients with relapsed or refractory non-Hodgkin's lymphoma, *J Clin Oncol* 13:588-595, 1995.

BEAC–CARMUSTINE-ETOPOSIDE-CYTARABINE-CYCLOPHOSPHAMIDE

Carmustine. 300 mg/m^2 intravenously on day -6.

Etoposide. 200 mg/m^2 intravenously on days -5, -4, -3, and -2.

Cytarabine. 100 mg/m^2 intravenously twice daily on days -5, -4, -3, and -2.

Cyclophosphamide. 35 mg/kg intravenously on days -5, -4, -3, and -2.

NOTE: Mesna may be given 50 mg/kg in divided doses on days -5, -4, -3, and -2. Bone marrow is given on day 0, after 2 days of no chemotherapy. In the report in Blood, *1991), there is a typographical error in Table 2 on p. 1590, indicating that etoposide is given for 6 days. It was given for only 4 days and this is clearly indicated in the final report (Philip et al, 1995). One should be very careful not to administer this high dose of cyclophosphamide if the patient has had a significant previous treatment with an anthracycline antibiotic such as doxorubicin or if the patient has had chest radiation that included the heart. If so, consider melphalan instead and use the BEAM regimen above.*

Selected Readings

Philip T et al: Parma international protocol: pilot study of DHAP followed by involved field irradiation and BEAC with autologous bone marrow transplantation, *Blood* 77:1587-1592, 1991.

Philip T et al: Autologous bone marrow transplantation as compared with salvage chemotherapy in relapses of chemotherapy sensitive non-Hodgkin's lymphoma, *N Engl J Med* 333:1540-1545, 1995.

BACT—CARMUSTINE-CYTARABINE-CYCLOPHOSPHAMIDE-THIOGUANINE

Carmustine. 200 mg/m^2 intravenously on day -6.

Cytarabine. 200 mg/m^2 intravenously on days -5,-4, -3, and -2.

Cyclophosphamide. 50 mg/kg intravenously on days -5, -4, -3, and -2.

Thioguanine. 200 mg/m^2 orally on days -5, -4, -3, and -2.

NOTE: Bone marrow infusion is given on day 0. Use of mesna should be considered for uroprotection.

Selected Reading
Philip T et al: Massive chemotherapy with autologous bone marrow transplantation in 50 cases of bad prognosis non-Hodgkin's lymphoma, *Br J Haematol* 60:599-609, 1985.

CBV—CYCLOPHOSPHAMIDE-CARMUSTINE-ETOPOSIDE

Cyclophosphamide. 1800 mg/m^2 intravenously on days -5, -4, -3, and -2.

Carmustine. 100 mg/m^2 intravenously on days -5, -4, -3, and -2.

Etoposide. 400 mg/m^2 every 12 hours on days -8, -7, and -6.

NOTE: Bone marrow is infused day 0. Reece et al (1991) give 600 mg/m^2 of carmustine but note increased toxicity and a higher early death rate. Jagannath et al (1989) give total doses of cyclophosphamide 6000 mg/m^2 (1500/day for 4 days), carmustine 300 mg/m^2, and etoposide 900 mg/m^2 (300/day for 3 days). Use of mesna should be considered for uroprotection.

Selected Readings
Demirer T et al: High-dose cyclophosphamide, carmustine, and etoposide followed by allogeneic bone marrow transplantation in patients with lymphoid malignancies who had received prior dose-limiting radiation therapy, *J Clin Oncol* 13:596-602, 1995.

Jagannath S et al: Prognostic factors for response and survival after high-dose cyclophosphamide, carmustine, and etoposide with autologous bone marrow transplantation for relapsed Hodgkin's disease, *J Clin Oncol* 7:179-185, 1989.

Reece DE et al: Intensive chemotherapy with cyclophosphamide, carmustine and etoposide followed by autologous bone marrow transplantation for relapsed Hodgkin's disease, *J Clin Oncol* 9:1871-1879, 1991.

ICE—IFOSFAMIDE-CARBOPLATIN-ETOPOSIDE

Ifosfamide. 4000 mg/m^2 intravenously on days -6, -5, -4, and -3.

Carboplatin. 600 mg/m^2 intravenously on days -6, -5, and -4.

Etoposide. 500 mg/m^2 intravenously on days -6, -5, and -4.

NOTE: Ifosfamide infusion is begun after morning etoposide. Mesna uroprotection is essential. Bone marrow is infused on day 0.

Selected Reading

Wilson WH et al: Phase I and II study of high-dose ifosfamide, carboplatin, and etoposide with autologous bone marrow rescue in lymphomas and solid tumors, *J Clin Oncol* 10:1712-1722, 1992.

CBVP–CYCLOPHOSPHAMIDE-CARMUSTINE-ETOPOSIDE-CISPLATIN

Cyclophosphamide.   1800 mg/m^2 intravenously on days -6, -5, -4, and -3.

Carmustine.   500 mg/m^2 intravenously on day -2.

Etoposide.   2400 mg/m^2 continuous IV infusion for 34 hours beginning on day -7.

Cisplatin.   50 mg/m^2 intravenously on days -7, -6, and -5.

NOTE: Doses are calculated on the basis of the lower value of ideal or actual body weight. Bone marrow is infused on day 0. Adequate hydration is essential before, during, and after therapy. Use of mesna should be considered for uroprotection.

Selected Reading

Reece DE et al: Intensive therapy with cyclophosphamide, carmustine, etoposide ± cisplatin, and autologous bone marrow transplantation for Hodgkin's disease in first relapse after combination chemotherapy, *Blood* 83:1193-1199, 1994.

MULTIPLE MYELOMA

TBC–THIOTEPA-BUSULFAN-CYCLOPHOSPHAMIDE

Thiotepa.   250 mg/m^2 intravenously on days -9, -8, and -7.

Busulfan.   1 mg/kg orally every 6 hours for 10 doses on days -6, -5, and -4.

Cyclophosphamide.   60 mg/kg intravenously on days -3 and -2.

NOTE: Mesna 250 mg/m^2 is given 30 minutes before and every 4 hours for six doses after each cyclophosphamide infusion. Bone marrow infusion is given on day 0 preceded by methylprednisolone 100 mg IV and diphenhydramine 50 mg IV. Consider use of mesna for uroprotection.

Selected Reading

Dimopoulos MA et al: Thiotepa, busulfan, and cyclophosphamide: a new preparative regimen for autologous marrow or blood stem cell transplantation in high-risk multiple myeloma, *Blood* 82:2324-2328, 1993.

DOUBLE-DOSE MELPHALAN AND SECOND TRANSPLANT

Melphalan.   100 mg/m^2 intravenously on days -3 and -2.

NOTE: Both bone marrow and peripheral blood stem cells are infused on day 0. On day +1, start daily subcutaneous injections of GM-CSF 250 µg/m^2 until granulocyte counts are greater than 2000/µL on 3 successive days. Three to 6 months later, a second autotransplant is given, usually using the same melphalan preparative regimen. However, for the second regimen, some patients were given total doses of busulfan 14 mg/kg and cyclophosphamide 120 mg/kg.

Selected Reading

Vesole DH et al: High-dose therapy for refractory multiple myeloma: improved prognosis with better supportive care and double transplants, *Blood* 84:950-956, 1994.

BREAST CANCERS

CTCB (OR TCC)–CYCLOPHOSPHAMIDE-THIOTEPA-CARBOPLATIN

Cyclophosphamide. 6000 mg/m^2 continuous IV infusion over 96 hours.

Thiotepa. 500 mg/m^2 continuous IV infusion over 96 hours.

Carboplatin. 800 mg/m^2 continuous IV infusion over 96 hours.

NOTE: Drugs are given on days -7, -6, -5, and -4 so that cyclophosphamide 1500 mg/m2, thiotepa 125 mg/m2, and carboplatin 200 mg/m^2 are the daily doses. Bone marrow is infused on day 0. Consider use of mesna for uroprotection.

Selected Reading

Antman K et al: A phase II study of high-dose cyclophosphamide, thiotepa, and carboplatin with autologous marrow support in women with measurable advanced breast cancer responding to standard-dose therapy, *J Clin Oncol* 10:102-110, 1992.

CCB (OR BCC)–CYCLOPHOSPHAMIDE-CISPLATIN-CARMUSTINE

Cyclophosphamide. 1875 mg/m^2 intravenously on days -6, -5, and -4.

Cisplatin. 55 mg/m^2 intravenously on days -6, -5, and -4.

Carmustine. 600 mg/m^2 intravenously on day -3.

NOTE: Cisplatin is given by continuous 72-hour IV infusion. Bone marrow infusion is given on day +1. The entire high-dose preparative regimen is predicated on a response to four courses of an induction regimen with the standard FAC (fluorouracil, doxorubicin, and cyclophosphamide) regimen. In another report, this group used AFM (doxorubicin, fluorouracil, and methotrexate with leucovorin rescue) as an induction regimen. Consider use of mesna for uroprotection.

Selected Reading

Peters WP et al: High-dose chemotherapy and autologous bone marrow support as consolidation after standard-dose adjuvant therapy for high-risk primary breast cancer, *J Clin Oncol* 11:1132-1143, 1993.

CT (TC)–CYCLOPHOSPHAMIDE-THIOTEPA

Cyclophosphamide. 2500 mg/m^2 intravenously on days -6, -4, and -2.

Thiotepa. 225 mg/m^2 intravenously on days -6, -4, and -2.

NOTE: Bone marrow is infused on day 0. Consider use of mesna for uroprotection.

Selected Reading

Williams SF et al: High-dose consolidation therapy with autologous stem cell rescue in stage IV breast cancer, *J Clin Oncol* 7:1824-1830, 1989.

Williams SF et al: High-dose consolidation therapy with authologous stem cell rescue in stage IV breast cancer: follow-up report, *J Clin Oncol* 10:1743-1747, 1992.

GERM CELL TUMORS

CBVP–CARBOPLATIN-ETOPOSIDE

Carboplatin. 500 mg/m^2 intravenously on days -7, -5, and -3.

Etoposide. 400 mg/m^2 intravenously on days -7, -5, and -3.

NOTE: Bone marrow infusion is given on day 0. Motzer et al,1993, gave both drugs on days -8, -6, and -4.

Selected Readings

Motzer RJ et al: Phase II trial of high-dose carboplatin and etoposide with autologous bone marrow transplantation in first-line therapy for patients with poor-risk germ cell tumors, *J Natl Cancer Inst* 85:1828-1835, 1993.

Nichols CR et al: High-dose carboplatin and etoposide with autologous bone marrow transplantation in refractory germ cell cancer: an Eastern Cooperative Oncology Group protocol, *J Clin Oncol* 10:558-563, 1992.

ICE–IFOSFAMIDE-CARBOPLATIN-ETOPOSIDE

Ifosfamide. 1500 mg/m^2 intravenously on days 1 to 5.

Carboplatin. 200 mg/m^2 intravenously on days 1 to 5.

Etoposide. 250 mg/m^2 intravenously on days 1 to 5.

NOTE: Bone marrow infusion is given five days after the completion of the chemotherapy drug administration. Consider use of mesna for uroprotection.

Selected Reading

Lotz JP et al: Phase I-II study of two consecutive courses of high-dose epipodophyllotoxin, ifosfamide and carboplatin with autologous bone marrow transplantation for treatment of adult patients with solid tumors, *J Clin Oncol* 9:1860-1870, 1991.

GENERAL REFERENCES

Armitage JO, Antman KH, eds: *High-dose cancer therapy*, ed 2, Baltimore, 1995, Williams & Wilkins.

Cooper DL: Peripheral blood stem cell transplantation. In DeVita VT Jr, Hellman S, Rosenberg SA, eds: *PPO updates* 8(12):1-12, 1994.

Elfenbein GJ, ed: Bone marrow transplantation in the 1990's: controversies and consensus, *Semin Oncol* 20(5 suppl 6):1-109, 1993.

Forman SJ, ed: Bone marrow transplantation, *Hematol Oncol Clin North Am* 4:507-714, 1990.

Forman SJ, Blume KG, Thomas ED, eds: *Bone marrow transplantation*, Boston, 1994, Blackwell Scientific.

Krigel RL, ed: Peripheral blood stem cell support, *Semin Oncol* 22:201-300, 1995.

Treleaven J, Wiernik P, eds: *Color atlas and text of bone marrow transplantation*, St. Louis, 1995, Mosby-Wolfe.

Williams SF, ed: Autologous bone marrow transplantation, *Hematol Oncol Clin North Am* 7:501-752, 1993.

10

Assessment and Management of Organ System Toxicity

The effects on the stem cells and the kinetics of the cell line in the peripheral blood compartment determine the degree and timing of suppression on each of the three major cell lines (Gastineau and Hoagland, 1992). The resultant clinical manifestations of anemia, granulocytopenia, and thrombocytopenia can be a direct result of treatment with cytotoxic drugs but may also be related to an underlying disease process.

ANEMIA

The etiology of anemia in the cancer patient is multifactorial and includes blood loss, diminished or absent nutritional stores, marrow infiltration by tumor, cumulative marrow suppression associated with prior treatment, anemia of chronic disease, decreased erythropoietin production, and direct effects of cytotoxic drugs (Henry, 1996; Bociek and Armitage, 1996). Altretamine, cisplatin, cytarabine, docetaxel (especially with higher doses), paclitaxel, and topotecan are the most common chemotherapeutic drugs associated with anemia. Many other cytotoxic agents have anemia listed as a toxicity but cited as infrequently observed or an uncommon side effect. A thorough laboratory assessment with a complete blood count, including a reticulocyte count, serum ferritin, vitamin B12, folic acid, and a direct Coombs' test is recommended to identify the cause of the anemia and enable the clinician to chose an appropriate therapy (Henry, 1996). In addition, assessment factors that may identify patients at high risk for clinically significant anemia should be considered. Such factors would include poor performance status, multiple metastatic sites, older age, underlying heart disease, altered nutritional status, and rate of fall of hemoglobin after initial chemotherapy (Henry, 1996). Blood loss as the etiology should be immediately assessed, particularly in the thrombocytopenic patient. In any man or postmenopausal woman with anemia, gastrointestinal (GI) bleeding should be suspected. In the premenopausal woman, there may be increased menstrual bleeding.

Management of anemia is determined by laboratory values, the underlying cause, and the patient's symptom profile. Red blood cell transfusions (see Chapter 11) , recombinant erythropoietin (see Chapter 4), and supportive interventions to manage symptoms such as dyspnea and fatigue represent the therapeutic alternatives for the patient with anemia.

NEUTROPENIA

Neutropenia is defined as an absolute neutrophil count (ANC) that is less than 1500 cells/mm^3. ANC is determined by multiplying the white blood cell count by the percentage of granulocytes (usually neutrophils and bands) in the differential cell count. When this number is less than 1500 cells/mm^3, the patient is at increased risk of developing an infection. Serious infection is inversely related to the degree and duration of the granulocytopenia. Significant risk exists for patients with prolonged granulocyte counts less than 500 cells/mm^3 (Bodey et al, 1966). Under these circumstances, infection with opportunistic, frequently endogenous organisms may occur when normal organisms are introduced into areas where they are not normally found, especially the pharynx, distal esophagus, gums, sinuses, anus, colon, lungs, urinary tract, venipuncture sites, marrow aspiration sites, vascular access sites, and biopsy sites. Careful patient assessment, selected preventive strategies, early detection, and prompt treatment are the key elements to reduce serious complications from treatment-induced neutropenic infection.

Assessment, Prevention, and Early Detection of Infection in the Neutropenic Patient

Assessment, prevention, and early detection are collaborative activities shared by health care professionals, the patient, and the patient's family. With the shift of oncology care from the hospital to the ambulatory setting, patient education has become critical. Not only is it important for the patient to be adequately informed, he should also be an active participant in his care. Patient and family education should include content on the susceptibility of patients and methods of infection transmission. Education should include an explanation of white blood cells, nadir counts, and time of predicted nadir; temperature taking; signs and symptoms of infection (Box 10-1); hygiene practices emphasizing hand washing; identification and assessment of high-risk areas for infection; care of access devices; risk-reduction activities, such as a low-microbial diet and avoidance of exposure to persons with communicable or infectious illnesses; and specific directions for access to their health care system 24 hours a day, 7 days a week (Dean, Hauber, and Rivera, 1996).

BOX 10-1
Signs and Symptoms of Infection

Instruct the patient and family about the following signs and symptoms of infection.
- Temperature more than 38° C (100.4° F)
- Chills
- Inflammation
- Rash
- Increased respiration
- General malaise
- Tenderness
- Swelling
- Headache
- Inability to bend head forward
- Urinary frequency with or without pain
- Cough with or without sputum

More than a decade ago, Pizzo and Schimpff (1983) identified four general principles to prevent or minimize the risk of infection in the patient with cancer: bolstering the host defense mechanisms, preserving the body's natural barriers of defense, reducing environmental organisms, and minimizing the endogenous microflora of the patient as a source of infection. These general principles remain relevant today even though there have been many factors that affect the application of the principles, such as treatment advances, new knowledge, and changes in the prevalence of infectious organisms.

The availability of hematopoietic growth factors represents the most recent advance in bolstering host defenses. Although a number of immunomodulating agents have been evaluated in the management of neutropenia and fever (Pizzo, 1993), the use of granulocyte colony-stimulating factors to reduce the duration and severity of neutropenia in patients with a moderate to high risk of infection has become common practice. The use of these growth factors has been associated with fewer infections, a decreased incidence of febrile neutropenia, a decreased incidence of oral mucositis in selected populations, and a decreased number of days in the hospital (Crawford et al, 1991; Gabrilove et al, 1988).

Preserving the body's natural barriers of defense for the neutropenic patient includes maintaining the integrity of mechanical barriers and supporting the integrity of the intestinal mucosa. Interventions to promote mechanical barrier integrity include avoidance of injections whenever possible; strategies to prevent skin breakdown; avoidance of bladder catheterization unless absolutely necessary (if necessary, intermittent catheterization is preferred over an indwelling catheter); perineal and rectal care guidelines (stress the importance of good personal hygiene, cleanliness, lubrication, and prevention of cross-contamination from sexual activity; avoid enemas, rectal thermometers, and rectal medications; prevent constipation with laxatives and stool softeners); daily baths; cleansing of puncture sites with iodophor solution twice a day until healed; oral care after meals and before bed or more frequently depending on level of risk; keeping fingernails and toenails short and clean; and emphasizing the importance of thorough and frequent hand washing.

Supporting the integrity of the intestinal mucosa and preventing infection also encompass the principle of minimizing the patient's endogenous flora as a source of infection. There is an overgrowth of intestinal pathogens that increases the susceptibility to infection from orally ingested pathogens when the normal gut flora is altered by antibiotics and/or immunosuppression (Carter, 1994). A low-microbial diet (Table 10-1) introduces minimal numbers of endogenous bacteria into the gut and a high-fiber diet minimizes the risk of colonic stasis, which may contribute to the risk of bacterial translocation (Carter, 1993). The diet should also be high in calories, protein, and vitamins and include an adequate fluid intake. Implementation of the low-microbial diet is recommended when the neutrophil count is predicted to fall, and the diet is maintained until neutrophil recovery (Carter, 1993). The use of selective decontamination with antibiotics appears to be associated with increased rather than decreased infectious risks (Pizzo, 1993), but innovative approaches with dietary and nutritional factors such as glutamine, fiber, and albumin offer new alternatives to risk reduction (Carter, 1994).

Interventions to reduce environmental organisms are applicable to the patient's home environment, but the risk of infection is greater in the hospital setting and is related to nosocomial infection and the number of personnel who are in contact with the patient. Many of the following guidelines to minimize or eliminate sources of infection from the hospital environment also apply to the ambulatory health care setting and to the patient's home. Suggested guidelines for care of the hospitalized neutropenic patient include the following:

- Wash hands frequently and thoroughly; this is the single most important measure in preventing infection. Use clean, disposable gloves with each patient.
- Place patient in a private room.
- Teach patients to avoid persons with viral or contagious illnesses; screen visitors for contagious diseases. Personnel who are ill, particularly with a respiratory or viral infection, should avoid direct patient care. Patients should avoid contact with persons recently vaccinated with live or attenuated virus vaccines.
- Do not allow stagnant water, fresh flowers, plants, humidifiers, or vaporizers in the patient's room; change water pitcher every day; avoid use of bar soap.
- Clean and disinfect equipment before patient contact and after each use with solution of one part bleach to nine parts water.
- Use a separate stethoscope for the patient and disinfect after each use.

TABLE 10-1
Low-Microbial Diet

Food category	Foods permitted	Foods omitted
Meat, fish, and poultry	Hot, well-cooked meat, fish, poultry, bacon, sausage, hot dogs, chicken/beef pot pies, beef stroganoff, spaghetti with meat sauce, gravies, and sauces	Raw or rare meat Meat or fish salads Deli or dried meats Processed lunch meats Lasagna Pizza
	Canned meat, fish, and shellfish Frozen dinners	
Vegetables and starch substitutes	Canned vegetables	Raw vegetables or salads
	Cooked fresh or frozen vegetables	Onion rings
	Canned bean salad	Au gratin potatoes
	Baked fresh squash	Potato salad
	Instant mashed potatoes	Macaroni salad
	Rice and pasta	
	Chow mein noodles	
Fruits	Canned fruit	Fresh fruits
	Cooked fruit	Dried fruits, including raisins
	Baked apples	Frozen fruits
Eggs	Well-cooked eggs: scrambled, boiled, or fried until yolk is firm	Uncooked eggs Semicooked eggs
Breads/cereals	All breads, rolls, muffins, buns, and bagels, except as noted	Breads/cereals containing nuts or raisins
	All hot and cold cereals, except as noted	Cinnamon/sweet rolls
	Tortillas	

Continued

TABLE 10-1
Low-Microbial Diet—cont'd

Food category	Foods permitted	Foods omitted
Bread/cereals (cont'd)	Pancakes, waffles, and French toast Crackers served in single wrapper	Doughnuts Onion bagels
Soups	All hot canned/dehydrated soups, broths, or bouillons	Homemade soups Commercial refrigerated soups Frozen soups Cold vegetable soups
Fats and oils	Margarine or shortening Shortening Single packets of mayonnaise or tartar sauce Canned gravy/sauces	Butter Homemade gravy Hollandaise sauce Mayonnaise/tartar sauce from multiserving containers
Beverages	Instant/brewed coffee or tea Instant/canned/bottled fruit drinks or juices Canned fruit or vegetable juices Carbonated beverages Pasteurized beer Bottled seltzer water Sterile water ice	Instant iced tea Bottled distilled water Nonpastuerized beer Wine Fresh fruit/vegetable juices
Milk/milk products	Heat-treated pasteurized milk Canned milk Instant hot cocoa Sterile milkshake products American cheese slices Creamed cheese in single packets	Outdated pasteurized milk Powdered instant breakfast mixes Whipped or sour cream Nondairy whipped topping Natural or cottage cheese Yogurt

	Processed pasteurized cheese and cheese food spreads	Buttermilk
	Canned puddings	Ice cream, ice cream bars, or sherbet
		Refrigerated puddings
Desserts/sweets	Pound or angel food cakes	All other cakes, pies, or cookies
	Gelatin	Cream-filled candy
	Honey, syrup, or sugar	Candy made with nuts or dried fruit
	Canned chocolate syrup	Candy bars
	Commercial cookies without filling, fruit, or nuts	
	Homemade custard	
	Candy: hardtack, gumdrops, jellybeans, lemon drops, marshmallows, peanut butter cups, or plain chocolate	
	Chewing gum	
Snacks	Corn or tortilla chips	All nuts
	Crackers	Candy-coated popcorn
	Popcorn	Pretzels
	Canned dips	Potato chips
	Smooth peanut butter	
	Flavor ices (on a stick)	
Condiments/spices	Single packets of mustard, ketchup, taco sauce, lemon juice, salad dressings, jam, or jelly	Condiments from multiserving containers
	Dill pickles	Green olives
	Canned black olives	Sweet pickle relish
	Seasonings, spices, or pepper added before cooking	Seasonings, spices, or pepper added after cooking
Nutritional supplements	Glucose polymers	
	All canned supplements	
	Powdered supplements mixed with sterile water	

From Carter LW: Influences of nutrition and stress on people at risk for neutropenia: nursing implications, *Oncol Nurs Forum*, 20:1241-1250, 1993.

Management of Fever and Infection in the Neutropenic Patient

The development of fever in a neutropenic patient represents an urgent clinical problem requiring prompt assessment and intervention. General principles for the management of the neutropenic patient with fever (i.e., temperature greater than 38.5° C, 101° F) are presented in Box 10-2. Empirical antibiotic therapy *must* be initiated without delay. Urgent care and emergency personnel in the patient's health care system must be well educated and fully understand the critical nature of the febrile neutropenic patient. The choice of specific antibiotics for the initial empirical therapy depends on a variety of factors (Pizzo, 1993), but the need to modify or add drugs to the initial antibiotic therapy is common (Table 10-2). Most patients with febrile neutropenia require hospitalization, but there may be a low-risk group, such as those patients with nonhematological malignancies with a predicted short duration of neutropenia, that may be successfully treated at home with antibiotics (Malik et al, 1994).

BOX 10-2

General Principles for the Management of Fever in Patients With Neutropenia

1. Instruct the patient to seek medical help if a fever develops when the neutrophil count is low or declining.
2. Evaluate the patient at least daily.
3. Initiate prompt therapy with broad-spectrum antibiotics when a patient with neutropenia (neutrophil count, <500/mm^3) becomes febrile (single elevation in oral temperature to >38.5° C, or three elevations to >38° C during a 24-hour period).
4. If the patient has an indwelling intravenous catheter, obtain cultures from each catheter port and lumen as well as from a peripheral vein. Rotate antibiotic therapy through each lumen of multiple-lumen catheters.
5. Monitor the patient closely for secondary infections requiring additions or modifications to the initial antibiotic regimen.
6. Continue empirical antibiotic therapy if the patient has prolonged (>1 week) neutropenia, particularly if there is persistent fever.
7. Add empirical antifungal therapy if a patient with neutropenia remains febrile after a week of broad-spectrum antibiotic therapy or has recurrent fever.
8. Discontinue antibiotic therapy when the neutrophil count rises above 500/mm^3 in a patient at high risk or is increasing in a patient at low risk.
9. Although 10 to 14 days of treatment is adequate in most patients with neutropenia, prolonged therapy is necessary for a patient with a residual focus of infection or invasive mycoses (e.g., hepatosplenic candidiasis).
10. All those caring for a febrile patient with neutropenia should wash their hands carefully before any contact with the patient.

From Pizzo PA: Management of fever in patients with cancer and treatment-induced neutropenia, *New Engl J Med,* 328:1323-1332, 1993.

TABLE 10-2
Common Modifications or Additions to Initial Empirical Antibiotic Therapy in Patients With Neutropenia and Fever

Status or symptoms	Modifications of primary regimen
Fever	
Persistent for >1 week	Add empirical antifungal therapy with amphotericin B
Recurrence after 1 week or later in patient with persistent neutropenia	Add empirical antifungal therapy
Persistent or recurrent fever at time of recovery from neutropenia	Evaluate liver and spleen by CT, ultrasonography, or MRI for hepatosplenic candidiasis, and evaluate need for antifungal therapy
Blood stream	
Cultures before antibiotic therapy	
Gram-positive organism	Add vancomycin pending further identification
Gram-negative organism	Maintain regimen if patient is stable and isolate if sensitive; if *P. aeruginosa*, *Enterobacter*, or *Citrobacter* is isolated, add an aminoglycoside or an additional β-lactam antibiotic
Organism isolated during antibiotic therapy	
Gram-positive organism	Add vancomycin
Gram-negative organism	Change to new combination regimen (e.g., imipenem plus gentamicin or vancomycin, or gentamicin plus piperacillin)

Continued

TABLE 10-2
Common Modifications or Additions to Initial Empirical Antibiotic Therapy in Patients With Neutropenia and Fever—cont'd

Status or symptoms	Modifications of primary regimen
Head, eyes, ears, nose, throat	
Necrotizing or marginal gingivitis	Add specific antianaerobic agent (clindamycin or metronidazole) to empirical therapy
Vesicular or ulcerative lesions	Suspect herpes simplex infection; culture and begin acyclovir therapy
Sinus tenderness or nasal ulcerative lesions	Suspect fungal infection with Aspergillus or Mucor
Gastrointestinal tract	
Retrosternal burning pain	Suspect Candida, herpes simplex, or both; add antifungal therapy and, if no response, acyclovir; bacterial esophagitis also a possibility; for patients who do not respond within 48 hours, endoscopy should be considered
Acute abdominal pain	Suspect typhlitis, as well as appendicitis, if pain in right lower quadrant; add specific antianaerobic coverage to empirical regimen and monitor closely for need for surgical intervention
Perianal tenderness	Add specific antianaerobic drug to empirical regimen and monitor need for surgical intervention, especially when patient is recovering from neutropenia

Respiratory tract	
New focal lesion in patient recovering from neutropenia	Observe carefully, since this may be a consequence of inflammatory response in concert with neutrophil recovery
New focal lesion in patient with continuing neutropenia	Aspergillus is the chief concern; perform appropriate cultures and consider biopsy; if patient is not a candidate for procedure, administer high-dose amphotericin B (1.5 mg/kg/day)
New interstitial pneumonitis	Attempt diagnosis by examination of induced sputum or bronchoalveolar lavage; if not feasible, begin empirical treatment with trimethoprim–sulfamethoxazole or pentamidine; consider noninfectious causes and the need for open-lung biopsy if condition has not improved after 4 days of therapy
Central venous catheters	
Positive culture for organisms other than bacillus species or Candida	Attempt to treat; rotate antibiotic administration in patients with multiple-lumen catheters
Positive culture for bacillus species or Candida	Remove catheter and treat appropriately
Exit-site infection with Mycobacterium or Aspergillus	Remove catheter and treat appropriately
Tunnel infection	Remove catheter and treat appropriately

From Pizzo PA: Management of fever in patients with cancer and treatment-induced neutropenia, *N Eng J Med*, 328:1323-1332, 1993.

Careful selection and close monitoring of such patients are essential when considering ambulatory antibiotic therapy as an alternative to hospitalization.

THROMBOCYTOPENIA

There are multiple factors related to the underlying malignancy that may alter platelet function, but thrombocytopenia, a platelet count of less than $100,000/mm^3$, is a very common and predictable side effect of chemotherapy-induced myelosuppression. Thrombocytopenia is reported as a potential or actual dose-limiting side effect for standard doses of carboplatin, dacarbazine, fluorouracil, lomustine, mitomycin, prednimustine, suramin, thiotepa, and trimetrexate. Delayed onset of thrombocytopenia and a cumulative dosing effect have been observed with carmustine, fludarabine, lomustine, mitomycin, streptozocin, and thiotepa. Increased risk of bleeding is the most significant outcome of a reduced platelet count. A moderate risk of bleeding exists when the platelet count falls to less than 50,000 cells/mm^3 , and major risk is associated with platelet counts less than 20,000 cells/mm^3 (Erickson, 1990). Critical risk occurs when the count is under 10,000 cells/mm^3, because fatal CNS bleeding, massive GI hemorrhage, or respiratory tract hemorrhage is likely to occur. Impaired tissue integrity from trauma and infection increases the likelihood of hemorrhage. Clotting and platelet disorders that are drug or illness related can contribute to serious bleeding problems, and the patient may become symptomatic even though platelet numbers do not appear dangerously low. Careful assessment of the patient for potential signs and symptoms of bleeding is indicated. The skin, mucous membranes, and fundi are important areas to assess. Clinical manifestations include increased bruising, petechiae, purpura (most frequently found on lower extremities, in skin creases, and along scratch marks), oozing from mucosal surfaces, and hypermenorrhea. The stool, urine, and vomitus should be tested for blood in patients at high risk for bleeding.

Preventive Measures

To prevent bleeding in patients, the following guidelines for practice are recommended:

- Avoid trauma to the patient.
- Decrease the patient's level of activity.
- Increase the patient's amount of rest.
- Avoid drugs that alter platelet function or clotting (Box 10-3).
- Monitor the platelet count regularly and anticipate nadir. Treatment should be modified according to the laboratory values, degree of risk, and patient symptoms.
- Surgical procedures, bone marrow biopsies, and parenteral injections are relatively contraindicated in the thrombocytopenic patient. Invasive procedures that are deemed essential should be done with trepidation, and platelet coverage should be planned ahead of time and availability confirmed. If a parenteral injection is necessary, a small-gauge needle should be used for intravenous or subcutaneous administration.

BOX 10-3
Medication That May Affect Platelet Function

Antimicrobials
Penicillins (ampicillin, carbenicillin, ticarcillin, piperacillin, etc.)
Cephalosporins (cefoperazone, cefotaxime, cephalothin, moxalactam, etc.)
Pentamidine
Amphotericin-B
Nitrofurantoin
Hydroxycholoroquine
Miconazole
Antiinflammatory agents
Aspirin and aspirin-containing combination products
Nonsteroidal antiinflammatory drugs (diclofenac, diflunisal, ibuprofen,
    indomethacin, naproxen, phenylbutazone, piroxicam, sulfinpyrazone,
    sulindac, tolmetin)
Cardiovascular drugs

Diltiazem	Propranolol
Isosorbide dinitrate	Quinidine
Nifedipine	Sodium nitroprusside
Nitroglycerine	Verapamil

Chemotherapy drugs

Carboplatin	Doxorubicin
Carmustine	Melphalan
Cyclophosphamide	Mitomycin
Dactinomycin	Plicamycin
Daunorubicin	Vincristine

Psychotropic drugs
Phenothiazines (chlorpromazine, fluphenazine, haloperidol, promethazine,
    trifluoperazine)
Antidepressants (amitriptyline, imipramine, nortriptyline)
Anesthetics
Local (butacaine, cocaine, dibucaine, procaine, tetracaine)
General (halothane)
Anticoagulants (heparin, warfarin sodium)
Thrombolytic agents (alteplase, streptokinase, urokinase)
Miscellaneous agents
Ticlopidine
Dextran
Lipid lowering agents (clofibrate)
ε-Aminocaproic acid
Antihistamines
Ethanol
Vitamin E
Radiographic contrast agents
Dipyridamole
Methylxanthines (caffeine, theophylline, aminophylline)
Prostaglandins I_2, S_2, E_1

- Pressure should be applied for at least 5 minutes with a pressure bandage for all IV injections, venipunctures, and bone marrow procedures.
- Patients should avoid blowing their noses and sneezing. For shaving, an electric razor is recommended. Blood pressure should be taken only when necessary.

Management of Bleeding and Moderate to Severe Thrombocytopenia

Transfusion of platelets is a common therapeutic intervention for platelet counts below 15,000 to 20,000/mm^3, although it is often dependent on the patient's symptoms. Indications, risks, and benefits of supportive blood component therapy for thrombocytopenia and the patient at risk of bleeding are discussed in Chapter 11.

Any sites of actual bleeding that develop in a patient should be kept clean, and measures should be taken to encourage clot formation. Ice application, nasal packing, or topical epinephrine may be necessary to stop epistaxis. Absorbable gelatin sponge (Gelfoam) or liquid thrombin applied to the site may be helpful in controlling bleeding gums.

GASTROINTESTINAL TOXICITY

Nausea, Vomiting, and Antiemetic Therapy

Clinical practice and patient outcomes have been dramatically influenced by advances in the understanding of the physiology of chemotherapy-induced nausea and vomiting and the role of serotonin in the process; the development and clinical application of serotonin antagonists to prevent emesis; and clinical research on the incidence, intensity, and perceived symptom distress of nausea and vomiting. The patterns of nausea and vomiting are more clearly defined, and subjective evaluation of symptoms is valued as an assessment parameter. Some general level of agreement has evolved regarding guidelines for first-line pharmacological management according to the drug or regimen's emetic potential.

Assessment

The first goal of assessment is to determine the learning needs of the patient and family. Information should be clear, as factual as possible, and related to the predicted occurrence and severity of chemotherapy-induced emesis and measures for relief and control.

Pharmacological management is the major intervention for treatment-induced nausea and vomiting. Antiemetic trials frequently assess the number of emetic episodes as the outcome measure for effectiveness of the drug or combination-drug regimen. Although these trials have provided strong evidence of the drug's activity, this restricted outcome measure fails to identify important clinical information, such as intensity of the experienced symptom, which could dramatically alter the plan of care (Cubeddu, 1992). An adequate evaluation of the effectiveness of antiemetic therapy should include the onset, duration, and intensity of nausea and vomiting, as well as the degree of distress each symptom produces for an individual patient.

Nausea, vomiting, and *retching* are conceptually separate terms and it is important to define them in language that is understood by the patient and family for accurate assessment (Rhodes, Johnson, and McDaniel, 1995). Nausea is an unpleasant sensation that is difficult to describe, but the term usually refers to a vague uneasiness or discomfort located in the epigastrium, throat region, or diffusely throughout the abdomen. It is characterized by a revulsion to food and is commonly referred to as "feeling sick to your stomach." Mild nausea may be relieved by eating, but moderate to severe nausea may prevent normal food intake and interfere with an individual's ability to carry on normal activities. Retching is a rhythmic, spasmodic movement involving the chest, diaphragm, and abdominal muscles that occurs before vomiting or alternately with vomiting. Vomiting is the forceful expulsion of the contents of the stomach, duodenum, or proximal jejunum through the mouth or nose, accompanied by somatic changes. Vomiting can be objectively measured or assessed by self-report. Nausea is usually subjectively reported, although severe nausea may have some objective elements to assess (Rhodes, Johnson, and McDaniel, 1995). Quantitative measurements of subjective ratings of nausea and vomiting are recommended to document as accurately as possible the patient's response and to provide documentation for reevaluation and management of subsequent treatments. Assessment using Likert-type or visual analog scales is user friendly, quick to complete, and practical for clinical and home settings. Such scales help discriminate among symptoms and identify patterns, as well as capture the level of perceived symptom distress. Monitoring the patient's weight and nutritional intake provides additional clinical parameters to assess, especially for patients who are not fully protected against treatment-induced nausea and vomiting.

Patterns of nausea and vomiting

There are three patterns of nausea and vomiting associated with chemotherapy: acute, delayed, and anticipatory. Acute nausea and vomiting occurs within the first 24 hours of treatment. The incidence and severity of nausea and vomiting are related to the emetogenic potential of the drug (Table 10-3), dose, route of administration, schedule, infusion rate, time of day the drug is given, patient characteristics, and combination of drugs. Knowledge of the onset and duration of symptoms of individual drugs (Table 10-4) and patterns for combination drug therapy is also essential for planning appropriate antiemetic therapy.

Delayed nausea and vomiting is defined by timing, specifically development (or continuation) of symptoms 24 hours after treatment with cisplatin or other highly emetogenic combination chemotherapy. Delayed nausea and vomiting associated with cisplatin is reported to occur in 21% to 81% of patients, lasts from 1 to 7 days, peaks around day 3, and is followed by a gradual decrease in incidence and severity (Lindley, Bernard, and Fields, 1989; Kris et al, 1985). Delayed or residual nausea and vomiting occurs even when antiemetics are effective in preventing acute symptoms within the first 24 hours (Cubeddu, 1992; Kris et al, 1992). Persistent nausea is more common than vomiting after treatment and appears to respond less well to antiemetic treatment. The effects on patient distress,

TABLE 10-3
Emetic Potential of Chemotherapy Drugs as Single Agents

Very high (>90%)	High (60%–90%)	Moderate (30%–60%)	Low (0%–30%)
Cisplatin	Azacytidine	Altretamine	Bleomycin
Cyclophosphamide*	Carboplatin	Amsacrine	Busulfan
Cytarabine*	Carmustine	L-Asparaginase	Cladribine
Dacarbazine	Cyclophosphamide	Daunorubicin	Chlorambucil
Mechlorethamine	Dactinomycin	Doxorubicin	Cytarabine
Melphalan*	Lomustine	Epirubicin	Docetaxel
Streptozocin		Idarubicin	Edatrexate
		Ifosfamide	Etoposide
		Mitomycin	5-Fluorouracil
		Mitoxantrone	Floxuridine
		Pentostatin	Fludarabine
		Plicamycin	Hydroxyurea
		Procarbazine	Irinotecan
		Topotecan	Melphalan
			Methotrexate
			Paclitaxel
			6-Mercaptopurine
			Thioguanine
			Thiotepa
			Tomudex
			Trimetrexate
			Vinblastine
			Vincristine
			Vinorelbine

*High dose.

nutritional intake, and weight loss may be clinically significant for some patients. Careful and routine posttreatment assessment is essential. Delayed symptomatology is no longer restricted to high-dose cisplatin therapy but is frequently observed in practice with non-cisplatin emetogenic regimens, especially those containing high-dose alkylating agents.

Anticipatory nausea and vomiting is the experiencing of one or both of these symptoms before receiving another chemotherapy treatment. It is a conditioned or learned response to previous effects from therapy and associated environmental stimuli. Approximately 20% to 65% of patients will develop anticipatory symptoms, with nausea occurring much more commonly (24% to 65%) than vomiting (9% to 18%) (Coons et al, 1987; Nerenz et al, 1986; Morrow, 1984). Clinical predictors for the development of these symptoms are moderate to severe postchemotherapy nausea and vomiting, increased anxiety levels, and younger age. Precipitating environmental factors include odors such as rubbing alcohol, certain substances and colors referable to particular cytotoxic drugs,

TABLE 10-4
Emetic Potential of Antineoplastic Agents

Agent	% of time agent induces emesis	Onset of emesis (hr)	Duration of emesis (hr)
Cisplatin*	>90	1-4	12-20
Dacarbazine*	>90	1-3	1-8
Mechlorethamine*	>90	0.5-2	2-24
Cytarabine* high dose	>90	1-3	3-8
Carboplatin	60-90	1-6	4-24
Carmustine*	60-90	2-4	4-12
Cyclophosphamide*	60-90	4-8	4-24
Dactinomycin	60-90	2-5	4-24
Procarbazine	30-60	24-27	Varies
Daunorubicin	30-60	1-3	4-24
Doxorubicin	30-60	1-3	4-24
Ifosfamide	30-60	2-3	4-24
Mitoxantrone	30-60	2-6	6-24
5-Fluorouracil	10-30	3-6	2-12
Mitomycin	30-60	1-2	3-4
Bleomycin	10-30	3-6	1-4
Cytarabine* low dose	10-30	6-12	3-5
Etoposide	10-30	3-8	1-4
Methotrexate*	10-30	4-12	3-12
Vinblastine	10-30	4-8	1-4
Vincristine	<10	4-8	1-4
Paclitaxel	<10	4-8	1-2
Docetaxel	<10	4-8	1-2

Modified from Rhodes VA, Johnson MH, McDaniel RW: Nausea, vomiting, and retching: the management of the symptom experience, *Semin Oncol Nurs* 11(4):256-265, 1995. Adapted from Borison HL, McCarthy LE: Neuropharmacology of chemotherapy-induced emesism, *Drugs* 25(suppl 1):8-17, 1993 and Dorr RT, Fritz WL: *Chemotherapy handbook*, Stamford, Conn, 1980, Appleton & Lange, pp 143-150.
*Dose-related; potential for emesis increases with higher doses.

personnel involved in drug administration, tastes, the drive to the office or hospital, anxiety about the potential success of venipuncture, and the actual physical treatment setting.

Management: pharmacological therapy

General principles for successful antiemetic therapy for chemotherapy-induced nausea and vomiting include aggressive therapy for chemotherapy-naive patients; adequate duration of coverage with antiemetics for the predicted risk period of symptoms; appropriate selection of agents and dosing according to the emetic potential of the chemotherapy; and consideration of nonpharmacological therapy such as distraction, meditation, or relaxation.

TABLE 10-5
Actions of Antiemetics

Drug type	Mechanism of action	Type of nausea controlled
Antihistamines	Act in neural pathways originating in the labyrinth	Motion sickness, Meniere's syndrome, vestibular sensitivity from narcotics, pregnancy-induced nausea, some postanesthetic vomiting
Benzodiazepines	Act centrally by depressing cerebral cortex or vomiting center	Nausea and vomiting with anxiety component, pregnancy-induced nausea, and postanesthetic vomiting
Anticholinergic drugs	Depress conduction in the vestibular cerebellar pathways and decrease excitability of labyrinth receptors	Little antiemetic activity, but scopolamine is of some value in motion sickness
Dopamine inhibitors Phenothiazines, butyrophenones	Reduce the effect of dopamine in the CTZ and in high doses may suppress the vomiting itself; potent inhibitor of the CTZ by blocking synaptic transmission of dopamine	All types of nausea and vomiting, excluding motion sickness Suggested activity with some chemotherapy-induced vomiting
Cannabinoids	Unknown Cerebral cortex?	Some activity with low emetogenic chemotherapy
Corticosteroids	Unknown Inhibition of enkephalins? Inhibition of prostaglandins?	Most effective in combination with other antiemetic drugs
Metoclopramide	Same as phenothiazines; also a 5-HT$_3$ inhibitor; may inhibit GI-induced nausea and vomiting	Most effective against cisplatin and combination chemotherapy regimens with moderate to high emetogenic potential
Serotonin antagonists	Binds to type 3 serotonin receptor 5-HT$_3$	Chemotherapy-induced; most effective for acute nausea and vomiting

CTZ, Chemoreceptor trigger zone; *5-HT$_3$*, 5-hydroxytryptamine, type 3; *GI*, gastrointestinal.

The past decade has increased our knowledge about the physiology of treatment-related nausea and vomiting and the mechanisms by which chemotherapeutic drugs induce nausea and emesis (Cubeddu, 1992; Kris, 1994). Management of nausea and vomiting is dependent on knowledge of the underlying physiological processes, the onset and duration of nausea and vomiting of chemotherapy drugs (Table 10-4), the pharmacology and the spectrum of activity of the antiemetic drugs (Table 10-5), and the profile of dose, schedule, duration of action, and side effects of the antiemetic and adjunct drugs for the prevention and management of nausea and vomiting (Table 10-6). New knowledge, the development and clinical application of serotonin antagonists, and other clinical research focused on prevention/management of chemotherapy-induced nausea and vomiting in the past decade provide data to support some general clinical guidelines to manage the various patterns of nausea and vomiting (Kris, 1994; Cleri, 1995).

Therapy to prevent acute nausea and vomiting should be chosen based on emetogenic risk of the chemotherapy. For highly or moderately emetogenic chemotherapy, a serotonin antagonist in combination with dexamethasone is recommended. Until further information is gained from trials and clinical practice, intravenous antiemetic drug administration is preferable for optimal effectiveness in preventing nausea and vomiting from chemotherapy with *very high* emetogenic potential. For moderately emetogenic therapy, oral administration of serotonin antagonists appears equally effective. For low-risk emetogenic chemotherapy, prochlorperazine or a serotonin antagonist (oral) are alternatives, and dexamethasone alone may be adequate for chemotherapy associated with a very low risk of nausea or vomiting.

Highly emetogenic chemotherapy is associated with delayed symptomatology, and treatment beginning on day 2 and extending for 3 to 5 days is recommended. A delayed regimen should also be prescribed for patients who develop residual symptoms, which may occur after several cycles of drugs or with lower emetogenic chemotherapy. Prochlorperazine, metoclopramide, ondansetron, dexamethasone, and the combination of any one of those antiemetics with dexamethasone have been reported as delayed regimens. Common adjuncts to these delayed regimens include diphenhydramine, primarily to control extrapyramidal symptoms associated with prochlorperazine and metoclopramide, and lorazepam, which can control extrapyramidal symptoms but is generally indicated to reduce anxiety. Although none of these therapies has been universally successful, the combination of an antiemetic and dexamethasone in controlling residual nausea and vomiting is superior to an antiemetic drug alone. The pathophysiology of delayed emesis is unknown but appears to be mediated by serotonin-independent mechanisms. The serotonin antagonists have been very successful in preventing acute emesis but have been relatively unsuccessful in controlling delayed symptoms (Kris et al, 1992; Gandara et al, 1992; Roila et al, 1991), further supporting the theory that serotonin receptors may have a minor role in delayed symptomatology. These data support the use of antiemetic drugs with different mechanisms of action for prevention of delayed symptoms, such as metoclopramide with

TABLE 10-6
Antiemetic Administration Guides

Drug	Route/Dose	Common side effects/ Special precautions
Phenothiazines		
Chlorpromazine	PO: 25-50 mg q4-6h IM: 12.5-50 mg q4-6h IV: 12.5-50 mg q4-6h	Postural hypotension, drowsiness, dizziness, blurred vision, extra-pyramidal symptoms
Prochlorperazine	PO: tablets: 10 mg q4h PO spansules: 10-30 mg q6-8h IV: 10-12 mg q4h PR: 25 mg q8-12h	Extrapyramidal symptoms, akathisia
Thiethylperazine	PO: 10 mg q4-6h PR: 10 mg q4-6h	Extrapyramidal symptoms
Perphenazine	PO: 2-4 mg q4-6h	Extrapyramidal symptoms
Serotonin antagonists		
Ondansetron	IVPB: 0.15 mg/kg q2-4h × 3 doses or 32-mg dose PO: 4-8 mg q8h	Give higher doses over at least 30 minutes to prevent dizziness; headache, constipation, diarrhea, transient increase in liver enzymes
Granisetron	IVP: 10 mg × 1 dose before chemotherapy PO: 1 mg 1 h before chemotherapy; repeat in 12 h	Headache, constipation, dizziness

Corticosteroids

Dexamethasone
- IV: 10-20 mg as a single dose before chemotherapy, then 10 mg q6h
- PO: 4-8 mg q6h

Hyperglycemia, perineal itching/burning with rapid IV infusion (usually given in combination with other antiemetics)

Benzamides

Metoclopramide
- IV: 1-3 mg/kg IVPB, before chemotherapy, then 1-3 mg/kg q2-3h × 3-5 doses
- PO: 1 mg/kg q2-4h

Diarrhea, drowsiness, extrapyramidal symptoms (may be combined with diphenhydramine to lower), akathisia

Benzodiazepines

Lorazepam
- PO: 0.5-2 mg q4h
- SL: 0.5-2 mg q4h
- IV: 0.5-2 mg q4h

Drowsiness, amnesia; use with caution in the elderly or with patients with renal or respiratory dysfunction

Diazepam
- PO: 2-4 mg q4-6h
- IV: 2-5 mg q4-6h

Sedation, amnesia; use with caution in the elderly and patients with impaired hepatic or renal function

Butyrophenones

Droperidol
- IV: 0.5-2 mg q4h

Extrapyramidal symptoms, drowsiness, akathisia, tachycardia, alterations in blood pressure

Haloperidol
- PO: 1-2 mg q3-6h
- IV: 1-2 mg q3-6h

Extrapyramidal symptoms, drowsiness, akathisia, tachycardia, alterations in blood pressure

Antihistamines

Diphenhydramine
- PO: 25-50 mg q4h
- IV: 1-2 mg q3-6h

May be given in combination with other antiemetic drugs to prevent extrapyramidal side effects; give IVP slowly; may cause drowsiness

Continued

TABLE 10-6
Antiemetic Administration Guides—cont'd

Drug	Route/Dose	Common side effects/ Special precautions
Cannabinoids		
Dronabinol	5 mg/m² 2 hours before chemotherapy, then q 2-4hr after chemotherapy for a total of 4-6 doses/1 day	Hypotension tachycardia, dysphoria; tolerated poorly by the elderly
Miscellaneous		
Promethazine	PO: 25 mg q4h PR: 25 mg q4h IV: 25 mg q4h	Phenothiazine derivative; may cause drowsiness; do not give Subq but give IVP slowly and well diluted
Hydroxyzine pamoate	PO: 25-30 mg q4h	**NEVER GIVE IV:** may cause hemolysis

PO, oral; *IM,* intramuscular; *IV,* intravenous; *PR,* per rectum; *IVP,* intravenous push; *IVPB,* intravenous piggyback; *SL,* sublingual; *Subq,* subcutaneous.

From Rhodes VA, Johnson MH, McDaniel RW: Nausea, vomiting, and retching: the management of the symptom experience, *Semin Oncol Nurs* 11:256-265, 1995.

dexamethasone or a dopamine antagonist (Kris, 1994; Herrstedt et al, 1993; Cleri, 1995). Declining protection from nausea and vomiting with multiple-day therapy could possibly be explained by the differing mechanisms responsible for acute and delayed symptomatology. As we await data from ongoing trials, use of drugs with different mechanisms of action for patients on multiple-day regimens who progress with symptoms of nausea and vomiting may be a reasonable clinical practice approach.

Anticipatory nausea and vomiting are strongly associated with post-treatment emesis, and therefore adequate control of acute posttreatment nausea and vomiting is critical. Once anticipatory symptoms develop, combining drugs with amnesic and antianxiety properties, such as lorazepam, with antiemetics has been recommended by some as preventive strategy (Laszlo, 1985), but confirmation of the clinical efficacy of this strategy has never been established. Behavioral treatment using progressive muscle relaxation and guided imagery instituted before chemotherapy can reduce anxiety levels and may have a role in reducing or preventing these conditioned responses (Burish et al, 1983; Burish et al, 1987).

Serotonin antagonists

The antiemetic effectiveness of the drug metoclopramide was known to be related to its effects on dopamine receptors and, to some degree, antagonism of 5-HT_3 receptors when given at high doses. The hypothesized role of serotonin in chemotherapy-induced nausea and vomiting led to further research and development of a new class of antiemetic agents in cancer therapy, the serotonin antagonists, of which ondansetron was the first to be marketed. Ondansetron hydrochloride (Zofran) and granisetron (Kytril) are competitive inhibitors of serotonin at the 5-HT_3 receptors at peripheral and central sites. The actions of serotonin (5-hydroxytryptamine), a neurotransmitter found in the central and peripheral nervous systems and enterochromaffin cells in the small intestine, are mediated by 5-HT receptors. There are several types of serotonin receptors—5-HT_1, 5-HT_2, and 5-HT_3. Binding of serotonin to the 5-HT_3 serotonin receptor is believed to be a major factor explaining cisplatin-induced emesis. Ondansetron is thought to act centrally in the area postrema, where there is a high density of 5-HT_3 receptors, and peripherally in the intestinal mucosa. Ondansetron is 70 to 125 times more potent than metoclopramide at peripheral 5-HT_3 receptors. Ondansetron has no effect on dopamine, acetylcholine, histamine, or endorphin receptors.

For acute nausea and vomiting associated with high-dose cisplatin (>100 mg/m^2), ondansetron prevents emesis in 20% to 58% of patients (Cleri, 1995; Kris, 1994). For lower doses of cisplatin and high to moderate emetogenic non-cisplatin therapy, ondansetron produces complete emesis control in 60% to 70% of patients. The addition of dexamethasone improves the response rate, which ranges from 61% to 91% complete protection (Hesketh et al 1994; Roila et al, 1991). For multiple-day chemotherapy, the response rate declines with progressive therapy days. The overall 5-day complete protection rate for ondansetron alone is 21% to 33% and increases to 38% to 66% if dexamethasone is administered in combination (Kris, 1994). The current recommendation for intravenous administration is a single 32-mg dose of ondansetron before chemotherapy.

Oral ondansetron at a dose of 8 mg 3 times a day produces complete response rates of 66% to 85% in moderately emetogenic chemotherapy, which are superior to metoclopramide and equivalent or superior to the combination of metoclopramide and dexamethasone (Beck, 1992; Campora et al, 1994; Fraschini et al, 1991). The optimal dose and schedule of oral ondansetron, however, has not yet been determined.

Ondansetron has been used for management of delayed or residual nausea and vomiting with disappointing results, which may be related to different mechanism from the acute emetic event (Hainsworth and Hesketh, 1992; Kris et al, 1992). Navarri et al (1995a) compared ondansetron with placebo in a group of cisplatin-treated patients who were free of emesis at 24 hours after chemotherapy. There were no differences in complete emesis protection for days 2 to 3 (36% versus 26%), but if complete and major responses were combined, ondansetron was associated with fewer emetic episodes (56% versus 37%). Although this study and others suggest some protection offered against delayed emesis, data to indicate use of serotonin antagonists after the first 24 to 48 hours have not been adequately demonstrated (Kris, 1994; Cleri, 1995; Campora et al, 1994). Metoclopramide in combination with dexamethasone provides better protection for delayed symptomatology than ondansetron (Kris et al, 1992; Levitt et al, 1993; Cleri, 1995).

The side effects of ondansetron are relatively mild and include headache (more common with a single high dose), transient liver function abnormalities, dizziness, tiredness, constipation, and diarrhea. Headache is commonly reported in 10% to 15% of patients treated and is relieved by acetaminophen. Transient liver function abnormalities, specifically elevated levels of alanine aminotransferase (SGPT), aspartate aminotransferase (SGOT), and bilirubin are reported in about 25% of patients. These abnormalities do not yet appear to have any clinical significance, but patients should be carefully monitored.

Granisetron (Kytril) is a potent selective 5-HT$_3$ serotonin antagonist. It has a longer half life than ondansetron (Table 10-6) but is similar in action (Ignoffo, 1994). At a dose of 10 µg/kg administered intravenously, complete protection for highly emetogenic chemotherapy is achieved in 40% to 60% of patients, with improved protection in the range of 75% to 80% against moderately emetogenic therapy and consistently better protection (>80%) when combined with dexamethasone (Cleri, 1995; Italian Group for Antiemetic Research, 1995). Oral granisetron at a dose of 1 mg twice daily produces complete protection in the range of 58% to 82% for moderately emetogenic chemotherapy (Hacking et al, 1992; Johnsonbaugh et al, 1994) and, in combination with dexamethasone, is superior to high-dose metoclopramide/dexamethasone therapy for cisplatin-based treatment (Heron et al, 1994).

In summary, the serotonin antagonists, ondansetron and granisetron, produce superior results when compared with other antiemetic drugs for acute emesis control, especially when combined with dexamethasone. Response rates and the side-effect profile are comparable (Ruff et al, 1994; Jantunen et al 1993; Navarri et al, 1995b), although cost differs and should be evaluated based on dose, number of prescribed doses, route, and individual patient factors (Cleri, 1995).

Phenothiazines and butyrophenones

The phenothiazines have been used for drug-induced nausea and vomiting for nearly 30 years (Moertel et al, 1963). Their effectiveness for chemotherapy-induced symptoms is restricted to those regimens with moderately low emetogenic potential. The intravenous route and higher doses (e.g., prochlorperazine 30 to 60 mg every 4 hours) have greater antiemetic activity but are also associated with more frequent and severe side effects, such as sedation, hypotension, and extrapyramidal side effects (akathisia, dystonia, parkinsonian symptoms, and rarely, oculogyric crisis). The incidence of akathisia, even with standard dosing, may be higher than expected and underreported by patients (Fleishman et al, 1994). Diphenhydramine or benztropine are recommended for preventing or managing extrapyramidal side effects. Patients, in particular those of younger age, need to be aware of the signs and symptoms of extrapyramidal side effects related to antiemetic therapy. Health care providers need to accurately assess patients to better discriminate antiemetic-induced akathisia from anxiety so that appropriate therapy is prescribed (Fleishman et al, 1994).

The phenothiazines are metabolized by the liver as glucuronides and sulfoxides and should be used with caution in patients with liver dysfunction.

The antiemetic effect is influenced by the route of administration. The same dose administered orally is predictably less effective than intravenous or intramuscular administration because of variable interpatient bioavailability. The onset of action also varies by route; the onset of action of tablets is within 30 to 40 minutes, the rectal route may take up to 1 hour to provide relief, and intramuscular injections generally take 10 to 20 minutes before they are effective.

Metoclopramide

At doses of 1 to 3 mg/kg, metoclopramide has been reported to completely prevent nausea and vomiting in up to 40% of patients receiving high-dose cisplatin (Sagar, 1990).

Greater efficacy (complete response, 70% to 80%) has been reported for lower-dose cisplatin and other moderate to high emetic regimens.

Optimal dose and schedule are controversial. For highly emetogenic chemotherapy, 2 to 3 mg/kg for two to six doses beginning at 30 minutes before chemotherapy and repeated every 2 hours appears to be the most effective (Kris et al, 1985), whereas a lower dose (1 mg/kg) may be adequate for moderately emetogenic therapy. Adverse effects include sedation, drowsiness, diarrhea, restlessness, dizziness, dysphoria, extrapyramidal reactions, and changes in blood pressure (Sheridan et al, 1982; Aapro et al, 1984). The incidence of extrapyramidal reactions has been observed to be significantly higher in patients younger than 30 years (Kris et al, 1983) and can usually be prevented with the administration of an anticholinergic drug such as diphenhydramine hydrochloride, scopolamine, or benztropine. Lorazepam is more effective at reducing the severity of akathisia.

Oral metoclopramide at comparable high doses appears equivalent to metoclopramide administered intravenously for acute nausea and vomiting

(Anthony et al, 1986). The combination of low-dose metoclopramide (e.g. 20 mg 3 times a day) and dexamethasone is a first-line therapy choice for delayed or residual nausea and vomiting (Cleri, 1995).

Benzodiazepines

The benzodiazepine drugs vary somewhat in their pharmacological spectrum, but as a class they are effective as a sedative, hypnotic, anxiolytic drug, muscle relaxant, and preanesthetic. Sedative effects can be achieved with lorazepam at doses of 0.5 to 3.0 mg, with minimal effect on respiratory and cardiovascular systems.

Lorazepam has minimal antiemetic activity but appears to have a role as an adjunct in combination antiemetic regimens because of its sedative and antianxiety effects and its ability to reduce extrapyramidal reactions. Kris et al (1987) compared diphenhydramine hydrochloride to lorazepam for prevention of metoclopramide-induced side effects. Although there was no reported difference in patient preference, lorazepam was associated with less restlessness, less recall and anxiety, fewer dystonic reactions, and increased sedation. Consideration of use should be based on assessment of the patient's anxiety level, the clinical setting, the risk of extrapyramidal reactions, and patient knowledge of the side effects. Patient acceptance of the sedative effects of this drug varies considerably, and treatment should be individualized based on the cited assessment parameters.

Cannabinoids

Delta-9-Tetrahydrocannabinol (THC, dronabinol, Marinol) and nabilone (Cesemet) have demonstrated activity against chemotherapy-induced nausea and vomiting, including patients refractory to conventional antiemetics. It is generally equal to or better than standard phenothiazines and may have greater effect (and less adverse effects) when combined with a phenothiazine (Lane et al, 1990).

Effect and outcome appear to be influenced by the age of the patient, attitudes and expectations, drug tolerance, dose, schedule, and administration.

Oral absorption is very slow (peak plasma concentrations may not occur until $1\frac{1}{2}$ to 3 hours after dosing) and erratic and may explain the findings that patients who experience a "high" achieve better antiemetic control than those who do not (Sallan, Zinberg, and Frei, 1975). In addition to the absorption problems, the other major limitation is toxicity. Sedation, dizziness, dry mouth, euphoria, dysphoria, anxiety, tachycardia, headache, ataxia, disorientation, and hallucinations limit the usefulness of the cannabinoids, especially in elderly patients.

Corticosteroids

Dexamethasone, the most commonly used steroid in antiemetic control of nausea and vomiting from chemotherapy, is effective alone for acute symptoms associated with drugs with low emetic potential and for delayed nausea after treatment. The most significant contribution of dexamethasone in preventing acute and delayed symptomatology is in combination with other antiemetic drugs (Kris et al, 1987; Roila et al, 1991; Cleri, 1995).

Although the primary focus is control of chemotherapy-induced nausea and vomiting, it is important to remember that hormonal therapy (e.g. estramustine and tamoxifen) as well as prescribed chemotherapy by the oral route may be associated with mild to moderate nausea. Patients should be routinely assessed for severity of symptoms and compliance with therapy.

Nonpharmacological Approaches to Nausea and Vomiting

Despite research efforts and advances in antiemetic therapy, drug therapy has failed to effectively control chemotherapy-induced nausea and vomiting in many patients. Many alternative approaches to drug therapy have been explored, including massage, distraction with music or art, and behavioral therapy (e.g., hypnosis, progressive muscle relaxation, biofeedback, systemic desensitization). These interventions have been shown to decrease the duration and frequency of nausea and vomiting and reduce anxiety levels (Cotanch and Strum, 1987; Frank, 1985; Burish et al, 1983).

Interest in behavioral therapy has grown, and many nurses and physicians are learning the techniques. It is hoped that continued research in this area will define the future role and benefit of behavioral treatment for chemotherapy-induced nausea and vomiting.

Consequences of Nausea and Vomiting

Nausea and vomiting can have debilitating effects on the patient's condition, especially when these effects occur in combination with already altered homeostatic function. Three major areas are affected by these problems: energy requirements, nutritional status, and fluid and electrolyte balance.

Energy requirements and nutritional status

The act of vomiting creates increased demands on the cardiovascular system. Inadequate oral intake and increased energy requirements are also obstacles in the process of rehabilitation of the cancer patient. Because of the systemic effects of nausea and vomiting, not only is ingested material unable to be retained, but the spontaneous desire to ingest food is impaired. Thus during a time when the promotion of healing and tissue repair is needed most, nutritional intake is often far below the necessary requirements. Patients who are malnourished are less likely to respond to chemotherapy and are less able to tolerate the side effects of antineoplastic therapy. Vomiting can impair the patient's ability to take oral medications such as leucovorin or dilantin, which can have serious consequences.

Fluid and electrolyte balance

Persistent nausea and vomiting cause severe disturbances in fluid and electrolyte balance. Metabolic alkalosis, resulting in hypokalemia and dehydration, causes an increased burden on the host nutritionally, physiologically, and emotionally. Dehydration can also increase the toxicity of nephrotoxic drugs. It is important to maintain accurate records of fluid loss, noting the time of onset of emesis and the frequency and intensity of emetic episodes.

Patients who experience nausea and vomiting must be made as comfortable as possible. Assessment should include the patient's previous experience and what has been helpful in the past so that care can be individualized.

The following suggestions may aid in decreasing the severity of this unpleasant GI toxicity:

- Provide a calm, reassuring environment
- Avoid foul smells
- Provide adequate room ventilation
- Use distraction techniques
- Offer antianxiety medications, if indicated
- Suggest peppermint oil (1 to 2 drops in water or soak a gauze pad for the aroma [Spross, 1987])
- Have emesis basin available, but out of sight
- Administer antiemetics prophylactically for acute and delayed emetic symptoms.

Anorexia and Taste Changes

Anorexia is simply the loss of appetite, although patients often may describe it in much stronger statements, such as "I can't stand the thought of food." Anorexia is the major cause of decreased dietary intake, and many factors contribute to this common patient symptom (Fig. 10-1). The duration of anorexia in a patient depends on the underlying cause. Transient anorexia is commonly associated with emotional distress, such as the initial diagnosis or diagnosis of a recurrence. This short-term anorexia is less likely to affect the patient's nutritional status as significantly as the anorexia associated with treatment or advanced disease, which is often chronic.

Changes in taste sensation and aversions to certain foods and food odors contribute to a decreased appetite in the cancer patient. Abnormalities include increased and decreased thresholds to sweet, sour, salty, and bitter tastes; a general loss of taste for food; metallic taste after drug therapy; and aversions to specific foods or liquids (Strohl, 1984).

Interventions for anorexia include pharmacological (e.g., steroids, megestrol) and nonpharmacological approaches, specifically dietary counseling, symptom management, psychosocial support, and nutritional support (Grant, 1987). The importance of eating despite anorexia should be emphasized, with food intake identified as a component of the treatment plan. Persuasion should never be used, nor should anger be shown with the patient for not eating. Satisfactory approaches often need to be discussed and reinforced with the family members.

For patients who experience a loss of sense of taste, a variety of pleasant food aromas may be substituted to stimulate appetite. A soothing aroma may pacify an unsettled stomach; therefore it is essential to know smells the patient likes or dislikes. Steam is aromatic, so food should be very hot when served. Also, sauces with a vanilla aroma or other essences may enhance certain desserts.

The interventions in Table 10-7 are recommended to enhance protein and caloric intake, maintain nutritional balance, and combat common problems.

Stomatitis

Oral toxicity from cancer chemotherapy is a significant treatment complication. Goals for minimizing oral toxicity and maintaining optimal

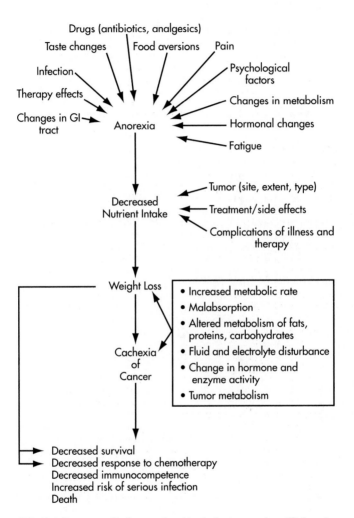

FIG. 10-1 Factors contributing to malnutrition in the cancer patient. *GI,* Gastrointestinal.

TABLE 10-7
Guidelines to Improve Food Intake

Alteration	Intervention
Taste changes	Suck on a sour candy or peppermint; rinse mouth before meals; avoid foods that are disliked; spice foods with mint, lemon, or basil; tart foods and seasonings may enhance flavor; marinate poultry and meats with sweet and sour sauces, Italian dressing, or sweet wines; use aromas to stimulate taste and appetite; suggest high-protein foods (eggs, cottage cheese, yogurt) for meat aversions
Loss of appetite	Try favorite foods, especially those high in calories; eat small meals more often; avoid greasy and fried foods; encourage patients to eat with family and friends; provide high-calorie, high-protein snacks; keep patients out of the kitchen during food preparation if possible; concentrate on calories; exercise for 5 to 10 min about 30 min before meals; avoid stress at mealtimes
Fatigue	Encourage eating the most nutritious meal in the morning; plan rest periods; avoid meals being served directly after a treatment or procedure; offer foods that do not require a lot of chewing
Dry mouth	Provide moist foods; use gravies and sauces to thin consistency; supply sugarless gum or candy to stimulate saliva, especially lemon drops; drink liquids throughout the day; avoid alcoholic beverages; avoid spicy or acidic foods; use artificial saliva
Bloating	Avoid greasy, fried foods; avoid carbonated beverages and gas-producing foods (beans, broccoli, carrots) and milk; provide small, frequent meals; encourage the patient to eat slowly
Dehydration	Supply juices, fruitades, soft drinks, broth; serve fruits with high water content (e.g., grapes and watermelon); offer jello, sherbet, and popsicles
Indigestion	Serve small, frequent meals; avoid spicy and greasy foods; avoid milk and milk products; give antacid 1 to 2 hours before meals and at bedtime; avoid alcohol and smoking; do not lie down immediately after eating
Nausea and vomiting	Take antiemetic medication before usual mealtimes; avoid favorite foods at this time; assess contributing factors (e.g., chemotherapy, narcotics, antibiotics); perform frequent oral care
Mucositis	Avoid acidic, grainy, raw foods; avoid very hot or cold temperatures; use pain-control measures before eating; eat soft-textured, bland foods
Difficulty swallowing	Use butter, gravy, and cream sauces; follow soft diet; cut food into small pieces; have small, frequent meals; avoid smoking and drinking alcoholic beverages; eat in an upright position, preferably in a chair; eat custards and puddings and drink milkshakes; avoid coarse, rough foods and bread

oral health focus on decreasing periodontal disease and oral infections, promoting adequate nutrition, facilitating verbal communication, and continuing treatment.

Poor oral hygiene is an important predisposing factor to oral complications of chemotherapy. Lack of regular, daily oral hygiene results in increased plaque buildup and calculus, producing short-term effects of gum irritation and dental caries and long-term effects of infection and periodontal disease with potential tooth loss. Contributing risk factors include poor nutrition, history of chronic oral infections, old age, alcohol consumption, smoking, and stress.

All patients should have an oral examination before myelosuppressive therapy. Routine dental hygiene procedures are recommended before chemotherapy with predicted neutropenia, and dental work should be performed for existing problems such as periodontal disease, extensive dental caries, or defective dental restorations (Peterson, 1992).

Preventive oral care

Dental hygiene practices and instructions for self-oral examination with a mirror should be reviewed with each patient. Preventive oral care should begin at the start of treatment in an attempt to prevent or minimize superinfection of the ulcerated lesions. Health care providers should perform routine oral assessments (Table 10-8).

The toothbrush is the most effective instrument for mechanical cleansing and plaque removal. Rinsing and flossing provide additional cleansing activity and aid in removal of food particles. Brushing is recommended after meals and before bed. For proper brushing, the toothbrush is held at a 45-degree angle at the junction of the tooth and gum. With a back-and-forth motion, 10 strokes are used for each two teeth. Unwaxed dental floss should be wrapped around the side of the tooth and carefully brought into the space between the tooth and gum with a gentle up-and-down motion 3 or 4 times. Flossing straight up and down should be avoided since that will injure the gum. Two alternatives to unwaxed dental floss are waxed dental tape and a double strand of waxed floss (Carter, 1992).

If the patient has dental prostheses, they should be brushed and placed in water until rinsing and cleansing of the oral cavity is completed. Mouthwash is an additional cleanser, but a commercial mouthwash is generally contraindicated because of the alcohol content and subsequent drying effect on the oral mucosa. The alcohol content of some common mouthwashes ranges from 9% to 27%. Patient education should include reminding patients and family members to check labels for content. Sodium chloride 0.9% solution, which is isotonic, nonirritating, and inexpensive, is preferred (Daeffler, 1980).

Dentures or denturelike appliances create an excellent harbor not only for fungus but for bacteria, since the denture usually contains porous and crazed areas of recessed sanctuaries (Toth and Frame, 1983). Prosthodontic appliances may also cause further mucosal injury, especially if the appliance does not fit well. Some dentists involved in oncological care recommend keeping all prosthodontic appliances out of the mouth during chemotherapy.

TABLE 10-8
Oral Assessment

Rating	Voice	Swallow	Lips	Tongue	Saliva	Mucous membranes	Gingiva	Teeth, dentures
1	Normal	Normal	Smooth, pink, moist	Pink, moist, papillae present	Watery	Pink, moist	Pink, firm	Clean, no debris present
2	Deep or raspy	Some pain	Dry or cracked	Coated or loss of papillae, with/without redness	Thick or ropy	Reddened or coated	Edematous	Plaque or debris in localized areas
3	Difficulty talking, painful	Unable to swallow	Ulcerated or bleeding	Blistered or cracked	Absent	Ulcerations with or without bleeding	Bleeding	Generalized plaque or debris

Modified from University of Nebraska Medical Center, Educational Services Department of Halbrand, Inc., 1985.

Chemotherapy-induced stomatitis

The cells of the oral mucosa are highly proliferative, with a life span of 10 to 14 days, and are susceptible to the damaging effects of some of the antineoplastic agents. Actual cell loss occurs with ulceration and denuded mucosa. As early as 3 days after the initiation of chemotherapy, oral erythematous mucositis may be evident (Toth and Frame, 1983). Early subjective symptoms may be increased sensitivity to hot and cold foods and intolerance to citrus juices.

Histological changes may be evident after 7 days of treatment, with signs of atrophic epithelium and loss of basal cell surfaces. The ulcerative form of mucositis then becomes clinically apparent and persists for 4 to 7 days (Daeffler, 1980). Signs and symptoms of mucositis often parallel the myelosuppressive pattern.

Ulcerations occur most frequently on the buccal mucosa and tongue but may appear anywhere on the mucosal surface from the lips to the esophagus. The cell-cyclespecific agents are more likely to produce this toxicity, with antibiotics and antimetabolites as major offenders. The drugs most frequently associated with stomatitis are bleomycin, dactinomycin, daunorubicin, docetaxel, doxorubicin, edetrexate, 5-fluorouracil, methotrexate, tomudex, and high-dose therapy with busulfan, etoposide, melphalan, and thiotepa. Less commonly associated drugs include cytarabine, plicamycin (mithramycin), mitomycin, 6-mercaptopurine, paclitaxel, 6-thioguanine, vinblastine, and vincristine.

The occurrence and severity of stomatitis are influenced by dose, schedule of drugs, combination drug therapy, and impairment of renal and hepatic function.

Prophylaxis

Performance of routine, systematic oral care appears to be a significant factor in reducing the degree of stomatitis and infectious complications (Beck, 1979; Graham et al, 1993). Although many cleansing and rinsing solutions have been studied for their role in preventing or reducing complications from stomatitis, water, saline, sodium bicarbonate, and hydrogen peroxide remain the most commonly used in practice (Madeya, 1996). Research on the prevention of mucositis with chlorhexidine (Peridex) in hospitalized patients who receive high-dose therapy has produced conflicting results (Ferretti et al, 1990; Epstein et al, 1992; Weisdorf et al, 1989). In a study of 227 outpatients receiving chemotherapy who followed a systematic oral assessment and management protocol, no differences in incidence, onset, or severity of mucositis were observed between those who used chlorhexidine versus those who used water (Dodd et al, 1996). Disadvantages of chlorhexidine include complaints of burning and staining of teeth and dental prostheses. The burning may be related to the alcohol content (11.6%), and further work is needed to confirm efficacy, any long-term toxicity to the oral tissues, and the cost effectiveness.

Treatment of stomatitis

The goal of oral care for the patient at risk or with stomatitis is to maintain the integrity of the oral mucosa, prevent secondary infection, provide pain relief, and maintain dietary intake. Prevention and management strategies begin with oral assessment. A variety of oral assessment guides are available (Iwamoto, 1996), and one example is provided in Table 10-8. Choice of a specific assessment guide should be based on the patient population and risk of the severity and predicted complications of stomatitis. General principles of care include brushing, rinsing, use of fluoride (toothpaste, dental floss), lip lubricants, and routine oral care, the frequency of which is influenced by the presence and severity of stomatitis (Table 10-9). There are multiple instruments, cleansing agents, rinsing solutions, and lubricants with cited advantages and disadvantages for use in clinical practice (Goodman et al, 1993; Iwamoto, 1996; Madeya, 1996). The most commonly accepted care includes a toothbrush as the instrument of choice.

If a toothbrush cannot be used, a foam brush soaked with chlorhexidine is an alternative, but a foam brush alone will not provide the same effectiveness in reducing plaque and gingivitis (Ransier et al, 1995). Cleansing agents include saline, sodium bicarbonate, or a combination of the two. Hydrogen peroxide has been used, but the efficacy and safety continue to be questioned (Iwamoto, 1996; Madeya, 1996). No superior topical agent for the relief of discomfort and pain associated with stomatitis has been identified, but a variety are available (Table 10-10) and should be selected based on the individual patient and practical application in the patient's care plan. Oral care should also include assessment for infection, especially in high-risk patients, and the stomatitis oral care program must be integrated into the infection-management plan (Peterson, 1992).

Diarrhea

Diarrhea in cancer patients may be related to a number of causes, such as anxiety, a change in diet, medication, infection, radiation, tumor, obstruction, and chemotherapy. The GI tract is susceptible to chemotherapy toxicity because of the rapid turnover of the mucosal cells, particularly with cell-cyclespecific agents. Diarrhea has been observed in as many as 75% of patients who receive chemotherapy. The agents most commonly associated with diarrhea are aminocamptothecin, cytarabine, dactinomycin, 5-azacytidine, 5-fluorouracil (especially in combination with high-dose leucovorin), hydroxyurea, irinotecan, methotrexate, mitotane, tomudex, and topotecan.

As with other chemotherapy-related toxicity, the dose, schedule, and combination of drugs influence the incidence and severity of a side effect, such as diarrhea. Knowledge of the significance of this symptom, consistent and reliable assessment parameters, and standard interventions are limited. The Oncology Nursing Society's Working Group on Diarrhea Management has begun to develop such a database to identify content areas for patient and family education and to target management interventions for specific patient populations (Engelking and Rutledge, 1996).

Persistent diarrhea requires intervention to minimize complications of dehydration, electrolyte imbalance, weakness, decreased caloric intake, and weight loss. The bowel must be allowed to rest and recuperate, and a regular diet should not be maintained during symptomatic periods. Suggestions for control of diarrhea include the following (Fedak, 1981):

Nutrition
- Eat a low-residue diet high in protein and calories

TABLE 10-9
Guide for Management of Stomatitis

Assessment	Sign or symptom	Intervention	Goal and rationale
Mild	Erythema, oral discomfort, burning, dryness	Brush teeth every 4 hr while awake using a nonabrasive fluoride toothpaste and soft-bristled brush; rinse with a solution of normal saline, baking soda (1 tsp in 500 mL of water) or a combination (1000 mL water with 1 tsp salt and 1 tsp baking soda); floss teeth with unwaxed dental floss or tape every day; apply lubricating jelly or artificial saliva to lips if dry or cracked; avoid irritants to the oral mucosa such as alcohol, spicy foods, and cigarette smoking	Maintain optimal condition and integrity of oral tissues; deterioration of the oral mucosa can begin within 6 hr if no oral care is performed; prevention of infection; normal saline rinse—it is isotonic, nonirritating, has no unpleasant taste, and is inexpensive; it is thought to aid in promoting healing and granulation of tissue; baking soda rinse—it is a good cleanser, particularly effective for thick saliva, mucous crusts, debris, and odor; patients may complain of an unpleasant taste; combining it with a normal saline rinse or flavoring it with a non-alcohol mouthwash may help; warn patients on sodium restriction about potential absorption

Continued

TABLE 10-9
Guide for Management of Stomatitis—cont'd

Assessment	Sign or symptom	Intervention	Goal and rationale
Moderate-severe	Burning, pain, difficulty swallowing, sensitivity to hot and cold, ulceration, bleeding, inflammation	Oral care every 1-3 hr; continue to use a soft toothbrush and floss unless it is too painful or bleeding occurs; a toothette or a 4 × 4-in. piece of gauze soaked in a rinsing solution can be used as an alternative; rinse with normal saline, baking soda, or a combination of the two; for patients who have trouble swishing or gargling, irrigate the mouth using a WaterPic, Asepto syringe, or an irrigating bag with tubing	Prevent infection and maintain integrity of oral mucosa; the toothbrush is superior to the toothette for oral hygiene, but one must weigh the risk of trauma with brushing and flossing, especially for the neutropenic and thrombocytopenic patient; the rationale for a normal saline or sodium bicarbonate rinse has been described; a Hibiclens 0.12% chlorhexidine gluconate mouthwash (Peridex, or 0.2% solution of 1:19 Hibiclens; alcohol-free mouthwash) as a mouth rinse used three times daily for patients is an alternative rinse
		Use lubricating jelly or artificial saliva on the lips; if the lips are crusted, cleanse with a 4 × 4-in. piece of gauze soaked in baking soda first	Artificial saliva aids in maintaining a normal pH of the oral cavity (6.6-6.9); minimize discomfort and maximize nutritional intake
		Apply local analgesics before meals, at bedtime, and as needed (see Table 10-10); consider systemic analgesia if pain relief is inadequate with local treatment	Application of local analgesics before meals will optimize comfort while eating or drinking; although there is a known sensitivity to hot and cold, refrigeration of cleansing or local analgesic preparations frozen into popsicles can create a numbing effect and vasoconstriction that may decrease bleeding complications and intake problems

TABLE 10-10
Topical Analgesia for Stomatitis

Treatment	Administration	Advantages and disadvantages
COATING AGENTS		
Orabase	Apply small amounts directly to tissues	Contains mineral oil, so aspiration is a potential concern, but it does provide protection to the mucosa; fast onset of action but short duration (<15 minutes)
Oratect-gel	Apply to dry lesions up to four times daily	Provides protective film for up to 2 hours
Kaopectate	10 mL to coat oral tissues	Kaopectate can provide relief by coating mucosa; the
Kaopectate/Benadryl Elixir		combination may increase local comfort by maintaining prolonged-contact analgesic with the oral tissues
Milk of magnesia	10 mL to coat oral tissues	Effect is short term and if not fully rinsed out, remaining solutions will dry out the oral mucosa.
Stomafate suspension	Swish/spit or swish/swallow	Sucralfate known to promote healing of ulceration, and combination of agents may enhance comfort by coating of tissues (suspension = sucralfate, 12 g; sterile water, 60 mL; Benylin syrup, 60 mL; Maalox suspension, 180 mL qs, good for 1 mo)
Vitamin E	Puncture capsule and apply directly on lesions	Benefit unknown; may provide relief and promote healing
Zilactin	Apply to lesions up to 4 times daily	Provides protective film coating over oral ulcers; patients may experience mild burning on application

Continued

TABLE 10-10
Topical Analgesia for Stomatitis—cont'd

Treatment	Administration	Advantages and disadvantages
TOPICAL ANESTHETIC AGENTS		
Dyclone 0.5%	5-10 mL swish/spit every 3-4 hr	Onset of pain relief within 10 min lasting up to 1 hr; contains no alcohol, but many patients complain of local discomfort on contact with the oral tissues
Benadryl Elixir	5-10 mL swish/spit every 3-4 hr	Request a low-alcohol content elixir, since the alcohol may cause burning; an alternative is to dissolve Benadryl capsules in water and add something with a strong flavor to reduce the bitter taste from the content of the capsule
Dyclone 0.5%/Benadryl Elixir	5-10 mL swish/spit every 3-4 hr	The combination of the analgesic and antithistamine may enhance the effect (30 mL of Dyclone 0.5% and 60 mL of Benadryl Elixir); analgesia may be enhanced by pouring over crushed ice in a 30-mL medicine cup and sipped
Ulcerase	Rinse or gargle every 2-3 hr, then expectorate	Patients report effect lasting up to 1 hr; free of alcohol and sugars
Xylocaine 2% Viscous	5-10 mL swish/spit	Duration is short term (20 min), and it may cause numbness of the tongue and interfere with swallowing

- Eliminate irritating or stimulating foods and beverages (e.g., whole-grain products, fried or greasy foods, fresh fruits, vegetables, products containing caffeine, and citrus juices)
- Eat foods and drink liquids high in potassium (e.g., baked potato, asparagus, bananas, Gatorade, and Kool-aid)
- Drink at least 3000 mL of noncarbonated fluid each day (bouillon, apple or grape juice, noncarbonated beverages, and Gatorade); avoid cola drinks (Weizman, 1986)
- Eat small, frequent meals
- Avoid extremes in food temperature
- Avoid milk and milk products; restart milk intake slowly after symptoms subside
- Use antidiarrheal medications

Comfort
- Use local heat to abdomen to minimize discomfort caused by cramping
- Rest to conserve energy
- Take a warm-water sitz bath
- Use topical applications of an anesthetic or ointment on the rectal area to enhance comfort and promote healing (e.g., Tucks, Desitin, Benzocaine, A and D ointment)
- Minimize stress and anxiety
- Use antidiarrheal medications (e.g., bulk-forming agents, narcotics)

Constipation

Constipation is defined as the infrequent, difficult passage of hard, dry stool. Frequency, size, consistency, and ease of passage of stool are the major criteria for assessment of bowel function (Cimprich, 1985). Symptoms include excessive straining, sensation of incomplete evacuation, abdominal cramping, discomfort with or without distention, and a feeling of fullness or pressure in the rectum. Prevention is the major therapeutic goal. Assessment should include a dietary history, age, usual elimination patterns, history of bowel alterations and management, mobility, and drugs.

General guidelines for prevention of constipation include the following (Gross, 1994):

1. Increase fiber in the diet (e.g., vegetables, fruits, nuts, raisins, and bran)
2. Add prunes or prune juice to the diet
3. Drink adequate amounts of fluid daily—at least eight glasses
4. Engage in light exercise
5. Plan a regular time every day, about 20 minutes, to sit on the toilet or commode, uninterrupted, in an attempt to defecate
6. Drink hot liquids that may stimulate bowel activity
7. Use bulk producers (Metamucil, Mitrolan), a stool softener, or both
8. Consider laxative use for patients who do not respond to these measures. Decreased mobility, older age, diuretics, anticholinergics, phenothiazines, antidepressants, iron preparations, laxative abuse, low-fiber diet, depressed mood, ignoring of the body's signal to defecate,

narcotics, and hemorrhoids are potential causes of constipation. Any or all of these causes may be present in the cancer patient. High-risk factors for the patient with cancer include tumor location, narcotics, immobility, older age, decreased oral intake, metabolic abnormalities (hypercalcemia, hypokalemia, hypomagnesemia), and chemotherapy with vinca alkaloids (Portenoy, 1987; Wrenn, 1989).

9. Narcotic analgesics predictably produce constipation, and the effect is dose related. Dietary changes and a bulk laxative are usually insufficient, and a stool softener with a gentle laxative should be included in a prophylactic bowel program for any patient receiving narcotic medication (Levy, 1985). The senna compounds, anthraquinone cathartics that stimulate the longitudinal peristalsis in the colon, have been shown to regularly reverse narcotic-induced constipation (Maguire, Yon, and Miller, 1981). For optimal results, the cathartic should be taken at the same time as the narcotic or on a similar schedule. Senokot tablets are the standardized senna concentrate, and dosing varies from one to two tablets every day up to four tablets twice daily. For patients who need a stool softener, Senokot-S includes the standardized senna concentrate and a stool softener, dioctyl sodium sulfosuccinate. Although there is great individual variety, the general goal should be a bowel movement every 2 to 3 days. If no bowel movement occurs after that time, a more aggressive approach, such as saline laxatives, sorbitol, lactulose (Table 10-11), or suppositories, is indicated, with careful monitoring for potential impaction (Levy, 1985). Protecting the integrity of the rectal mucosa of the patient who is leukopenic or thrombocytopenic is a priority, and a prophylactic bowel regimen is essential to prevent the need for suppositories or enemas, which are contraindicated in this patient population.

DERMATOLOGICAL TOXICITY

Antineoplastic therapy can produce both local and systemic dermatological toxicities. Local toxicity occurs in the tissues surrounding the site of drug administration and is described by a variety of venous and cutaneous responses: phlebitis, urticaria, pain, erythema, vein discoloration, and tissue necrosis secondary to extravasation of a drug.

Systemically, hair loss is the most common manifestation, but erythematous rashes, pruritus, dermatitis, and hyperpigmentation are reported with chemotherapy toxicity. Although most cutaneous reactions are short lived and associated with minimal physical morbidity, nurses and physicians must be alert to potential reactions, keep the patient informed, institute prompt interventions, and continually assess for potential psychological morbidity associated with alterations in body image.

Alopecia

Fear and anxiety are common responses for patients who learn that they may lose their hair as a result of treatment. The actual experience of complete or nearly complete hair loss has often been described by patients as

TABLE 10-11
Prevention and Management of Constipation

Category	Agents	Onset of action (hr)	Mechanism	Side effects	Comments
Bulk producers	Methylcellulose, polycarbophil, psyllium	12–24 (up to 72)	Hydrophilic agents absorb water from the gut; softens and increases the size of stool	Bloating, flatulence, or abdominal cramping may develop; increase bulk gradually	Dietary fiber is the single best source of bulk; the effect of bulk laxatives may not be apparent for a few days; adequate fluid intake is essential; avoid administering psyllium with salicylates, nitrofurantoin, and digitalis; may decrease action of these drugs
Saline laxatives	Magnesium sulfate, milk of magnesia, magnesium citrate, sodium phosphate, Phospho-soda	0.5–3	Unabsorbed solutes retain water and increase fluid in the colon; fluid accumulation distends bowel and induces peristaltic movement	Strong cathartic effect; may be associated with abdominal cramping, flatulence, and liquid stools	Do not promote return of normal bowel function; are most useful as a preparation for diagnostic tests; avoid magnesium laxatives with renal dysfunction; avoid sodium laxatives in patients with edema, congestive heart failure, and hypertension

Continued

TABLE 10-11
Prevention and Management of Constipation—cont'd

Category	Agents	Onset of action (hr)	Mechanism	Side effects	Comments
Stimulant laxatives	Cascara sagrada, casanthranol, senna, phenolphthalein,	6–10	Stimulates peristalsis in the colon	Electrolyte disturbances and bowel changes with prolonged use	The senna compounds are effective in reversing narcotic-induced constipation; results are best if taken with the narcotic or on a similar schedule (Maguire and Yon, 1981); phenolphthalein and bisacodyl may be excreted in the bile to be active; not effective in biliary obstruction or diversion
	Castor oil	2–6			
	Bisacodyl suppository 0.25–1				
Softeners	Docusate, polaxer	24–72	Promotes water retention, softens stool; no laxative action	—	Good to prevent straining; most beneficial when stool is hard
Miscellaneous	Sorbitol, lactulose	24–48	Lactulose and sorbitol are osmotic cathartics, are effective in treatment of resistant vincristine-induced constipation; act only in the colon with no evidence of tolerance	Diarrhea; may cause electrolyte disturbance with prolonged use in the elderly	Use with caution in diabetics because it contains galactose and lactose; patient compliance may be enhanced if it is mixed with water, milk, or juice; is good for long-term treatment and protects against laxative abuse
	Mineral oil	6–8			
	Glycerin suppository	0.25–0.5			

Modified from the National Cancer Institute: *PDQ cancer information, supportive care statement: constipation, impaction and bowel obstruction,* 1992.

the most devastating side effect of chemotherapy. Hair is an integral part of physical appearance, and its loss may negatively affect self-image, body image, coping skills, and social interactions. The degree of distress may be minimized by adequate preparation for the loss, possible interventions, and ongoing support from health care professionals and family members.

The cells and tissues responsible for hair differentiation and growth have very high mitotic and metabolic rates. The germinative tissue of an average hair root produces 0.35 mm of hair shaft every 24 hours, and in doing so, each day the majority of the cell population is duplicated.

The chemotherapy drugs that act in the DNA synthesis and mitosis phases of the cell cycle do not differentiate between actively replicating normal cells and malignant cells. Therefore the hair is sacrificed either by partial or complete damage to the hair shaft or root. Cell destruction of the hair root is associated with complete or nearly complete alopecia. The hair either falls out spontaneously or is lost when combing, usually in large clumps. If the hair shaft is damaged, resulting in constriction caused by the resulting atrophy or necrosis, the hair will break off easily at the point of constriction. If the root is not destroyed, a patchy, thinning pattern of hair loss will result. Hair loss can be described as minimal, moderate, or severe, which corresponds to toxicity criteria of Grades 1, 2, and 3 as follows:

1. *Minimal loss:* Less than 25% of hair; obvious to the patient but not necessarily to others.
2. *Moderate loss:* 25% to 50% of hair; obvious thinning of scalp hair but not enough to indicate the use of a wig or alternative head covering.
3. *Severe loss:* More than 50% of hair; extensive hair loss generally indicating the need for a wig or alternative head covering.

Hair loss from chemotherapy is reversible. Many times hair begins to regrow despite continued therapy, and it is not unusual for new hair to reappear 2 to 3 months later. Hair growth during treatment can be explained by a certain percentage of the hair being in a "resting" phase when the initial insult from chemotherapy was received. Drugs mainly affect growing hairs (anagen phase), which accounts for 85% of the hair follicles on the human scalp. Since the anagen phase is approximately 3 months for scalp hair, it is common not to see hair regrowth for 3 to 5 months.

Chemotherapeutic agents most frequently associated with hair loss are aminocamptothecin, cyclophosphamide, doxorubicin, dactinomycin, daunorubicin, etoposide, idarubicin, ifosfamide, irinotecan, mechlorethamine, paclitaxel, topotecan, and vincristine. Drugs described as less frequently associated because of a lower incidence and/or a lesser degree of alopecia include bleomycin, carmustine, epirubicin, 5-fluorouracil, methotrexate, melphalan, mitomycin, mitoxantrone, teniposide, and vinorelbine.

Although we know the drugs most likely to produce hair loss, the dose, scheduling, route of administration, pharmacokinetics, and combination drug therapy significantly challenge our predictive accuracy. For example, the route of cyclophosphamide (oral versus intravenous) is an important factor in predicting the incidence and degree of hair loss when used in combination with 5-fluorouracil, methotrexate, and/or doxorubicin (CMF, CAF). The risk of hair loss and degree of severity is more predictable with intravenous as opposed to oral cyclophosphamide when administered with methotrexate and fluorouracil, and complete hair loss is virtually certain with the combination of doxorubicin and cyclophosphamide. High-dose alkylating-agent therapy is also associated with a very predictable complete hair loss risk.

The impact of hair loss and acceptance of potential alternatives should be carefully assessed for each patient. Preparatory information is an important component in minimizing distress associated with potential hair loss. We must strive to be as accurate as possible in predicting the risk, degree of severity, and timing of drug-induced hair loss.

There are a wide variety of non–cancer-therapy drugs and patient conditions that can produce alopecia. Examples include heparin, propranolol, high doses of vitamin A, androgens, hypothyroidism, iron deficiency, and malnutrition (Keller and Blausey, 1988).

Prevention

The scalp is supplied by superficial blood vessels that can be fairly easily occluded for a short time by pressure without local tissue damage. Strategies to prevent toxicity to the hair follicles were based on the use of local pressure or hypothermia to reduce or prevent blood supply to the hair follicles until the plasma concentration of the drug has decreased or disappeared. Early reports described the use of tightly tied tourniquets, but this method is not recommended because of the difficulty of equalizing the pressure on underlying tissues and concern about potential nerve damage.

In the 1970s, clinical research on scalp cooling began with patients receiving doxorubicin and was based on the findings that tissue uptake of the drug was a temperature-sensitive process (Luce et al, 1973). Early attempts with bags of crushed ice secured to the head to form a turban were followed by more sophisticated products such as cryogel bags, cold packs, and thermocirculators. The primary indication for scalp cooling is with drugs that are administered over a short period and that disappear rapidly from the bloodstream, such as doxorubicin, vincristine, vinblastine, dactinomycin, and mechlorethamine. Scalp hypothermia is contraindicated for patients with hematological malignancies who are at high risk for central nervous system dissemination and patients with cutaneous T-cell lymphoma. For patients with solid tumors who may be at greater risk for scalp metastases, this intervention has become very controversial (Keller and Blausey, 1988; Siepp, 1983). Even though patients at risk for scalp metastases constitute a very small percentage of all those treated who might benefit, the Food and Drug Administration (FDA) halted commercial sale of scalp-cooling devices until additional clinical data are submitted ensuring their safety and efficacy (Camp-Sorrell, 1991). The FDA action, combined with variable results of the efficacy of scalp cooling as a preventive strategy and the time for nurses to implement the intervention, has almost eliminated its use in clinical practice. In practice, a percentage of patients remain very distressed about potential hair loss and desire some protective intervention. Several institutions have decided to respond to patient requests for scalp hypothermia as a preventive measure, provided that the risks and benefits are clearly presented and an informed consent is obtained (Camp-Sorrell, 1991).

Management

Nurses, physicians, and pharmacists should make every effort to correct misconceptions and provide accurate information. Patients are shocked when they experience hair loss unexpectedly, and the purchase of a wig or head covering before loss of more than 50% of hair occurs may decrease the distress. Interventions to help maximize patient adjustment and minimize the distress associated with hair loss include the following:

1. Explain to the patient the rationale for the occurrence of alopecia, the relative incidence, and the degree of hair loss expected specific to the chemotherapy drug(s) prescribed.
2. Encourage the patient to express emotions regarding the information provided.
3. Reiterate the fact that hair regrows and that changes in color or texture may occur. It is common for hair to grow back in curly, whereas a change of color (e.g., to gray) is uncommon.
4. Suggest the use of wigs, colorful scarves, and hats. Explore insurance coverage for the use of wigs as prosthetic devices for the head. Patients should purchase wigs before total hair loss occurs. Consultation with the patient's hairdresser for styling is recommended. Information about supportive programs such as the "Look Good, Feel Better Program" should also be provided. Check with your local program for the scope of services offered for men, women, and children. For treatment associated with a very high risk of hair loss, some patients have chosen to have their heads shaved, which they report as less stressful than dealing with hair continuously falling out.
5. Discourage the use of dryers, hot rollers, and curling irons, since they may facilitate increased hair loss.
6. Protect the head from the sun with a hat or sunscreen if complete or nearly complete alopecia has occurred. Maintain scalp cleanliness and conditioning after total alopecia.

Drugs with potential for local toxicity

Potential local toxic effects from chemotherapeutic drugs range from transient local discomfort during administration to severe tissue necrosis with potential damage to tendons and nerves. There is a lack of uniformity in the literature classifying drugs according to their toxic potential. Chemotherapeutic drugs have been described as irritants, vesicants, and those associated with acute local reactions such as erythema, phlebitis, urticaria, and pain.

An irritant is a drug that often produces a local venous response with or without a skin reaction. Complaints of tenderness along the vein and burning are common and may be accompanied by erythema. These symptoms are usually short lived, subsequent tissue damage is uncommon, and necrosis does not occur. Some irritant drugs, such as doxorubicin, also have well-known vesicant properties. Others, such as vinorelbine may have suspected vesicant potential (ONS, 1996). A vesicant is a drug that produces an irritant reaction so severe that plasma escapes from the extracellular space, blisters are formed, and tissue destruction results. Drugs have been described as vesicants by degree (i.e., severe, moderate), as a potential vesicant, or as having vesicant properties. The lack of knowledge and consistent

TABLE 10-12
Local Tissue Injury of Selected Chemotherapeutic Drugs

Long-term injury	Short-term injury
Dactinomycin	Carmustine
Daunorubicin	Cisplatin
Doxorubicin	Etoposide
Epirubicin	5-Fluorouracil
Idarubicin	Mechlorethamine
Mitomycin	Plicamycin
	Vinblastine
	Vincristine
	Vinorelbine

terminology about which drugs will produce tissue necrosis makes decisions about management of drug extravasations a practice challenge (Boyle and Engelking, 1996). Rudolph and Larson (1987) suggest classifying drugs according to their tissue nucleic acid binding affinity. Drugs that do not bind to DNA cause tissue damage immediately, but are either inactivated or quickly metabolized and followed by the normal healing process. Drugs that bind to DNA also produce immediate tissue damage, but in contrast, they remain in the tissues, resulting in long-term injury (Table 10-12). This proposed concept, supported by laboratory data, demonstrates that anthracycline levels can persist in the tissues for several months and supports the clinical observations of lack of spontaneous healing, progressive ulceration, delayed skin reactions, recall phenomena, and the necessity of complete surgical excision for cure (Argenta and Manders, 1983; Duray, Cuono, and Madri, 1986; Wood and Ellerhorst-Ryan, 1984).

Extravasation prevention

Extravasation is the escape of a chemotherapeutic drug from a vessel to the surrounding tissues, either by leakage or direct infiltration. Morbidity from extravasation depends on the particular drug being administered, the amount extravasated, its concentration, and the delay in recognition and treatment.

The onset of symptoms may occur immediately or several days to weeks after drug administration. Immediate symptoms commonly described are discomfort, burning, and erythema. Pain, edema, induration, ulceration, and necrosis often occur later.

For peripheral drug administration, the risk of extravasation can be minimized by prudent site selection, good venipuncture technique, and careful drug administration. Cancer patients at high risk for complications from chemotherapy administration include those with preexisting vascular disease, malnutrition, small or fragile veins, previous chemotherapy, combination chemotherapy, axillary lymphadenectomy, and prior radiation to potential infusion sites. Recent skin testing may also limit vein choice, since infusions passing over the site of skin testing may result in extravascular leakage (Welch-McCaffrey and Kenneally, 1983).

The general principle in site selection is to choose an area that will offer the best protection to tendons and nerves and cause the least loss of function if extravasation occurs. Generally, one should avoid areas of recent chemotherapy administration and prior irradiation and extremities with lymphedema or prior axillary dissection. Venipuncture sites that are 24 hours old or less should be noted and infusion sites distal to these avoided (Harwood, 1986). An area in the forearm, preferably the upper part of the forearm, is the optimal site because of the presence of extensive soft tissue. The dorsum of the hand and joints are not recommended because of the potential damage to tendons and neurovascular structures, the potential for contractures or functional loss, and the difficulty posed by these sites for successful surgical interventions (Rudolph and Larson, 1987).

Ignoffo and Friedman (1980) recommend an ordered preference for site selection: forearm, dorsum of the hand, wrist, and then antecubital fossa. Although the antecubital fossa is recognized for its large veins that often are easily accessible, it is the least favorable alternative because important arteries and veins are located there. Extravasation may be more difficult to detect there because of the amount of subcutaneous tissue, resulting in a greater concentration of drug infiltration and subsequent functional loss of a major joint temporarily, or perhaps permanently, from contractures.

The following general guidelines regarding venipuncture and infusion are provided to minimize the risk of extravasation:

1. Select a small-gauge (e.g., 21-gauge) cannula, either a steel needle or a polyethylene catheter.
2. Begin a new infusion for drug administration.
3. If venipuncture is unsuccessful, make a second attempt in the opposite arm. If the same arm must be used, choose a site proximal to the first venipuncture and make sure it is not the same vein.
4. Infuse normal saline or an appropriate IV solution to test vein patency.
5. Instruct the patient to report immediately any changes in sensation, particularly pain, burning, or stinging.
6. Administer vesicant drugs one at a time through the side arm or Y connection of the IV line (ONS, 1996). Administer the drug slowly, checking for continued patency by allowing IV fluid to flow in freely or by withdrawing blood. Observe constantly for signs of infiltration. Do *not* pinch the IV tubing while administering the drug because it may increase the pressure, especially in a small vein, and cause extravascular leakage.
7. Infuse at least 20 mL of solution after drug administration.

Central venous access devices are recommended for continuous infusion of vesicant chemotherapy because of the decreased risk of extravasation. The risk of extravasation is not eliminated, however, with peripherally placed or centrally placed catheters. Backflow caused by fibrin sheath formation, needle dislodgement from port reservoir, and catheter damage or malposition have been causative factors in drug extravasation (Camp-Sorrell, 1992; Mayo and Pearson, 1995;

ONS, 1996). The guidelines used to ensure patency of central devices serve as the basis for proceeding with drug administration, especially regarding the ability to withdraw blood. If a blood return is not established, a chest radiograph or dye study is indicated before administration of a vesicant. These studies will confirm catheter placement and identify any fibrin sheath formation that may cause potential backtracking of the drug (Mayo and Pearson, 1995).

Extravasation management

Early recognition of an extravasation may help prevent serious toxicity. Signs and symptoms of an infiltration include slowing or cessation of IV flow, increased resistance when administering the drug, patient complaints, swelling or erythema, and poor or no blood return. For patients with central venous catheters, the chest wall or port pocket should be observed for any swelling; the ease of administration should be evaluated, as well as withdrawal of blood; and the patient assessed for symptoms of pain, burning sensations, discomfort, or pressure.

Once an extravasation is recognized, delay because of lack of knowledge or policy about treatment can affect the outcome. It is important to have a written protocol established for the staff to treat extravasation immediately and with consistency. The following guidelines should be followed if an extravasation is suspected:

1. Stop the infusion.
2. Disconnect the intravenous tubing and attempt to aspirate residual medication from the access needle.
3. For all drugs except the vinca alkaloids: during the first 24 to 48 hours, apply ice for 15 to 20 minutes at least 4 times a day and elevate the extremity if it is a peripheral site (Harwood, 1986; Rudolph and Larson, 1987; ONS, 1996).
4. For the vinca alkaloids, apply heat.
5. Consider an antidote. Hyaluronidase and local heat are recommended by the manufacturer for the vinca alkaloids and are standard practice interventions. For all other drugs, standard practice is the application of ice, although not all manufacturers specifically recommend cold application (Goodman et al, 1996). Local injection of steroids to reduce the inflammatory response has been proposed and studied in animals and humans, but no definitive advantage to healing has been established. Clinical reports on the benefits are even lacking for the clinically accepted instillation of one sixth molar sodium thiosulfate for mechlorethamine infiltration (Ignoffo and Friedman, 1980).
6. Document the incident. Documentation records for venipuncture sites and reactions provide valuable information and legal protection (Boyle and Engelking, 1996). Photograph the site if possible.
7. Follow the patient closely for at least 2 weeks, carefully observing the site. This should include an early consultation with a plastic surgeon and, if symptoms are present, with a physical therapist.

BOX 10-4
Drugs Associated With Venous Cutaneous Reactions

Amsacrine	Epirubicin
Carboplatin	5-Fluorouracil
Carmustine	Idarubicin
Dacarbazine	Mechlorethamine
Daunorubicin	Mitomycin
Docetaxel	Paclitaxel
Doxorubicin	Vinorelbine

Venous reactions

Although extravasation of drugs that may produce tissue necrosis and functional impairment is a serious complication, it is important to recognize other local venous and cutaneous responses to drug administration. These reactions can be acute or occur weeks after treatment. Burning, pain, erythema, tenderness along the vein, urticaria, and pruritus are common immediate reactions, whereas thrombosed veins, persistent phlebitis, hyperpigmentation of veins, or discoloration of affected tissues may be observed weeks to months after drug administration (Box 10-4).

The anthracyclines are associated with local urticaria, streaking erythema, pain, and complaints of a stinging sensation, commonly referred to as a *flare reaction.* These reactions occur in probably less than 20% of patients treated, are transient, and usually resolve within 1 to 2 hours (Curran, Luce, and Page, 1990). Reconstitution with an isotonic diluent, slowing the rate of administration, and dilution of the drug concentration with the IV solution may minimize or prevent recurrence of flare reactions with subsequent doses. Pretreatment with diphenhydramine alone or with dexamethasone may be considered as well.

Carmustine and dacarbazine often produce significant burning and discomfort. Placing ice along the venous pathway above the insertion site and adequate dilution of the drug may provide some pain relief. Vinorelbine produces venous irritation reported as tenderness along the vein and erythema in about one third of patients (Brogden and Nevidjon, 1995). The incidence and severity of this venous reaction can be significantly reduced by administering the drug over 6 to 10 minutes rather than a 20- to 30-minute infusion (Rittenberg, Gralla, and Rehmeyer, 1995).

Systemic Dermatological Effects

Skin changes not caused by extravasation of chemotherapeutic drugs include dermatitis, nail changes, hyperpigmentation, urticaria, acral erythema, photosensitivity reactions, and radiation-enhancing reactions (DeSpain, 1992). Many of these cutaneous reactions are self-limited, lasting only for the duration of therapy. Rash formation and erythema can occur with a variety of chemotherapeutic drugs (Table 10-13).

TABLE 10-13
Dermatitis Associated With Chemotherapeutic Drugs

Chemotherapeutic drug	Type of reaction
Aminoglutethimide	Erythematous maculopapular rash
Azacytidine	Pruritic rash (rare)
Bleomycin	Rash, urticaria, erythematous swelling, hyperkeratosis
Carboplatin	Rash (rare)
Carmustine	Transient facial and neck flush, rash, pruritis
Chlorambucil	Occasional dermatitis
Cytarabine	Rash
Dacarbazine	Transient facial and neck flush
Dactinomycin	Acneiform rash, folliculitis
Daunorubicin	Rash, urticaria
Doxorubicin	Local erythemia, urticaria, and pruritus along the vein
Edatrexate	Rash
Epirubicin	Dermatitis
5-Fluorouracil	Dermatitis
Floxuridine	Rash, pruritus (rare)
Leuprolide	Erythema, skin rash
Hydroxyurea	Rash
Isotretinoin	Dry skin, pruritus, exfoliation
Mechlorethamine	Topical: contact allergy
Methotrexate	Rash, urticaria
Mitomycin	Rash, photosensitivity
Pentostatin	Rash, dry skin
Plicamycin	Dermatitis, facial flushing
Procarbazine	Facial flushing associated with alcohol intake, skin rash, photosensitivity
Tomudex	Rash
Tretinoin	Dry skin, pruritus, mild exfoliation
Trimetrexate	Rash (dose-limiting)

Nail changes during chemotherapy include pigmentation, brittleness, and slowed growth (Table 10-14). Pigmentation is the most frequent change and seems to affect dark-skinned patients more commonly than Caucasian patients. Pigment appears at the base of the nail as horizontal or vertical bands and grows out distally with the nail (DeSpain, 1992). This change in nail pigmentation usually is correlated with increased pigmentation in the fingers. Banding may also occur.

Drug-induced hyperpigmentation of the skin and mucous membranes (Table 10-15) can be focal or diffuse and generally resolves with time, although occasionally it may be permanent (DeSpain, 1992; Knobf and Kalm, 1990).

Acral erythema is a syndrome of demarcated, tender erythematous plaques on the soles of the feet and palms of the hands of patients that

TABLE 10-14
Nail Changes

Drug	Effect
Bleomycin	Nail loss
Cyclophosphamide	Hyperpigmentation
Doxorubicin	Hyperpigmentation
5-Fluorouracil	Nail cracking and loss
Hydroxyurea	Brittle nails

TABLE 10-15
Pigmentation Changes Associated With Chemotherapy

Drug	Pigmentation change
Bleomycin	Linear hyperpigmented streaks across the trunk, hyperpigmentation over small joints
Busulfan	Generalized skin darkening, hyperpigmentation
Carmustine	Hyperpigmentation after erythema
Cyclophosphamide	Hyperpigmentation in sun-exposed areas (nails, teeth, gingivae)
Dactinomycin	Hyperpigmentation
Doxorubicin	Oral mucosa hyperpigmentation
5-Fluorouracil	Photosensitivity, hyperpigmentation
Methotrexate	Photosensitivity, hyperpigmentation
Thiotepa	Hyperpigmentation (areas occluded by bandages)

can range from mild to extremely painful. This toxicity, also referred to as *palmar-plantar erythrodysesthesia syndrome*, is most often associated with cytarabine, doxorubicin, and fluorouracil, but has also been observed in patients who received cyclophosphamide, hydroxyurea, methotrexate, mitotane, and 6-mercaptopurine (DeSpain, 1992). In patients whose acute leukemia is treated with cytarabine, the skin reactions associated with this toxicity may be quite severe, painful, and transiently debilitating. The patient initially may complain of tingling sensations of the hands and feet that generally progress to swelling, pain, tenderness to touch, intense erythema with blanching between joints, and finally, desquamation (Richards and Wujcik, 1992). The cause of the syndrome from onset to symptoms to healing is 1 to 2 weeks. Management is focused on pain relief (systemic and local measures), elevation of extremities, and prevention of infection.

Enhanced Skin Reactions With Multimodality Therapy

Multimodality therapy is the established approach for many hematological and nonhematological malignancies. The use of combination therapy with chemotherapy and radiation has increased over the last 20 years, resulting in an increased incidence of cutaneous toxicity. Radiation skin reactions are defined as *enhancement* or *recall reactions* (DeSpain, 1992). Enhancement is related to the combined effect of the chemotherapy and radiation and is dependent on the drug dosage, time, and sequence of radiotherapy and the pharmacology of the chemotherapeutic agents. Dry and moist desquamation are the most common skin reactions. Nurses and physicians must be aware of potential enhanced cutaneous responses and adequately prepare patients and family members to recognize side effects early to allow for prompt interventions (O'Rourke, 1987).

The recall reaction phenomenon was first described with administration of dactinomycin after a course of radiotherapy. A skin reaction can be observed after drug administration in the areas of previous radiation. Recall reactions may occur within several weeks of treatment with radiotherapy, but have been observed up to months or years later. Recall reactions are most frequently observed with dactinomycin and doxorubicin, but may also be associated with bleomycin, etoposide, hydroxyurea, methotrexate, triazinate, trimetrexate, and vinblastine (DeSpain, 1992). Reactions should be carefully documented and followed for each patient.

RENAL TOXICITY

Major risk factors for renal toxicity in patients with cancer include nephrotoxic chemotherapy drugs, age, nutritional status, concurrent use of other nephrotoxic drugs, and preexisting renal dysfunction (Lydon, 1989; Lydon, 1986; Patterson and Reams, 1992). Drugs most commonly associated with renal toxicity include L-asparaginase, azacytadine, carboplatin, cisplatin, hydroxyurea, ifosfamide, methotrexate, mitomycin, nitrosoureas, pentostatin, plicamycin, streptozocin, and suramin.

Before initiating therapy with any potentially renal-toxic drug, it is essential to assess renal function and evaluate risk factors. There are several laboratory tests to assess chemotherapy drug–induced glomerular or tubular damage (Table 10-16) that will aid in monitoring renal function, the significance of which is dependent on the acuity of the patient and risk factors for serious renal sequelae (Lydon 1989; King, Hoffart, and Murray, 1992).

Plasma concentrations of blood urea nitrogen (BUN) and creatinine are common assessment parameters, but their use is very limited because damage to the kidney may be quite significant before elevations in serum levels are detected. The most reliable method to assess renal function that will reflect glomerular function with reasonable accuracy is the creatinine clearance (see Appendix A, Table A-5). A 24-hour collection of urine for creatinine clearance is recommended to monitor patients and alter drug doses to prevent or minimize renal toxicity. Patient teaching about the urine-collection process and the need for adequate hydration is *essential*. Written instructions should be provided and translated into appropriate languages for

TABLE 10-16
Assessment of Renal Function

Test	Purpose	Normal values	Procedure
Blood urea nitrogen	Gross index of glomerular function	7–18 mg/dL	Venous sample
Creatinine	Assess glomerular filtration ability of kidney	F: 0.6–1.2 mg/dL M: 0.7–1.3 mg/dL	Venous sample
Creatinine clearance	Determines glomerular filtration rate	F: 75–115 mg/min M: 85–125 mg/min	Timed urine specimen (12 or 24 hr), venous blood sample for serum creatinine
Protein	Glomerular and tubular function assessment	1–14 mg/dL	Dipstick AM void; if positive, collect 24-hr specimen
Specific gravity	Measures kidney's ability to concentrate/dilute urine; assesses tubular or medullary damage	1.010–1.025	Random urine sample, measure with urinometer, refractometer, or dipstick
Osmolality	Measures kidney's ability to concentrate and dilute urine; assesses tubular or medullary damage	Random sample: 500–800 mOsm/kg Fluid restriction sample: 850 mOsm/kg	Fluid deprivation (12 hr) preferred
pH	Measures free hydrogen ion (H^+) concentration in urine	4.6–8.0 pH <7 = acid urine pH >7 = alkaline urine	Dipstick on freshly voided specimen
Casts	Assesses tubular damage	Red, white, and fatty casts = 0/LPF	Urinalysis
Cytology	Assesses tubular damage	RBCs = 1–2/LPF, 0–1/HPF, WBCs: 0–4/HPF Epithelial cells: occasional	Clean-catch urine sample

Continued

TABLE 10-16
Assessment of Renal Function—cont'd

Test	Purpose	Normal values	Procedure
Glucose glycosuria	Determines reabsorptive capacity of renal tubules	Random sample: negative Quantitative sample (24 hr): <0.5 g/day	Random urine specimen or 24-hr specimen
Amino acids	Determines reabsorptive capacity of renal tubules	Random sample: none 24-hr sample: 0–200 mg/24 hr	Freshly voided specimen or 24-hr collection
Enzymes β_2-microglobulin, n-acetyl B, and aminotransferases	Determines renal tubular cell damage	None or trace amounts	Timed urine collection; check with individual laboratory

Modified from Lydon J: Assessment of renal function in the patient receiving chemotherapy, *Cancer Nurs* 12:133-143, 1989.
LPF, Low-power field; *HPF,* high-power field.

the population served. Inadequate or inaccurate collections may result in erroneous values with unexpected toxicities, delays in treatment, and alterations in planned hospitalizations.

Of the major risk factors for nephrotoxicity, impaired renal function is a significant one. Repeated courses of nephrotoxic drugs may result in decreased renal function demonstrated by subclinical or clinically obvious renal impairment. For example, prior treatment with cisplatin has been reported to increase myelosuppression and gastrointestinal and renal toxicity with subsequent methotrexate administration (Pitman et al, 1979) and effect the pharmacokinetics of other renally excreted drugs such as bleomycin and paclitaxel (Kintzel and Dorr, 1995). Toxicity to other organ systems may result when kidney function is altered, such as an increased risk of neurotoxicity associated with the administration of ifosfamide and cytarabine in patients with impaired renal function. Thus renal clearance of chemotherapy drugs is a very important factor in potential toxicity, either to the renal or other organ systems (Durivage and Burnham, 1991). Chemotherapy drugs with a renal clearance of ≥30% of the administered dose in patients with impaired renal function may result in a higher dose intensity and thus a greater toxicity (Kintzel and Dorr, 1995). Recommendations for dose adjustments based on the patient's renal function with chemotherapy drugs that have a ≥30% renal clearance are provided in Table 10-17. Risk factors for specific agents, the type of damage, clinical abnormalities, and basic management strategies are presented in Table 10-18 (Durivage and Burnham, 1991; Kintzel and Dorr, 1995; Lydon, 1986; Patterson and Reams, 1992).

High-dose therapy, especially high doses of drugs in conditioning regimens for bone marrow or peripheral stem cell transplantation, may result in a greater incidence of and more severe renal toxicity. Acute renal failure and hemolytic uremic syndrome are potentially serious and fatal complications (Fields et al, 1995; van der Lelie et al, 1995). These complications involve many factors, not just the chemotherapeutic agent. King, Hoffart, and Murray (1992) provide a comprehensive review of acute renal failure in bone marrow transplantation with specific guidelines for identifying patients at risk, differential diagnosis of renal impairment, and management of the patient at risk or in acute renal failure.

Bladder Toxicity

Hemorrhagic cystitis is associated with ifosfamide and cyclophosphamide, and an increased incidence of bladder carcinoma has been associated with prolonged use of these drugs. Standard doses of cyclophosphamide, especially with oral administration, produce bladder toxicity in ≥10% of patients (Patterson and Reams, 1992). High-dose cyclophosphamide, like its structural analogue ifosfamide, presents a major risk for the development of hemorrhagic cystitis. Contact of the bladder wall with toxic metabolites, primarily acrolein, produces mucosal erythema, inflammation, ulceration, necrosis, diffuse small-vessel hemorrhagic oozing, and a reduced bladder capacity (Stillwell and

TABLE 10-17
Guidelines for Dosage Adjustment of Renally Cleared Antitumor Drugs

Agent	Fraction of normal dose based on patient's creatinine clearance		
	60 mL/min	45 mL/min	30 mL/min
Alkylating agents			
Carmustine	0.80	0.75	NR[b]
Lomustine	0.75	0.70	NR[b]
Semustine	0.75	0.70	NR[b]
Cisplatin[a]	0.75	0.50	NR[b]
Carboplatin[c]	Adjust carboplatin using formula		
Ifosfamide	0.80	0.75	0.70
Melphalan (IV)	0.85	0.75	0.70
Antimetabolites			
Cytarabine (1–3 g/m^2)	0.60	0.50	NR[b]
Fludarabine	0.80	0.75	0.65
Methotrexate	0.65	0.50	NR[b]
Pentostatin	0.70	0.60	NR[b]
Topoisomerase inhibitors			
Etoposide	0.85	0.80	0.75
Topotecan	0.80	0.75	0.70
Miscellaneous			
Bleomycin	0.70	0.60	NR[b]
Dacarbazine	0.80	0.75	0.70
Hydroxyurea	0.85	0.80	0.75
PALA	0.60	0.50	0.35

Modified from Kintzel PE, Dorr RT: Anticancer drug renal toxicity and elimination: dosing guidelines for altered renal function, *Cancer Treatment* Rev 21:33-64. 1995.
[a]Empiric adjustment due to nephrotoxicity.
[b]NR, consider use of alternative drugs if feasible.
[c]See carboplatin dosing in Chapter 3 and in Appendix A, Table A-6.

Benson, 1988). Symptoms include hematuria (microscopic or gross) and dysuria. The uroprotective agent 2-mercaptoethane sulfonate sodium (mesna) acts by binding to acrolein to result in a nontoxic thioether (Durivage and Burnham, 1991). The use of mesna and hydration with ifosfamide or high-dose cyclophosphamide significantly reduces the incidence of bladder toxicity (Hows et al, 1984; Zalupski and Baker, 1988). If hemorrhagic cystitis develops, discontinuation of treatment with the drug and vigorous hydration are indicated. Depending on the degree of toxicity, bladder irrigation, fulguration, and in rare instances cystectomy may be warranted (Patterson and Reams, 1992; Stillwell and Bensen, 1988).

TABLE 10-18
Alterations in Renal Function of Selected Chemotherapeutic Drugs

Drug	Alteration	Risk factors	Abnormalities	Management
Cisplatin	Damage to proximal and distal tubules	Concurrent use of other nephrotoxic drugs	Azotemia	Prevention: hydration (2–3 L) and diuresis (>100 mL/hr)
	Decreased renal tubular reabsorption	Existing renal dysfunction	↑BUN	Magnesium supplement (Evans et al, 1995)
			↑Serum creatinine	Supportive: electrolyte replacement, dose adjustment, discontinuation of drug therapy
			↑Uric acid	
			↓Creatinine clearance	
			↓Serum magnesium	
			↓Serum calcium	
			Proteinuria	
			↓Potassium	
Cyclophosphamide	SIADH	High dose and hydration with free water (i.e., D_5W)	Hyponatremia	Prevention: monitor electrolytes, hydration with normal saline
			↓Urine output	
			↑Urine osmolality	Supportive: discontinue drug therapy
			↓Serum osmolality	
Ifosfamide	Proximal tubular defect	High-dose administration	↑BUN	Prevention: adequate hydration, monitor for early signs of toxicity; may be reversible
		Existing renal dysfunction	↑Serum creatinine	
			↓Creatinine clearance	
			Proteinuria	

Continued

TABLE 10-18
Alterations in Renal Function of Selected Chemotherapeutic Drugs—cont'd

Drug	Alteration	Risk factors	Abnormalities	Management
Methotrexate	Injury to proximal and distal convoluted tubules	High-dose therapy Dehydration Existing renal dysfunction Concurrent use of other nephrotoxic drugs Existing effusions or ascites Prior treatment with cisplatin	↑BUN ↑Serum creatinine ↓Creatinine clearance Hematuria Azotemia Oliguria Hypokalemia Aminoaciduria Electrolyte abnormalities	Prevention (high dose): hydration, adequate urine output, alkalinization to maintain pH ≥ 7.0 Supportive: hydration Administer leucovorin if serum methotrexate levels are elevated (see Chapter 3)
Mitomycin	Mild, reversible renal insufficiency Hemolytic-uremic syndrome (uncommon)	Prolonged therapy Cumulative doses >60–100 mg	↑BUN ↑Serum creatinine ↓Platelets Anemia Proteinuria Hematuria Hypertension	Prevention: none Supportive: ? plasma pheresis

Drug	Mechanism	Risk factors	Signs	Prevention/Management
Nitrosoureas	Glomerular and tubular damage	Cumulative doses ≥ 1.2 g/m²	↑BUN ↑Serum creatinine	Prevention: adjust dose for renal impairment Supportive: monitor cumulative dose and renal function
Plicamycin	Damage to proximal and distal tubules	Daily schedule with cumulative doses >25–50 µg/kg	↑BUN ↑Serum creatinine Proteinuria Azotemia ↓Serum electrolytes	Prevention: avoid high doses; monitor for early signs toxicity
Streptozocin	Damage to renal tubules	Doses >1–1.5 g/m²/wk Concurrent use of other nephrotoxic drugs Existing renal dysfunction	↑BUN ↑Serum creatinine Proteinuria ↓Creatinine clearance Glucosuria Hypokalemia Renal tubular acidosis Hypophosphatemia	Prevention: monitor early signs of toxicity; protein, amino acids in urine, phosphate, potassium in serum Adequate hydration

SIADH, Syndrome of inappropriate antidiuretic hormone; *D₅W,* 5% dextrose in water.

PULMONARY TOXICITY

Chemotherapy drugs can directly or indirectly produce lung-tissue damage. Regardless of a direct or indirect action, the resulting toxicity is damage to both endothelial and epithelial cells (pneumocytes) (Cooper and Matthay, 1987; Kriesman and Wolkove, 1992). The clinical presentations of pulmonary toxicity associated with chemotherapy fall into three major categories: pneumonitis/fibrosis, hypersensitivity pneumonitis, and noncardiogenic pulmonary edema (Cooper and Matthay, 1987). These are not exclusive categories, and many patients will exhibit symptoms and histological findings representative of more than one type of toxicity (Table 10-19).

The most common toxicities observed clinically are pneumonitis and pulmonary fibrosis. Bleomycin can be used as a prototype for this type of pulmonary toxicity (Kriesman and Wolkove, 1992). Symptoms include dyspnea, nonproductive cough, fatigue, and weight loss and may occur acutely but, more commonly, over a period of several weeks. Chest radiography often shows pulmonary infiltrates, and treatment is discontinuation of treatment with the drug and administration of corticosteroids (Cooper and Matthay, 1987; Kriesman and Wolkove, 1992). There is a wide incidence range even for an individual drug (i.e., bleomycin, up to 50%; mitomycin, 3% to 36%), and the time of onset of symptoms is difficult to predict with accuracy (Cooper and Matthay, 1987; Kriesman and Wolkove, 1992; Limper and McDonald, 1990; O'Driscoll et al, 1990).

Although bleomycin can be used as a prototype for most chemotherapy drug–induced lung damage, methotrexate represents a drug with a broad range of pulmonary toxicity: endothelial injury, capillary leak, pulmonary edema, and pulmonary fibrosis (Kriesman and Wolkove, 1992; Shapiro et al, 1991). Symptoms may be acute and precipitate acute respiratory distress syndrome or may be gradual, with their onset varying from days to years. Recovery generally occurs, although fatal cases of pulmonary fibrosis have been reported (van der Veen et al, 1995).

Hypersensitivity pneumonitis has been associated with azathioprine, bleomycin, methotrexate, and procarbazine (Cooper and Matthay, 1987). Symptoms of dyspnea, cough, chills, myalgia, and headache are reported with physical findings of fever, pulmonary crackles, and a skin rash in up to half of patients. The chest radiograph shows diffuse infiltrates, and a pleural effusion may be present. Treatment is discontinuation of treatment with the drug and administration of corticosteroids. The outcome of treatment is generally good, although the condition can be potentially life threatening (Hilliquin et al, 1996).

Noncardiogenic pulmonary edema is associated with an acute onset of respiratory symptoms and is likely related to capillary leak syndrome. Drugs associated with this uncommon toxicity include cytarabine, cyclophosphamide, methotrexate, mitomycin, and teniposide (Cooper and Matthay, 1987).

Early detection of pulmonary toxicity is limited. Pulmonary function tests are routinely used for high-risk patients, but sensitivity to early changes is variable. Diffusing capacity for carbon monoxide (DLCO) appears to be a relatively sensitive indicator of early pulmonary changes,

TABLE 10-19
Pulmonary Toxicity Associated With Chemotherapy

Drug	Frequency			Comment
	Common (0%–50%)	Uncommon (<30%)	Rare (<5%)	
L-Asparaginase			✓	
Azathioprine			✓	
Bleomycin	✓			Dose relationship; increased risk with elderly
Busulfan		✓		Long latent period more common for onset of symptoms
Carmustine	✓			Dose relationship; may have delayed onset up to years
Chlorambucil			✓	
Cyclophosphamide		✓		Incidence may increase with higher doses
Cytarabine		✓		Increased risk with higher doses
Dactinomycin		✓		Documented with radiotherapy only
Doxorubicin		✓		Documented with radiotherapy only
Edatrexate			✓	
Etoposide			✓	
Fludarabine		✓		
Ifosfamide			✓	
Lomustine		✓		
Melphalan			✓	
Methotrexate		✓		Role may increase with etoposide therapy

Continued

ABLE 10-19
Pulmonary Toxicity Associated With Chemotherapy—cont'd

Drug	Frequency			Comment
	Common (0%–50%)	Uncommon (<30%)	Rare (<5%)	
Mitomycin	√			May interact with oxygen, cyclophosphamide, radiotherapy
Pentostatin			√	
Procarbazine			√	
Semustine		√		
Teniposide			√	
Vincristine		√		Only observed when administered with mitomycin
Vinblastine		√		Only observed when administered with mitomycin
Vindesine		√		Only observed when administered with mitomycin
Vinorelbine		√		Only observed when administered with mitomycin

but it is relatively nonspecific. Although the role of DLCO in chemotherapy drug–induced damage is controversial, it continues to be used in clinical practice (Cooper and Matthay, 1987; Kriesman and Wolkove, 1992). Chest radiographs often indicate extensive or irreversible pulmonary fibrosis, and the role of computed tomography (CT) and magnetic resonance imaging (MRI) as sensitive predictors of early changes is yet to be defined.

CARDIAC TOXICITY

Congestive heart failure and cardiomyopathy associated with anthracycline drugs are the most common cardiac toxicities. Myocardial ischemia, pericarditis, arrhythmias, miscellaneous electrocardiogram (ECG) changes, and angina occur much less frequently (Allen, 1992). Cardiac effects of anthracycline therapy can be acute, chronic, or late onset. Acute effects (arrhythmias, ECG changes, sinus tachycardia) occur within hours of bolus administration, are transient, and do not appear to be related to dose, schedule, or future development of cardiomyopathy (Allen, 1992). Chronic anthracycline cardiomyopathy may present during or weeks to months after therapy, but most commonly occurs within 1 year of treatment (Shan, Lincoff, and Young, 1996). Late-onset cardiac toxicity (more than 1 year after treatment) increases with length of follow-up and occurs in previously asymptomatic patients, emphasizing the need for continued assessment of cardiac function in long-term survivors (Postma et al, 1996; Steinherz, Steinherz, and Tan, 1995). Observed abnormalities include arrhythmias, ventricular dysfunction, decreased ejection fraction, fractional shortening on echocardiogram, and cardiac failure.

The cumulative anthracycline drug dose and mediastinal radiation are the two most significant risk factors. Other risk factors, identified in Table 10-20, have been proposed to influence the risk or severity of cardiac toxicity, but remain somewhat controversial (Allen, 1992; Shan, Lincoff, and Young, 1996; Steinherz and Steinherz, 1991).

The cause of anthracycline cardiac toxicity is multifactorial, including free radicalmediated myocardial injury, myocyte damage from calcium overload, myocardial adrenergic function disturbances, release of vasoactive amines, and cellular-induced toxicity from the metabolites of doxorubicin (Shan, Lincoff, and Young, 1996). The myofibrils (contractile structures of the myocyte) are the critical organelles damaged, and the varying degrees of loss of those structures directly affect the ability of the heart to contract. The variation of myofibril loss presumably explains the range of cardiac toxicity from minor ECG changes to fatal congestive heart failure (Steinherz and Steinherz, 1991; Kaszyk, 1986).

The primary management strategy of anthracycline cardiac toxicity is early detection. Several methods have been evaluated to identify early changes over the years. Radionuclide angiocardiography (RNA) and echocardiograms are the noninvasive methods commonly used in practice, despite their relative insensitivity for detecting early signs of cardiac toxicity (Shan, Lincoff, and Young, 1996). Because of the wide variation in individual sensitivity to anthracycline doses, patients should be

TABLE 10-20
Risk Factors for Anthracycline-Related Cardiac Toxicity

Risk factor	Comment
Cumulative dose	Risk <10% for doses <450 mg/m^2, increases linearly with doses ≥550 mg/m^2
Schedule	Peak plasma levels appear to be an important factor; less cardiac toxicity with lower doses, more frequent administration, and continuous infusions
Mediastinal radiation	Strong risk factor
Preexisting cardiac disease	Mechanism not fully understood but appears to influence incidence
Age	Young children and older adults (>70 yr) appear at greater risk
Concurrent chemotherapy	Limited data (Allen, 1992), but cyclophosphamide, etoposide, dactinomycin, mitomycin, melphalan, vincristine, bleomycin, and dacarbazine suspected
Individual sensitivity	Wide variation of toxicity

routinely monitored during therapy, with attention to proposed risk factors. Long-term follow-up monitoring is also recommended based on the increased incidence of cardiac toxicity over time (Steinherz, Steinherz, and Tan, 1995) and the reported 4.5% to 7% incidence of cardiac failure in patients previously treated with anthracycline therapy (Shan, Lincoff, and Young, 1996).

Endomyocardial biopsy is a reliable method for assessing cardiac toxicity, but it is an invasive and expensive procedure that is restricted to experienced physicians and used only for selected patients.

Management of cardiac dysfunction secondary to anthracycline damage is conventional treatment of heart failure. Because of the limited value of this intervention and the number of cardiac fatalities, prevention of cardiac toxicity has been a focus for clinicians and researchers. Altering the method of drug delivery (i.e., schedule, use of liposomal anthracyclines), evaluation of less cardiotoxic structural analogs of the anthracyclines, and cardioprotectants represent the three major strategies employed (Shan, Lincoff, and Young, 1996). Although there is enthusiasm for the role of cardioprotectants, the antitumor effect of the anthracycline therapy must be maintained. Thus each strategy must be carefully and critically evaluated for outcome measures related to tumor response *and* toxicity.

Several other chemotherapeutic drugs are reportedly associated with cardiac toxicity (Allen, 1992), but except for cyclophosphamide, 5-fluorouracil, and paclitaxel, most represent single case reports. High-dose cyclophosphamide-induced cardiac toxicity has become a more significant clinical problem with the increased use of high-dose therapy and transplantation. Cyclophosphamide appears to have a direct effect on the endothelium, which can lead to hemorrhagic cardiac necrosis with high-dose therapy (Shuey, 1994). Transient pericardial effusion, arrhythmias, and ECG changes have been reported, but cardiomyopathy associated with pericarditis is the most common outcome, presenting as heart failure.

NEUROLOGICAL TOXICITY

There is a wide range of CNS symptoms related to chemotherapy-induced neurological toxicity (Table 10-21). Symptoms may be transient and mild or severe with significant dysfunction and risk of mortality. The CNS toxic

TABLE 10-21
Central Nervous System Function and Neurotoxicity

Functional area	Normal	Abnormal
Cerebrum		
Mental status	Intellect	Confusion
	Memory	Memory loss
	Judgment	Change in level of consciousness
	Abstract thinking	Delirium/psychoses
		Seizures
		Cognitive dysfunction
Peripheral nerves		
Sensory	Reflex arc	Diminished deep tendon reflexes
	Touch	Numbness/tingling
	Temperature	Decreased sensation
	Vibration	Decreased sensation
	Pain	Jaw or abdominal pain
	Proprioception	Sensory ataxia
Motor	Voluntary movement	Foot drop
		Muscle weakness
Autonomic system	Bowel and bladder function	Constipation/ileus
		Urinary incontinence
		Bladder atony
		Colicky pain
Cerebellum	Maintenance of muscle tone	
	Equilibrium	Ataxia
	Coordinating movement and position sense	Dysarthria
		Dysmetria
		Dysdiadochokinesia
		Horizontal nystagmus

Continued

TABLE 10-21
Central Nervous System Function and Neurotoxicity—cont'd

Functional area	Normal	Abnormal
Meninges	Cover and protect brain brain and spinal cord	Meningismus
		Paraplegia
		Blindness
Cranial nerves		
Olfactory	Smell	—
Optic	Vision	Optic neuritis
		Papilledema
		Blurred vision/blindness
		Retrobulbar neuritis
Oculomotor	Regulates eye movements	Diplopia
Trochlear abducens	Extraocular movements	Nystagmus
		Ptosis
Trigeminal	Mastication	Jaw pain
Facial	Facial expression	Facial palsy
	Taste	Taste changes?
Auditory	Hearing	Tinnitus
	Equilibrium	Hearing loss
		Nystagmus
		Vertigo
Glossopharyngeal	Swallowing	Dysphagia
	Taste	Taste changes?
Vagus	Voice	Hoarseness
	Swallowing	Dysphagia
		Dysphonia

From Meehan J, Johnson B: The neurotoxicity of antineoplastic agents. In Hubbard S, Greene P, Knobf M, eds: *Current issues in cancer nursing practice*, Philadelphia, 1991, JB Lippincott, pp 1-11.

effects associated with chemotherapeutic drugs have been categorized by the functional area affected and the toxicity produced (Kaplan and Wiernik, 1982; Patchell and Posner, 1985; Meehan and Johnson, 1991). Encephalopathy, peripheral neuropathy, cerebellar syndromes, autonomic neuropathy, and cranial nerve toxicity represent the range of neurological complications associated with systemic drug treatment (Box 10-5). Although the range of CNS side effects is quite broad, the incidence of clinically significant neurological toxicity is relatively low to moderate for the majority of the chemotherapy drugs. Dose, route of administration, age of the patient, hepatic and renal function, concomitant use of other neurotoxic drugs, and concurrent use of cranial or CNS radiotherapy can each influence the incidence rate and severity of neurological symptoms associated with selected chemotherapy drugs.

BOX 10-5
Neurotoxicity Associated With Cytotoxic Drugs

Acute myelopathy	Cladribine
Intrathecal methotrexate	Cisplatin
Intrathecal cytarabine	Cyclophosphamide
Intrathecal thiotepa	5-Fluorouracil
Autonomic neuropathy	Fludarabine
Cisplatin	Ifosfamide
Procarbazine	Methotrexate
Paclitaxel	Mitotane
Vinblastine	PALA
Vincristine	Pentostatin
Vinorelbine	Procarbazine
Cerebellar syndromes	**Peripheral neuropathy**
Altretamine	Altretamine
Cytarabine	Azacytidine
5-Fluorouracil	Carboplatin
Procarbazine	Cladribine
Cranial nerve toxicity	Cisplatin
Carmustine	Cytarabine
Cisplatin	Didanosine
5-Fluorouracil	Etoposide
Ifosfamide	Fludarabine
Vinblastine	Paclitaxel
Vincristine	Procarbazine
Encephalopathy (cerebral)	Suramin
L-Asparaginase	Thiotepa (high dose)
Azacytidine	Teniposide
Busulfan (high dose)	Vinblastine
Cytarabine (high dose)	Vincristine
Carmustine	Vinorelbine

The mechanisms of CNS insult are not fully understood for all drugs, and several drugs produce more than one type of neurological toxicity (Box 10-5). As an example, ifosfamide is associated with a wide variety of symptoms including confusion, restlessness, lethargy, somnolence, mental status changes, seizures, motor cerebellar alterations, and cranial nerve dysfunction (Cain and Bender, 1995). Comprehensive assessment is indicated, including review of potential risk factors such as renal and hepatic function and a careful neurological screening examination each day the patient is receiving therapy. Establishing the patient's baseline cognitive function is a critical assessment parameter. Patients and family should be well educated about potential symptoms. Changes may be subtle or more pronounced, the latter of which can be quite alarming to patients and family, especially if the changes occur in the home setting. Neurological symptoms associated with ifosfamide usually resolve in 2 to 3 days for the majority of patients (Cain and Bender, 1995; Cameron, 1993). High-dose cytarabine is another example of a chemotherapy drug that mandates careful and routine screening of patients at each dose because of the potential for acute cerebellar toxicity. Relating drug dose to potential organ system toxicity has become a critical factor in today's oncology environment of dose-intense therapy. As higher doses of therapy are administered, assessment of systems must be thorough and comprehensive to identify early signs of predictable drug effects and to document unsuspected organ system toxicity. The potential risk factors, such as previous drug treatment, alterations in drug clearance because of renal or hepatic dysfunction, or concurrent radiotherapy, may significantly alter the toxicity profile of the patient who receives high-dose therapy.

Acute encephalopathies and cerebellar syndromes are serious CNS toxicities, but they are fairly limited to a few drugs and select patient populations. In contrast, peripheral neuropathy is associated with many chemotherapeutic agents (Box 10-5), and the expanded indications and use of cisplatin, paclitaxel, and high doses of drugs in transplant conditioning regimens has further increased the incidence. Mild distal sensory paresthesias are common, represent early signs of neuropathy, and are tolerable for most patients. However, more severe sensory alterations (i.e., painful paresthesias, loss of deep-tendon reflexes, sensory ataxia, perceptual alterations), Lhermitte's sign, muscle cramps, and motor symptoms can significantly alter a patient's functional ability, comfort, and overall quality of life (Ostchega, Donohue, and Fox, 1988; Rowinsky et al, 1993). Symptoms may stabilize or worsen after therapy is completed but have been reported to persist in 31% to 73% of patients several years after treatment (Siegal and Haim, 1990; Hansen, Helweg-Larsen, and Trojaborg, 1989; Stoter et al, 1989). Physical and subjective assessments of the patient's distress and perceived functional impairment are critical to therapeutic decisions and plan of care. Management with narcotic analgesics for drug-induced dysesthesias or a trial of a drug such as amitriptyline for relief of neuropathic pain may be indicated for symptomatic patients (Rowinsky et al, 1993).

In addition to chemotherapy-induced neurological toxicity, cytokines are associated with a wide variety of neurological symptoms. Acute, subacute, and chronic neurological side effects have been reported with interferon, interleukin-2, and tumor necrosis factor (Meyers, 1995). Of these cytokines, interferon is more commonly administered, and thus the neurotoxicity profile is more well defined. Onset of symptoms may be within a week of beginning therapy, the severity of symptoms appears to be dose dependent, and symptoms generally resolve with dose reductions or discontinuation of therapy, although some patients have evidence of chronic symptomatology. Difficulty concentrating, memory problems, slowed thinking, impaired motor coordination, impaired visuomotor skills, trouble with calculations, depression, apathy, and confusion are reported symptoms (Meyers, 1995). Baseline neurological assessment of the patient is an essential pretreatment parameter. Ongoing neurological assessment, including subjective patient and family reports of cognitive function, is critical to early identification of neurological toxicity so that appropriate and timely interventions, such as dose adjustments, can be considered (Bender, Monti, and Kerr, 1996). The differential diagnosis of impairment of neurobehavioral changes from emotional reactions to illness is difficult and emphasizes the importance of assessment. For most patients, careful evaluation of their behavior, attentiveness, ability to converse logically and to comprehend and follow instructions, and short-term memory provides a practical ongoing assessment, which can identify patients who should be seen for a more formal neurological examination (Meyers, 1995).

GONADAL TOXICITY

The effects of chemotherapy and hormone therapy on gonadal function, sexuality, and reproductive capability have been extensively reviewed (Kreuser et al, 1990; Chamorro, 1991; Myers and Schilsky, 1992; Averette, Boike, and Jarrell, 1990). Gonadal dysfunction as a consequence of treatment with alkylating agents was reported in the early 1970s, and these drugs remain the most significant gonadal toxins. Several factors influence the risk of gonadal injury and can result in testicular atrophy and primary ovarian failure (Box 10-6). Patients with Hodgkin's disease, because of their age and curability potential, have been a major focus for evaluating chemotherapy effects on fertility and sexuality (Whitehead et al, 1983; Waxman et al, 1982; Chapman, Sutcliffe, and Malpas, 1979b; Ramona et al, 1981). The initiation of adjuvant systemic therapy in the mid 1970s to its current widespread use in premenopausal women with breast cancer has intensified the focus of drug-induced gonadal dysfunction and the consequences of related symptom distress and quality-of-life issues (Knobf, 1996; Rose and David, 1980; Samaan et al, 1978; Young-McGaughan, 1996).

Age and the corresponding gonadal activity at the time of treatment are major factors in outcome (Whitehead et al, 1983; Waxman et al, 1982; Chapman, Sutcliff, and Malpas, 1979a; Gershenson, 1988; Mehta, Beattie, and DasGupta, 1991; Rivkees and Crawford, 1988). In women younger than 30 years of age, the risk of gonadal dysfunction resulting in menstrual changes is very low. As age increases in women, there is an

---

BOX 10-6

Factors Influencing Gonadal Damage and Recovery Associated With Chemotherapy Treatment

Age
Gonadal activity at the time of treatment
Drug dose
Duration of treatment
Underlying malignancy
Specific drugs/regimens

inverse relationship between the incidence of ovarian dysfunction and time to occurrence. In a sample of 70 women with breast cancer receiving cyclophosphamide-methotrexate-fluorouracil (CMF) adjuvant therapy, 77% developed amenorrhea, and the time to amenorrhea was age dependent, averaging 5.5 months for women younger than 35 years, 2 to 3 months for women older than 35 but younger than 45 years, and only 1 month if a woman was older than 45 years (Mehta, Beattie, and Das-Gupta, 1991).

The underlying malignancy appears to be an important factor, particularly for males diagnosed with Hodgkin's disease. Gonadal dysfunction, observed as impotence and inadequate sperm counts, has been reported before initiation of therapy. Assessment of pretreatment gonadal function is very important in predicting outcome and for counseling patients regarding fertility options after completion of therapy (Sweet, Servy, and Karow, 1996).

Specific drug treatment is also a factor when discussing fertility. Combination chemotherapy for Hodgkin's disease, using doxorubicin, bleomycin, vinblastine, and dacarbazine (ABVD), is associated with significantly less gonadal toxicity for both males and females than therapy with mustargen, oncovin, procarbazine, and prednisone (MOPP) (Santoro et al, 1987). High-dose therapy, especially with alkylating agents in the majority of conditioning regimens for transplantation, also results in a more predictable and irreversible gonadal dysfunction.

Although fertility is a major issue for most younger patients, symptoms associated with gonadal dysfunction and the impact on sexuality are important issues for both young and older patients. In premenopausal women treated with chemotherapy, the drug-induced ovarian failure producing menopausal symptoms (i.e., hot flashes, irritability, nervousness, decreased vaginal lubrication) may be very distressful and affect daily function, sleep patterns, and sexual relationships (Chapman, Sutcliffe, and Malpas, 1979b; Young-McGaughan, 1996).

In addition to chemotherapy, there is a wide variety of symptoms associated with hormonal therapy, including diminished or lost libido, hot flashes, mood changes and vaginal discharge in women and gynecomastia and impotence in men. These are important side effects related to quality of life and should be assessed and managed according to the patient's perceived distress.

Pretreatment considerations for preservation of fertility options have focused on sperm banking and gonadal protection (Kreuser et al, 1990; Chamorro, 1991; Averette, Boike, and Jarrell, 1990). Attempts to preserve gonadal function by using oral contraceptives and gonadotropin-releasing hormone (GnRH) analogues have not been universally successful, and results are in general disappointing. Cryopreservation of sperm has some limitations but remains a viable and potentially successful intervention for male patients (Koeppel, 1995). It is important for oncology professionals to maintain current knowledge of the technology in this area as well as the available resources for patients related to the procedure, cost, storage, and legal issues (Sweet, Servy, and Karow, 1996).

OTHER ORGAN SYSTEM TOXICITY

Vascular (Doll and Yarbro, 1992), ocular (Burns, 1992), and hepatic (Perry, 1992) are additional organ system toxicities that have been associated with chemotherapeutic agents. In general, vascular and ocular toxicities are uncommon or represent minor alterations in system function. Although this is also generally true for hepatotoxicity, there are selected drugs that have been associated with hepatocellular damage and with venoocclusive disease in high-dose therapy. Patients who receive drugs that are metabolized primarily through the liver and those patients with compromised liver function require careful attention and monitoring. Perry (1992) offers dose-reduction guidelines for patients with hepatic dysfunction, defined as elevated serum bilirubin levels (>1.5) and elevated SGOT levels (>60) for the following drugs: doxorubicin, daunorubicin, vinblastine, vincristine, etoposide, cyclophosphamide, methotrexate, 5-fluorouracil, and amsacrine. Although there are data directly associating chemotherapy with liver toxicity, multiple factors must be considered in the differential diagnosis of abnormal liver function tests in a patient with cancer, such as preexisting liver disease, other hepatotoxic medications, comorbid conditions, and liver metastases. With all organ system toxicity, all potential causes of the observed abnormality must be considered and evaluated before a management plan is designed for the symptoms or toxicity and before any treatment alterations are planned.

REFERENCES

Bone marrow suppression

Bociek RG, Armitage JO: Hematopoietic growth factors, *CA, Cancer J Clin* 46:165-184, 1996.

Bodey GP et al: Quantitative relationships between circulating leukocytes and infection in patients with acute leukemia, *Ann Intern Med* 64:328-340, 1966.

Carter LW: Influences of nutrition and stress on people at risk for neutropenia: nursing implications, *Oncol Nurs Forum* 20:1241-1250, 1993.

Carter LW: Bacterial translocation: nursing implications in the care of patients with neutropenia, *Oncol Nurs Forum* 21:857-865, 1994.

Crawford J et al: Reduction by granulocyte colony-stimulating factor of fever and neutropenia induced by chemotherapy in patients with small cell lung cancer, *N Engl J Med* 325:164-170, 1991.

Dean GE, Hauber D, Rivera LM: Infection. In McCorkle R et al, eds: *Cancer nursing: a comprehensive textbook,* Philadelphia, 1996, WB Saunders, pp 963-978.

Erickson JM: Blood support for the myelosuppressed patient, *Semin Oncol Nurs* 6:61-66, 1990.

Gabrilove JL et al: Effect of granulocyte colony-stimulating factor on neutropenia and associated mortality due to chemotherapy for transitional cell carcinoma of the urothelium, *N Engl J Med* 318:1414-1422, 1988.

Gastineau DA, Hoagland HC: Hematologic effects of chemotherapy, *Semin Oncol* 19:543-550, 1992.

Henry DH: Recombinant human erythropoietin treatment of anemic cancer patients, *Cancer Practice* 4(4):180-184, 1996.

Malik IA et al: Self-administered antibiotic therapy for chemotherapy-induced, low risk febrile neutropenia in patients with non-hematologic neoplasms, *Clin Infect Dis* 19:522-527, 1994.

Pizzo PA: Management of fever in patients with cancer and treatment-induced neutropenia, *N Engl J Med* 328:1323-1332, 1993.

Pizzo PA, Schimpff SC: Strategies for the prevention of infection in the myelosuppressed cancer patient, *Cancer Treat Rep* 67:223-234, 1983.

Gastrointestinal toxicity

Aapro MS et al: Double blind crossover study of the antiemetic efficacy of high-dose dexamethasone vs high-dose metoclopramide, *J Clin Oncol* 2:466-471, 1984.

Anthony LB et al: Antiemetic effect of oral doses versus intravenous metoclopramide in patients receiving cisplatin: a randomized double blind trial, *J Clin Oncol* 4:98-103, 1986.

Beck S: Impact of a systematic oral care protocol on stomatitis after chemotherapy, *Cancer Nurs* 2:185-199, 1979.

Beck TM: Efficacy of ondansetron tablets in the management of chemotherapy induced emesis: review of clinical trials, *Semin Oncol* 19:20-25, 1992.

Burish TG et al: Behavioral relaxation techniques in reducing the distress of cancer chemotherapy patients, *Oncol Nurs Forum* 10:32-35, 1983.

Burish TG et al: Conditioned side-effects induced by cancer chemotherapy: prevention through behavioral treatment, *J Consult Clin Psychol* 55:42-48, 1987.

Campora E et al: Ondansetron and dexamethasone versus standard combination antiemetic therapy, *Am J Clin Oncol* 17: 522-526, 1994.

Carter LW: Alternatives to unwaxed floss and peroxide rinses recommended, *Oncol Nurs Forum* 19:939-940, 1992.

Cimprich B: Symptom management: constipation, *Cancer Nurs* 8(suppl):39-43, 1985.

Cleri LB: Serotonin antagonists, *Oncol Nurs Patient Treatment and Support* 2(1):1-19, Philadelphia, 1995, Lippincott-Raven.

Coons HL et al: Anticipatory nausea and emotional distress in patients receiving cisplatin-based chemotherapy, *Oncol Nurs Forum* 14:31-35, 1987.

Cotanch PH, Strum S: Progressive muscle relaxation as antiemetic therapy for cancer patients, *Oncol Nurs Forum* 14:33-37, 1987.

Cubeddu LX: Mechanisms by which cancer chemotherapeutic drugs induce emesis, *Semin Oncol* 19(suppl 15):2-13, 1992.

Daeffler RJ: Oral hygiene measures for patients with cancer. Parts I-III, *Cancer Nurs* 3:347-356, 1980; 3:427-432, 1980; 4:29-35, 1981.

Dodd ML et al: Randomized clinical trial for chlorhexidine versus placebo for prevention of oral mucositis in patients receiving chemotherapy, *Oncol Nurs Forum* 23:921-927, 1996.

Engelking C, Rutledge D: Cancer-related diarrhea: oncology nurse perceptions of a neglected symptom and its management, *Oncol Nurs Forum* 23:352, 1996 (abstract).

Epstein JB et al: Efficacy of chlorhexidine and nystatin rinses in the prevention of oral complications in leukemia and bone marrow transplantation, *Oral Surg Oral Med Oral Pathol* 73:682-689, 1992.

Fedak MK: Nutrition and cancer. In Donovan MI, ed: *Cancer care: a guide for patient education,* New York, 1981, Appleton-Century-Crofts, pp 149-175.

Ferretti GA et al: Chlorhexidine prophylaxis for chemotherapy and radiotherapy induced stomatitis: a randomized double blind trial, *Oral Surg Oral Med Oral Pathol* 69:331-338, 1990.

Fleishman SB et al: Antiemetic-induced akathisia in cancer patients receiving chemotherapy, *Am J Psychiatry* 151:763-765, 1994.

Frank J: The effects of music therapy and guided visual imagery on chemotherapy induced nausea and vomiting, *Oncol Nurs Forum* 12:47-52, 1985.

Fraschini G et al: Evaluation of three oral dosages of ondansetron in the prevention of nausea and emesis associated with cyclophosphamide-doxorubicin chemotherapy, *J Clin Oncol* 9:1268-1274, 1991.

Gandara DR et al: The delayed emesis syndrome from cisplatin: phase III evaluation of ondansetron versus placebo, *Semin Oncol* 19(4 suppl 10):67-71, 1992.

Goodman M et al: Integumentary and mucous membrane alterations. In Groenwald S et al, eds: *Cancer nursing principles and practice*, Boston, 1993, Jones & Bartlett, pp 777-778.

Graham KM et al: Reducing the incidence of stomatitis using a quality assessment and improvement approach, *Canc Nurs* 16:117-122, 1993.

Grant M: Nausea, vomiting and anorexia, *Semin Oncol Nurs* 3:277-286, 1987.

Gross J: Functional alterations—bowel. In Johnson BL, Gross J, eds: *Handbook of oncology nursing*, ed 2, Boston, 1994, Jones & Bartlett, pp 517-528.

Hacking A et al: Oral granisetron—simple and effective: a preliminary report, *Eur J Cancer* 28A:S28-S32, 1992.

Hainsworth JD, Hesketh PJ: Single-dose ondansetron for the prevention of cisplatin-induced emesis: efficacy results, *Semin Oncol* 19:14-19, 1992.

Heron JF et al: Oral granisetron alone and in combination with dexamethasone: a double-blind randomized comparison against high dose metoclopramide plus dexamethasone in prevention of cisplatin-induced emesis, *Ann Oncol* 5:579-584, 1994.

Herrstedt J et al: Ondansetron plus metopimazine compared with ondansetron alone in patients receiving moderately emetogenic chemotherapy, *N Engl J Med* 328:1076-1080, 1993.

Hesketh PJ et al: A randomized double-blind comparison of intravenous ondansetron alone and in combination with intravenous dexamethasone in the prevention of high dose cisplatin-induced emesis, *J Clin Oncol* 12: 596-600, 1994.

Ignoffo RJ: Granisetron, *Cancer Practice* 2:229-231, 1994.

Italian Group for Antiemetic Research: Persistence of efficacy of three antiemetic regimens and prognostic factors in patients undergoing moderately emetogenic chemotherapy, *J Clin Oncol* 13:2417-2426, 1995.

Iwamoto R: Alterations in oral status. In McCorkle R et al, eds: *Cancer nursing: a comprehensive textbook*, ed 2, Philadelphia, 1996, WB Saunders, pp 944-962.

Jantunen IT et al: 5-HT3 receptor antagonists in the prophylaxis of acute vomiting induced by moderately emetogenic chemotherapy—a randomised study, *Eur J Cancer* 29: 1669-1672, 1993.

Johnsonbaugh RE et al: Oral granisetron once daily provides effective antiemesis in patients receiving moderately emetogenic chemotherapy, *Ann Oncol* 5(suppl):205, 1994.

Kris MG: Ondansetron: a specific serotonin antagonist for the prevention of chemotherapy-induced vomiting. In DeVita VT Jr, Hellman S, Rosenberg SA, eds: *Principles and practice of oncology, PPO updates* 8(2):1-11, 1994.

Kris MG et al: Extrapyramidal reactions with high-dose metoclopramide, letter, *N Engl J Med* 309:433-434, 1983.

Kris MG et al: Incidence, course and severity of delayed nausea and vomiting following the administration of high-dose cisplatin, *J Clin Oncol* 3:1379-1384, 1985.

Kris MG et al: Antiemetic control and prevention of side effects of anticancer therapy with lorazepam or diphenhydramine when used in combination with metoclopramide plus dexamethasone, *Cancer* 60:2816-2822, 1987.

Kris MG et al: Oral ondansetron for the control of delayed emesis after cisplatin, *Cancer* 70:1012-1016, 1992.

Lane M et al: Dronabinol and prochlorperazine alone and in combination as antiemetic agents for cancer chemotherapy, *Am J Clin Oncol* 13:480-484, 1990.

Laszlo J et al: Lorazepam in cancer patients treated with cisplatin: a drug having antiemetic, amnesic and anxiolytic effects, *J Clin Oncol* 3:864-869, 1985.

Levitt M et al: Ondansetron compared with dexamethasone and metoclopramide as antiemetics in the chemotherapy of breast cancer with cyclophosphamide, methotrexate and fluorouracil, *N Engl J Med* 328:1081-1083, 1993.

Levy MH: Pain management in advanced cancer, *Semin Oncol* 12:394-410, 1985.

Lindley CM, Bernard S, Fields SM: Incidence and duration of chemotherapy-induced nausea and vomiting in the outpatient oncology population, *J Clin Oncol* 7:1142-1149, 1989.

Madeya ML: Oral complications from cancer therapy. Part II. Nursing implications for assessment and treatment, *Oncol Nurs Forum* 23:808-819, 1996.

Maguire LC, Yon JL, Miller E: Prevention of narcotic induced constipation, letter, *N Engl J Med* 305:1651, 1981.

Moertel CG et al: A controlled clinical evaluation of anti-emetic drugs, *JAMA* 186:116-118, 1963.

Morrow GR: Clinical characteristics associated with the development of anticipatory nausea and vomiting in cancer patients undergoing chemotherapy treatment, *J Clin Oncol* 2:1170-1176, 1984.

Navarri RM et al: Oral ondansetron for the control of cisplatin-induced delayed emesis: a large multicenter trial of ondansetron versus placebo, *J Clin Oncol* 13:2408-2416, 1995a.

Navarri RM et al: Comparative clinical trial of granisetron and ondansetron in the prophylaxis of cisplatin induced emesis, *J Clin Oncol* 13:1242-1248, 1995b.

Nerenz DR et al: Anxiety and drug taste as predictors of anticipatory nausea in cancer chemotherapy, *J Clin Oncol* 4:224-233, 1986.

Peterson DE: Oral complications of chemotherapeutic agents, *Semin Oncol* 19:478-491. 1992.

Portenoy RK: Constipation in the cancer patient: causes and management, *Med Clin North Am* 71:303-310, 1987.

Ransier A et al: A combined analysis of a toothbrush, foam brush and a chlorhexidine-soaked foam brush in maintaining oral hygiene, *Canc Nurs* 18(5):393-396, 1995.

Rhodes VA, Johnson MH, McDaniel RW: Nausea, vomiting and retching: the management of the symptom experience, *Semin Oncol Nurs* 11:256-265, 1995.

Roila F et al: Prevention of cisplatin-induced emesis: a double blind multicenter randomized cross-over study comparing ondansetron and ondansetron plus dexamethasone, *J Clin Oncol* 9:675-678, 1991.

Ruff R et al: Ondansetron compared with granisetron in the prophylaxis of cisplatin-induced acute emesis: a multicentre double-blind randomised parallel group study, *Oncology* 51:113-118, 1994.

Sagar SM: The current role of anti-emetic drugs in oncology: a recent revolution in patient symptom control, *Cancer Treat Rev* 18:95-135, 1990.

Sallan SE, Zinberg NE, Frei E III: Antiemetic effect of delta-9-tetrahydrocannabinol in patients receiving cancer chemotherapy, *N Engl J Med* 293:795-797, 1975.

Sheridan C et al: Transient hypertension after high doses of metoclopramide, letter, *N Engl J Med* 307:1346, 1982.

Spross J: Peppermint oil for nausea and vomiting, *Oncol Nurs Forum* 14:103, 1987.

Strohl R: Understanding taste changes, *Oncol Nurs Forum* 11:81-84, 1984.

Toth BB, Frame RT: Dental oncology: the management of disease and treatment related oral/dental complications associated with chemotherapy, *Curr Probl Cancer* 7:7-35, 1983.

Weisdorf DJ et al: Oropharyngeal mucositis complicating bone marrow transplantation: prognostic factors and the effect of chlorhexidine mouth rinse, *Bone Marrow Transplant* 4:89-95, 1989.

Weizman Z: Cola drinks and rehydration in acute diarrhea, letter, *N Engl J Med* 315:768, 1986.

Wrenn K: Fecal impaction, *N Engl J Med* 321:658-662, 1989.

Dermatological toxicity

Argenta LC, Manders EK: Mitomycin C extravasation injuries, *Cancer* 51:1080-1082, 1983.

Boyle DM, Engelking C: Vesicant extravasation: myths and realities, *Oncol Nurs Forum* 22:57-67, 1996.

Brogden JM, Nevidjon B: Vinorelbine tartrate (Navelbine): drug profile and nursing implications of a new vinca alkaloid, *Oncol Nurs Forum* 22:635-646, 1995.

Camp-Sorrell D: Scalp hypothermia devices: current status, *ONS News* 6:1-5, 1991.

Camp-Sorrell D: Implantable ports, *J Intrav Nurs* 15:262-273, 1992.

Curran CF, Luce JK, Page JA: Doxorubicin-associated flare reactions, *Oncol Nurs Forum* 17:387-389, 1990.

DeSpain JD: Dermatologic toxicity of chemotherapy, *Semin Oncol* 19:501-507, 1992.

Duray PH, Cuono CB, Madri JA: Demonstration of cutaneous doxorubicin extravasation by rhodamine filtered fluorescence microscopy, *J Surg Oncol* 31:21-25, 1986.

Goodman M et al: Use caution when managing paclitaxel and taxotere infiltrations, *Oncol Nurs Forum* 23:541-542, 1996.

Harwood KV: Prevention of mitomycin extravasation at prior venipuncture sites, *Oncol Nurs Forum* 13:70, 1986.

Ignoffo RJ, Friedman MA: Therapy of local toxicities caused by extravasation of cancer chemotherapeutic drugs, *Cancer Treat Rev* 7:17-27, 1980.

Keller JF, Blausey LA: Nursing issues and management in chemotherapy-induced alopecia, *Oncol Nurs Forum* 15:603-607, 1988.

Knobf M, Kalm D: Enhanced hyperpigmentation with combination chemotherapy, *Oncol Nurs Forum* 17:762, 1990.

Luce JK et al: Prevention of alopecia by scalp cooling of patients receiving Adriamycin, *Cancer Chemother Rep* 57:108, 1973.

Mayo DJ, Pearson DC: Chemotherapy extravasation: a consequence of fibrin sheath formation around venus access devices, *Oncol Nurs Forum* 22:675-680, 1996.

Oncology Nursing Society: *Cancer chemotherapy guidelines and recommendations for practice,* Pittsburgh, 1996, Oncology Nursing Press.

O'Rourke ME: Enhanced cutaneous effects in combined modality therapy, *Oncol Nurs Forum* 14:31-35, 1987.

Richards C, Wujcik D: Cutaneous toxicity associated with high-dose cytosine arabinoside, *Oncol Nurs Forum* 19:1191-1195, 1992.

Rittenberg CN, Gralla RJ, Rehmeyer TA: Assessing and managing venous irritation associated with vinorelbine tartrate (Navelbine), *Oncol Nurs Forum* 22:707-710, 1996.

Rudolph R, Larson DL: Etiology and treatment of chemotherapeutic agent extravasation injuries: a review, *J Clin Oncol* 5:1116-1126, 1987.

Siepp CA: Scalp hypothermia: indications for precaution, *Oncol Nurs Forum* 10:12, 1983.

Welch-McCaffrey D, Kenneally B: Skin testing and extravasation, *Oncol Nurs Forum* 10:80, 1983.

Wood H, Ellerhorst-Ryan JM: Delayed adverse skin reactions associated with mitomycin-C administration, *Oncol Nurs Forum* 11:14-18, 1984.

Renal toxicity

Durivage HJ, Burnham NL: Prevention and management of toxicities associated with antineoplastic drugs, *J Pharm Pract* 4:27-48, 1991.

Evans TR et al: A randomised study to determine whether routine intravenous magnesium supplements are necessary in patients receiving cisplatin chemotherapy with continuous infusion 5-fluorouracil, *Eur J Cancer* 31A:174-178, 1995.

Fields KK et al: Maximum tolerated doses of ifosfamide, carboplatin, and etoposide given over 6 days followed by autologous stem-cell rescue: toxicity profile, *J Clin Oncol* 13:323-332, 1995.

King CR, Hoffart N, Murray ME: Acute renal failure in bone marrow transplantation, *Oncol Nurs Forum* 19:1327-1335, 1992.

Kintzel PE, Dorr RT: Anticancer drug renal toxicity and elimination: dosing guidelines for altered renal function, *Cancer Treat Rev* 21:33-64, 1995.

Lydon J: Nephrotoxicity of cancer treatment, *Oncol Nurs Forum* 13:68-77, 1986.

Lydon J: Assessment of renal function in the patient receiving chemotherapy, *Cancer Nurs* 12:133-143, 1989.

Patterson WP, Reams GP: Renal toxicities of chemotherapy, *Semin Oncol* 19:521-528, 1992.

Pitman S et al: Sequential methotrexate-leucovorin (MTX-LCV) and cisplatin (CDDP) in head and neck cancer, *Proc Am Soc Clin Oncol* 20:419, 1979.

van der Lelie H et al: Hemolytic uremic syndrome after high dose chemotherapy with autologous stem cell support, *Cancer* 76(11):2338-2342, 1995.

Bladder toxicity

Hows JM et al: Comparison of mesna with forced diuresis to prevent cyclophosphamide induced hemorrhagic cystitis in marrow transplantation: a prospective randomized study, *Br J Cancer* 50:753-756, 1984.

Patterson WP, Reams GP: Renal toxicities of chemotherapy, *Semin Oncol* 19:521-528, 1992.

Stillwell TJ, Benson RC: Cyclophosphamide-induced hemorrhagic cystitis, *Cancer* 61:451-457, 1988.

Zalupski M, Baker LH: Ifosfamide, *J Natl Cancer Inst* 80:556-566, 1988.

Pulmonary toxicity

Cooper JA, Matthay R: Drug-induced pulmonary disease, *Dis Mon* 33:61-120, 1987.

Hilliquin P et al: Occurrence of pulmonary complications during methotrexate therapy in rheumatoid arthritis, *Br J Rheumatol* 35:441-445, 1996.

Kriesman H, Wolkove N: Pulmonary toxicity of antineoplastic therapy, *Semin Oncol* 19:508-520, 1992.

Limper AH, McDonald JA: Delayed pulmonary fibrosis after nitrosourea therapy, *N Engl J Med* 323:407-409, 1990.

O'Driscoll BR et al: Active lung fibrosis up to 17 years after chemotherapy with carmustine (BCNU) in childhood, *N Engl J Med* 323:378-382, 1990.

Shapiro CL et al: Drug-related pulmonary toxicity in non-Hodgkin's lymphoma, *Cancer* 68:699-705, 1991.

van der Veen MJ et al: Fatal pulmonary fibrosis complicating low dose methotrexate therapy for rheumatoid arthritis, *J Rheumatol* 22:1766-1768, 1995.

Cardiac toxicity

Allen A: The cardiotoxicity of chemotherapeutic drugs, *Semin Oncol* 19:529-542, 1992.

Kaszyk LK: Cardiac toxicity associated with cancer therapy, *Oncol Nurs Forum* 13:81-88, 1986.

Postma A et al: Late cardiotoxicity after treatment for a malignant bone tumor, *Med Pediatr Oncol* 26:230-237, 1996.

Shan K, Lincoff M, Young JB: Anthracycline-induced cardiotoxicity, *Ann Intern Med* 125:47-58, 1996.

Shuey KM: Heart, lung and endocrine complications of solid tumors, *Semin Oncol Nurs* 10:117-188, 1994.

Steinherz LJ, Steinherz PG: Delayed anthracycline cardiac toxicity. In DeVita VT Jr, Hellman S, Rosenberg SA, eds: *Principles and practice of oncology, PPO updates* 5(4):1-15, 1991.

Steinherz LJ, Steinherz PG, Tan C: Cardiac failure and dysrhythmias 6-19 years after anthracycline therapy: a series of 15 patients, *Med Pediatr Oncol* 24:352-361, 1995.

Neurological toxicity

Bender CM, Monti EJ, Kerr ME: Potential mechanisms of interferon toxicity, *Cancer Practice* 4:35-39, 1996.

Cain JW, Bender CM: Ifosfamide-induced neurotoxicity: associated symptoms and nursing implications, *Oncol Nurs Forum* 22:659-666, 1995.

Cameron JC: Ifosfamide neurotoxicity, *Cancer Nurs* 16:40-46,1993.

Hansen SW, Helweg-Larsen S, Trojaborg W: Long term neurotoxicity in patients treated with cisplatin, vinblastine and bleomycin for metastatic germ cell cancer, *J Clin Oncol* 7:1457-1461, 1989.

Kaplan RS, Wiernik PH: Neurotoxicity of antineoplastic drugs, *Semin Oncol* 9:103-130, 1982.

Meehan JL, Johnson BL: The neurotoxicity of antineoplastic agents. In Hubbard SM, Greene P, Knobf MT, eds: *Current issues in cancer nursing practice,* Philadelphia, 1991, JB Lippincott, pp 1-11.

Meyers CA: Mental status changes. In Reiger PT, ed: *Biotherapy: a comprehensive overview,* Boston, 1995, Jones & Bartlett, pp 259-270.

Ostchega Y, Donohue M, Fox N: High-dose cisplatin-related peripheral neuropathy, *Cancer Nurs* 11:23-32, 1988.

Patchell RA, Posner JB: Neurologic complications of systemic cancer, *Neurol Clin* 3:729-750, 1985.

Rowinsky EK et al: Clinical toxicities encountered with paclitaxel (Taxol), *Semin Oncol* 20(4 suppl 3):1-15, 1993.

Siegel T, Haim N: Cisplatin-induced peripheral neuropathy, *Cancer* 66:1117-1123, 1990.

Stoter G et al: Ten-year survival and late sequelae in testicular cancer patients treated with cisplatin, vinblastine and bleomycin, *J Clin Oncol* 7:1099-1104, 1989.

Gonadal toxicity

Averette HE, Boike GM, Jarrell MA: Effects of cancer chemotherapy on gonadal function and reproductive capacity, *CA, Cancer J Clin* 40:199-210, 1990.

Chamorro T: Gonadal and reproductive sequelae of cancer therapy. In Hubbard S, Greene P, Knobf M, eds: *Current issues in cancer nursing practice,* Philadelphia, 1991, JB Lippincott, pp 1-14.

Chapman RM, Sutcliffe SB, Malpas JS: Cytotoxic-induced ovarian failure in women with Hodgkin's disease. I. Hormone function, *JAMA* 242:1877-1881, 1979a.

Chapman RM, Sutcliffe SB, Malpas JS: Cytotoxic-induced ovarian failure in women with Hodgkin's disease. II. Effects on sexual function, *JAMA* 242:1882-1884, 1979b.

Gershenson DM: Menstrual and reproductive function after treatment with combination chemotherapy for malignant ovarian germ cell tumors, *J Clin Oncol* 6:270-275, 1988.

Knobf MT: Menopausal symptoms. In Hassay Dow K, ed: *Contemporary issues in breast cancer,* Boston, 1996, Jones & Bartlett, pp 85-97.

Koeppel KM: Sperm banking and patients with cancer, *Cancer Nurs* 18:306-312, 1995.

Kreuser ED et al: Gonadal toxicity following cancer therapy in adults: significance, diagnosis, prevention and treatment, *Cancer Treat Rev* 17:169-175, 1990.

Mehta RR, Beattie CW, DasGupta TK: Endocrine profile in breast cancer patients receiving chemotherapy, *Breast Cancer Res Treat* 20:125-132, 1991.

Myers SE, Schilsky RL: Prospects for fertility after cancer chemotherapy, *Semin Oncol* 19:597-604, 1992.

Ramona MJ et al: Male gonadal dysfunction in Hodgkin's disease, *JAMA* 245:1323-1328, 1981.

Rivkees SA, Crawford JD: The relationship of gonadal activity and chemotherapy-induced gonadal damage, *JAMA* 259:2123-2125, 1988.

Rose DP, David TE: Effects of adjuvant chemohormonal therapy on the ovarian and adrenal function of breast cancer patients, *Cancer Res* 40:4043-4047, 1980.

Samaan NA et al: Pituitary-ovarian function in breast cancer patients on adjuvant chemoimmunotherapy, *Cancer* 41:2084-2087, 1978.

Santoro A et al: Long term results of combined chemotherapy-radiotherapy approach in Hodgkin's disease: superiority of ABVD plus radiotherapy versus MOPP plus radiotherapy, *J Clin Oncol* 5:27-37, 1987.

Sweet V, Servy EJ, Karow AM: Reproductive issues for men with cancer: technology and nursing management, *Oncol Nurs Forum* 23:51-58, 1996.

Waxman JH et al: Gonadal function in Hodgkin's disease: long term follow-up of chemotherapy, *BMJ* 285:1612-1613, 1982.

Whitehead E et al: The effect of combination chemotherapy on ovarian function in women treated for Hodgkin's disease, *Cancer* 52:933-988, 1983.

Young-McGaughan S: Sexual functioning in women with breast cancer after treatment with adjuvant therapy, *Cancer Nurs* 19:308-319, 1996.

Other organ system toxicity

Burns LJ: Ocular toxicities of chemotherapy, *Semin Oncol* 19:492-500, 1992.

Doll DC, Yarbro JW: Vascular toxicity associated with antineoplastic agents, *Semin Oncol* 19:580-596, 1992.

Perry MC: Chemotherapeutic agents and hepatotoxicity, *Semin Oncol* 19:551-565, 1992.

11

Blood Transfusion Therapy for the Cancer Patient

EDWARD L. SNYDER, MD

The professional oncology health care worker needs a general working knowledge of modern transfusion practice. This chapter will discuss basic blood component therapy, including indications for use of components and derivatives. Further, it will provide the reader with an understanding of how to recognize and treat transfusion reactions.

BLOOD COMPONENTS

Red blood cell (RBC) components comprise over 50% of the total transfused blood components. Although previously it was standard practice to transfuse whole blood (WB) to anemic oncology patients, this practice has changed completely (Ness and Rothko, 1995). WB is usually not available in most blood centers. In modern transfusion medicine, RBCs, either in the form of (packed) RBCs or additive solution red blood cells (AS-RBCs), are the preferred form of therapy. RBCs are prepared by collecting whole blood and removing sufficient plasma to prepare a unit with a hematocrit of about 75%. AS-RBCs are prepared by removing most of the plasma, leaving a hematocrit of about 90%, but replacing the volume with a crystalloid solution containing a variety of blood additives including, depending on the manufacturer, glucose or mannitol, and adenine. Thus the AS-RBC unit has a lower hematocrit of approximately 55% and, because of the extra adenine, an increased shelf life from the 35 days for RBC to 42 days for the AS-RBC units. It is important for the oncologist to remember that all three products (WB, RBCs, and AS-RBCs) vary only in the amount and type of supernatant plasma; all have the *same* red cell mass. RBCs or AS-RBCs are the components of choice for treatment of anemia in medical or surgical, pediatric or adult oncology patients. If indicated, these units can be further processed (i.e., leukocyte reduced, washed, irradiated, or cytomegalovirus [CMV] seronegative), depending on a patient's needs.

TYPES OF DONATIONS

There are a variety of types of blood donations, including **autologous** donations, where a surgical patient preoperatively donates a unit of his or her own blood. This type of donation is not often feasible for oncology patients but should be offered if the patient has an acceptable hematocrit (>33%), is not septic, and is clinically capable of donating a unit of blood. Other types of blood donations include **directed donor**, where patients have relatives or friends donate for them, and **designated donor**, where a unit of blood either from a directed donor or from the regular blood bank supply is selected and set aside for a specific patient. In this way, multiple requests for small aliquots of blood can be filled from that single product. This approach is most appropriate for pediatric oncology patients in whom multiple aliquots from a single unit may be requested, thus decreasing concern over multiple-donor exposures. Frozen red blood cells (FRBCs), another red cell component, can be stored frozen up to 10 years. There is little need for FRBCs for oncology patients, because liquid storage suffices in most cases.

Indication for RBC Transfusion

It is generally agreed that the indication for RBC transfusion should be based on the clinical status of the patient (NHLBI, 1993). No longer are RBC triggers, such as a hemoglobin of less than 10 g/dL or a hematocrit <30%, used as appropriate indications for a transfusion. The current approach stresses that transfusion is less often indicated when the hemoglobin is greater than 7 g/dL or when the hematocrit is greater than 21%, and that below those values, transfusion is more often indicated. The decision to transfuse, however, should primarily be based on clinical symptomatology in conjunction with the laboratory data. Clinical symptoms to consider include fatigue, headache, tachycardia, hypotension, cardiac arrhythmia, dizziness, chest pain, and syncope. Patients with cardiopulmonary dysfunction are of special concern. For oncology patients, RBCs should be administered through a leukoreduction blood filter (see p. 561). One unit of RBCs raises the hemoglobin in an average adult by 1 g/dL and the hematocrit by 3%.

PLATELETS

Platelets are given to patients with thrombocytopenia or thrombocytopathy (Slichter, 1995; NHLBI, 1993). The most common indication in oncology patients is an aplastic or hypoplastic marrow caused by chemotherapy, radiation therapy, or a myelophthisic process. The standard platelet transfusion product is a random-donor platelet (RDP) unit prepared from an individual WB donation prepared by differential centrifugation techniques. Platelets contain a minimum dose of 5.5×10^{10} platelets per bag (Klein, 1996; Code of Federal Regulations, 1995). They have a shelf life of 5 days when stored at 20° to 24° C. The usual dose of platelets is about 1 unit/10 kg of body weight (up to 6 to 10 units at most hospitals). Assuming that there is no reason for decreased platelet survival, this usually raises the recipient's platelet count by 5000 to 10,000/μL per unit infused. Other types of platelets include single-donor platelets (SDPs) prepared by apheresis techniques, which contain more than 3×10^{11} platelets per bag. Generally, SDPs contain the equivalent of 5 or 6 units of pooled RDPs. SDPs can be prepared from a platelet apheresis donor chosen at random. These random single-donor platelets (RSDPs) may be the standard platelet product at some institutions. In addition to RDP and RSDP, platelets can be prepared from specially selected human leukocyte antigen (HLA)–matched donors (HLA-matched SDPs).

Cross-matched platelets also can be used to provide therapy for individuals who have become refractory to platelet transfusion. *Platelet refractoriness* is defined as a failure to manifest an increment in the posttransfusion platelet count. Causes of platelet refractoriness include bone marrow transplantation, disseminated intravascular coagulation (DIC), hypersensitivity to drugs, HLA alloantibody, sepsis, immune complexes, viremia, platelet autoantibody, or an inflammatory process. The following formula is used to determine whether the platelet increment is appropriate for the dose of platelets and the patient's body size:

$$\text{CCI} = \frac{[\text{Posttransfusion platelet count}] - [\text{Pretransfusion platelet count}] \times \text{BSA}}{\text{total platelets transfused} \times 10^{-11}}$$

NOTE: CCI, Corrected count increment; platelet count is in μL; BSA, body surface area in m².

A CCI of over 7500, measured at 1 to 4 hours after transfusion, is considered acceptable and is a sign that the platelets are surviving appropriately. Although standard practice varies among institutions, it is recommended that a posttransfusion platelet count be obtained soon after the platelet transfusion has finished to determine the outcome of the blood-product infusion. Preferably, a platelet count should be obtained within 4 hours of termination of the platelet transfusion. In patients with a shortened platelet survival, a count taken at 24 hours or later may miss the peak platelet count; indeed, if the posttransfusion platelet count had returned to the patient's baseline by 24 hours, one would not know if the count had ever increased. This is important in determining the need for special HLA-matched or cross-matched platelet products. A platelet count taken 10 minutes after a platelet transfusion has been shown to be equivalent to a count taken 1 to 4 hours after transfusion (O'Connell, Lee, and Schiffer, 1988). This is useful if a posttransfusion count needs to be obtained from a patient who needs to leave the clinic or office shortly after the platelet transfusion has finished. Patients who become refractory will not show an increase in their posttransfusion platelet count. Such patients should have HLA antibody typing performed and may be considered candidates for HLA-matched or cross-matched platelets.

For patients who fail to respond to either of these modalities, a platelet drip may be useful. A platelet drip as practiced at some institutions consists of infusing 1 unit of platelets each hour for a total of 24 units each day. The equivalent in RSDP would be 4 to 5 units per day. The platelets can be infused through an electromechanical pump to ensure an infusion rate of approximately 50 mL/hr. Platelet drips ensure that platelets are continually infused, which may be of some benefit to the refractory oncology patient. Even though a platelet drip provides multiple units of RDPs or RSDPs, this practice is not likely to appreciably increase the patient's platelet count. There is little evidence that this practice is substantially better than bolus infusions. However, a drip may be useful when there is a shortage of platelets in the blood center by helping to spread out the platelet usage for some refractory patients over a 24-hour period. For treatment of patients with severe refractoriness to platelet transfusion, the oncologist should consult the institution's blood transfusion director.

Indication for Platelet Transfusion

The use of triggers to gauge the need for a platelet transfusion has become as problematic as the use of triggers for RBC transfusions. Although some physicians use low platelet values (e.g., 5000 to 10,000/µL) as the value at which they transfuse platelets, other physicians prefer to transfuse at higher platelet counts (e.g., 15,000 to 20,000/µL) (Beutler, 1993; Pisciotto et al, 1995). Again, it is generally believed that the decision to provide platelet transfusions should be based not only on the patient's platelet count, but on the patient's clinical status as well (Slichter, 1995). For an individual who has had a recent operation and who has a platelet count of 25,000/µL, the risk of bleeding is greater than that for a patient with a similar platelet count but who has not just had surgery. Other factors to consider include the presence of any intercurrent diseases that may affect platelet function, such as hypersplenism or drug-induced thrombocytopathies. Platelets are collected by relatively inefficient centrifugation techniques and are often contaminated with donor RBCs. Accordingly, Rh-negative oncology patients who receive units of Rh positive platelets may be candidates for a dose of Rh immune globulin. Although there are no Rh antigens on platelets themselves, Rh antigens are present on any Rh-positive red cells, which may contaminate the platelet product. One 300-µg dose of Rh immune globulin is sufficient to protect against over 75 units of Rh-positive platelets because the units contain very small amounts of RBCs.

GRANULOCYTES

Granulocyte transfusions are infrequently used in modern oncology practice. However, when they are requested, it is primarily for the treatment of gram-positive or gram-negative bacterial sepsis in neutropenic oncology patients who are unresponsive to appropriate antibiotics (Strauss, 1995). There are insufficient data to recommend use of granulocyte transfusions for fungal infections. Although in the past granulocyte collections resulted in a dose of 1×10^{10} neutrophils per bag, a dose of 5 to 10 µg/kg of G-CSF given to normal donors can permit collection of 50 to 60 times this amount of neutrophils from a single G-CSF–stimulated donor (Bensinger et al, 1993). This advance in treatment, when approved by the FDA, could well increase the clinical usefulness of granulocyte transfusions. Though infrequently requested by the oncologist, granulocyte transfusion should be restricted to use in individuals with an absolute neutrophil count less than 500/µL, evidence of myeloid hypoplasia (usually the result of chemotherapy, radiation therapy, or a myelophthisic process), an infection that has been shown to be nonresponsive to antibiotics for a minimum of 24 to 48 hours, and a reasonable chance for recovery. Granulocytes should be provided for a patient on a daily basis; they cannot be stored beyond 24 hours. Although granulocytes are not usually HLA matched, because of the large number of red cells contained in the granulocyte concentrates (hematocrit of 1% to 2%), the product must be crossmatched. Although the data are equivocal, because of the few anecdotal reports of pulmonary reactions, it is generally believed that granulocytes should not be transfused in close proximity to infusion of amphotericin. The oncologist health care worker should bear in mind that although granulocyte transfusions are available, many clinicians believe that they provide minimal benefit beyond that achieved with use of appropriate antibiotic therapy. Administration of G-CSF to the *patient* has also decreased the need to initiate granulocyte transfusions.

PLASMA AND CRYOPRECIPITATE

The indications for transfusion of fresh frozen plasma (FFP) to oncology patients are limited to those patients with DIC, hypofibrinogenemia, or a coagulopathy of some other cause (Hillyer and Berkman, 1995; NHLBI, 1993). FFP is a biohazardous human fluid and should *never* be infused as a volume replacement; albumin, plasma protein fraction, crystalloid, or nonplasma colloid solutions such as hydroxyethyl starch should be used to simply expand the plasma volume. Cryoprecipitate is prepared by thawing FFP at 4° C. It contains fibrinogen and factor VIII. Cryoprecipitate does not contain factor V. Thus for patients with DIC, cryoprecipitate is indicated only to increase the level of factor VIII or fibrinogen. To increase the level of factor V during the treatment of DIC, FFP must also be given. There are few, if any, indications for use of cryoprecipitate in noncoagulopathic oncology patients.

TRANSFUSION REACTIONS

A *transfusion reaction* is defined as any adverse effect that occurs that is causally related to a blood transfusion (Snyder, 1995). This includes immunological reactions as well as transfusion-transmitted diseases (Table 11-1).

Hemolytic Reactions

There are four characteristics of hemolytic transfusion reactions; two are related to time—acute and delayed reactions—and two are related to location and type of hemolysis, intravascular and extravascular. **Acute** reactions occur when blood is given and antibodies against some of the RBC antigens are already present in the recipient; the patient reacts within minutes. This occurs with reactions to the ABO system. Delayed reactions occur when the patient is transfused and since no antibody or a very low titer of antibody exists, time for the antibodies to be synthesized must

TABLE 11-1
Differential Diagnosis of Acute Transfusion Reactions

Reaction type	Presenting signs and symptoms
Acute intravascular hemolytic	Fever, chills, dyspnea, hypotension, tachycardia, flushing, vomiting, back pain, hemoglobinuria, hemoglobinemia, shock
Acute extravascular hemolytic	Fever, indirect hyperbilirubinemia, posttransfusion hematocrit increment lower than expected
Febrile reaction	Fever, chills
Allergic (mild)	Urticaria, pruritus, rash
Anaphylactic	Dyspnea, bronchospasm, hypotension, tachycardia, shock
Hypervolemic	Dyspnea, tachycardia, hypertension, headache, jugular venous distention
Septic	Fever, chills, hypotension, tachycardia, vomiting, shock

From Snyder EL: Transfusion reactions. In Hoffman R et al, eds: *Hematology: basic principles and practice,* ed 2, New York, 1995, Churchill Livingstone.

pass before the reaction can occur. The delay varies from 3 to 7 days for anamnestic or recall responses to 2 to 3 weeks after transfusion for a primary immunization. **Delayed** responses are characteristic of reactions to non-ABO RBC antigens. Serologically, hemolytic transfusion reactions are associated with a new positive direct antiglobulin (Coombs') test (DAT). The clinician should remember that the DAT-positive RBCs coated with antibody are the *donor's* RBCs, *not* the patients.

Acute Intravascular Hemolytic Transfusion Reactions (AIHTR)

Transfusion reactions can also be classified by location (that is, whether they occur in the intravascular or the extravascular space). **Intravascular** reactions occur when an RBC antibody binds the entire complement cascade to the erythrocyte membrane, including the C5b-9 complex. When the C5b-9 (membrane attack) complex binds to the RBC membrane, it literally results in a formation of a hole in the membrane, forming a water channel. The water channels (holes) in the RBC membrane result in osmotic hemolysis. This also is associated with generation of complement, fragments C3a and C5a, which causes hypotension, shock, tachycardia, dyspnea, renal dysfunction, and often a coagulopathy. The sine qua non of an AIHTR is red plasma and red urine. Chest pain, nausea, and bronchospasm can also occur. Renal failure often occurs because of hypoperfusion of the renal tubules secondary to the drop in cardiac output, and also because of renal vasoconstriction caused by release of free hemoglobin, which binds nitric oxide. Nitric oxide induces vasodilation, and if blocked, renal vasodilation cannot occur (Capon and Goldfinger, 1995). The complement activation also stimulates leukocytes, resulting in activation and generation of adhesive molecules. These adhesive molecules permit the neutrophils to stick to the pulmonary capillary bed and impede gas exchange across the alveolar epithelium. A diagnosis

---

BOX 11-1
Approach to Workup of an Acute Intravascular Hemolytic Transfusion Reaction

If an acute transfusion reaction occurs:

1. *Stop blood component infusion immediately*
2. Maintain intravenous access with a suitable crystalloid or colloid solution
3. Maintain blood pressure, heart rate
4. Maintain an adequate airway
5. Give a diuretic or institute a fluid diuresis, or both
6. Obtain blood/urine for transfusion reaction workup

 Blood bank workup of suspected transfusion reaction:
 Check paperwork to ensure correct blood component was transfused to the right patient
 Observe plasma for hemoglobinemia
 Perform direct antiglobulin test
 Repeat compatibility testing (crossmatch)
 Repeat other serologic testing as needed (ABO, Rh)
 Analyze urine for hemoglobinuria

If intravascular hemolytic reaction confirmed:

7. Monitor renal status (BUN, creatinine)
8. Monitor coagulation status (prothrombin time, partial thromboplastin time, fibrinogen)
9. Monitor for signs of hemolysis (LDH, bilirubin, haptoglobin)
10. If sepsis is suspected, culture as appropriate

From Snyder EL: Transfusion reactions. In Hoffman R et al, eds: *Hematology: basic principles and practice,* ed 2, New York, 1995, Churchill Livingstone.

of an AIHTR is made in the blood bank by serotyping the patient and the donor unit and documenting the development of a positive new DAT.

 Treatment of an AIHTR is a medical emergency (Box 11-1). It may require maintenance of airway, blood pressure, and renal function. The patient may require intubation and pressors such as low-dose dopamine (<5 µg/kg/min, higher doses can cause renal vasoconstriction). Renal damage can be minimized by use of diuretics and maintenance of a diuresis of >100 mL/hour until pigmenturia has stopped; renal failure may require dialysis. Mannitol can be used if treatment of the AIHTR starts immediately. If a prolonged delay in initiating therapy occurs, furosemide or another diuretic is preferred. This is to avoid pulmonary edema caused by fluid overload if mannitol is infused after anuric renal failure has occurred. Laboratory monitoring of an AIHTR includes evaluation of lactic dehydrogenase (LDH), indirect bilirubin levels, and the DAT. DIC can be followed with monitoring of the prothrombin time and partial thromboplastin time; renal failure can be evaluated by measurement of BUN and creatinine levels.

Acute Extravascular Hemolytic Transfusion Reactions (AEHTR)

An acute **extravascular** reaction occurs when a unit is transfused and either no complement is fixed (IgG bound only) or complement is fixed only to C3a. This results in the removal of the IgG-coated RBCs by extravascular sites such as the spleen or the C3b-coated RBCs by the liver, all without generation of clinically significant amounts of C3a or C5a. Although patients will also develop a new positive DAT and show an elevation in LDH and indirect bilirubin levels, in contrast to the medical emergency of an AIHTR, patients with AEHTR are usually asymptomatic because of the lack of complement activation. The only standard therapy for an AEHTR is observation. Patients usually recover without acute intervention, and when the incompatible donor cells are cleared from the patient's circulation, the DAT will return to negative. Delayed intravascular (DIHTR) and delayed extravascular (DEHTR) hemolytic reactions also occur. The DIHTR is not as life threatening as an AIHTR because of the slow onset of hemolysis and minimal biological response modifier generation seen with DIHTRs. DEHTRs are not uncommon. They may not be detected during the patient's hospital stay. When the transfused patient returns months or years later, however, a new antibody may be detected in the serum, an antibody that occurred in response to the prior transfusion(s).

Febrile Reactions

Febrile reactions are caused by an interaction between donor (or recipient) leukocytes and recipient (or donor) leukocyte antibodies (leukoagglutinins). The formation of leukocyte antigen-antibody complexes results in complement binding and release of endogenous pyrogens such as cytokines IL-1, IL-6, and TNF-α. This inflammatory response results in the release of prostaglandin E$_2$ by the hypothalamus, which causes an increase in patient temperature and produces a fever, often accompanied by chills or rigors. Inflammatory cytokines can also be produced in the blood bag during storage (Stack and Snyder, 1994; Stack et al, 1995). Most patients tolerate febrile reactions without major problems. However, severe febrile reactions may be life threatening for individuals with impaired cardiac reserves or an intercurrent illness (Dinarello, Cannon, and Wolff, 1988). Severe rigors can be controlled by use of small doses of subcutaneous or intramuscular meperidine (Demerol).

Premedication

Patient premedication before blood transfusion is a somewhat controversial issue. Many physicians routinely premedicate all pretransfusion patients with acetaminophen and diphenhydramine. Other physicians do not believe in giving prophylactic medications and reserve such pharmacotherapy for patients with a history of recurrent febrile or allergic reactions. Still others use medication only if a reaction occurs. Use of aspirin is contraindicated for control of fever in thrombocytopenic individuals because aspirin can block the enzyme cyclooxygenase, which is required for normal platelet function. Diphenhydramine has *no* value in the treatment or prevention of a febrile reaction. The health care worker should remember that it is very unlikely that 650 mg acetaminophen will block or mask a serious febrile reaction. Similarly, neither will 50 mg of diphenhydramine mask a serious allergic reaction. Leukoreduced RBCs or platelets should be used for patients with recurrent febrile reactions; washed RBCs could be used but are not as effectively leukoreduced as are the filtered products.

Septic Transfusions

Individuals who receive blood transfusions can develop hypotension and shock secondary to bacterial contamination of the unit of blood (Goldman and Blajchman, 1991; Ness, 1996). Blood cultures should be taken from individuals who spike very high temperatures with or without hypotension; it is recommended that the implicated blood product bag(s) be cultured as well. Organisms range from gram-positive, such as *Staphylococcus* species, to gram-negative bacteria, including *Enterobacter* and *Pseudomonas* species. It is often difficult to distinguish febrile from septic transfusion reactions. Febrile reactions are usually self-limiting, and patients usually do not develop shock. For an individual with a severe septic reaction, however, shock is quite common. Such reactions may be fatal unless rapidly treated with broad-spectrum antibiotics. The risk of infection in a unit of blood is approximately 1 in 1500.

Allergic Reactions

Allergic reactions occur commonly. The patients have no fever but are subject to pruritus and urticaria. Allergic complications can also manifest as anaphylaxis, with bronchospasm and cardiovascular collapse. Medication for mild reactions is usually 25 mg to 50 mg of diphenhydramine. Although mild urticarial reactions are common, they do not extend to become anaphylactic reactions. If an individual has an allergic reaction, the transfusing unit should be stopped. If the reaction is mild, it is acceptable to restart the unit provided the hives fade and *only* if the patient has no fever and no signs of pulmonary dysfunction or vasomotor instability. Anaphylactic reactions such as those caused by IgA deficiency are rare but should be treated as one would any anaphylactic reaction, including use of steroids and pressors.

OTHER ADVERSE CONDITIONS

Transfusion-transmitted diseases remain a constant concern. The risk of acquiring the human immunodeficiency virus (HIV) from a unit of blood is now approximately 1 in 450,000; human T-cell leukemia/lymphoma virus (HTLV-I) is 1 in 640,000; hepatitis B, 1 in 67,000; and hepatitis C 1 in 100,000 (Dodd, 1992; Lackritz et al, 1995). Modern transfusion services provide special products for cancer patients, including use of leukoreduction filters to remove large numbers of viable white cells. These filters are indicated for prevention of febrile reactions. Furthermore, since cancer patients are often transfused and are thus at risk for developing HLA alloimmunization, leukoreduction filters may be employed to decrease the incidence of HLA antibody formation. These filters remove over 3 $\log_{10}$ leukocytes. At these levels, the incidence of alloimmunization drops dramatically. Many oncologists believe that individuals with cancer are immunosuppressed, and if they are CMV seronegative, they should receive CMV-seronegative products. Data now show that units of blood leukoreduced with a 3 $\log_{10}$ removal filter are likely to be equivalent to CMV-seronegative blood products (Bowden et al, 1995). Since CMV is carried inside neutrophils, leukoreduction is a useful means of preventing CMV transmission. Blood transfusion into immunosuppressed cancer patients can also produce posttransfusion graft-versus-host disease (GVHD). All cellular blood products for oncology patients should be irradiated with a minimum of 2500 cGy (rads) to prevent posttransfusion GVHD (Quinnan, 1993). It is important to remember that leukoreduction filters must *never* be used in place of irradiation to prevent GVHD. Irradiation is the only acceptable method to prevent posttransfusion GVHD.

ADMINISTRATION OF BLOOD PRODUCTS

Among the most important aspect of a transfusion is ensuring that the correct patient gets the correct product. Thus not only a check, but a double check of the wrist band and the label on the blood bag(s) must be performed by the transfusionist to be absolutely certain that the intended recipient has been correctly identified. It is equally as important to ensure that the label on the tube of blood initially sent for crossmatching was also correctly labeled. Other caveats to remember when administering blood include that all blood or components must be transfused through an administration set containing a filter; blood or components should not be warmed over 42° C, preferably in an approved blood warmer with temperature-monitoring devices; any blood component should be administered within 4 hours (the blood bank can aliquot the product if longer infusion times are planned); the only intravenous crystalloid solution to use for diluting blood or components is normal (0.9%) saline; and last, blood must be stored under monitored, temperature-controlled conditions. Do not store blood in refrigerators containing food or in non–blood bank-monitored refrigerators or incubators.

Modern transfusion practice has changed dramatically. The oncologist or oncology health care professional faced with any transfusion problem should consult the hospital or blood center medical director for further information on any of the topics discussed in this brief review.

REFERENCES

Bensinger WI et al: The effects of daily recombinant human granulocyte colony-stimulating factor administration on normal granulocyte donors undergoing leukapheresis, *Blood* 81:1883-1888, 1993.

Beutler E: Platelet transfusions: the 20,000/μL trigger, *Blood* 81:1411-1413, 1993.

Bowden RA et al: A comparison of filtered leukocyte-reduced and cytomegalovirus (CMV) seronegative blood products for the prevention of transfusion-associated CMV infection after marrow transplant, *Blood* 78:246-250, 1995.

Capon SM, Goldfinger D: Acute hemolytic transfusion reaction, a paradigm of the systemic inflammatory response: new insights into pathophysiology and treatment, *Transfusion* 35:513-520, 1995. Published erratum appears in *Transfusion* 35:7941, 1995.

Code of Federal Regulations, 21 CFR 600-799, Washington, DC, April 1995, U.S. Government Printing Office.

Dinarello CA, Cannon JG, Wolff SM: New concepts on the pathogenesis of fever, *Rev Infect Dis* 10:168-189, 1988.

Dodd RY: The risk of transfusion transmitted infection, editorial, *N Engl J Med* 327:419-421, 1992.

Goldman M, Blajchman M: Blood product associated bacterial sepsis, *Transf Med Rev* 5:73-83, 1991.

Hillyer CD, Berkman EM: Transfusion of plasma derivatives: fresh frozen plasma, cryoprecipitate, albumin and immunoglobulins. In Hoffman R et al, eds: *Hematology: basic principles and practice*, ed 2, New York, Churchill Livingstone, 1995, pp 2011.

Klein H, ed: *Standards for blood banks and transfusion services*, ed 17, Bethesda, Md, 1996, American Association of Blood Banks.

Lackritz EM et al: Estimated risk of transmission of the human immunodeficiency virus by screened blood in the United States, *N Engl J Med* 333:1721-1725, 1995.

Ness PM: Bacterial transmission by transfusion. In Rossi EC et al, eds: *Principles of transfusion medicine*, ed 2, Baltimore, 1996, Williams & Wilkins, pp 739.

Ness PM, Rothko K. Principles of red blood cell transfusion. In Hoffman R et al, eds: *Hematology: basic principles and practice*, ed 2, New York, 1995, Churchill Livingstone, pp 1981.

NHLBI, National Blood Resource Education Program Expert Panel: *Transfusion alert: indications for the use of red blood cells, platelets and fresh frozen plasma*, NHLBI-NIH Publication 93-2974a, August 1993.

O'Connell B, Lee EJ, Schiffer CA: The value of 10 minute posttransfusion platelet counts, *Transfusion* 28:66-67, 1988.

Pisciotto PT et al: Prophylactic versus therapeutic platelet transfusion practices in hematology and/or oncology patients, *Transfusion* 35:498-502, 1995.

Quinnan GV: *Recommendations regarding license amendments and procedures for gamma irradiation of blood products*, Washington, DC, July 22, 1993, Office of the Director, Center for Biologics Evaluation and Research, Food and Drug Administration.

Slichter S: Principles of platelet transfusion therapy. In Hoffman R et al, eds: *Hematology: basic principles and practice*, ed 2, New York, 1995, Churchill Livingstone, pp 1987.

Snyder EL: Transfusion reactions. In Hoffman R et al, eds: *Hematology: basic principles and practice*, ed 2, New York, 1995, Churchill Livingstone, pp 2045.

Stack G, Snyder EL: Cytokine generation in stored platelet concentrates, *Transfusion* 34:20-25, 1994.

Stack G et al: Cytokine generation in stored, white cell–reduced and bacterially contaminated units of red cells, *Transfusion* 35:199-203, 1995.

Strauss R: Principles of white blood cell transfusion. In Hoffman R et al, eds: *Hematology: basic principles and practice*, ed 2, New York, 1995, Churchill Livingstone, pp 2006.

12

Principles of Pediatric Cancer Therapy

DIANE M. KOMP, MD

Although cancer is a relatively rare event in children in comparison to adults, no other group of cancer patients has more fully realized the benefits of modern chemotherapy and combined modality therapy. Many of the principles that now benefit adults with diverse cancers were first learned in the treatments of Wilms' tumor and acute leukemia of childhood. Although most children diagnosed with cancer are and should be treated by pediatric oncologists, medical oncologists would be well served by a familiarity with the treatment principles and long-term consequences of cancer treatment in childhood.

The success in treating children with cancer is reflected in the mortality rates of patients under 15 years of age, rates that have dropped by 68% in the last 3 decades. Many of these surviving young adults will seek follow-up care from medical oncologists.

CLINICAL COOPERATIVE GROUPS

It has been estimated that 80% of children in the United States with cancer are treated under protocols of the two pediatric cooperative groups sponsored by the National Cancer Institute—the Pediatric Oncology Group (POG) and the Children's Cancer Study Group (CCSG). Most of the group protocols are "front-line" studies appropriate for newly diagnosed, untreated patients (Vietti et al, 1992). With the exception of diseases with poor prognosis, front-line studies are phase III studies that incorporate the best-known aspects of standard proven therapy (Meyers, 1987). Randomized studies frequently compare two regimens that could be selected individually as nonstudy treatment choices (D'Angio et al, 1989).

A major thrust of contemporary pediatric front-line studies is the inclusion of tumor biology studies performed in collaborative reference laboratories. Thus the value of the studies exceeds the relative merit of the chemotherapy question asked in the randomized comparisons (Brodeur et al, 1987). Access to large numbers of patients with acute lymphoblastic leukemia and neuroblastoma, to name only two examples, has accelerated the basic understanding of these diseases in patients.

EARLY SIDE EFFECTS OF THERAPY

Because of the anticipated long survival of most children diagnosed with cancer and the number of years at risk for delayed consequences, it is worth dividing side effects into early and late groupings. This division is also of value in discussions with parents because the types of side effects that evoke emotional responses and problems with acceptance of therapy are more likely to be observable and early (Gaes, 1987). On the other hand, the types of side effects that are of more importance to physicians are both unseen and delayed. For purposes of this chapter, only those side effects with important adult-child differences will be addressed.

Nausea and Vomiting

In general, the younger the child, the less nausea and vomiting is noted, given a weight-equivalent dosing of chemotherapy. Furthermore, the younger the children, the less they are disturbed by vomiting when it does occur and the more likely they are to just vomit and get back to happily doing whatever they want to do. Anticipatory vomiting is usually not seen until 9 years of age. When it does occur, it has the same implications as it does in adults. As with adults, serotonin inhibitors are the most useful agents for drugs causing moderate to severe nausea and vomiting. Our agent of choice is ondansetron (Zofran). Granisetron may be substituted but should not be given in doses less than 20 µg/kg or when morphine is also in use and contributing to nausea and vomiting. The efficacy of both ondansetron and granisetron is augmented by corticosteroids, but the following are disease situations in which steroids may be relatively contraindicated:

1. Brain tumors where the patient is not already on steroids for increased intracranial pressure. Since steroids increase the integrity of the blood-brain barrier, the chemotherapy may not cross as effectively.
2. Bone tumor patients with bone allografts. Wound and graft healing are impaired by corticosteroids. Some orthopedic oncologists consider this an absolute contraindication; others permit the treating chemotherapist to make judgments about patients quality of life.

Hair Loss

In general, younger children are not as concerned about hair loss as are teenagers and adults. As one wise child said, "It's what's on a person's inside that counts." This does not mean that parents won't be distressed by impending hair loss. Both child and parents benefit to know that all chemotherapy-related and most radiation-associated hair loss is temporary. As of the time of writing, health insurers are still covering hair transplantation for patients whose permanent hair loss is secondary to cancer treatment.

DELAYED CONSEQUENCES OF TREATMENT

Infertility

Before puberty, both the male spermatogonia and female ova are in a more resting state and not undergoing rapid division. For this reason, there may be less impact on fertility than is usually seen in postpubertal males and females. For example, prepubertal males are not expected to have universal permanent azoospermia from MOPP chemotherapy nor do prepubertal females so treated experience a hastening of their biological clocks towards menopause. Since fecundity is multifactorial and not simply dependent on the number of ova or sperm, the exact risks of impaired fertility cannot yet be estimated for children treated at various prepubertal ages. Nonetheless, studies to date show lower fertility rates of children treated for cancer than in their siblings (Byrne et al, 1987).

Secondary Malignancy

Although children in general are as or more subject as adults to secondary malignancy after cancer treatment, the type of secondary malignancy seen may differ. For example, prepubescent children treated for Hodgkin's disease with combined-modality therapy are more likely to develop an in-port radiation-associated malignancy than acute nonlymphocytic leukemia. Pubescent females run a higher risk of breast cancer from in-port radiation therapy. For this reason and the fertility issues raised above, modern protocols for children with Hodgkin's disease differ from adult protocols in their strategy, with chemotherapy and lower doses of radiation used even in lower-stage disease (Tucker et al, 1984).

Neurotoxicity

One of the most difficult problems facing the oncologist treating children today is the strategies for brain tumor patients. Radiation to the brain under 6 years of age is likely to cause intellectual deficits. Radiation to the brain under 1 year of age can cause devastating deficits. For this reason, current "baby brain tumor" protocols rely on the use of chemotherapy—which is *not* curative—to keep the tumor under control until the brain has a chance to further develop.

Although the elimination of routine use of prophylactic cranial irradiation has dramatically reduced the risk of leukoencephalopathy in children with acute lymphoblastic leukemia under 6 years of age, similar effects can be seen from intrathecal therapy with or without intermediate-dose intravenous methotrexate. Seizures and learning disabilities continue to be reported and their cause and prevention are areas of active investigation.

ETHICAL CONSIDERATIONS

Consent

From a legal point of view, informed consent for minor children must be obtained from the parent or legal guardian. When parents are separated, divorced with joint custody, or have expressed conflicting opinions about treatment, it is wise to have both parents sign. When they are in agreement and are married and living together, one signature suffices. Although minor children are not legally required to sign, children over 9 years of age, and especially teenagers, may *assent* to their treatment and may choose to cosign. Parents may guide caregivers as to the appropriate level of the child's involvement in the consent procedure.

Disclosure of Diagnosis and Prognosis

Pediatric oncologists generally advise parents that children should be informed about their illness and treatment in an age-appropriate fashion, but this should be a merciful version of the truth. Children are highly discerning about falsehood, will lose confidence in parents and caregivers when lied to, and possibly imagine worse scenarios than the actual situation. It is important to remember that *at some level* and *in some way* there is always something to be hopeful about and to include this early in any conversation with parents. Most parents prefer to be the ones to tell their children, with the assistance of caregivers (Komp, 1995).

Childhood cancer is for most affected patients a chronic and not an acute disease, even when the outcome is a fatal one. This has particular importance to "age-appropriate" revelations because the patient will evolve through different age phases while in treatment. This is a relatively simple matter in treatment settings where there are many other children, as they will consult with and learn from each other.

"Do Not Resuscitate" Orders

As with consent for treatment, the parent or legal guardian is the appropriate discussion partner and legal signator when it comes to Do Not Resuscitate (DNR) orders. With the exception of teenagers, and in contrast to the treatment assent process, young children are rarely involved in these discussions that are difficult and painful enough for adults. It is highly unusual for a teenager to ask for or permit discussion of life-limiting measures, even when quadriplegic. Typically, these physician-parent discussions disclose the normal feelings of ambivalence that parents experience in regard to letting go. Unlike adult patients, the discussion of advanced directives has not been addressed before hospitalization as a matter of routine. Hospital ward staff members may push physicians about DNR status to increase their own level of comfort. It is important for all of us to remember that advanced directives and DNR orders are designed to meet the needs of the patient, not those of the hospital's staff.

Hospice

Although home hospice services are commonly used in the terminal management of children with cancer, inpatient hospice beds are rarely used. Most children with cancer have a warm, trusting relationship with at least their nurses, if not their doctors. If they cannot be at home, they want to be with people they know and love rather than well-meaning strangers.

It is always sad when a child dies, even when it becomes inevitable. Ironically, despite the proliferation of hospice services with home care programs, fewer children are dying at home today than a decade ago. In an era when the cure rates are so high, it is hard for many parents (and even their children) to believe that the medical miracle is not there for them as well. Parents may reject home care that is called "hospice," even when it provides a higher quality of palliative care, because of the association of hospice with death. Although managed care may change what is available to families as alternatives to the hospital, it is important that continuity be provided when care is provided away from the familiar medical site. A single house call may be more worthwhile than a dozen phone calls, both for assessing the situation and keeping the commitment that is essential in the care of children—to care and give care to the bitter end.

REFERENCES

Brodeur GM et al: Consistent N-*myc* copy number in simultaneous or consecutive neuroblastoma samples from sixty individual patients, *Canc Res* 47:4248-4253, 1987.

Byrne J et al: Effects of treatment on fertility in long-term survivors of childhood or adolescent cancer, *N Engl J Med* 317:1315-1321, 1987.

D'Angio GJ et al: Treatment of Wilms' tumor: results of the third national Wilms' Tumor Study, *Cancer* 64:349-360, 1989.

Gaes J: *My book for kids with cansur: a child's autobiography of hope*, Aberdeen, Texas, 1987, Melius & Peterson.

Komp DM: *A child shall lead them: lessons in hope from children with cancer in images of grace: a pediatrician's trilogy of faith, hope, and love*, Grand Rapids, Mich, 1995, Zondervan.

Meyers PA: Malignant bone tumors in children: osteosarcoma, *Hem Oncol Clin North Am* 1:655-665, 1987.

Tucker MA et al: Cancer risk following treatment of childhood cancer. In Boice JD, Fraumeni JF Jr, eds: *Radiation carcinogenesis: epidemiology and biological significance*, New York, 1984, Raven, pp 211-224.

Vietti TJ et al: Progress against childhood cancer: the Pediatric Oncology Group experience, *Pediatrics* 89:597-600, 1992.

APPENDIX A

TABLE A-1
Calculation of Body Surface Area

Mostellar	Du Bois	Haycock
BSA (m²) = $\sqrt{\dfrac{\text{height} \times \text{weight}}{3600}}$	BSA (m²) = (wt$^{0.425}$) $\times$ (ht$^{0.725}$) $\times$ 71.84	BSA (m²) = (wt$^{0.5378}$) $\times$ (ht$^{0.3964}$) $\times$ 0.024265

From Mostellar RD: Simplified calculation of body-surface area, *N Engl J Med* 317:1098, 1987; Du Bois D, Du Bois EF: A formula to estimate the approximate surface area if height and weight be known, *Arch Intern Med* 17:863-871, 1916; and Haycock GB, Schwartz GJ, Wisotsky DH: Geometric method for measuring body surface area: a height-weight formula validated in infants, children, and adults, *J Pediatr* 93:62-66, 1978.
BSA, Body surface area; *m²*, meters squared; *ht*, height in centimeters; *wt*, weight in kilograms.

TABLE A-2
Calculation of Body Surface Area in Adult Amputees*

Body parts	Women (%)	Men (%)
Hand plus five fingers	2.65	2.83
Lower part of arm	3.80	4.04
Upper part of arm	5.65	5.94
Foot	2.94	3.15
Lower part of leg	6.27	5.99
Thigh	12.55	11.80

NOTE: Dose reductions may not be necessary in all amputee patients. Metabolism and clearance of a drug does not necessarily change in amputee patients. Use professional judgment when deciding to reduce drug doses.

From Colangelo PM et al: Two methods for estimating body surface area in adult amputees, *Am J Hosp Pharm* 41:2650-2655, 1984.
*BSA (m²) = BSA - [(BSA) $\times$ (%BSA$_{part}$)], where *BSA* is body surface area, *m²* is meters squared, and *BSA$_{part}$* is body surface area of amputated body part.

TABLE A-3
Ideal Body-Weight Charts*

Height (cm)	Weight (kg)	Height (cm)	Weight (kg)	Height (cm)	Weight (kg)
MALES					
145	51.9	159	59.9	173	68.7
146	52.4	160	60.5	174	69.4
147	52.9	161	61.1	175	70.1
148	53.6	162	61.7	176	70.8
149	54.0	163	62.3	177	71.6
150	54.5	164	62.9	178	72.4
151	55.0	165	63.5	179	73.3
152	55.8	166	64.0	180	74.2
153	56.1	167	64.6	181	75.0
154	56.6	168	65.2	182	75.6
155	57.2	169	65.9	183	76.5
156	57.9	170	66.6	184	77.3
157	57.9	171	67.3	185	78.1
158	59.3	172	68.0	186	78.9
FEMALES					
140	44.9	150	50.4	160	56.2
141	45.4	151	51.0	161	56.9
142	45.9	152	51.5	162	57.6
143	46.4	153	52.0	163	58.3
144	47.0	154	52.5	164	58.9
145	47.5	155	53.1	165	59.5
146	48.0	156	53.7	166	60.1
147	48.6	157	54.3	167	60.7
148	49.2	158	54.9	168	61.4
149	49.8	159	55.5	169	62.1

Modified from Jellife DB: *The assessment of the nutritional status of the community*, Geneva, 1986, WHO.
*Ideal body weight for height. This table corrects the 1960 Metropolitan Standards to nude weight without shoe heels.

TABLE A-4
Performance Scale (Karnofsky and ECOG)

	ECOG		Karnofsky
0	Fully active, able to carry on all predisease performance without restriction	100%	Normal, no complaints, no evidence of disease
		90%	Able to carry on normal activity; minor signs or symptoms of disease
1	Restricted in physically strenuous activity but ambulatory and able to carry out work of a light or sedentary nature, e.g., light housework, office work	80%	Normal activity with effort; some signs or symptoms of disease
		70%	Cares for self; unable to carry on normal activity or to do active work
2	Ambulatory and capable of all self-care but unable to carry out any work activities; up and about more than 50% of waking hours	60%	Requires occasional assistance, is mostly able to care for himself
		50%	Requires considerable assistance and frequent medical care
3	Capable of only limited self-care, and confined to bed or chair more than 50% of waking hours	40%	Disabled, requires special care assistance
		30%	Severely disabled, hospitalization indicated; death not imminent
4	Completely disabled; cannot carry on any self-care; totally confined to bed or chair	20%	Very sick, hospitalization necessary; active supportive treatment necessary
		10%	Moribund, fatal processes progressing rapidly
5	Dead	0%	Dead

Modified from Karnofsky DA et al: The use of the nitrogen mustards in the palliation treatment of carcinoma with particular reference to bronchogenic carcinoma, *Cancer* 1:634-656, 1948, and Oken MM et al: Toxicity and response criteria of the Eastern Cooperative Oncology Group, *Am J Clin Oncol* 5:649-655, 1982.

TABLE A-5
Methods Used To Calculate Creatinine Clearance*

Calculated from a timed urine collection

$$\text{Creatinine Clearance} = \frac{\text{Urine Creatinine}}{\text{Serum Creatinine}} \times \frac{\text{Urine Volume}}{\text{Time}^\dagger}$$

Estimated from age, weight, serum of creatinine

Cockcroft and Gault method [‡]:

$$\text{Creatinine Clearance}_{men} = \frac{(140 - \text{age}) \times (\text{Lean Body Wt})}{(\text{Serum Creatinine}) \times 72}$$

$$\text{Creatinine Clearance}_{women} = 0.85 \times \text{Creatinine Clearance}_{men}$$

Jeliffe method [§]: (For an individual with BSA of 1.73 m^2)

$$\text{Creatinine Clearance} = \frac{100}{\text{Serum Creatinine}} - 12$$

---

*Units used in calculations are as follows: creatinine clearance (mL/min); age (yr); serum creatinine (mg/dL); time (min); urine creatinine (mg/dL); weight (kg); urine volume (mL).

[†]Time = duration of urine collection; 24 hours = 1440 minutes; 12 hours = 720 minutes; 8 hours = 480 minutes; less than 20% variability with 8, 12, and 24 hour collection times. (From Baumann TJ et al: Minimum urine collection periods for accurate determination of creatinine clearance in critically ill patients, *Clin Pharm* 6:393-398, 1987.)

[‡]From Cockcroft DW, Gault MH: Prediction of creatinine clearance from serum creatinine, *Nephron* 16:31-41, 1976.

[§]From Jeliffe RW: Estimation of creatinine clearance when urine cannot be collected, *Lancet* 1:975-976, 1971.

BSA, Body surface area.

TABLE A-6
Carboplatin Dosing Calculations

PLATELET NADIR METHOD*

Previously Untreated Patients

Dose (mg/m²) = 0.091 × (CrCl/BSA) × (Pre PC − Desired Nadir PC/Pre PC × 100) + 86

Previously Treated Patients

Dose (mg/M²) = 0.091 × (CrCl/BSA) × [(Pre PC − Desired Nadir PC/Pre PC × 100) − 17] + 86

AREA UNDER THE CURVE METHOD†

Dose (mg) = Target AUC × (CrCl + 25)

Previously Untreated Patients

Target AUC = 6 to 8 mg/mL/min

Previously Treated Patients

Target AUC = 4 to 6 mg/mL/min

*From Egorin MJ et al: Prospective validation of a pharmacologically based dosing scheme for the *cis*-diamminedichloroplatinum(II) analogue diamminecyclobutanedicarboxylatoplatinum, *Cancer Res* 45:6502-6506, 1985.
†From Calvert AH et al: Carboplatin dosage: prospective evaluation of a simple formula based on renal function, *J Clin Oncol* 7:1748-1756, 1989. *BSA*, Body surface area; *CrCl*, creatinine clearance; *Pre PC*, pretreatment platelet count; *PC*, platelet count; *AUC*, Area Under the [plasma concentration] Curve.

TABLE A-7
National Cancer Institute Common Toxicity Criteria

Toxicity	Grade			
	0	1	2	3	4
Blood/bone marrow					
WBC	≥4.0	3.0–3.9	2.0–2.9	1.0–1.9	<1.0
PLT	WNL	75.0–normal	50.0–74.9	25.0–49.9	<25.0
Hgb	WNL	10.0–normal	8.0–10.0	6.5–7.9	<6.5
Granulocytes/bands	≥2.0	1.5–1.9	1.0–1.4	0.5–0.9	<0.5
Lymphocytes	≥2.0	1.5–1.9	1.0–1.4	0.5–0.9	<0.5
Hemorrhage (clinical)	None	Mild, no transfusion	Gross, 1-2 units transfusion per episode	Gross, 3-4 units transfusion per episode	Massive, >4.0 units transfusion per episode
Infection	None	Mild	Moderate	Severe	Life threatening
Gastrointestinal					
Nausea	None	Able to eat reasonable intake	Intake significantly decreased but can eat	No significant intake	—
Vomiting	None	1 episode in 24 hr	2–5 episodes in 24 hr	6–10 episodes in 24 hr	>10 episodes in 24 hr, or requiring parenteral support

Diarrhea	None	Increase of 2–3 stools/day over pre-Rx	Increase of 4–6 stools/day, or nocturnal stools, or moderate cramping	Increase of 7–9 stools/day, or incontinence, or severe cramping	Increase of ≥10 stools/day or grossly bloody diarrhea, or need for parenteral support
Stomatitis	None	Painless ulcers, erythema, or mild soreness	Painful erythema, edema, or ulcers, but can eat	Painful erythema, edema, or ulcers, and cannot eat	Requires parenteral or enteral support
Liver					
Bilirubin	WNL	—	<1.5 × N	>1.5–3.0 × N	>3.0 × N
Transaminase (SGOT, SGPT)	WNL	≤2.5 × N	2.6–5.0 × N	5.1–20.0 × N	>20.0 × N
Alkaline phosphatase or 5' nucleotidase	WNL	≤2.5 × N	2.6–5.0 × N	5.1–20.0 × N	>20.0 × N
Clinical	No change from baseline	—	—	Precoma	Hepatic coma
Kidney, bladder					
Creatinine	WNL	<1.5 × N	1.5–3.0 × N	3.1–6.0 × N	>6.0 × N
Proteinuria	No change	1+ or <0.3 g% or <3 g/L	2–3+ or 0.3–1.0 g% or 3–10 g/L	4+ or >1.0 g% or >1.0 g/L	Nephrotic syndrome
Hematuria	Negative	Micro only	Gross, no clots	Gross + clots	Requires transfusion
Alopecia	No loss	Mild hair loss	Pronounced or total hair loss	—	—

Continued

TABLE A-7
National Cancer Institute Common Toxicity Criteria—cont'd

Toxicity	Grade				
	0	1	2	3	4
Pulmonary	None or no change	Asymptomatic, with abnormality in PFTs	Dyspnea on significant exertion	Dyspnea at normal level of activity	Dyspnea at rest
Heart					
Dysrhythmias	None	Asymptomatic, transient, requiring no therapy	Recurrent or persistent, no therapy required	Requires treatment	Requires monitoring; hypotension, ventricular tachycardia, or fibrillation
Function	None	Asymptomatic, decline of resting ejection fraction by less than 20% of baseline value	Asymptomatic, decline of resting ejection fraction by more than 20% of baseline value	Mild CHF, responsive to therapy	Severe or refractory CHF
Ischemia	None	Nonspecific T-wave flattening	Asymptomatic, ST and T-wave changes suggesting ischemia	Angina without evidence for infarction	Acute myocardial infarction
Pericardial	None	Asymptomatic effusion, no intervention required	Pericarditis (rub, chest pain, ECG changes)	Symptomatic effusion; drainage required	Tamponade; drainage urgently required

Blood pressure				
Hypertension	None or no change	Asymptomatic, transient increase by greater than 20 mm Hg (D) or to >150/100 mm Hg if previously WNL; no treatment required	Recurrent or persistent increase by greater than 20 mm Hg (D) or to >150/100 mm Hg if previously WNL; no treatment required	Requires therapy	Hypertensive crisis
Hypotension	None or no change	Changes requiring no therapy (including transient orthostatic hypotension)	Requires fluid replacement or other therapy but no hospitalization	Requires therapy and hospitalization; resolves within 48 hr of stopping the agent	Requires therapy and hospitalization for >48 hrs after stopping the agent
Neurological				
Sensory	None or no change	Mild paresthesias, loss of deep tendon reflexes	Mild or moderate objective sensory loss; moderate paresthesias	Severe objective sensory loss or paresthesias that interfere with function	—
Motor	None or no change	Subjective weakness; no objective findings	Mild objective weakness without significant impairment of function	Objective weakness with impairment of function	Paralysis

Continued

TABLE A-7
National Cancer Institute Common Toxicity Criteria—cont'd

Toxicity	Grade			
	0	1	2	3	4
Neurological (cont'd)					
Cortical	None	Mild somnolence or agitation	Moderate somnolence or agitation	Severe somnolence, agitation, confusion, disorientation, or hallucinations	Coma, seizures, toxic psychosis
Cerebellar	None	Slight incoordination, dysdiadochokinesis	Intention tremor, dysmetria, slurred speech, nystagmus	Locomotor ataxia	Cerebellar necrosis
Mood	No change	Mild anxiety or depression	Moderate anxiety or depression	Severe anxiety or depression	Suicidal ideation
Headache	None	Mild	Moderate or severe but transient	Unrelenting and severe	—
Constipation	None or no change	Mild	Moderate	Severe	Ileus >96 hr
Hearing	None or no change	Asymptomatic, hearing loss on audiometry only	Tinnitus	Hearing loss interfering with function but correctable with hearing aid	Deafness not correctable

Vision	None or no change	—	—	Symptomatic subtotal loss of vision	Blindness
Skin	None or no change	Scattered macular or papular eruption or erythema that is asymptomatic	Scattered macular or papular eruption or erythema with pruritus or other associated symptoms	Generalized symptomatic macular, papular, or vesicular eruption	Exfoliative dermatitis or ulcerating dermatitis
Allergy	None	Transient rash, drug fever <38° C 100.4° F	Urticaria, drug fever equal to 38° C or 100.4° F, mild bronchospasm	Serum sickness, bronchospasm, requires parenteral medication	Anaphylaxis
Fever in absence of infection	None	37.1–38.0° C or 98.7–100.4° F	38.1–40.0° C or 100.5–104.0° F	>40.0° C or >104.0° F for less than 24 hr	>40.0° C (104.0° F) for more than 24 hr, or fever accompanied by hypotension
Local	None	Pain	Pain and swelling, with inflammation or phlebitis	Ulceration	Plastic surgery indicated
Weight gain/loss	<5.0%	5.0–9.9%	10.0–19.9%	≥20.0%	—

Continued

TABLE A-7
National Cancer Institute Common Toxicity Criteria—cont'd

Toxicity	Grade				
	0	1	2	3	4
Metabolic					
Hyperglycemia (mg/dL)	<116	116–160	161–250	251–500	>500 or ketoacidosis
Hypoglycemia (mg/dL)	>64	55–64	40–54	30–39	<30
Amylase	WNL	<1.5 × N	1.5–2.0 × N	2.1–5.0 × N	>5.1 × N
Hypercalcemia (mg/dL)	<10.6	10.6–11.5	11.6–12.5	12.6–13.5	≥13.5
Hypocalcemia (mg/dL)	>8.4	8.4–7.8	7.7–7.0	6.9–6.1	≤6.0
Hypomagnesemia (mg/dL)	>1.4	1.4–1.2	1.1–0.9	0.8–0.6	≤0.5
Coagulation					
Fibrinogen	WNL	0.99–0.75 × N	0.74–0.50 × N	0.49–0.25 × N	≤0.24 × N
Prothrombin time	WNL	1.01–1.25 × N	1.26–1.50 × N	1.51–2.00 × N	>2.00 × N
Partial thromboplastin time	WNL	1.01–1.66 × N	1.67–2.33 × N	2.34–3.00 × N	>3.00 × N

NOTE: *Modifications of these criteria have been developed by U.S. Cooperative Oncology Groups (e.g., ECOG, SWOG, CALGB), the World Health Organization, and pharmaceutical firms.*

WBC, white blood cell; *PLT,* platelet; *Hgb,* hemoglobin; *Rx,* therapy; *WNL,* within normal limits; *PFT,* pulmonary function test; *CHF,* congestive heart failure; *ECG,* electrocardiogram.

TABLE A-8
Autologous Bone Marrow Transplant Studies, Supplemental Toxicity Criteria

Grade 5	Death caused by bacterial or fungal infection or hemorrhage with neutrophils <500/mm^3 or platelets <10,000/mm^3 more than 8 weeks after marrow transplantation
Grade 4	Neutrophils <500/mm^3 and/or platelets <10,000/mm^3 for a duration in excess of 8 weeks
Grade 3	Neutrophils <500/mm^3 and/or platelets <10,000/mm^3 for a duration of 4 to 8 weeks
Grade 2	Neutrophils <500/mm^3 and/or platelets <10,000/mm^3 for a duration up to 4 weeks
Grade 1	Neutropenia and/or thrombocytopenia, but neutrophils never <500/mm^3 and platelets never <10,000/mm^3

NOTE: All other nonhematological toxicities should be graded by the Common Toxicity Criteria.

TABLE A-9
Temperature Conversion Chart

Fahrenheit	Celsius (Centigrade)
94	34.4
95	35.0
96	35.5
97	36.1
98	36.6
98.6	37.0
99	37.2
100	37.7
101	38.3
102	38.8
103	39.4
104	40.0
105	40.5
106	41.1
107	41.6
108	42.2

ACRONYMS AND THE DRUGS THEY REPRESENT

Medicine is now in a period of abbreviation. We have standard abbreviations that everyone understands (e.g., mg, cm, kg), and we have abbreviations that are specific to an institution or an individual that almost no one else understands. In between, there are the abbreviations known to an "in group" of a specialty, that are moderately well understood by those experienced in the area, but are a mystery to those new to the field. Drug abbreviations fall into this in-between area as do drug acronyms for combinations. Usually, the acronyms use the first letter of the drug's generic name (e.g., CVP for cyclophosphamide, vincristine, and prednisone) or the drug's trade name (e.g., ABVD where the A represents Adriamycin (doxorubicin), or a hybrid such as the drug's chemical/generic name (e.g., CHOP, where H represents hydroxydaunorubicin [doxorubicin] and O represents Oncovin [vincristine]). Occasionally, the letter represents an old code name or abbreviation from the time the drug was investigational and had no generic or trade name (e.g., VP-16-213 [etoposide], sometimes shortened to VP-16 and then to V as in VIP for etoposide, ifosfamide, Platinol [cisplatin]).

To help navigate through the alphabet soup of chemotherapy acronyms and jargon names (ara-C for cytarabine, DDP or cDDP for cisplatin, VM-26 for teniposide, CBDCA for carboplatin, CPT-11 for irinotecan, JM-8 for carboplatin), Table A-10 has been provided to alert the uninitiated to some of the possibilities of interpretation.

TABLE A-10
Drug Acronyms

Letter	Potential drug represented	
A	Actinomycin D (dactinomycin)	Ara-A (vidarabine)
	Adriamycin (doxorubicin)	Ara-C (cytarabine)
	Aldesleukin	Asparaginase
	Alkeran (melphalan)	Azacytidine
	Amsacrine	Azathioprine
B	BCNU (carmustine)	Busulfan
	Bleomycin	
C	Carboplatin	Citrovorum factor (leucovorin)
	Carmustine	Cladribine
	CBDCA (carboplatin)	Cosmegen (Dactinomycin)
	CCNU (lomustine)	CPT-11 (irinotecan)
	CdA (cladribine)	Cyclophosphamide
	CDDP (cisplatin)	Cytarabine
	Cisplatin	Cytosar-U (cytarabine)
	Cis-retinoic acid	

TABLE A-10
Drug Acronyms—cont'd

Letter	Potential drug represented	
D	Dacarbazine	Dibromodulcitol
	Daunomycin (daunorubicin)	Diethylstilbestrol
	Daunorubicin	Docetaxel
	DDP (cisplatin)	Doxorubicin
	Deoxycoformycin (pentostatin)	DTIC (dacarbazine)
	Dexamethasone	
E	Emcyt (estramustine)	Etoposide
	Epirubicin	Etretinate
	Estramustine	Eulexin (flutamide)
F	Floxuridine	Flutamide
	Fludarabine	Folinic acid (leucovorin)
	Fluorouracil	FUDR (floxuridine)
G	Gallium nitrate	Gemzar (gemcitabine)
	Gemcitabine	Goserelin
H	Halotestin (fluoxymesterone)	Hydrea (hydroxyurea)
	Hexamethylmelamine (altretamine)	Hydroxydaunorubicin (doxorubicin)
	High-dose	Hydroxyurea
	HN_2 (mechlorethamine)	
I	Idamycin (idarubicin)	Interferon
	Idarubicin	Interleukin-2
	Ifex (ifosfamide)	Irinotecan
	Ifosfamide	Isotretinoin
	Imuran (azathioprine)	
J	JM-8 (carboplatin)	
L	L-PAM (melphalan)	Levamisole
	Leucovorin	Lomustine
	Leukeran (chlorambucil)	Lupron (leuprolide)
	Leuprolide	Lysodren (mitotane)
	Leustatin (cladribine)	
M	Matulane (procarbazine)	Mithracin (plicamycin)
	Melphalan	Mitomycin
	Mercaptopurine	Mitotane
	Mesna	Mitoxantrone
	MethylGAG (mitoguazone)	Mustard (mechlorethamine)
	Methotrexate	Mutamycin (mitomycin)
N	Navelbine (vinorelbine)	Nolvadex (tamoxifen)
	Neutrexin (trimetrexate)	Novantrone (mitoxantrone)
	Nitrogen mustard (mechlorethamine)	
O	Octreotide	Oncovin (vincristine)

Continued

TABLE A-10
Drug Acronyms—cont'd

Letter	Potential drug represented	
P	Paclitaxel	Plicamycin
	PAM (melphalan)	Platinol (cisplatin)
	Paraplatin (carboplatin)	Prednimustine
	Peg-asparaginase	Prednisone
	Pentostatin	Procarbazine
	Platinum (cisplatin)	
S	Sandostatin (octreotide)	Stilbestrol (diethylstilbestrol)
	Solumedrol (methylprednisolone)	Streptozocin
T	Tamoxifen	Thioguanine
	Taxol (paclitaxel)	Thiotepa
	Taxotere (docetaxel)	Topotecan
	Tegison (etretinate)	Tretinoin
	Teniposide	Trimetrexate
U	Uracil	Uracil mustard
V	Velban (vinblastine)	Vindesine
	Vepesid (etoposide)	Vinorelbine
	Vesanoid (tretinoin)	VM-26 (teniposide)
	Vinblastine	VP-16 (etoposide)
	Vincristine	
Z	Zanosar (streptozocin)	Zoladex (goserelin)
	Zidovudine	

APPENDIX B

General References

Abeloff MD et al, eds: *Clinical oncology*, New York, 1995, Churchill Livingstone.

Ahlgren J, Macdonald J, eds: *Gastrointestinal oncology*, Philadelphia, 1992, JB Lippincott.

Aisner J et al, eds: *Comprehensive textbook of thoracic oncology*, Baltimore, 1996, Williams & Wilkins.

Armitage JO, Antman KH, eds: *High-dose cancer therapy: pharmacology, hematopoietins, stem cells*, ed 2, Baltimore, 1995, Williams & Wilkins.

Balducci L, Lyman GH, Ershler WB, eds: *Geriatric oncology*, Philadelphia, 1992, JB Lippincott.

Beahrs OH et al, eds, for American Joint Committee on Cancer: *Manual for staging of cancer*, ed 4, Philadelphia, 1992, JB Lippincott.

Bell WR: *Hematologic and oncologic emergencies*, New York, 1995, Churchill Livingstone.

Berek JS, Hacker NF, eds: *Practical gynecologic oncology*, ed 2, Baltimore, 1994, Williams & Wilkins.

Beutler E et al, eds: *Williams' hematology*, ed 5, New York, 1995, McGraw-Hill.

Bland KI, Copeland EM III, eds: *The breast: comprehensive management of benign and malignant diseases*, Philadelphia, 1991, WB Saunders.

Brain MC, Carbone PP, eds: *Current therapy in hematology-oncology*, ed 5, St. Louis, 1995, Mosby.

Broder S, ed: *Molecular foundations of oncology*, Philadelphia, 1991, JB Lippincott.

Broder S, Merigan TC Jr, Bolognesi D, eds: *Textbook of AIDS medicine*, Baltimore, 1994, Williams & Wilkins.

Burke MB, Wilkes GM, Ingwersen K, eds: *Cancer chemotherapy: a nursing process approach*, ed 2, Boston, 1995, Jones & Bartlett.

Calabresi P, Schein PS, eds: *Medical oncology*, ed 2, New York, 1993, McGraw-Hill.

Canellos GP, Lister A, Sklar JL, eds: *The lymphomas*, Philadelphia, 1996, WB Saunders.

Carey DN, ed: *Lung cancer*, Boston, 1995, Arnold.

Chabner BA, Longo DL, eds: *Cancer chemotherapy and biotherapy: principles and practice*, ed 2, Philadelphia, 1996, Lippincott-Raven.

Cohen AM, Winawer SJ, eds: *Cancer of the colon, rectum and anus*, New York, 1995, McGraw-Hill.

Cohen PT, Sande MA, Volberding PA, eds: *The AIDS knowledge base*, ed 2, Boston, 1994, Little, Brown.

Cox JD, ed: *Moss' radiation oncology*, ed 7, St Louis, 1994, Mosby.

DeVita VT Jr, Hellman S, Rosenberg SA, eds: *AIDS: etiology, diagnosis, treatment and prevention*, ed 4, Philadelphia, 1996, Lippincott-Raven.

DeVita VT Jr, Hellman S, Rosenberg SA, eds: *Cancer: principles and practice of oncology*, ed 5, Philadelphia, 1997, Lippincott-Raven.

DeVita V Jr, Hellman S, Rosenberg SA, eds: *Biologic therapy of cancer*, ed 2, Philadelphia, 1995, Lippincott-Raven.

DiSaia PJ, Creasman WT, eds: *Clinical gynecologic oncology*, ed 4, St. Louis, 1993, Mosby.

Donegan WL, Spratt JS, eds: *Cancer of the breast*, ed 4, Philadelphia, 1995, WB Saunders.

Dorr RT, Von Hoff DD: *Cancer chemotherapy handbook*, ed 2, Norwalk, Conn, 1994, Appleton & Lange.

Foley JF, Vose JM, Armitage JO, eds: *Current therapy in cancer*, Philadelphia, 1994, WB Saunders.

Forman SJ, Blume KG, Thomas ED, eds: *Bone marrow transplantation*, Cambridge, Mass, 1994, Blackwell.

Freireich EJ, Stass SA, eds: *Molecular basis of oncology*, Cambridge, Mass, 1995, Blackwell.

Gale RP, Juttner C, Henon P, eds: *Blood stem cell transplants*, New York, 1994, Cambridge University Press.

Griffiths K et al: *Nutrition and cancer*, St. Louis, 1996, Mosby.

Groenwald SL et al, eds: *Cancer symptom management*, Boston, 1996, Jones & Bartlett.

Gross J, Johnson B, eds: *Handbook of oncology nursing*, ed 2, Boston, 1994, Jones & Bartlett.

Handin RI, Lux SE, Stossel TP, eds: *Blood: principles and practice of hematology*, Philadelphia, 1995, JB Lippincott.

Harris JR et al, eds: *Diseases of the breast*, Philadelphia, 1996, JB Lippincott.

Harvey JC, Beattie EJ, eds: *Cancer surgery*, Philadelphia, 1996, WB Saunders.

Haskell C, ed: *Cancer treatment*, ed 4, Philadelphia, 1995, WB Saunders.

Henderson ES, Lister TA, Greaves MF, eds: *Leukemia*, ed 6, Philadelphia, 1996, WB Saunders.

Hoffman R et al, eds: *Hematology: basic principles and practice*, ed 2, New York, 1995, Churchill Livingstone.

Holland JF et al, eds: *Cancer medicine*, ed 4, Philadelphia, 1996, Lea & Febiger.

Horwich A, ed: *Combined radiotherapy and chemotherapy in clinical oncology*, Boston, 1992, Little, Brown.

Horwich A, ed: *Oncology: a multidisciplinary textbook*, New York, 1995, Chapman & Hall.

Hoskins WJ, Perez CA, Young RC, eds: *Principles and practice of gynecologic oncology*, ed 2, Philadelphia, 1996, JB Lippincott.

Jandl JH: *Textbook of hematology*, ed 2, Boston, 1996, Little, Brown.

Johnson BE, Johnson DH, eds: *Lung cancer*, New York, 1995, Wiley-Liss.

Kirkwood JM, Lotze MT, Yasko JM, eds: *Current cancer therapeutics*, ed 2, New York, 1996, Churchill Livingstone.

Knapp R, Berkowitz RS, eds: *Gynecologic oncology*, ed 2, New York, 1993, McGraw-Hill.

Lanzkowsky P, ed: *Manual of pediatric hematology and oncology*, New York, 1994, Churchill Livingstone.

Lee GR et al, eds: *Wintrobe's clinical hematology*, ed 9, Philadelphia, 1993, Lea & Febiger.

Levin VA, ed: *Cancer in the nervous system*, New York, 1996, Churchill Livingstone.

Libman H, Witzburg RA, eds: *HIV infection: a clinical manual*, ed 3, Boston, 1996, Little, Brown.

Liebman MC, Camp-Sorrell D, eds: *Multimodal therapy in oncology nursing*, St. Louis, 1996, Mosby.

Love RR, ed: *UICC manual of clinical oncology*, ed 6, Berlin, 1994, Springer-Verlag.

Macdonald J, Haller D, Mayer R, eds: *Manual of oncologic therapeutics*, ed 3, Philadelphia, 1995, JB Lippincott.

Magrath IT, Shad AT, eds: *Non-Hodgkin's lymphoma*, ed 2, Boston, 1996, Little, Brown.

Markman M, Hoskins WJ, eds: *Cancer of the ovary*, Philadelphia, 1993, JB Lippincott.

McCorkle R et al, eds: *Cancer nursing: a comprehensive text*, ed 2, Philadelphia, 1994, WB Saunders.

McKenna RJ Sr, Murphy GP, eds: *Cancer surgery*, Philadelphia, 1994, JB Lippincott.

Mendelsohn J et al, eds: *The molecular basis of cancer*, Philadelphia, 1995, WB Saunders.

Miller DR, Baehner RL, eds: *Blood diseases of infancy and childhood*, ed 7, St. Louis, 1995, Mosby.

Million RR, Cassisi NJ, eds: *Management of head and neck cancer: a multidisciplinary approach*, ed 2, Philadelphia, 1994, JB Lippincott.

Mitchell MS, ed: *Biological approaches to cancer treatment*, New York, 1993, McGraw-Hill.

Moosa AR, Schimpff SC, Robson MC, eds: *Comprehensive textbook of oncology*, ed 2, Baltimore, 1991, Williams & Wilkins.

Murphy GP, Lawrence W Jr, Lenhard RE Jr, eds: *Textbook of clinical oncology*, Atlanta, 1995, American Cancer Society.

Myers EN, Suen JY, eds: *Cancer of the head and neck*, Philadelphia, 1996, WB Saunders.

Niederhuber JE, ed: *Current therapy in oncology*, St. Louis, 1993, Mosby.

Omoigui S: *The pain drugs handbook*, St. Louis, 1995, Mosby.

Pass H et al, eds: *Lung cancer: principles and practice*, Philadelphia, 1996, Lippincott-Raven.

Patt RB, ed: *Cancer pain handbook*, Philadelphia, 1993, JB Lippincott.

Peckham M, Pinedo HM, Veronesi U, eds: *Oxford textbook of oncology*, New York, 1995, Oxford University Press.

Perez C, ed: *Principles and practice of radiation oncology*, Philadelphia, 1996, Lippincott-Raven.

Perry MC, ed: *Chemotherapy source book*, ed 2, Baltimore, 1996, Williams & Wilkins.

Pizzo PA, Poplack DG, eds: *Principles and practice of pediatric oncology*, ed 3, Philadelphia, 1996, Lippincott-Raven.

Raaf JH, ed: *Soft tissue sarcomas*, St. Louis, 1993, Mosby.

Rieger PT, ed: *Biotherapy: a comprehensive overview*, Boston, 1995, Jones & Bartlett.

Roth J, Ruckdeschel JC, Weisenburger TH, eds: *Thoracic oncology*, Philadelphia, 1995, WB Saunders.

Roth JA, Cox JD, Hong WK, eds: *Lung cancer*, Cambridge, Mass, 1993, Blackwell.

Rubin P, ed: *Clinical oncology: a multidisciplinary approach for physicians and students*, ed 7, Philadelphia, 1993, WB Saunders.

Rubin SC, ed: *Chemotherapy of gynecologic cancers*, Philadelphia, 1996, Lippincott-Raven.

Rubin SC, Sutton GP, eds: *Ovarian cancer*, New York, 1993, McGraw-Hill.

Saunders CM: *Management of terminal malignant diseases*, Boston, 1993, Little, Brown.

Saunders CM: *Living with dying: a guide to palliative care*, ed 3, New York, 1995, Oxford University Press.

Skeel RT, Lachant NA, eds: *Handbook of cancer chemotherapy*, ed 4, Boston, 1995, Little, Brown.

Souhami R, Tobias J: *Cancer and its management*, Cambridge, Mass, 1995, Blackwell.

Stamatoyannopoulos G et al, eds: *The molecular basis of blood diseases*, ed 2, Philadelphia, 1994, WB Saunders.

Stomper PC: *Cancer imaging manual*, Philadelphia, 1993, JB Lippincott.

Tannock IF, Hill RP, eds: *The basic science of oncology*, ed 2, New York, 1992, McGraw-Hill.

Tennenbaum L, ed: *Cancer chemotherapy and biotherapy: a reference guide*, ed 2, Philadelphia, 1994, WB Saunders.

Treleaven J, Wiernik P, eds: *Color atlas and text of bone marrow transplantation*, St. Louis, 1995, Mosby-Wolfe.

Twycross R: *Pain relief in advanced cancer*, Edinburgh, 1994, Churchill Livingstone.

Twycross: *Symptom management in advanced cancer*, New York, 1995, Radcliff.

Vogelzang NJ et al, eds: *Comprehensive textbook of genitourinary oncology*, Baltimore, 1996, Williams & Wilkins.

Waller A, Caroline NL: *Handbook of palliative care in cancer*, Boston, 1996, Butterworth-Heinemann.

Wanebo HJ, ed: *Colorectal cancer*, St. Louis, 1993, Mosby.

Wasserman LR, Berk PD, Berlin NI, eds: *Polycythemia vera and the myeloproliferative disorders*, Philadelphia, 1994, WB Saunders.

Wiernik PH et al, eds: *Neoplastic diseases of the blood*, ed 3, New York, 1996, Churchill Livingstone.

Wiley RG, ed: *Neurological complications of cancer*, New York, 1995, Dekker.

INDEX

A

A-8103, 178

8103-Abbott, 178

ABC-P for multiple myeloma, 406-407

ABDIC for Hodgkin's disease, 376

Abitrexate, 159-162

ABMT; see Autologous bone marrow transplant

ABPP, 230-232

Absolute neutrophil count (ANC), 476

ABV for Kaposi's sarcoma, 348

ABVD for Hodgkin's disease, 376-377

ABVD for Hodgkins' disease, 544

9-AC, 53-54

AC for breast carcinoma, 318

Accutane, 140-142

Accutane Roche, 140-142

Acetaminophen
   for pain, 454
   premedication and, 560

ACOB for non-Hodgkin's disease, 385-386

ACOMLA for non-Hodgkin's disease, 386

Acquired immunodeficiency syndrome (AIDS), Kaposi's sarcoma of, alfa interferons for, 239

Acral erythema, 524-525

4'-(9-Acridinylamino) methanesulfon-*m*-anisidide, 56-58

Acridinylanisidide, 56-58

Acrolein, bladder toxicity and, 529

Acronyms, 582-584

ACT-D, 94-95

Actimmune, 244-246

Actinomycin-C, 94-95

Actinomycin-D, 94-95

Acute extravascular hemolytic transfusion reactions (AEHTR), 558, 560

Acute hemolytic transfusion reactions, 557

Acute intravascular hemolytic transfusion reactions (AIHTR), 558-560

Acute lymphoblastic leukemia (ALL), combination chemotherapy for, 349-354

Acute myelopathy, cytotoxic drugs and, 541

Acute nonlymphocytic leukemia (ANLL), combination chemotherapy for, 354-361

Acute promyelocytic leukemia (APL), combination chemotherapy for, 355

Acyclovir (Zovirax), postherpetic neuralgia and, 460

AD for sarcoma, 425

Ad Hoc Committee on Cancer Pain of the American Society of Clinical Oncology, 449-450

Additive solution red blood cells (AS-RBCs), 553

Adenocarcinoma, gastric, combination chemotherapy for, 339-342

Adenocarcinoma regimen for cervical carcinoma, 331

Adherence immunoaffinity columns, 466

Adjuvant BEP for ovarian germ cell cancer, 418

Adjuvant fluorouracil-leucovorin for colon carcinoma, 333

Adjuvant fluorouracil-levamisole for colon carcinoma, 334

Adjuvant VAC for ovarian germ cell cancer, 417-418

ADOC for thymoma, 432

ADR-529, 99-101

Adrenal cortical carcinoma, combination chemotherapy for, 310-311

Adria, 105-109

Adriamycin, 105-109

Adriamycin MDV, 105-109

Adriamycin PFS, 105-109

Adriamycin RDF, 105-109

ADRs; see Adverse drug reactions

Adrucil, 121-123

Advanced directives, 441

Adverse drug reactions (ADRs), reporting, in clinical trials, 36-37

AEHTR; see Acute extravascular hemolytic transfusion reactions

Agency for Health Care Policy and Research, 450

Agrelin, 58-59

AIDS; *see* Acquired immunodeficiency syndrome
AIDS-related infusional regimen for non-Hodgkin's disease, 387
AIDS-related intravenous regimen for non-Hodgkin's disease, 387
AIDS-related oral regimen for non-Hodgkin's disease, 386-387
AIHTR; *see* Acute intravascular hemolytic transfusion reactions
Airway reactions, anaphylactic, 271-272
Akathisia, phenothiazines and, 499
Alanine aminotransferase (SGPT), 498
Alcohol content of mouthwashes, 505
Aldesleukin, 222, 225-228
  for renal cell cancer, 237
Alferon, 236-242
Alkaban AQ, 212-214
Alkeran, 154-155
Alkeran IV, 154-155
Alkylating agents, 4-5
  gonadal toxicity and, 542
ALL; *see* Acute lymphoblastic leukemia
All transretinoic acid (ATRA), 207-209
  for promyelocytic leukemia, 355-356
Allergic transfusion reactions, 558, 561
Allogeneic bone marrow transplant, 462-466
All-trans-retinoic acid, 207-209
Alopecia, 514-523
  management of, 519
  prevention of, 518
Alpha interferons, 236-242
Alpha-Tamoxifen, 191-193
ALT; *see* Autolymphocyte therapy
Altretamine, 50-51
  drug interactions and, 10
  indications for, 43
  for ovarian carcinoma, 413, 414-415
AMA; *see* American Medical Association
Ambulatory infusion pumps for delivery of antineoplastic drugs, 276, 303, 304
Amen, 151-152
American Board of Internal Medicine, 438
American College of Physicians, 438
American Medical Association (AMA), 437-438
American Pain Society, 449-450
American Society
  of Clinical Oncology (ASCO), 450, 465

  of Hematology (ASH), 466
  of Hospital Pharmacists, 261
Amethopterin, 159-162
Amifostine, 43, 51-53
2-Amino-5-bromo-6-phenyl-4(3H)-pyrimidone, 230-232
Aminocamptothecin, 53-54
9-Aminocamptothecin, 53-54
2-[(3-aminopropyl)amino]-dihydrogen phosphate, 51-53
Aminoglutethimide, 55-56
  drug interactions and, 10
  indications for, 43
Aminohydroxypropylidene biphosphonate, 174-176
Aminopurine-6-thiolhemihydrate, 198-200
Amitriptyline
  for neuropathic pain, 542
  postherpetic neuralgia and, 460
Amputees, adult, calculating body surface area in, 569
AMSA, 56-58
AMSA-AZA for acute nonlymphycytic leukemia, 356
Amsacrine, 56-58
  for acute lymphoblastic leukemia, 350, 352-353
  for acute nonlymphycytic leukemia, 356, 360
  indications for, 43
  for leukemias, 469
Anagrelide, 58-59
Anal carcinoma, combination chemotherapy for, 311-312
Analgesic ladder, 449-450
Analgesics
  for mild pain, 451-454
  for moderate pain, 454-455
  narcotic, constipation and, 514
  oral, 452-453
  for severe pain, 455-458
  topical, for stomatitis, 511-512
Anaphylaxis, 561
  systemic, in adults, 271-273
Anastrozole, 43, 59-61
ANC; *see* Absolute neutrophil count
Anemia, 475-476
Anesthetics, platelet function and, 487
ANLL; *see* Acute nonlymphocytic leukemia
Anorexia, 502, 503, 504
Anthracycline
  cardiac toxicity from, 537-538
  venous reactions and, 523

Antibiotics, antitumor, 6
Anticholinergic drugs for nausea and
  vomiting, 492
Anticipatory vomiting, 565
Anticoagulants, platelet function and,
  487
Anticonvulsants, drug interactions and,
  10-13
Antidepressants, postherpetic neuralgia
  and, 460
Antiemetic therapy, 488-501
Antihistamines for nausea and
  vomiting, 492, 495
Antiinflammatory agents, platelet
  function and, 487
Antimetabolites, 7, 8
Antimicrobials, platelet function and,
  487
Antineoplastic drugs, 41-218, 260-306
  administration of, 42, 260-306
  ambulatory infusion pumps for
    delivery of, 303, 304
  availability of, 42
  cellular kinetics and, 2
  classification of, 41
  combination, 307-435
    for acute lymphoblastic leukemia,
      349-354
    for acute nonlymphocytic
      leukemia, 354-361
    for adrenal cortical carcinoma,
      310-311
    for anal carcinoma, 311-312
    for bladder carcinoma, 312-315
    for brain tumors, 316-317
    for breast carcinoma, 317-327
    for carcinoid syndrome, 327-329
    for carcinoma of unknown
      primary, 329-330
    for cervical carcinoma, 330-332
    for chronic granulocytic leukemia,
      362-364
    for chronic lymphocytic leukemia,
      364-365
    for chronic myelocytic leukemia,
      362-364
    for colon carcinoma, 332-336
    for elderly, 400-402
    for endometrial cancer, 336
    for esophageal carcinoma, 337-339
    for extragonadal germ cell cancer,
      428-432
    for gastric adenocarcinoma,
      339-342

  for gestational trophoblastic
    disease, 342-343
  for head and neck squamous cell
    carcinoma, 344-347
  for Hodgkin's disease, 375-382
  for islet cell carcinoma, 327-329
  for Kaposi's sarcoma, 347-349
  for leukemia, 349-365
  for lung cancer, 365-375
  for lymphoma, 375-400
  for malignant mesothelioma,
    404-406
  for melanoma, 402-404
  for multiple myeloma, 406-409
  for non-Hodgkin's disease,
    382-399
  for non–small-cell carcinoma,
    365-370
  for osteosarcoma, 409-411
  for ovarian carcinoma, 411-417
  for ovarian germ cell cancer,
    417-418
  for pancreatic carcinoma, 418-420
  for primary non-Hodgkin's
    lymphoma of central nervous
    system, 400-402
  for prostatic carcinoma, 420-423
  for renal cell carcinoma, 423-425
  for sarcoma, 425-428
  for small-cell lung cancer, 370-375
  for testicular germ cell cancer,
    428-432
  for thymoma, 432-434
  for thyroid carcinoma, 434-435
  for transitional cell carcinoma,
    312-315
  compatibilities of, 42
  controlling exposure to, 261-262,
    263-267
  dose of, 42, 268-269
  drug interactions with, 8-17
  drug resistance and, 3-4
  emetic potential of, 490, 491
  hypersensitivity reactions to, 269-274
  incompatibilities of, 42
  indications for, 41-42, 43-49
  intravenous delivery of; *see*
    Intravenous administration
    of antineoplastic drugs
  local tissue injury and, 520
  OSHA guidelines for handling,
    261-262
  pharmacology, 1-20
  platelet function and, 487

preparation of, 42
regional delivery of; *see* Regional
 administration of
 antineoplastic drugs
routes of administration of, 274,
 275-277
stability of, 42
storage of, 42
toxicity of, 42
Antitumor antibiotics, 6
Antitumor immunity, biological
 response modifiers and, 220
Antrypol, 189-191
APD, 174-176
APE for gestational trophoblastic
 disease, 342
Apheresis catheters, 280-282
APL; *see* Acute promyelocytic leukemia
Ara-C, 88-91
Ara-C syndrome, cytarabine for, 90
Area under the curve method, 573
Areas under the plasma concentration-
 time curves (AUCs), 14, 17
Aredia, 174-176
Arimidex, 59-61
ASH; *see* American Society of
 Hematology
Asparaginase, 43, 61-63
L-Asparaginase, 61-63
 for acute lymphoblastic leukemia,
  350-351, 352-354
 anaphylactic reactions and, 270
 drug interactions and, 13
Aspartate aminotransferase (SGOT), 498
Aspirin
 for pain, 451-454
 premedication and, 560-561
AS-RBCs; *see* Additive solution red
 blood cells
ATC for breast carcinoma, 319
ATRA; *see* All transretinoic acid
Atypical multidrug resistance, 3-4
AUCs; *see* Areas under the plasma
 concentration-time curves
Autologous Blood and Marrow
 Transplantation Registry of
 North America, 466
Autologous blood donations, 554
Autologous bone marrow transplant
 (ABMT), 462-466, 581
Autolymphocyte therapy (ALT) for
 prostatic carcinoma, 424
Autonomic neuropathy, cytotoxic
 drugs and, 541

Autonomy, medical ethics and, 436
AVM for breast carcinoma, 319
AZA-CR, 63-65
Azacytidine, 63-65
 for acute nonlymphycytic leukemia,
  356, 361
 for chronic granulocytic (myleocytic)
  leukemia, 363
 indications for, 43
5-Azacytidine, 63-65
 for acute nonlymphycytic leukemia,
  356
 for chronic granulocytic (myleocytic)
  leukemia, 363
Azathioprine, hypersensitivity
 pneumonitis and, 534
5-AZC, 63-65

B

BA-16038, 55-56
"Baby brain tumor" protocols in
 pediatric cancer therapy, 566
Bacillus Calmette-Guérin, 219, 228-230
BACOP for non-Hodgkin's disease, 388
BACT for lymphomas, 471
BAP for multiple myeloma, 407
BAP for thyroid carcinoma, 434
BAPP for thymoma, 432-433
BAVC for leukemias, 469
Bay Area Leukemia Study Group for
 acute lymphoblastic
 leukemia, 350-351
Bayer 205, 189-191
B-CAVe for Hodgkin's disease, 377
BCC for breast cancers, 473
B-cell growth factor, 248-250
B-cell stimulating factor, 248-250
BCG, 228-230
 for carcinoma in situ of bladder,
  237
BCGF, 248-250
BCNU, 75-77
 for brain tumors, 316
BEAC for lymphomas, 470-471
BEAM for lymphomas, 470
Benadryl Elixir for stomatitis, 512
Beneficence, medical ethics and, 436
Benzamides for nausea and vomiting,
 495
Benzodiazepines for nausea and
 vomiting, 492, 495, 500
Benztropine for extrapyramidal side
 effects, 499

BEP
  for ovarian germ cell cancer, 418
  for testicular and extragonadal germ
      cell cancer, 428-429
Betaseron, 242-244
BIC for cervical carcinoma, 331
Bicalutamide, 65-67
  drug interactions and, 13
  indications for, 43
  for prostatic carcinoma, 423
BiCNU, 75-77
Bilirubin, 498
Biological response modifiers (BRMs),
      219-259
  antitumor immunity, 220
  clinical development of, 220
  hematopoietic growth factors,
      220-221
  interferons, 221, 236-240
  interleukins, 222
  prevention and management of
      toxicities, 222-225
Biological safety cabinet (BSC), OSHA
      guidelines for, 263
BIP for cervical carcinoma, 331
BL4126A, 58-59
Bladder carcinoma, combination
      chemotherapy for, 312-315
Bladder toxicity, 529-530
Blenoxane, 67-69
Bleomycin, 67-69
  for carcinoma of unknown primary,
      330
  for cervical carcinoma, 331
  drug interactions and, 13
  for gestational trophoblastic disease,
      343
  for head and neck squamous cell
      carcinoma, 344-346
  for Hodgkin's disease, 376-377, 380,
      381, 382, 544
  hypersensitivity pneumonitis and, 534
  indications for, 43, 44
  for Kaposi's sarcoma, 348
  for non-Hodgkin's disease, 385-386,
      387, 388, 389, 390, 395,
      396-399
  for osteosarcoma, 411
  for ovarian germ cell cancer, 418
  for primary non-Hodgkin's
      lymphoma of central nervous
      system, 400-401, 402
  pulmonary toxicity and, 534
  for testicular and extragonadal germ
      cell cancer, 428-429, 430-431

  for thymoma, 432-433
  for thyroid carcinoma, 434, 435
BLM, 67-69
Blood components, blood transfusion
      therapy and, 553
Blood donations, types of, 554
Blood transfusion reactions; *see*
      Transfusion reactions
Blood transfusion therapy, 553-563
  administration of blood products in,
      562
  adverse conditions in, 561-562
  blood components, 553
  cryoprecipitate, 557
  granulocytes, 556-557
  plasma, 557
  platelets, 554-556
  transfusion reactions, 557-561
  types of blood donations, 554
BMC for head and neck squamous cell
      carcinoma, 344
BMY26538-01, 58-59
Body surface area (BSA), 569
  in adult amputees, 569
  drug doses and, 268-269
Body weight, 269, 570
Bone marrow transplants, 462-466, 581
  high-dose chemotherapy and,
      469-474
Brain tumors, combination
      chemotherapy for, 316-317
Breast carcinoma
  combination chemotherapy for,
      317-327
  high-dose chemotherapy for, 473-474
BRMs; *see* Biological response
      modifiers
5-Bromo-6-phenylisocytosine, 230-232
Brompton cocktail, 457-458
Bropirimine, 230-232
  for carcinoma in situ of bladder, 237
BSA; *see* Body surface area
BSC; *see* Biological safety cabinet
BSF, 70-72, 248-250
BSO, 72-73
BUCY for leukemias, 469
Bulk producers for constipation, 515
Buserelin, 69-70
Buserelin acetate, 69-70
Busulfan, 70-72
  indications for, 44
  for leukemias, 469-470
  for multiple myeloma, 472
Buthionine sulfoxime, 72-73
Buthionine sulfoximine, 72-73

DL-Buthionine-[S,R]-sulfoxime, 72-73
Butyrophenones for nausea and
vomiting, 492, 495, 499
BUVP for leukemias, 469-470
BVAM for primary non-Hodgkin's
lymphoma of central nervous
system, 400
BVCPP for Hodgkin's disease, 377

C

CABO for head and neck squamous
cell carcinoma, 344-345
Cachectin, 256-258
CAD for sarcoma, 425-426
CAE for small-cell lung cancer,
370-371
CAF
for breast carcinoma, 319
high-dose, for breast carcinoma,
319-320
Calcitrol
for bladder carcinoma, 315
for transitional cell carcinoma, 315
Calvert formula, 268-269
Camptosar, 138-140
Camptothecin-11, 138-140
Cancer; *see also* Carcinoma
blood transfusion therapy and; *see*
Blood transfusion therapy
brain, combination chemotherapy
for, 316-317
breast; *see* Breast carcinoma
combination chemotherapy for, 336
ethical considerations in; *see* Ethics
extragonadal germ cell, combination
chemotherapy for, 428-432
lung, combination chemotherapy
for, 365-375
ovarian germ cell, combination
chemotherapy for, 417-418
testicular germ cell, combination
chemotherapy for, 428-432
Cancer Information Service, National
Cancer Institute network of,
24, 450
Cancer therapy, pediatric; *see* Pediatric
cancer therapy
Cannabinoids for nausea and
vomiting, 492, 496, 500
CAP
for adrenal cortical carcinoma, 310
for endometrial cancer, 336
for non–small-cell lung carcinoma,
366

CAP/BOP
for non-Hodgkin's disease, 388
for primary non-Hodgkin's
lymphoma of central nervous
system, 400-401
Capsaicin (Zostrix), postherpetic
neuralgia and, 460
Carbamazepine (Tegretol), postherpetic
neuralgia and, 460
Carboplatin, 73-75
for bladder carcinoma, 315
for breast carcinoma, 324, 473
for carcinoma of unknown primary,
330
for cervical carcinoma, 331, 332
for esophageal carcinoma, 337
for germ cell tumors, 474
for head and neck squamous cell
carcinoma, 345
indications for, 44
for lymphomas, 471-472
for melanoma, 403
for non-Hodgkin's disease, 393
for non–small-cell lung carcinoma,
366, 367, 368
for ovarian carcinoma, 412-414, 416,
417
for small-cell lung cancer, 371, 373,
374
for testicular and extragonadal germ
cell cancer, 429
for transitional cell carcinoma, 315
Carboplatin dosing, 268-269, 573
Carboplatinum, 73-75
Carcinoid syndrome, combination
chemotherapy for, 327-329
Carcinoma; *see also* Cancer
adrenal cortical, combination
chemotherapy for, 310-311
anal, combination chemotherapy
for, 311-312
bladder, combination chemotherapy
for, 312-315
breast; *see* Breast carcinoma
cervical, combination chemotherapy
for, 330-332
colon, combination chemotherapy
for, 332-336
esophageal, combination
chemotherapy for, 337-339
head and neck squamous cell,
combination chemotherapy
for, 344-347
islet cell, combination
chemotherapy for, 327-329

Carcinoma *(cont.)*
  non–small-cell lung, combination
    chemotherapy for, 365-370
  ovarian, combination chemotherapy
    for, 411-417
  pancreatic, combination
    chemotherapy for, 418-420
  prostatic, combination
    chemotherapy for, 420-423
  renal cell, combination
    chemotherapy for, 423-425
  small-cell, combination
    chemotherapy for, 370-375
  thyroid, combination chemotherapy
    for, 434-435
  transitional cell, combination
    chemotherapy for, 312-315
  of unknown primary (CUP),
    combination chemotherapy
    for, 329-330
Cardiac toxicity, 537-539
Cardiovascular drugs, platelet function
  and, 487
Cardiovascular reactions, anaphylactic,
  272-273
Carmustine, 75-77
  for brain tumors, 316-317
  for breast cancers, 473
  drug interactions and, 13
  for Hodgkin's disease, 377
  indications for, 44
  for leukemias, 469
  for lymphomas, 470-471, 472
  for melanoma, 403-404
  for multiple myeloma, 406-407, 408,
    409
  for primary non-Hodgkin's
    lymphoma of central nervous
    system, 400
  venous reactions and, 523
Casodex, 65-67
Catapres; *see* Clonidine
Catheter care, 285-288
Catheter occlusion, 294
CAV for small-cell lung cancer, 372
CBCP for multiple myeloma, 407
CBDCA, 73-75
CBV for lymphomas, 471
CBVP
  for germ cell tumors, 474
  for lymphomas, 472
CCB for breast cancers, 473
CCNU, 147-149
  for brain tumors, 316
  for non-Hodgkin's disease, 386-387

CCRG 81045, 195-196
CCSG; *see* Children's Cancer Study
  Group
CD
  for acute nonlymphycytic leukemia,
    356
  for malignant mesothelioma, 405
2-CdA, 81-83
CDDP, 78-81
CE for adrenal cortical carcinoma,
  310-311
CEB for testicular and extragonadal
  germ cell cancer, 429
CEE
  for prostatic carcinoma, 420-421
  for thymoma, 433
CeeNU, 147-149
Cell cycle, phases of, 2
Cell kill hypothesis, 307
Cellular kinetics, antineoplastic drugs
  and, 2
Celsius, conversion to Fahrenheit,
  581
Central nervous system
  neurotoxicity and, 539-540
  primary non-Hodgkin's lymphoma
    of, combination
    chemotherapy for, 400-402
Central venous catheters, 279-288
  complications of, 291-295
  tunneled, 280-282, 284-285, 286-287
CEP for Hodgkin's disease, 377-378
Cephalotaxine, 131-132
Cerebellar syndromes, cytotoxic drugs
  and, 541, 542
Cerubidine, 95-97
Cervical carcinoma, combination
  chemotherapy for, 330-332
Cesemet; *see* Nabilone
CFBM for head and neck squamous
  cell carcinoma, 345-346
CFM for prostatic carcinoma, 421
CFP for breast carcinoma, 320
CHAD for ovarian carcinoma, 413
CHAP-5 for ovarian carcinoma, 413
Chemoimmunotherapy for melanoma,
  403
Chemoradiotherapy for primary
  non-Hodgkin's lymphoma
  of central nervous system,
  400-402
Chemotherapy; *see* Antineoplastic
  drugs
Children's Cancer Study Group
  (CCSG), 564

Chlorambucil, 77-78
  for chronic lymphocytic leukemia,
    364-365
  for Hodgkin's disease, 378, 379
  indications for, 44
Chlordeoxyadenosine, 81-83
2-Chlordeoxyadenosine, 81-83
Chlorhexidine (Peridex) for mucositis,
    507
2-Chloro-2-deoxyadenosine, 81-83
bis-Chloronitrosourea, 75-77
Chlorpromazine for nausea and
    vomiting, 494
CHLVPP for Hodgkin's disease, 378
CHOD for primary non-Hodgkin's
    lymphoma of central nervous
    system, 400
CHOEP for non-Hodgkin's disease,
    388-389
CHOP for non-Hodgkin's disease, 389
CHOP-BLEO for non-Hodgkin's
    disease, 389
Choriocarcinoma, 307
Chronic granulocytic leukemia,
    combination chemotherapy
    for, 362-364
Chronic hepatitis B, alfa interferons
    for, 239
Chronic hepatitis non-A, non-B/C,
    alfa interferons for, 239
Chronic lymphocytic leukemia (CLL),
    combination chemotherapy
    for, 364-365
Chronic myelocytic leukemia (CML),
    combination chemotherapy
    for, 362-364
Chronic myelogenous leukemia, alfa
    interferons for, 239
CIC for ovarian carcinoma, 413-414
Cigarette smoking as cause of cancer, 1
Cimetidine
  anaphylactic reactions and, 270
  for non-Hodgkin's disease, 399
  for primary non-Hodgkin's
    lymphoma of central nervous
    system, 401, 402
  for small-cell lung cancer, 373
CISCA
  for bladder carcinoma, 313
  for transitional cell carcinoma, 313
Cisdiamminedichloroplatinum, 78-81
Cisplatin, 78-81
  for adrenal cortical carcinoma,
    310-311
  for bladder carcinoma, 313-315

  for brain tumors, 316
  for breast carcinoma, 323, 326, 473
  for carcinoid (malignant) and islet
    cell carcinoma, 327, 328
  for carcinoma of unknown primary,
    330
  for cervical carcinoma, 331, 332
  drug interactions and, 13-14
  for endometrial cancer, 336
  for esophageal carcinoma, 337-339
  for gastric adenocarcinoma, 340, 341
  for gestational trophoblastic disease,
    342, 343
  for head and neck squamous cell
    carcinoma, 344-347
  indications for, 44
  for lymphomas, 472
  for malignant mesothelioma,
    405-406
  for melanoma, 403-404, 404
  for multiple myeloma, 407
  for non-Hodgkin's disease, 391-393,
    397
  for non–small-cell lung carcinoma,
    366-367, 368, 369-370
  for osteosarcoma, 410, 411
  for ovarian carcinoma, 412-416
  for ovarian germ cell cancer, 418
  for pancreatic carcinoma, 419
  for prostatic carcinoma, 420-421
  renal function and, 531
  for small-cell lung cancer, 372-374,
    375
  for testicular and extragonadal germ
    cell cancer, 428-432
  for thymoma, 432-434
  for thyroid carcinoma, 434-435
  for transitional cell carcinoma,
    313-315
Citrovorum factor, 142-145
Cladribine, 44, 81-83
CldAdo, 81-83
Clinical cooperative groups, pediatric
    cancer therapy and, 564-565
Clinical equipoise in clinical trials, 23
Clinical oncology trials, 22-25
Clinical trials, 21-40
  adverse drug reactions in, reporting,
    36-37
  conducting, 29-37
  data retrieval in, 35
  drug development and, 25-29
  patient enrollment in, 23, 30-34
  phase I, 27, 28
  phase II, 28

Clinical trials *(cont.)*
phase III, 28
phase IV, 29
preclinical evaluation of drugs in,
25-27
prospective monitoring in, 35-36
protocols in; *see* Protocols in clinical
trials
quality assurance in, 37
reasons for not enrolling patients
onto, 23
serious adverse events in, reporting,
36-37
source documents in, 34-35
CLL; *see* Chronic lymphocytic
leukemia
Clonidine (Catapres), 457
CM for adrenal cortical carcinoma, 311
CMF adjuvant therapy; *see*
Cyclophosphamide-
methotrexate-fluorouracil
adjuvant therapy
CMF for breast carcinoma, 322
intravenous 21-day, 320-321
intravenous 28-day, 321
CMFP for breast carcinoma, 321
CML; *see* Chronic myelocytic leukemia
C-MOPP for non-Hodgkin's disease,
389
CMV
for bladder carcinoma, 313
for transitional cell carcinoma, 313
CNOP for non-Hodgkin's disease, 390
Coating agents for stomatitis, 511
Cocktail, Brompton, 457-458
CODE for small-cell lung cancer,
372-373
Colon carcinoma, combination
chemotherapy for, 332-336
Colony-stimulating factor, 221
COLP for thymoma, 433
Combination chemotherapy; *see*
Antineoplastic drugs,
combination
Communication, hazard, OSHA
guidelines for, 267
Community Clinical Oncology
Program (COOP), 22
Condylomata acuminata, alfa
interferons for, 239
Consent, informed; *see* Informed
consent
Constipation, 513-514, 515-516
Coombs' test, 558

COOP; *see* Community Clinical
Oncology Program
Cooper regimen for breast carcinoma,
307, 321-322
COP-BLAM for non-Hodgkin's
disease, 390
COP-BLAM III for non-Hodgkin's
disease, 390
COPP for non-Hodgkin's disease, 391
Cordotomy, 459
Corticosteroids
for nausea and vomiting, 492, 495,
500-501
postherpetic neuralgia and, 460
Cortisone acetate for adrenal cortical
carcinoma, 311
Cosmegen, 94-95
Cotrimoxazole
for non-Hodgkin's disease, 386, 396,
399
for primary non-Hodgkin's
lymphoma of central nervous
system, 401, 402
for small-cell lung cancer, 373
Co-vidarabine, 176-177
CP for chronic lymphocytic leukemia,
364-365
CPE for small-cell lung cancer, 373
CPM, 83-86
CPT-11, 138-140
13-CRA, 140-142
Cranial nerve toxicity, cytotoxic drugs
and, 541
Creatinine clearance, 269, 572
Cryoprecipitate, blood transfusion
therapy and, 557
Cryopreservation of sperm, 544
CsA, 86-88
CT for breast cancers, 473-474
CTCB for breast cancers, 473
CTX, 83-86
CUP; *see* Carcinoma of unknown
primary
Curretab, 151-152
Cutaneous reactions
anaphylactic, 271-272
venous, 523
CVAD for chronic granulocytic
(myelocytic) leukemia,
362-363
CVP
for chronic lymphocytic leukemia,
364-365
for non-Hodgkin's disease, 391

CVPP for Hodgkin's disease, 378
Cyclooxygenase, premedication and,
        560-561
Cyclophosphamide, 83-86
    for acute lymphoblastic leukemia,
        352, 353-354
    for adrenal cortical carcinoma,
        310
    for bladder carcinoma, 313
    bladder toxicity and, 529
    for brain tumors, 316
    for breast cancers, 473-474
    for breast carcinoma, 318, 319-322,
        323-324
    for carcinoid (malignant) and islet
        cell carcinoma, 328
    cardiac toxicity from, 538-539
    for chronic lymphocytic leukemia,
        364-365
    drug interactions and, 14
    employee exposure to, 261
    for endometrial cancer, 336
    for gestational trophoblastic disease,
        342-343
    for Hodgkin's disease, 377
    indications for, 44
    for leukemias, 469
    for lymphomas, 470-471, 472
    for malignant mesothelioma,
        405-406
    for multiple myeloma, 406-407, 408,
        409, 472
    for non-Hodgkin's disease, 385-387,
        388-389, 390, 391, 392,
        393-394, 395, 396-399
    for non–small-cell lung carcinoma,
        366-368
    for osteosarcoma, 411
    for ovarian carcinoma, 413, 414-416,
        417
    for ovarian germ cell cancer, 417-418
    for primary non-Hodgkin's
        lymphoma of central nervous
        system, 400-402
    for prostatic carcinoma, 421
    pulmonary toxicity from, 534, 535
    renal function and, 531
    for sarcoma, 425-426
    for small-cell lung cancer, 370-371,
        372, 373
    for testicular and extragonadal germ
        cell cancer, 430-431
    for thymoma, 432, 433-434
    for transitional cell carcinoma, 313

Cyclophosphamide-methotrexate-
        fluorouracil (CMF) adjuvant
        therapy, 544
Cyclosporin-A, 86-88
Cyclosporine, 44, 86-88
Cycrin, 151-152
L-Cysteinamide, 168-170
Cytadren, 55-56
Cytarabine, 88-91
    for acute lymphoblastic leukemia,
        350, 351-354
    for acute nonlymphycytic leukemia,
        356-359, 360, 361
    for chronic granulocytic (myelocytic)
        leukemia, 363
    drug interactions and, 14
    indications for, 45
    for leukemias, 469
    for lymphomas, 470-471
    for non-Hodgkin's disease, 386, 387,
        391, 394, 397, 398-399
    for ovarian carcinoma, 415
    for primary non-Hodgkin's
        lymphoma of central nervous
        system, 400
    pulmonary toxicity from, 534, 535
Cytokines, 220, 542
Cytosar, 88-91
Cytosar-U, 88-91
Cytosine arabinoside, 88-91
Cytotoxic drugs
    in hematopoietic transplantation,
        463
    neurotoxicity associated with, 541
Cytoxan, 83-86
Cytoxan Lyophilized, 83-86
CY-VA-DIC for sarcoma, 426

D

Dacarbazine, 91-93
    for Hodgkin's disease, 376-377,
        544
    indications for, 45
    for melanoma, 403-404
    for sarcoma, 425-428
    venous reactions and, 523
DACP, 78-81
Dactinomycin, 94-95
    for gestational trophoblastic disease,
        342-343
    indications for, 45
    for melanoma, 403
    for osteosarcoma, 411

Dactinomycin *(cont.)*
  for ovarian germ cell cancer, 417-418
  radiation skin reactions and, 526
  for testicular and extragonadal germ
      cell cancer, 430-431
DAT; *see* Direct antiglobulin test
DAT for acute nonlymphycytic
      leukemia, 356-357
Data retrieval in clinical trials, 35
Daunomycin, 95-97
Daunorubicin, 95-97
  for acute lymphoblastic leukemia,
      350-351, 352, 353-354
  for acute nonlymphycytic leukemia,
      355-357, 358-359
  for chronic granulocytic (myelocytic)
      leukemia, 363
  indications for, 45
DaunoXome, 95-97
dCF, 176-177
*o,p'*DDD, 164-165
DDP, 78-81
Death with Dignity Act, 444
Decadron, 98-99
Delayed extravascular hemolytic
      transfusion reactions
      (DEHTRs), 560
Delayed hemolytic transfusion
      reactions, 557-558
Delayed intravascular hemolytic
      transfusion reactions
      (DIHTRs), 560
Deltasone, 183-184
4-Demethoxydaunorubicin, 134-135
2'-Deoxycoformycin, 176-177
2'-Deoxy-2',2'-difluorocytidine
      monohydrochloride, 127-129
Depo-Provera, 151-152
Dermatitis, 524
Dermatological toxicity, 514-526
  alopecia, 514-523
  multimodality therapy and, 525-526
  systemic, 523-525
DES, 101-102
Designated donor, blood donations
      and, 554
Dexamethasone, 98-99
  for acute lymphoblastic leukemia,
      351-352, 353-354
  anaphylactic reactions and, 270
  for chronic granulocytic (myelocytic)
      leukemia, 362-363
  for multiple myeloma, 408
  for nausea and vomiting, 495, 500

  for non-Hodgkin's disease, 387,
      391-393, 396-398
  for primary non-Hodgkin's
      lymphoma of central nervous
      system, 400
Dexone, 98-99
Dexrazoxane, 45, 99-101
DFCI-TCH Study III for
      osteosarcoma, 410
dFdC, 127-129
DHAD, 166-168
DHAP for non-Hodgkin's disease, 391
DHAQ, 166-168
Diagnosis, disclosure of, 439, 567
Dialysis, peritoneal, 300-301
Diarrhea, 508-513
Diazepam for nausea and vomiting,
      495
DIC, 91-93
DICE for non-Hodgkin's disease,
      391-392
DICEP for non-Hodgkin's disease, 392
Diet, low-microbial, 478, 479-481
Diethylstilbestrol, 45, 101-102
Diethylstilbestrol diphosphate, 101-102
Diffusing capacity for carbon
      monoxide (DLCO), 534-537
2',2' Difluorodeoxycytidine, 127-129
Digitalis glycosides, drug interactions
      and, 14
DIHTRs; *see* Delayed intravascular
      hemolytic transfusion
      reactions
Dihydrocodeine for pain, 454
N-(5-[N-(3,4-Dihydro-2-methyl-4-
      oxoguinazolin-6-ylmethyl)-N-
      methylamino]-2-thenoyl)-L-
      GLUTAMIC ACID-, 202-204
Dihydroxyanthracenedione, 166-168
Dimethyl triazeno imidazole
      carboxamide, 91-93
Diphenhydramine
  allergic reactions and, 561
  anaphylactic reactions and, 270
  for extrapyramidal side effects, 499
  for nausea and vomiting, 495
  premedication and, 560-561
Direct antiglobulin test (DAT), 558
Directed donor, blood donations and,
      554
Disclosure of diagnosis and prognosis,
      439
  in pediatric cancer therapy, 567
Discontinuing care, 440

DLCO; *see* Diffusing capacity for carbon monoxide
DLT; *see* Dose-limiting toxicity
DMBV for thyroid carcinoma, 435
DNA cross-linking agents, 4-5
DNR, 95-97
Do not resuscitate (DNR) orders, 439-440
  in pediatric cancer therapy, 567
Docetaxel, 45, 102-105, 309
Domains, multidrug resistance and, 3-4
Dopamine inhibitors for nausea and vomiting, 492
Dormant phase of cell cycle, 2
Dose calculation, 268-269
Dose intensity, 462
Dose-limiting toxicity (DLT), 463, 464
Double effect, indirect euthanasia and, 443
Double-dose melphalan for multiple myeloma, 472-473
Doxepin, postherpetic neuralgia and, 460
Doxil; *see* Doxorubicin hydrochloride liposomal injection
Doxorubicin, 105-109
  for acute lymphoblastic leukemia, 353-354
  for acute nonlymphycytic leukemia, 361
  for adrenal cortical carcinoma, 310, 311
  for bladder carcinoma, 313-314
  for breast carcinoma, 318, 319, 320, 322, 323-324, 326-327
  for carcinoid (malignant) and islet cell carcinoma, 328-329
  for cervical carcinoma, 331, 332
  for chronic granulocytic (myelocytic) leukemia, 362-363
  for endometrial cancer, 336
  for esophageal carcinoma, 338
  for gastric adenocarcinoma, 339-340, 341
  for Hodgkin's disease, 376-377, 379, 380, 381, 544
  indications for, 45
  for Kaposi's sarcoma, 348
  for malignant mesothelioma, 405-406
  for multiple myeloma, 406-407, 408-409
  for non-Hodgkin's disease, 385-386, 387, 388-389, 390, 393-394, 395, 396-397, 398-399

  for non–small-cell lung carcinoma, 366
  for osteosarcoma, 410, 411
  for ovarian carcinoma, 413, 414-416
  for pancreatic carcinoma, 419
  for primary non-Hodgkin's lymphoma of central nervous system, 400-402
  for prostatic carcinoma, 421
  for sarcoma, 425-428
  for small-cell lung cancer, 370-371, 372-373
  for thymoma, 432-434
  for thyroid carcinoma, 434-435
  for transitional cell carcinoma, 313-314
Doxorubicin hydrochloride liposomal injection (Doxil), 105-109
Dronabinol for nausea and vomiting, 496, 500
Droperidol for nausea and vomiting, 495
Drug acronyms, 582-584
Drug interactions, 8-17
  definition of, 8
  likelihood of, 9-10
  mechanisms of, 9
Drug resistance, 3-4
  atypical multidrug, 3-4
  multidrug, 3
  topoisomerases and, 3-4
Drugs
  antineoplastic; *see* Antineoplastic drugs
  development of, clinical trials and, 25-29
  evaluation of, clinical trials in; *see* Clinical trials
  preclinical evaluation of, 25-27
DS for prostatic carcinoma, 421
DTIC, 91-93
DTIC-Dome, 91-93
Duke high-dose intensity AFM for breast carcinoma, 322
Durable power of attorney for health care, advanced directives and, 441
Duragesic; *see* Fentanyl
DVIP for non-Hodgkin's disease, 392-393
DXM, 98-99
Dyclone 0.5% for stomatitis, 512

E

EAP for gastric adenocarcinoma, 340
EAP-II for gastric adenocarcinoma, 340
Eastern Cooperative Oncology Group (ECOG), 393, 448, 571
ECCO for small-cell lung cancer, 373
ECOG; *see* Eastern Cooperative Oncology Group
10-EDAM, 109-110
Edatrexate, 109-110
Efudex, 121-123
Elastomeric ambulatory infusion pump, 303
Elderly, combination chemotherapy in, 400-402
ELF, for gastric adenocarcinoma, 340-341
Elipten, 55-56
Elspar, 61-63
EMA-CO for gestational trophoblastic disease, 342-343
modified, 343
Emcyt, 111-113
Emesis; *see* Nausea and vomiting
Employee, prevention of exposure of, to hazardous drugs, OSHA guidelines for, 263-267
Encephalopathy, cytotoxic drugs and, 541, 542
Endometrial cancer, combination chemotherapy for, 336
Endomyocardial biopsy, 538
Endoxan, 83-86
Energy requirements, nausea and vomiting and, 501
Enhancement reactions, 526
Enzymes, 7
EPEG, 113-116
4'-Epiadriamycin, 110-111
EPIC for non-Hodgkin's disease, 393
4'-Epidoxorubicin, 110-111
Epidural administration of narcotics, 458
Epinephrine, anaphylactic reactions and, 274
Epipodophyllotoxin, 113-116
Epirubicin, 110-111
for bladder carcinoma, 314-315
for breast carcinoma, 323
for Hodgkin's disease, 382
for primary non-Hodgkin's lymphoma of central nervous system, 401-402
for prostatic carcinoma, 420-421
for thymoma, 433

for transitional cell carcinoma, 314-315
EPOCH for non-Hodgkin's disease, 393-394
Epoetin alfa, 232-233
for anemia, 237
Epogen, 232-233
Ergamisol, 250-252
Erwinia asparaginase, 61-63
Erythropoietin alfa, 232-233
ESHAP for non-Hodgkin's disease, 397
Esophageal carcinoma, combination chemotherapy for, 337-339
Estoposide phosphate (Etopophos), 113-116
Estracyt, 111-113
Estramustine, 111-113
drug interactions and, 14
indications for, 45
nausea and vomiting and, 501
for prostatic carcinoma, 420-422
Estramustine phosphate, 111-113
Ethanethiol, 51-53
Ethics, 436-447
advanced directives, 441
discontinuing care, 440
do not resuscitate orders, 439-440
hospice, 441-442
managed care, 437-438
in pediatric cancer therapy, 566-568
consent, 566-567
disclosure of diagnosis and prognosis, 567
do not resuscitate orders, 567
hospice, 567-568
physician-assisted suicide, 442-445
principles in medical ethics, 436-437
truthfulness, 438-439
Ethiofos, 51-53
10-Ethyl-10-deaza-aminopterin, 109-110
Ethyol, 51-53
Etopophos; *see* Estoposide phosphate
Etoposide, 113-116
for acute lymphoblastic leukemia, 351-353, 354
for acute nonlymphycytic leukemia, 359-360
for adrenal cortical carcinoma, 310-311
for breast carcinoma, 324
for carcinoid (malignant) and islet cell carcinoma, 327
for carcinoma of unknown primary, 330
for gastric adenocarcinoma, 340-341

for germ cell tumors, 474
for gestational trophoblastic disease, 342-343
for Hodgkin's disease, 377-378, 379, 382
indications for, 45
for leukemias, 469-470
for lymphomas, 470-472
for non-Hodgkin's disease, 386-387, 388-389, 391-394, 395, 397, 398-399
for non–small-cell lung carcinoma, 366, 367-368
for osteosarcoma, 411
for ovarian germ cell cancer, 418
for primary non-Hodgkin's lymphoma of central nervous system, 401-402
for prostatic carcinoma, 421
for sarcoma, 427
for small-cell lung cancer, 370-371, 372-374, 375
for testicular and extragonadal germ cell cancer, 428-429, 430, 431-432
for thymoma, 433
Euflex, 124-125
Eulexin, 124-125
Euthanasia, 442-445
Evaluation of drugs
clinical trials in; *see* Clinical trials
preclinical, 25-27
EVAP for Hodgkin's disease, 379
Extragonadal germ cell cancer, combination chemotherapy for, 428-432
Extravasation, 520-522, 523

F

FAC for pancreatic carcinoma, 419
FAC-S for carcinoid (malignant) and islet cell carcinoma, 328
Fahrenheit, conversion to Celsius, 581
FAM for gastric adenocarcinoma, 339-340
FAMP, 119-121
FAM-S for pancreatic carcinoma, 419
FAMTX for gastric adenocarcinoma, 341
FAP
for esophageal carcinoma, 338
for gastric adenocarcinoma, 341
for pancreatic carcinoma, 419
Fareston, 206-207

FC-1157a, 206-207
FDC for adrenal cortical carcinoma, 311
Febrile transfusion reactions, 558, 560
FEC for breast carcinoma, 323
Fentanyl (Duragesic) for pain, 457, 458
FEP for breast carcinoma, 323
Fertility; *see* Gonadal toxicity
Fever, neutropenia and, 482-486
FFP; *see* Fresh frozen plasma
Fibonacci method, modified, in clinical trials, 27, 28
Filgrastim, 233-236
for bladder carcinoma, 315
drug interactions and, 14-15
for esophageal carcinoma, 339
for neutropenia, 237
for non–small-cell lung carcinoma, 368
for small-cell lung cancer, 374
for transitional cell carcinoma, 315
Final Exit, 444
Finasteride, 46, 116-117
Five-Drug Cancer and Leukemia Group B Induction Regimen for acute lymphoblastic leukemia, 352
Flare reaction, 523
Floxuridine, 117-119
drug interactions and, 15
indications for, 46
Fludara, 119-121
Fludarabine, 119-121
indications for, 46
for non-Hodgkin's disease, 394-395
Fludarabine phosphate, 119-121
Fludrocortisone acetate for adrenal cortical carcinoma, 311
Fluid and electrolyte balance, nausea and vomiting and, 501-502
2-Fluoroadenine arabinoside-5-phosphate, 119-121
2-Fluoro-ara AMP, 119-121
5-Fluoro-2'-deoxyuridine, 117-119
Fluoroplex, 121-123
5-Fluorouracil, 121-123
drug interactions and, 15
for adrenal cortical carcinoma, 311
for anal carcinoma, 312
for breast carcinoma, 319, 320, 321-322, 323-324, 325, 326
for carcinoid (malignant) and islet cell carcinoma, 328, 329
cardiac toxicity from, 538
for cervical carcinoma, 331

5-Fluorouracil *(cont.)*
for colon carcinoma, 333, 334, 335, 336
for esophageal carcinoma, 337-338
for gastric adenocarcinoma, 339-340, 341-342
for head and neck squamous cell carcinoma, 345-347
indications for, 46
for non-Hodgkin's disease, 394
for ovarian carcinoma, 415
for pancreatic carcinoma, 419, 420
for prostatic carcinoma, 421
Fluoxymesterone, 123-124
for breast carcinoma, 326-327
indications for, 46
Flurbiprofen for pain, 454
Flutamide, 124-125
indications for, 46
for prostatic carcinoma, 422-423
F-MACHOP for non-Hodgkin's disease, 394
FMP for non-Hodgkin's disease, 394-395
Foam brush, toothbrushing and, 508
Folex, 159-162
Folex-Pfs, 159-162
Folinic acid, 142-145
Food intake, improving, 504
5-Formyltetrahydrofolate, 142-145
Fourneau 309, 189-191
FRBCs; *see* Frozen red blood cells
French Multicenter Study for acute lymphoblastic leukemia, 352-353
Fresh frozen plasma (FFP), 557
Frozen red blood cells (FRBCs), 554
Ftorafur, 193-195
5-FU, 121-123
FUDR, 117-119
5-FUDR, 117-119

G

"Gag rule," 437-438
Gallium nitrate, 125-127
for bladder carcinoma, 315
indications for, 46
for transitional cell carcinoma, 315
Gammaphos, 51-53
Ganciclovir OSHA guidelines for handling, 262
Ganite, 125-127
Gastric adenocarcinoma, combination chemotherapy for, 339-342

Gastrointestinal toxicity, 488-514
anorexia and, 502, 503, 504
antiemetic therapy and, 488-501
constipation and, 513-514, 515-516
diarrhea and, 508-513
nausea and vomiting and, 488-501
stomatitis and, 502-508
taste changes and, 502, 503, 504
GCP; *see* Good clinical practice
G-CSF; *see* Granulocyte colony-stimulating factor
Gelfoam, thrombocytopenia and, 488
Gemcitabine, 46, 127-129, 309
Gemzar, 127-129
Genetic engineering, 222
Germ cell tumors, high-dose chemotherapy for, 474
German Multistudy Group for acute lymphoblastic leukemia, 353-354
Germanin, 189-191
Gestational trophoblastic disease, combination chemotherapy for, 342-343
GGP 30693, 109-110
Glutathione (GSH), 4
Glutathione S-transferase (GST), 4
GnRH; *see* Gonadotropin-releasing hormone
Gonadal toxicity, 543-544
Gonadotropin-releasing hormone (GnRH), 544
Good clinical practice (GCP), 21-40
Goserelin, 129-131
for prostatic carcinoma, 422
Goserelin acetate
indications for, 46
for prostatic carcinoma, 423
Graft-versus-host disease (GVHD), 466
posttransfusion, 562
Granisetron (Kytril) for nausea and vomiting, 494, 497, 498-499, 565
Granulocyte colony-stimulating factor (G-CSF), 14, 222, 233-236, 477
Granulocyte-macrophage colony-stimulating factor, 253-255
Granulocytes, blood transfusion therapy and, 556-557
Groshong type of tunneled central venous catheter, 285
Growth factors, hematopoietic,

biological response modifiers and, 220-221
GSH; *see* Glutathione
GST; *see* Glutathioine S-transferase
GVHD; *see* Graft-versus-host disease

H

Hair loss, 514-523, 565
Hairy cell leukemia, 307
  alfa interferons for, 239
Haloperidol for nausea and vomiting, 495
Halotestin, 123-124
Hazard communication, OSHA guidelines for, 267
Hazardous drugs, prevention of employee exposure to, OSHA guidelines for, 263-267
H-CAP for ovarian carcinoma, 414-415
HCGF, 246-248
HD; *see* Hodgkin's disease
HDCT; *see* High-dose chemotherapy
Head and neck squamous cell carcinoma, combination chemotherapy for, 344-347
Health care agent, advanced directives and, 441
Health insurance, clinical trials and, 24-25
Health maintenance organizations (HMOs), clinical trials and, 24-25
Hematopoietic cell growth factor, 246-248
Hematopoietic growth factors, 220-221, 477
Hematopoietic transplantation, cytotoxic drugs in, 463
Hemolytic reactions, 557-558
Hepatic toxicity, 545
Hepatitis B, 561
  chronic, alfa interferons for, 239
Hepatitis C, 561
Hepatitis non-A, non-B/C, chronic, alfa interferons for, 239
Heroin, 457-458
Herpes zoster, 459-460
HEXA-CAF for ovarian carcinoma, 415
Hexadrol, 98-99
Hexalen, 50-51
Hexamethylmelamine, 50-51
Hexastat, 50-51

HHT, 131-132
High-dose chemotherapy (HDCT), 462-474
  for breast cancers, 473-474
  for germ cell tumors, 474
  for leukemias, 467, 469-470
  for lymphomas, 467, 470-472
  for multiple myeloma, 472-473
  with stem cell support, 462-474
High-dose fluorouracil/leucovorin for breast carcinoma, 326
High-dose leucovorin for breast carcinoma, 325
HIV; *see* Human immunodeficiency virus
HLA; *see* Human leukocyte antigen
HLA antibody formation, blood transfusion therapy and, 562
HMM, 50-51
HN_2, 4, 149-150
Hodgkin's disease (HD), 544
  alcohol-induced pain associated with, 451
  combination chemotherapy for, 375-382
HOE 766, 69-70
Holoxan, 135-138
Homoharringtonine, 131-132
HOP for testicular and extragonadal germ cell cancer, 429-430
Hopkins 16-week dose-intense regimen for breast carcinoma, 323-324
Hospice, 441-442
  in pediatric cancer therapy, 567
HTLV-I; *see* T-cell leukemia/lymphoma virus
Huber-point needles, implanted ports and, 290
Human immunodeficiency virus (HIV), 561
Human leukocyte antigen (HLA), 555
HXM, 50-51
Hycamptamine, 204-206
Hycamptin, 204-206
Hydrdocodone for pain, 454
Hydrea, 132-133
Hydrocortisone
  for non-Hodgkin's disease, 396
  for prostatic carcinoma, 422
Hydromorphone for pain, 457
Hydroxycarbamide, 132-133
Hydroxydaunomycin, 105-109
Hydroxydaunorubicin, 105-109
5-Hydroxytryptamine, 497

Hydroxyurea, 132-133
  for brain tumors, 317
  for chronic granulocytic (myeolocytic)
      leukemia, 363-364
  indications for, 46
Hydroxyzine pamoate for nausea and
    vomiting, 496
Hyperpigmentation of skin, 524, 525
Hypersensitivity pneumonitis, 534
Hypersensitivity reactions
  antineoplastic drugs and, 269-274
  signs and symptoms of, 270

I

Ibenzmethyzin, 184-186
Ibuprofen for pain, 454
ICE
  for germ cell tumors, 474
  for lymphomas, 471-472
  for testicular and extragonadal germ
      cell cancer, 430
ICI 176,334, 65-67
ICI 118630, 129-131
ICRF-187, 99-101
Idamycin, 134-135
Idarubicin, 134-135
  for acute nonlymphycytic leukemia,
      357-358
  indications for, 46
Idarubicin hydrochloride, 134-135
Ideal body-weight charts, 570
Ifex, 135-138
IFN alfa-2a, 236-242
IFN alfa-2b, 236-242
IFN alfa-n1, 236-242
IFN alfa-n3, 236-242
IFN-beta, 242-244
IFN-Bser, 242-244
IFN-gamma, 244-246
Ifosfamide, 135-138
  for acute lymphoblastic leukemia,
      354
  for bladder carcinoma, 315
  bladder toxicity and, 529
  for brain tumors, 316-317
  for breast carcinoma, 324
  for cervical carcinoma, 331, 332
  for germ cell tumors, 474
  indications for, 47
  for lymphomas, 471-472
  neurological toxicity and, 541-542
  for non-Hodgkin's disease, 391-393,
      395, 397, 399

  for non–small-cell lung carcinoma,
      366, 368, 369-370
  for ovarian carcinoma, 413-414
  renal function and, 531
  for sarcoma, 426-428
  for small-cell lung cancer, 371-372,
      373-374, 375
  for testicular and extragonadal germ
      cell cancer, 429-430, 431
  for transitional cell carcinoma, 315
IL-1; *see* Interleukin-1
IL-2; *see* Interleukin-2
IL-3, 246-248
IL-4, 248-250
Imidazole carboxamide, 91-93
ImmuCyst, 228-230
Immune surveillance, 220
Immunity
  antitumor, biological response
      modifiers and, 220
  natural, 220
Implanted ports, 276, 279, 280-282,
    288-291
IMVP-16 for non-Hodgkin's disease,
    395
Indirect euthanasia, 443
Infection
  central venous catheters and, 291-294
  neutropenia and, 476-478, 482-486
  reservoir usage and, 296-300
Infertility as delayed consequence of
    treatment, 566
Informed consent, 308, 439
  autologous bone marrow transplant
      and, 464
  in pediatric cancer therapy, 566-567
Infusaid implantable pump, 296, 297
Infusion and venipuncture, guidelines
    for, 521
Infusion pumps, ambulatory, for
    delivery of antineoplastic
    drugs, 276, 303, 304
Institutional Review Board (IRB), 308
Insurance, clinical trials and, 24-25
Intensive five-drug therapy for acute
    nonlymphycytic leukemia,
    358-359
Intercalation, antitumor antibiotics
    and, 6
Interferon alfa, drug interactions and,
    15
Interferon alfa-2a, 236-242
  for colon carcinoma, 334
  for esophageal carcinoma, 338

for hairy cell leukemia, 237
Interferon alfa-2b, 236-242
  for hairy cell leukemia, 237
Interferon alfa-2c, 238
Interferon alfa-n1, 236-242
Interferon alfa-n3, 236-242
  for condylomata acuminata, 237
Interferon alpha for melanoma, 403
Interferon beta, 242-244
Interferon beta-1b, 242-244
  for multiple sclerosis, 238
Interferon gamma, 244-246
Interferon gamma-1b, 244-246
  for ovarian carcinoma, 238
Interferons, 221, 236-240
Interleukin(s), biological response
    modifiers and, 222
Interleukin-1 (IL-1), 220
Interleukin-2 (IL-2), 220, 222, 225-228
  for melanoma, 403
Interleukin-3, 246-248
  for thrombocytopenia, 238
Interleukin-4, 248-250
  for melanoma, 238
Interleukin-6, 238
Interleukin-11, 238
International Bone Marrow Transplant
    Registry, 466
Intraarterial delivery of antineoplastic
    drugs, 275, 295-296, 297
Intramuscular administration of
    antineoplastic drugs, 275
Intraperitoneal cisplatin-cytarabine for
    ovarian carcinoma, 415
Intraperitoneal delivery of
    antineoplastic drugs, 276,
    300-301
Intrapleural delivery of antineoplastic
    drugs, 277, 301-302
Intrathecal administration of
    antineoplastic drugs, 276
Intrathecal administration of narcotics,
    458
Intravenous administration of
    antineoplastic drugs, 274-295
  central venous access, 279-288,
    291-295
  implanted ports, 288-291
  peripheral venous access, 274-279
Intraventricular delivery of
    antineoplastic drugs, 276,
    296-300
Intravesicular administration of
    antineoplastic drugs, 277

Intron-A, 236-242
Involuntary euthanasia, 443
IRB; *see* Institutional Review Board
Irinotecan, 47, 138-140, 309
Islet cell carcinoma, combination
    chemotherapy for, 327-329
Isoenzymes, glutathione S-transferase, 4
Isophosphamide, 135-138
Isotretinoin, 140-142
Italian study for colon carcinoma, 333

J
JM-8, 73-75
Judicial Council of American Medical
    Association, 440
Justice, medical ethics and, 436-437

K
Kaopectate for stomatitis, 511
Kaopectate/Benadryl Elixir for
    stomatitis, 511
Kaposi's sarcoma (KS)
  of AIDS, alfa interferons for, 239
  combination chemotherapy for,
    347-349
Karnofsky, 571
Ketoconazole
  for non-Hodgkin's disease, 386, 396,
    399
  for primary non-Hodgkin's
    lymphoma of central nervous
    system, 401, 402
  for prostatic carcinoma, 422
  for small-cell lung cancer, 373
Ketrax, 250-252
Kevorkian, Jack, 443
Kidney toxicity, 526-533
KS; *see* Kaposi's sarcoma
Kytril; *see* Granisetron

L
Lactic dehydrogenase (LDH), acute
    intravascular hemolytic
    transfusion reactions and,
    559-560
Ladakamycin, 63-65
Lanvis, 198-200
Laxatives
  saline, for constipation, 516
  stimulant, for constipation, 516
LCV, 142-145

LD10 in clinical trials, 27
LD-ACOP-B for primary non-Hodgkin's
lymphoma of central nervous
system, 401
LDH; *see* Lactic dehydrogenase
Left ventricular ejection fraction
(LVEF), 41
Leo 1031, 182
Leucocristine, 214-216
Leucovorin, 142-145
for acute lymphoblastic leukemia,
351, 352-353
for breast carcinoma, 318, 322,
323-324, 325, 326
for colon carcinoma, 333, 334,
335-336
drug interactions and, 15
for gastric adenocarcinoma, 340-342
for gestational trophoblastic disease,
342-343
for head and neck squamous cell
carcinoma, 346-347
high-dose, for breast carcinoma, 325
indications for, 47
for non-Hodgkin's disease, 386, 387,
394, 396-397, 398-399
for osteosarcoma, 410, 411
for primary non-Hodgkin's
lymphoma of central nervous
system, 400
Leucovorin calcium, 142-145
Leukemia
acute lymphoblastic, combination
chemotherapy for, 349-354
acute nonlymphocytic, combination
chemotherapy for, 354-361
acute promyelocytic, combination
chemotherapy for, 355
chronic granulocytic, combination
chemotherapy for, 362-364
chronic lymphocytic, combination
chemotherapy for, 364-365
chronic myelocytic, combination
chemotherapy for, 362-364
chronic myelogenous, alfa
interferons for, 239
hairy cell, 239, 307
high-dose chemotherapy for, 467,
469-470
Leukeran, 77-78
Leukine, 253-255
Leukoreduction filters, blood
transfusion therapy and, 562
Leuprolide
indications for, 47

for prostatic carcinoma, 422-423
Leuprolide acetate, 145-147
for prostatic carcinoma, 423
Leuprorelin acetate, 145-147
Leustatin, 81-83
Levamisole, 250-252
for colon carcinoma, 238, 334
drug interactions and, 15
Levorphanol for pain, 457
LHRH for prostatic carcinoma, 423
Liquid Pred, 183-184
Living will, medical ethics and, 440
LNH-80 for non-Hodgkin's disease,
395
LNH-84 for non-Hodgkin's disease,
395
Lomustine, 147-149
for brain tumors, 316, 317
for Hodgkin's disease, 376, 377-378,
381
indications for, 47
for melanoma, 404
for non-Hodgkin's disease, 386-387
for thymoma, 433
"Look Good, Feel Better Program,"
519
LOPP for Hodgkin's disease, 379
Lorazepam for nausea and vomiting,
495, 500
Low-microbial diet, 478, 479-481
Lung cancer, combination
chemotherapy for, 365-375
Lupron, 145-147
Lupron Depot, 145-147
Lupron Depot-3 Month, 145-147
LV, 142-145
LVEF; *see* Left ventricular ejection
fraction
Lymphoid blast crisis, chronic
granulocytic (myeleocytic)
leukemia and, 364
Lymphokines, 222
Lymphoma
high-dose chemotherapy for, 467,
470-472
Hodgkin's, combination
chemotherapy for, 375-382
non-Hodgkin's; *see* Non-Hodgkin's
lymphoma
Lysodren, 164-165

M

3M for breast carcinoma, 325
M-2 for multiple myeloma, 408

MAC
  for bladder carcinoma, 313
  for transitional cell carcinoma, 313
MACOP-B for non-Hodgkin's disease, 396
MAI for sarcoma, 427
MAID for sarcoma, 427-428
Malignancy, secondary, as delayed consequence of treatment, 566
Malignant melanoma, adjuvant treatment for, alfa interferons for, 239
Malignant mesothelioma, combination chemotherapy for, 404-406
Malnutrition in cancer patients, 502, 503, 504
m-AMSA, 56-58
Managed care, 437-438
Mannitol
  acute intravascular hemolytic transfusion reactions and, 559
  for non–small-cell lung carcinoma, 366
Marinol for nausea and vomiting, 500
Mast cell growth factor, 246-248
Matulane, 184-186
Maximally tolerated dose (MTD), 220
m-BACOD for non-Hodgkin's disease, 396-397
m-BNCOD for non-Hodgkin's disease, 397-398
MCGF, 246-248
MEC for acute nonlymphycytic leukemia, 359
Mechlorethamine, 4, 149-150
  for Hodgkin's disease, 379-381
  indications for, 47
Med Tamoxifen, 191-193
Medicaid, 437
Medical ethics, principles of, 436-437
Medical surveillance, OSHA guidelines for, 267
Medicare, 437
  clinical trials and, 24-25
MEDLARS, Physician's Data Query database and, 24
Medroxyprogesterone, 47
Medroxyprogesterone acetate, 151-152
Megace, 152-153
Megakaryocyte growth and development factor, 252
Megestrol, 152-153

  for prostatic carcinoma, 421
Megestrol acetate, 47, 152-153
Melanoma
  combination chemotherapy for, 402-404
  malignant, adjuvant treatment for, alfa interferons for, 239
Melphalan, 154-155
  double-dose, for multiple myeloma, 472-473
  drug interactions and, 15
  for Hodgkin's disease, 381
  indications for, 47
  for lymphomas, 470
  for multiple myeloma, 408, 409
  for thyroid carcinoma, 435
Meperidine for pain, 455
MER-BCG; *see* Methanol-extracted residue of BCG
2-Mercaptoethane sulfonate sodium, renal toxicity and, 530
Mercaptopurine, 155-157
  drug interactions and, 15-16
  indications for, 47
6-Mercaptopurine, 155-157
  for acute lymphoblastic leukemia, 353-354
  for acute nonlymphycytic leukemia, 361
Mesna, 157-159
  for acute lymphoblastic leukemia, 354
  for bladder carcinoma, 315
  for breast carcinoma, 324
  for cervical carcinoma, 331, 332
  indications for, 47
  for non-Hodgkin's disease, 392-393, 397
  for non–small-cell lung carcinoma, 366, 369-370
  for ovarian carcinoma, 413-414
  renal toxicity and, 530
  for sarcoma, 426, 427-428
  for small-cell lung cancer, 371-372, 374, 375
  for testicular and extragonadal germ cell cancer, 430, 431
  for transitional cell carcinoma, 315
Mesnex, 157-159
Mesnum, 157-159
Mesothelioma, malignant, combination chemotherapy for, 404-406
Methadone for pain, 457
Methanol-extracted residue of BCG (MER-BCG), 219

Methotrexate, 159-162
for acute lymphoblastic leukemia,
350-351, 352-354
for acute nonlymphycytic leukemia,
361
for bladder carcinoma, 313-315
for brain tumors, 316
for breast carcinoma, 318, 321-322,
323-324, 325
for cervical carcinoma, 332
for colon carcinoma, 335-336
drug interactions and, 16
for gastric adenocarcinoma, 341
for gestational trophoblastic disease,
342-343
for head and neck squamous cell
carcinoma, 344-346
for Hodgkin's disease, 382
hypersensitivity pneumonitis and,
534
indications for, 47, 48
for non-Hodgkin's disease, 386, 387,
394, 395, 396-399
for osteosarcoma, 410, 411
for ovarian carcinoma, 415
for primary non-Hodgkin's
lymphoma of central nervous
system, 400
pulmonary toxicity and, 534, 535
renal function and, 532
for transitional cell carcinoma,
313-315
Methotrexate LPF, 159-162
Methotrexate sodium, 159-162
N-Methylhydrazine, 184-186
4-Methyl-2-hydroxy-2-(4-hydroxy-4-
methylpentyl) butanedioate
ester, 131-132
Methylphenidate (Ritalin), 457
Methylprednisolone
for acute nonlymphycytic leukemia,
361
for chronic granulocytic (myeleocytic)
leukemia, 363
for non-Hodgkin's disease, 395, 397
Meticorten, 183-184
Metoclopramide for nausea and
vomiting, 492, 495, 497,
499-500
Mexate, 159-162
Mexate-AQ, 159-162
M-F for esophageal carcinoma, 338
MGDF, 252
for thrombocytopenia, 238

Midline vascular access devices,
280-282
Milk of magnesia for stomatitis, 511
MINE for non-Hodgkin's disease, 397
MINE-ESHAP for non-Hodgkin's
disease, 397
Mini-ICE for breast carcinoma, 324
MIP for non–small-cell lung
carcinoma, 368
Mithracin, 178-180
Mithramycin, 178-180
Mitomycin, 162-164
for anal carcinoma, 312
for breast carcinoma, 319, 325
drug interactions and, 16
for esophageal carcinoma, 338
for gastric adenocarcinoma, 339-340
indications for, 48
for malignant mesothelioma, 405
for non–small-cell lung carcinoma,
366-367, 368
for pancreatic carcinoma, 419, 420
pulmonary toxicity from, 534, 536
renal function and, 532
Mitomycin-C, 162-164
Mitotane, 164-165
for adrenal cortical carcinoma, 311
drug interactions and, 16
indications for, 48
Mitotic inhibitors, 7
Mitoxana, 135-138
Mitoxantrone, 166-168
for acute lymphoblastic leukemia,
351, 352-353, 354
for acute nonlymphycytic leukemia,
359-360
for bladder carcinoma, 315
for breast carcinoma, 324, 325
for chronic granulocytic (myeleocytic)
leukemia, 363
indications for, 48
for non-Hodgkin's disease, 390,
394-395, 397-398, 399
for prostatic carcinoma, 423
for transitional cell carcinoma, 315
Mitoxantrone hydrochloride, 166-168
MK-906, 116-117
MOF-STREP for colon carcinoma, 335
MOP-BAP for Hodgkin's disease, 380
MOPP for Hodgkin's disease, 307,
375-376, 379-380, 544
MOPP/ABV hybrid for Hodgkin's
disease, 380
Moranyl, 189-191

Morphine for pain, 455-458
Mostarinia, 182
Mouthwash in stomatitis oral care
        program, 505
6-MP, 155-157
MP for multiple myeloma, 408
MS for adrenal cortical carcinoma, 311
MTD; *see* Maximally tolerated dose
MTX, 159-162
Mucositis, 507
Multi-CSF, 246-248
Multidrug resistance, 3
Multimodality therapy, skin reactions
        and, 525-526
Multiple myeloma
    alfa interferons for, 239
    combination chemotherapy for,
        406-409
    high-dose chemotherapy for, 472-473
Multi-potential colony-stimulating
        factor, 246-248
Mustargen, 149-150
    for Hodgkins' disease, 544
Mutamycin, 162-164
MV for breast carcinoma, 325
M-VAC
    for bladder carcinoma, 313-314
    for transitional cell carcinoma,
        313-314
MVAC for cervical carcinoma, 332
M-VAV, high-dose, for bladder
        carcinoma, 314
M-VEC
    for bladder carcinoma, 314-315
    for transitional cell carcinoma,
        314-315
MVNC
    for bladder carcinoma, 315
    for transitional cell carcinoma, 315
MVP for non–small-cell lung
        carcinoma, 368
MVPP for Hodgkin's disease, 380-381
Myelogenous leukemia, chronic, alfa
        interferons for, 239
Myelopathy, acute, cytotoxic drugs
        and, 541
Myleran, 70-72
Myofibril cell loss, 537

N

Nabilone (Cesemet) for nausea and
        vomiting, 500
Naganin, 189-191

Naganol, 189-191
Nail changes, 524, 525
Naloxone, 457
Naltrexone, 457
Naphuride, 189-191
Naproxen for pain, 454
Narcotic analgesics, constipation and,
        514
Narcotics for pain, 455-457
National Cancer Institute (NCI), 22,
        23, 24, 25, 36-37, 307, 450,
        564
    Common Toxicity Criteria scale of,
        37, 574-580
National Cooperative Drug Discovery
        Group, 27
National Library of Medicine,
        Physician's Data Query
        database and, 24
Natulan, 184-186
Natural immunity, 220
Natural killer (NK) cells, 220
Natural products
    antineoplastic drugs and, 6
    plant alkaloids and, 6-7
Nausea and vomiting, 488-501
    consequences of, 501-502
    energy requirements and, 501
    fluid and electrolyte balance and,
        501-502
    nonpharmacological approaches to,
        501
    nutritional status and, 501
    as side effects of pediatric cancer
        therapy, 565
Navelbine, 216-218
Naxamide, 135-138
NCCTG study for colon carcinoma,
        333
NCI; *see* National Cancer Institute
Neoadjuvant fluorouracil-cisplatin for
        esophageal carcinoma,
        338-339
Neoral, 86-88
Neosar, 83-86
Nephrotoxic chemotherapy, 526-530
Nerve blocks, 459
Neupogen, 233-236
Neuralgia, postherpetic, 459-460
Neurological toxicity, 539-543
Neuropathy, autonomic, cytotoxic
        drugs and, 541
Neurosurgical analgesic interventions,
        459

Neurotoxicity
 cytotoxic drugs and, 541
 as delayed consequence of
  treatment, 566
Neutrexin, 209-211
Neutropenia, 476-486
 fever and, 482-486
 infection and, 476-478, 479-481,
  482-486
NHL; *see* Non-Hodgkin's lymphoma
Nipent, 176-177
Nitrogen mustard, 4, 149-150
Nitrosoureas, renal function and, 532
NK cells; *see* Natural killer cells
NOAC for non-Hodgkin's disease, 398
Nolvadex, 191-193
Nolvadex-D, 191-193
Noncardiogenic pulmonary edema,
  534
Non-Hodgkin's lymphoma (NHL)
 of central nervous system, primary,
  combination chemotherapy
  for, 400-402
 combination chemotherapy for,
  382-399
Noninvasive pain-relief measures, 458,
  459
Nonmaleficence, medical ethics and,
  436
Non–small-cell lung carcinoma
  (NSCLC), combination
  chemotherapy for, 365-370
Nonseminomatous tumors, 428-432
Nonsteroidal antiinflammatory drug
  (NSAID), 451-454
Nontunneled central venous catheters,
  279
Nonvoluntary euthanasia, 443
5'-Noranhydrovinblastine, 216-218
Normeperidine, 455
Novantrone, 166-168
Novo-Tamoxifen, 191-193
NSABP-CO3 trial for colon
  carcinoma, 333
NSAID; *see* Nonsteroidal
  antiinflammatory drug
NSC-740, 159-162
NSC-750, 70-72
NSC-752, 198-200
NSC-755, 155-157
NSC-762, 149-150
NSC-67574, 214-216
NSC-134087, 182
NSC-3053, 94-95
NSC-3088, 77-78

NSC-3590, 142-145
NSC-6396, 200-202
NSC-8806, 154-155
NSC-141540, 113-116
NSC-141633, 131-132
NSC-77213, 184-186
NSC-603071, 53-54
NSC-79037, 147-149
NSC-13875, 50-51
NSC-15200, 125-127
NSC-82151, 95-97
NSC-409962, 75-77
NSC-606864, 129-131
NSC-609699, 204-206
NSC-19893, 121-123
NSC-85998, 188-189
NSC-218321, 176-177
NSC-89199, 111-113
NSC-352122, 209-211
NSC-24559, 178-180
NSC-614629, 233-236
NSC-25154, 178
NSC-26271, 83-86
NSC-26980, 162-164
NSC-224131, 173-174
NSC-27640, 117-119
NSC-617589, 253-255
NSC-618085, 248-250
NSC-32065, 132-133
NSC-34462, 211-212
NSC-296961, 51-53
NSC-34936, 189-191
NSC-362856, 195-196
NSC-626715, 109-110
NSC-102816, 63-65
NSC-628503, 102-105
NSC-169780, 99-101
NSC-38721, 164-165
NSC-105014, 81-83
NSC-301739, 166-168
NSC-367982, 236-242
NSC-106977, 61-63
NSC-109724, 135-138
NSC-241240, 73-75
NSC-45388, 91-93
NSC-373361, 242-244
NSC-373364, 225-228
NSC-177023, 250-252
NSC-113891, 157-159
NSC-639186, 202-204
NSC-49842, 212-214
NSC-377523, 236-242
NSC-180973, 191-193
NSC-312887, 119-121
NSC-249992, 56-58

NSC-119875, 78-81
NSC-122758, 207-209
NSC-122819, 196-198
NSC-123127, 105-109
NSC-125066, 67-69
NSC-256439, 134-135
NSC-256942, 110-111
NSC-125973, 170-172
NSC-63878, 88-91
NSC-326231, 72-73
NSCLC; *see* Non–small-cell lung
        carcinoma
Nurses, research, as members of
        clinical trial team, 34
Nutrition
    diarrhea and, 508-513
    nausea and vomiting and, 501
NVB, 216-218

O
OBD; *see* Optimal biologic dose
Occupational Safety and Health
        Administration (OSHA), 261,
        262, 263-267
Octreotide, 48, 168-170
Octreotide acetate, 168-170
Octreotide pamoate, 168-170
Ocular toxicity, 545
Ommaya reservoir, 296, 298-299
Oncaspar, 61-63
Oncology Nursing Society, 261
Oncovin, 214-216
    for Hodgkin's disease, 544
Ondansetron (Zofran), 497-499
    for nausea and vomiting, 494, 565
Optimal biologic dose (OBD), 220
Orabase for stomatitis, 511
Oral administration of antineoplastic
        drugs, 275
Oral analgesics, 452-453
Oral care, preventive, 505, 506
Orasone, 183-184
Oratect gel for stomatitis, 511
Ora-testryl, 123-124
Oregon, welfare laws of, 437
Organ system toxicity, 475-552
    anemia, 475-476
    cardiac toxicity, 537-539
    dermatological toxicity, 514-526
    gastrointestinal toxicity, 488-514
    gonadal toxicity, 543-544
    hepatic toxicity, 545
    neurological toxicity, 539-543
    neutropenia, 476-486

    ocular toxicity, 545
    pulmonary toxicity, 534-537
    renal toxicity, 526-533
    thrombocytopenia, 486-488
    vascular toxicity, 545
OSHA; *see* Occupational Safety and
        Health Administration
Osteosarcoma, combination
        chemotherapy for, 409-411
Ovarian carcinoma, combination
        chemotherapy for, 411-417
Ovarian germ cell cancer,
        combination chemotherapy
        for, 417-418
Ovarian germ cell tumor, 412
Oxycodone for pain, 454
OxyContin, 454, 457

P
P glycoprotein (Pgp), 3
PAC
    for ovarian carcinoma, 415-416
    for thymoma, 433-434
Paclitaxel, 170-172, 309
    anaphylactic reactions and, 270
    for breast carcinoma, 319, 326
    for carcinoma of unknown primary,
        330
    cardiac toxicity from, 538
    for esophageal carcinoma, 339
    for head and neck squamous cell
        carcinoma, 346
    indications for, 48
    for non–small-cell lung carcinoma,
        368
    for ovarian carcinoma, 416, 417
    for prostatic carcinoma, 421-422
    for small-cell lung cancer, 373, 374
Pain, assessment of, 450-451
Pain management, 448-461
    additional measures for, 458-460
    analgesics; *see* Analgesics
    noninvasive, 458, 459
    underestimating need for, 448-450
PALA, 173-174
PALA disodium, 173-174
Palmar-plantar erythrodysesthesia
        syndrome, 525
L-PAM, 154-155
PAME for acute lymphoblastic
        leukemia, 352-353
Pamidronate, 48, 174-176
Pamidronate disodium, 174-176
Panasol-S, 183-184

Pancreatic carcinoma, combination chemotherapy for, 418-420
Papaver somniferum plant, 455
Paraplatin, 73-75
Passive euthanasia, 443
Patient enrollment in clinical trials, 23, 30-34
Patient Self-Determination Act, 441
Patient-controlled analgesia, 458
Patient's quality of life, 308
PAVe for Hodgkin's disease, 381
PBF for head and neck squamous cell carcinoma, 346
PC for ovarian carcinoma, 415-416
PCV plus radiotherapy for brain tumors, 317
P/DOCE for primary non-Hodgkin's lymphoma of central nervous system, 401-402
PDQ database; *see* Physician's Data Query database
PEB for carcinoma of unknown primary, 330
Pediatric cancer therapy, 564-568
  clinical cooperative groups, 564-565
  delayed consequences of, 566
  early side effects of, 565
  ethical considerations of, 566-568
Pediatric Oncology Group (POG), 564
Pegasparaginase, 61-63
PEG-asparagase, 61-63
Pentamidine, OSHA guidelines for handling, 262
Pentazocine for pain, 454-455
Pentostatin, 176-177
  drug interactions and, 16
  indications for, 48
Performance scale, 571
Peridex; *see* Chlorhexidine
Peripheral neuropathy, cytotoxic drugs and, 541
Peripheral venous access, 274-279
Peripherally inserted central catheter (PICC), 279-285
Peristaltic ambulatory infusion pump, 303
Peritoneal dialysis, 300-301
Perphenazine for nausea and vomiting, 494
PFL for head and neck squamous cell carcinoma, 346-347
Pgp; *see* P glycoprotein
Phase I clinical trials, 27, 28
Phase II clinical trials, 28
Phase III clinical trials, 28

Phase IV clinical trials, 29
Phenothiazines for nausea and vomiting, 492, 494, 499
L-Phenylalanine mustard, 154-155
Phenytoin, drug reactions and, 10-13
Phosphonacetyl-L-aspartic acid, 173-174
Photodegradation, dacarbazine and, 93
Photofrin, 180-182
Physician-assisted suicide, 442-445
Physicians as members of clinical trial team, 34
Physician's Data Query (PDQ) database, 23-24, 307
PICC; *see* Peripherally inserted central catheter
Pigmentation changes, 524, 525
Pipobroman, 48, 178
Piroxicam for pain, 454
Plant alkaloids, 6-7
Plasma
  blood transfusion therapy and, 557
  fresh frozen, 557
Platelet drips, 555-556
Platelet nadir method, 573
Platelet refractoriness, 555
Platelets, blood transfusion therapy and, 554-556
Platinol, 78-81
Platinol-AQ, 78-81
Platinum, 78-81
cis-Platinum, 78-81
Pleuroperitoneal shunt, 302
Plicamycin, 178-180
  for chronic granulocytic (myleocytic) leukemia, 363-364
  indications for, 48
  renal function and, 532
Pluripotential stem cell (PPSC), 466
Pneumocytes, 534
Pneumonitis, 534
POC for melanoma, 404
POG; *see* Pediatric Oncology Group
Poppy, 455
Porfimer sodium, 48, 180-182
Porton asparaginase, 61-63
Postherpetic neuralgia, 459-460
PPSC; *see* Pluripotential stem cell
Preclinical evaluation of drugs, 25-27
Prednimustine, 182
  for Hodgkin's disease, 377-378
Prednisolone
  for acute nonlymphycytic leukemia, 361

for Hodgkin's disease, 382
for non-Hodgkin's disease, 388-389,
393
Prednisone, 183-184
for acute lymphoblastic leukemia,
350-351, 352-354
for acute nonlymphycytic leukemia,
358-359
for breast carcinoma, 320, 321-322
for chronic granulocytic (myeleocytic)
leukemia, 364
for chronic lymphocytic leukemia,
364-365
for Hodgkin's disease, 376, 377,
378-381, 382, 544
for multiple myeloma, 406-407,
408-409
for non-Hodgkin's disease, 385-386,
388, 389, 390, 391, 393-395,
396, 398-399
for primary non-Hodgkin's
lymphoma of central nervous
system, 400-402
for prostatic carcinoma, 423
for small-cell lung cancer, 373
for thymoma, 432-433
Premedication, transfusion reactions
and, 560-561
President's Commission for the Study
of Ethical Problems in
Medicine and Biomedical
and Behavioral Research, 440
Primary non-Hodgkin's lymphoma of
central nervous system,
combination chemotherapy
for, 400-402
Procarbazine, 184-186
for brain tumors, 317
drug interactions and, 16
for Hodgkin's disease, 377, 378-381,
544
hypersensitivity pneumonitis and,
534
indications for, 48
for melanoma, 404
for non-Hodgkin's disease, 387, 388,
389, 390, 391
for primary non-Hodgkin's
lymphoma of central nervous
system, 400-401
Prochlorperazine for nausea and
vomiting, 494
Procrit, 232-233
Procytox, 83-86
Prognosis, disclosure of, 439, 567

Prokine, 253-255
Proleuken, 225-228
PRO-MACE-CYTABOM for
non-Hodgkin's disease,
398-399
Promethazine for nausea and vomiting,
496
Proscar, 116-117
Prospective monitoring in clinical
trials, 35-36
Prostate specific antigen (PSA) for
prostatic carcinoma, 420
Prostatic carcinoma, combination
chemotherapy for, 420-423
Protocols in clinical trials
development of, 30, 31-33
review checklist for, 31-33
team for, 30, 34
Provera, 151-152
PSA; *see* Prostate specific antigen
PSC-833, 186-188
Psychotropic drugs, platelet function
and, 487
PTG, 196-198
Pulmonary edema, noncardiogenic,
534
Pulmonary fibrosis, 534
Pulmonary toxicity, 534-537
Purinethol, 155-157
P-VABEC for primary non-Hodgkin's
lymphoma of central nervous
system, 402
PVB
for carcinoma of unknown primary,
330
for gestational trophoblastic disease,
343
for ovarian germ cell cancer,
418
for testicular and extragonadal germ
cell cancer, 430
Pyridoxine for acute nonlymphycytic
leukemia, 360

Q
Quality assurance in clinical trials,
37
Quality of life of patient, 308

R
Radiation, whole-brain, for brain
tumors, 317
Radiation skin reactions, 526

Radionuclide angiocardiography (RNA), 537-538
Radiotherapy
  for brain tumors, 316-317
  for esophageal carcinoma, 337
  for head and neck squamous cell carcinoma, 347
  PCV plus, for brain tumors, 317
Random single-donor platelets (RSDPs), 555
Random-donor platelets (RDPs), 554
Ranitidine, anaphylactic reactions and, 270
Rationing, medical ethics and, 436-437
RBCs; *see* Red blood cells
RDPs; *see* Random-donor platelets
Recall reactions, 526
Recombinant beta interferon, 242-244
Recombinant human IL-4, 248-250
Recombinant human thrombopoietin, 255-256
Recombinant IL-3, 246-248
Recombinant-methionyl human granulocyte-colony stimulating factor, 233-236
Record keeping, OSHA guidelines for, 267
Red blood cells (RBCs), transfusion of, 554
Regional administration of antineoplastic drugs, 295-302
  intraarterial, 295-296, 297
  intraperitoneal, 300-301
  intrapleural, 301-302
  intraventricular, 296-300
Remisar, 230-232
Renal cell carcinoma, combination chemotherapy for, 423-425
Renal function, assessment of, 526, 527-528, 529
Renal toxicity, 526-533
Research nurses as members of clinical trial team, 34
Resting phase of cell cycle, 2
Retching, 489
13-*cis*-Retinoic acid, 140-142
rG-CSF, 233-236
rGM-CSF, 253-255
rh GM-CSF
  for bladder carcinoma, 314
  for sarcoma, 426
  for transitional cell carcinoma, 314
Rheumatrex, 159-162
Rhizotomy, 459

rhTPO, 255-256
rhuIL-4, 248-250
rHuMGDF, 252
rIFN-B, 242-244
rIL-2, 225-228
Ritalin; *see* Methylphenidate
r-met HuG-CSF, 233-236
RNA; *see* Radionuclide angiocardiography
Roferon, 236-242
RP 56976, 102-105
RSDPs; *see* Random single-donor platelets
rTNF-alpha, 256-258
Rubex, 105-109
Rubidomycin, 95-97

S

SAEs; *see* Serious adverse events
Saline laxatives for constipation, 515
Salvage mitoxantrone-ifosfamide-etoposide for acute lymphoblastic leukemia, 354
Salvage regimen for acute nonlymphycytic leukemia, 360
Sandimmune, 86-88
Sandostatin, 168-170
L-Sarcolysin, 154-155
Sarcoma
  combination chemotherapy for, 425-428
  Kaposi's; *see* Kaposi's sarcoma
Sargramostim, 253-255
  for acute lymphoblastic leukemia, 354
  for bladder carcinoma, 314
  for chronic granulocytic (myelocytic) leukemia, 363
  for neutropenia, 238
  for transitional cell carcinoma, 314
SC for carcinoid (malignant) and islet cell carcinoma, 328
SCAB for Hodgkin's disease, 381
SCH 52365, 195-196
SCLC; *see* Small-cell lung cancer
SD for carcinoid (malignant) and islet cell carcinoma, 328-329
SDPs; *see* Single-donor platelets
SDZ PSC 833, 186-188
Secondary malignancy as delayed consequence of treatment, 566

Seminomas, 428-432

Semustine for colon carcinoma, 335

Septic transfusions, 558, 561

Serious adverse events (SAEs), reporting, in clinical trials, 36-37

Serotonin, 497

Serotonin antagonists for nausea and vomiting, 492, 494, 497-499, 565

SF for carcinoid (malignant) and islet cell carcinoma, 329

SGOT; *see* Aspartate aminotransferase

SGPT; *see* Alanine aminotransferase

Side effects of pediatric cancer therapy, 565

Simultaneous fluorouracil-cisplatin radiation for head and neck squamous cell carcinoma, 347

Single-donor platelets (SDPs), 555

SKF 104864-A, 204-206

Skin toxicity; *see* Dermatological toxicity

Small-cell lung cancer (SCLC), combination chemotherapy for, 370-375

SMF for pancreatic carcinoma, 420

Smoking as cause of cancer, 1

SMS 201-995, 168-170

SMS 201-995 LAR, 168-170

SMS 201-995 pa LAR, 168-170

Sodium thiosulfate for ovarian carcinoma, 415

Sodium-2-mercaptoethanesulphonate, 157-159

Softeners for constipation, 516

Source documents in clinical trials, 34-35

Sparfosate sodium, 173-174

Sperm, cryopreservation of, 544

Spills, OSHA guidelines for, 266

SQ-1089, 132-133

Squamous cell carcinoma, head and neck, combination chemotherapy for, 344-347

Stanford regimen for Hodgkin's disease, 381-382

Stem cell support, high-dose chemotherapy with, 462-474

Sterecyt, 182

Stilbestrol, 101-102

Stilphostrol, 101-102

for prostatic carcinoma, 421

Stimulant laxatives for constipation, 516

Stomafate suspension for stomatitis, 511

Stomatitis, 502-508

chemotherapy-induced, 507

preventive oral care and, 505, 506

prophylaxis for, 507

topical analgesia for, 511-512

treatment of, 507-508, 509-510

Streptozocin, 188-189

for adrenal cortical carcinoma, 311

for carcinoid (malignant) and islet cell carcinoma, 328-329

for colon carcinoma, 335

for Hodgkin's disease, 381

indications for, 49

for pancreatic carcinoma, 419, 420

renal function and, 532

Streptozotocin, 188-189

Study coordinators as members of clinical trial team, 34

Subcutaneous administration of antineoplastic drugs, 275

Suicide, physician-assisted, 442-445

Suprefact, 69-70

Suramin, 189-191

Suramin sodium, 189-191

Sympathectomy, 459

Syringe ambulatory infusion pump, 303

T

T-10 for osteosarcoma, 410

Tamofen, 191-193

Tamoplex, 191-193

Tamoxifen, 191-193

indications for, 49

for melanoma, 403-404

nausea and vomiting and, 501

pain and, 451

Tamoxifen citrate, 191-193

Tarabine Pfs, 88-91

Taste changes, 502, 503, 504

Taxol, 170-172

Taxotere, 102-105

TBC for multiple myeloma, 472

TC for breast cancers, 473-474

TCC for breast cancers, 473

T-cell growth factor, 225-228

T-cell growth factor II, 248-250

T-cell leukemia/lymphoma virus (HTLV-I), 561

T-cell replacing factor, 225-228
TCGF-II, 248-250
TdT; *see* Terminal deoxynucleotidyl transferase
Tegafur, 193-195
 drug interactions and, 17
Tegretol; *see* Carbamazepine
Temozolomide, 195-196
Temperature conversion chart, 581
Tenckoff catheter, 300
Teniposide, 196-198
 for acute lymphoblastic leukemia, 350-351, 353
 drug interactions and, 17
 indications for, 49
 pulmonary toxicity from, 534, 535
Terminal deoxynucleotidyl transferase (TdT), 362
Termizole, 250-252
TESPA, 200-202
Testicular germ cell cancer, combination chemotherapy for, 428-432
delta-9-Tetrahydrocannabinol for nausea and vomiting, 500
6-TG, 198-200
THC for nausea and vomiting, 500
T-helper cells, 220
Thenylidene-lignan-P, 196-198
Theracys, 228-230
Thiethylperazine for nausea and vomiting, 494
Thioguanine, 198-200
 for acute lymphoblastic leukemia, 353-354
 for acute nonlymphycytic leukemia, 356-357
 indications for, 49
 for lymphomas, 471
6-Thioguanine, 198-200
 for acute nonlymphycytic leukemia, 356-357, 358-359
Thioguanine Tabloid, 198-200
Thioplex, 200-202
Thiotepa, 200-202
 for breast carcinoma, 326-327, 473-474
 drug interactions and, 17
 indications for, 49
 for multiple myeloma, 472
Thoracentesis, 301
Thrombocytopenia, 486-488
 management of bleeding in, 488

 medications affecting platelet function, 486, 487
 preventive measures for, 486-488
Thrombolytic agents, platelet function and, 487
Thrombopoietin, 255-256
 for thrombocytopenia, 238
Thymoma, combination chemotherapy for, 432-434
Thyroid carcinoma, combination chemotherapy for, 434-435
Tice BCG, 228-230
T-lymphocytes, 220
TMQ, 209-211
TMTX, 209-211
TNF; *see* Tumor necrosis factor
TNF-alpha, 256-258
Tomudex, 202-204
Toothbrushing in stomatitis oral care program, 505, 508
Topical analgesia for stomatitis, 5 11-512
Topoisomerase inhibitors, 6-7
Topoisomerases, 3-4
Toposar, 113-116
Topotecan, 49, 204-206, 309
Topotecan AC/AF, 204-206
Topotecan hydrochloride, 204-206
Toremifene, 49, 206-207
Toremifene citrate, 206-207
Toremifenum, 206-207
Toxicity
 biological response modifiers and, 222-225
 bladder, 529-530
 cardiac, 537-539
 dermatological; *see* Dermatological toxicity
 gonadal, 543-544
 hepatic, 545
 National Cancer Institute criteria for, 574-580
 neurological, 539-543
 ocular, 545
 organ system; *see* Organ system toxicity
 pulmonary, 534-537
 renal, 526-533
 vascular, 545
TPO, 255-256
TRA, 207-209
Transfusion reactions, 557-561
 acute extravascular hemolytic, 558, 560

acute intravascular hemolytic,
558-560
allergic, 558, 561
febrile, 558, 560
hemolytic, 557-558
premedication, 560-561
septic, 558, 561
Transfusion therapy, blood; *see* Blood
transfusion therapy
Transitional cell carcinoma,
combination chemotherapy
for, 312-315
Tretinoin, 207-209
drug interactions and, 17
indications for, 49
TRF, 225-228
Trials, clinical; *see* Clinical trials
Triethylenephosphoramide, 200-202
N,N',N''-Triethylene-
thiophosphoramide, 200-202
Trimetrexate, 49, 209-211
Tris(1-aziridinyl)phosphine sulfide,
200-202
Truthfulness, 438-439
TSPA, 200-202
Tumor flare, goserelin and, 130
Tumor necrosis factor (TNF), 220,
256-258
for melanoma, 238
Tumors, brain, combination
chemotherapy for, 316-317
Tunneled central venous catheters,
279, 280-282, 284-285,
286-287
Typical multidrug resistance, 3

U

UFT, 193-195
Ulcerase for stomatitis, 512
Unknown primary, carcinoma of,
combination chemotherapy
for, 329-330
Uracil mustard, 49, 211-212
Uramustine, 211-212
Urine collection process, 526-529
Uromitexan, 157-159

V

VAB VI for testicular and extragonadal
germ cell cancer, 430-431
VAC for ovarian germ cell cancer,
417-418

VACOP-B for non-Hodgkin's disease,
399
VAD for multiple myeloma, 408
VAP for multiple myeloma, 408-409
VAPA for acute nonlymphycytic
leukemia, 361
Vascular access devices, 280-282
Vascular toxicity, 545
VATH for breast carcinoma, 326-327
VBAP for multiple myeloma, 409
VBM for Hodgkin's disease, 382
VCAP for multiple myeloma, 409
VCR, 214-216
VDP for melanoma, 404
VEEP for Hodgkin's disease, 382
VEIP for testicular and extragonadal
germ cell cancer, 431
Velban, 212-214
Velbe, 212-214
Velsar, 212-214
Venipuncture and infusion, guidelines
for, 521
Venous cutaneous reactions, 523
Venous infusion ports, 290
Venous reactions to drug
administration, 523
VePesid, 113-116
Vercyte, 178
Vesanoid, 207-209
Vesicants, 519-520
VICCE for small-cell lung cancer, 374
VIG
for bladder carcinoma, 315
for transitional cell carcinoma, 315
VIM for non-Hodgkin's disease, 399
Vinblastine, 212-214
for bladder carcinoma, 313-315
for breast carcinoma, 319, 325,
326-327
for carcinoma of unknown primary,
330
for cervical carcinoma, 332
for esophageal carcinoma, 337-338
for gestational trophoblastic disease,
343
for Hodgkin's disease, 376-377,
378-379, 380, 381, 382, 544
indications for, 49
for Kaposi's sarcoma, 348, 349
for melanoma, 404
for non–small-cell lung carcinoma,
367, 368, 369
for ovarian germ cell cancer, 418
for prostatic carcinoma, 422

Vinblastine *(cont.)*
  for testicular and extragonadal germ
      cell cancer, 430-432
  for transitional cell carcinoma,
      313-315
Vinblastine sulfate, 212-214
Vincaleukoblastine, 212-214
Vincasar Pfs, 214-216
Vincristine, 214-216
  for acute lymphoblastic leukemia,
      350-351, 352-354
  for acute nonlymphycytic leukemia,
      358-359, 361
  for brain tumors, 316, 317
  for breast carcinoma, 321-322,
      323-324
  for chronic granulocytic (myelocytic)
      leukemia, 362-363, 364
  for chronic lymphocytic leukemia,
      364-365
  for colon carcinoma, 335
  for gestational trophoblastic disease,
      342-343
  for head and neck squamous cell
      carcinoma, 344-345
  for Hodgkin's disease, 379-380, 381,
      382
  indications for, 49
  for Kaposi's sarcoma, 348, 349
  for melanoma, 404
  for multiple myeloma, 408-409
  for non-Hodgkin's disease, 385-386,
      387, 388-389, 390, 391,
      393-394, 396-399
  for osteosarcoma, 410
  for ovarian germ cell cancer, 417-418
  for primary non-Hodgkin's
      lymphoma of central nervous
      system, 400-402
  for sarcoma, 426
  for small-cell lung cancer, 371,
      372-373, 374
  for testicular and extragonadal germ
      cell cancer, 429-430
  for thymoma, 432, 433
  for thyroid carcinoma, 435
Vincristine sulfate, 214-216
Vindesine
  for non-Hodgkin's disease, 395
  for non–small-cell lung carcinoma,
      369
Vinorelbine, 216-218, 309
  for breast carcinoma, 327
  for head and neck squamous cell
      carcinoma, 347

  indications for, 49
  for non–small-cell lung
      carcinoma, 369-370
  venous reactions and, 523
Vinorelbine tartrate, 216-218
VIP
  for non–small-cell lung carcinoma,
      369-370
  for small-cell lung cancer, 375
  for testicular and extragonadal germ
      cell cancer, 431
Viral interferons, 221
Vitamin A acid, 207-209
Vitamin E for stomatitis, 511
VLB, 212-214
VM-26, 196-198
VMCP for multiple myeloma, 409
Voluntary active euthanasia, 443
Vomiting
  anticipatory, 565
  nausea and; *see* Nausea and
      vomiting
VP-16, 113-116
VP-16-213, 113-116
VP for chronic granulocytic
      (myleocytic) leukemia, 364
VPV for testicular and extragonadal
      germ cell cancer, 431-432
Vumon, 196-198

W

Warfarin, drug interactions and, 17
Waste disposal, OSHA guidelines for,
      266
WBRT; *see* Whole-body radiation
      therapy
Weight, drug doses and, 269
Weight charts, 570
Welfare laws, medical ethics and,
      437
Wellcovorin, 142-145
Wellferon, 236-242
WHO; *see* World Health
      Organization
Whole-body radiation therapy
      (WBRT), 467
Whole-brain radiation for brain
      tumors, 317
Will, living, medical ethics and, 440
World Health Organization (WHO),
      analgesic ladder of,
      449-450
WR-2721, 51-53
WR-83799, 132-133

X

Xylocaine 2% Viscous for stomatitis,
    512

Z

Zanosar, 188-189
Zavedos, 134-135
ZD 1694, 202-204
Zilactin for stomatitis, 511
Zinecard, 99-101
Zofran; *see* Ondansetron
Zoladex, 129-131
Zostrix; *see* Capsaicin
Zovirax; *see* Acyclovir